BSAVA Manual of Exotic Pets
Fourth edition

Editors:

Anna Meredith
MA VetMB CertLAS CertZooMed MRCVS

The R(D)SVS Hospital for Small Animals,
The University of Edinburgh,
Easter Bush, Veterinary Centre,
Roslin, Midlothian, EH25 9RG, UK

Sharon Redrobe
BSc BVetMed CertLAS CertZooMed MRCVS

Zoo Veterinary Officer,
Bristol Zoo Gardens, Clifton,
Bristol BS8 3HA, UK

Published by:

British Small Animal Veterinary Association
Woodrow House, 1 Telford Way, Waterwells
Business Park, Quedgeley, Gloucester GL2 2AB

A Company Limited by Guarantee in England.
Registered Company No. 2837793.
Registered as a Charity.

Figures 1.1, 17.1, 17.9, 17.10, 20.4, 22.2 and 22.16 were drawn by
S.J. Elmhurst BA Hons and are printed with her permission.

Figures 13.3, 13.4, 13.6 and 13.7 were drawn by Nigel Harcourt-Brown
BVSc DipECAMS FRCVS and are printed with his permission.

A catalogue record for this book is available from the British Library.

ISBN 0 905214 47 1

The publishers and contributors cannot take responsibility for information
provided on dosages and methods of application of drugs mentioned in
this publication. Details of this kind must be verified by individual users
from the appropriate literature.

Typeset by: Fusion Design, Fordingbridge, Hampshire, UK

Printed by: Grafos, Barcelona, Spain

Other titles in the BSAVA Manuals series:

For information on these and all BSAVA publications please visit our website: www.bsava.com

Contents

Contributors

Andreas Artmann DVM
Zoologischer Garten Schmieding, Schmieding 19, 4691 Krenglbach, Austria

Michelle G. Barrows BVMS BSc MRCVS
C.J. Hall Veterinary Surgeons, 15 Temple Sheen Road, Sheen, London SW14 7PY, UK

John Chitty BVetMed CertZooMed MRCVS
Strathmore Veterinary Clinic, London Road, Andover, Hampshire SP10 2PH, UK

Margaret E. Cooper LLB FLS
Wildlife Health Services, PO Box 153, Wellingborough, Northants NN8 2ZA, UK

David A. Crossley BVetMed FAVD MRCVS
24 Tudor Grove, Middleton, Manchester M24 5AJ, UK

Paul Flecknell MA VetMB PhD DLAS MRCVS
Comparative Biology Centre, The Medical School, Framlington Place,
Newcastle-upon-Tyne NE22 4HH, UK

Greg Fleming DVM
Box 100126, College of Veterinary Medicine, University of Florida, Gainesville, FL 32610-0126, USA

Simon J. Girling BVMS (Hons) CertZooMed CIBiol MIBiol MRCVS
Braid Veterinary Hospital, 171 Mayfield Road, Edinburgh EH9 3AZ, UK

Gidona Goodman DVM MSc MRCVS
Dept of Veterinary Clinical Studies, Royal (Dick) School of Veterinary Studies,
Hospital for Small Animals, Easter Bush Veterinary Centre, Roslin, Midlothian EH25 9RG, UK

Nigel H. Harcourt-Brown BVSc DipECAMS FRCVS
30 Crab Lane, Bilton, Harrogate, North Yorkshire HG1 3BE, UK

Darryl Heard BSc BVMS PhD DipACZM
Box 100126, College of Veterinary Medicine, University of Florida, Gainesville, FL 32610-0126, USA

Claudia Hochleithner
Tierklinik Strebersdorf, Mühlweg 5, 1210 Vienna, Austria

Manfred Hochleithner
Tierklinik Strebersdorf, Mühlweg 5, 1210 Vienna, Austria

Heidi L. Hoefer DVM
236 Beverly Road South, Huntington, NY 11746, USA

Elliott Jacobson DVM PhD DipACZM
Box 100126, College of Veterinary Medicine, University of Florida, Gainesville, FL 32610-0126, USA

Cathy A. Johnson-Delaney DVM
Attending Veterinarian, SNBL USA Ltd, 6605 Merrill Creek Parkway, Everett, WA 98203, USA

Emma Keeble BVSc CertZooMed MRCVS
Dept of Veterinary Clinical Studies, Royal (Dick) School of Veterinary Studies,
Hospital for Small Animals, Easter Bush Veterinary Centre, Roslin, Midlothian EH25 9RG, UK

Brad Lock DVM
Box 100126, College of Veterinary Medicine, University of Florida, Gainesville, FL 32610-0126, USA

Bruce Maclean BSc BVM&S MRCVS
Kelperland Veterinary Centre, Ascot Road, Touchen End, Nr Maidenhead, Berkshire SL6 3LA, UK

Stuart D.J. McArthur BVetMed MRCVS
Holly House Veterinary Surgery, 468 Street Lane, Leeds LS17 6HA, UK

Anna Meredith MA VetMB CertLAS CertZooMed MRCVS
Royal (Dick) School of Veterinary Studies, Hospital for Small Animals,
Easter Bush Veterinary Centre, Roslin, Midlothian EH25 9RG, UK

Hannah E. Orr BVM&S CertLAS MRCVS
Comparative Biology Centre, The Medical School, Framlington Place,
Newcastle-upon-Tyne NE2 4HH, UK

Paul Raiti DVM
Beverlie Animal Hospital, 171 West Grand Street, Mount Vernon, NY 10552, USA

Sharon Redrobe BSc BVetMed CertLAS MRCVS
Zoo Veterinary Officer, Bristol Zoo Gardens, Clifton, Bristol BS8 3HA, UK

Nico J. Schoemaker DVM DipECAMS DipABVP
Division of Avian and Exotic Animal Medicine, Utrecht University, Yalelaan 8,
3584 CM Utrecht, The Netherlands

Michael D. Stanford BVSc MRCVS
Birch Heath Veterinary Clinic, Tarporley, Cheshire CW6 9UU, UK

David J. Taylor MA VetMB PhD MRCVS
Department of Veterinary Pathology, University of Glasgow Veterinary School, Bearsden Road,
Bearsden, Glasgow G61 1QH, UK

Susan M. Thornton BSc BVetMed MRCVS
International Zoo Veterinary Group, Keighley Business Centre, South Street, Keighley,
West Yorkshire BD21 1AG, UK

Roger J. Wilkinson MA VetMB CertVD MRCVS
Thornbury Vet Group, 515 Bradford Road, Thornbury, Bradford BD3 7BA, UK

David L. Williams MA VetMB PhD CertVOphthal MRCVS
Department of Clinical Veterinary Medicine, University of Cambridge, Madingley Road,
Cambridge CB3 0ES

Foreword

The fourth edition of the *BSAVA Manual of Exotic Pets* is an essential purchase for the practice bookshelf. The previous edition has been an excellent source of information but has been so well used that many of us have given up trying to keep the pages together. This new text is just in time.

No single volume can cover the potential medical or surgical problems affecting the complete range of species we refer to as 'exotic pets' but demand has led to this entirely rewritten edition which, like its predecessor, provides an overview and guides those seeking more detailed help to the relevant texts.

A total of 30 international authors have written this manual under the editorial guidance of Anna Meredith and Sharon Redrobe, using the familiar problem-oriented format. Changes from the previous edition include chapters on clinical anatomy and imaging, a comprehensive formulary for each chapter, the inclusion of fancy pigs and some US pet species, and over 200 colour illustrations. Practitioners and nurses will find the tables of fluid or supportive therapy and laboratory values of particular use.

The BSAVA Publications Committee and management team are to be congratulated on the quality of this manual. Working in practice one relies on training, experience, common sense and, especially when dealing with unfamiliar species, the expertise of colleagues when making a diagnosis or deciding when a referral is appropriate. These pages will provide that expertise for veterinary surgeons, nurses, students and for enthusiastic owners wishing to expand their own knowledge.

Julian Wells BVSc MRCVS
BSAVA President 2001–2002

Preface

The 1991 Edition of the *Manual of Exotic Pets* has been the most successful of the BSAVA manual series. There can be few vets in practice in the UK that have not, at some time or other in their career, been grateful for some hastily read information when faced with an unfamiliar species in the consulting room. However, after ten years and with the huge increase in veterinary knowledge of exotic species, it was very much in need of an update. Even the term 'exotic' can be something of a misnomer nowadays, as many of the species covered are very common and make up a large proportion of many practice case loads.

When faced with the task of editing a new edition we asked ourselves what would be really useful to the practitioner. Thus, in addition to a wealth of background information that can be digested at leisure, we have asked the authors to provide easy-to-read tables, charts, tips and practical advice that can be quickly assimilated and used in the clinical environment. This new edition is different in several other respects too: it covers new species – fancy pigs and a range of new small mammals; it has wonderful new chapters on anatomy and imaging of mammals, birds and reptiles; and it is packed with illustrations, many in colour. The increase in depth of information means that exotic cases can be dealt with to a much higher standard, which is in line with increasing owner expectations of veterinary care.

We invited authors who we felt could provide the very best and most up-to-date coverage of their subjects and they have more than exceeded our expectations with the quality of their contributions. They have all done a wonderful job and we would like to thank them very sincerely for their hard work and dedication.

We would also like to thank Marion Jowett, BSAVA Publishing Manager, for her hard work, cajoling, patience, and expert advice and guidance.

No other text available covers the full range of exotic pets in this way, and we believe that this edition will rapidly earn its place as a 'must-have' book on every practice shelf. We are sure you will enjoy it and cannot fail to find it useful.

Anna Meredith
Sharon Redrobe
September 2001

Mammalian imaging and anatomy

Simon J. Girling

Introduction

The reasoning behind performing diagnostic imaging techniques in small or exotic mammals is the same as that propounded for any species. The desire is to detect internal foreign bodies and to diagnose fractures and dislocations, tumours, abscesses and organ enlargement/reduction as well as pregnancy. In addition, many contrast techniques are now becoming more routinely used, allowing greater amounts of detail and information to be elucidated from the digestive and urinary systems as well as such structures as lacrimal ducts. It can still, however, be a challenge to obtain diagnostic images from some of the smaller species. This is often due to their rapid respiratory rates and fine skeletal structures, which may push the routine resolution of screen cassette film to its limits. Thus non-screen films are being increasingly used.

The larger species have their own peculiar problems, with the need often for mobile or large animal radiography units for species such as the pot-bellied pig. Ultrasonography is now being used much more widely in veterinary medicine, and the exotic mammal field is no different. Units are now affordable and highly mobile as well as providing small enough sector transducer probes to make examination of the smallest mammal possible. Some practices and institutions are able to provide magnetic resonance imaging (MRI) and computed tomography (CT) scanning equipment, taking diagnostic imaging one stage further.

Considerations that need to be addressed for each patient include:

- Is the patient aggressive, highly mobile or stressed? If so, consideration should be given to the use of chemical restraint prior to diagnostic imaging
- Does the patient have serious respiratory distress or hypovolaemic shock? If so, prior oxygenation, circulatory support and minimal restraint techniques should be considered, or diagnostic procedures postponed until stabilization has been achieved
- What is the area to be imaged?
- What is the size/age of the patient to be examined?

Ultimately, the goal for any diagnostic procedure is to achieve safe immobility and positioning of the patient to obtain consistent and clear images. In reality, however, some patients are not good candidates for chemical or excessive physical restraint, and compromises may need to be made.

Positioning

Ideally, the patient should be immobilized chemically to provide optimal positioning and to allow staff and other personnel to vacate the immediate area in the case of radiography (as per health and safety guidelines). Details of anaesthetic and sedative regimens are given for individual species in each chapter. In general, for many healthy and debilitated individuals the use of the gaseous anaesthetic isoflurane is to be advocated for its wide margin of safety for both animals and anaesthetists. Some species may be sufficiently tame to be restrained by the use of weighted sandbags or, in the case of ultrasonography, manual restraint may be used, and indeed is helpful for orientating the patient. Some of the smaller species that may be too debilitated to sedate or restrain may be placed into small cardboard carry boxes and then placed on the radiographic cassette/film in emergency situations, although this results in an inevitable sacrifice in radiographic quality.

The positioning of exotic or small mammal patients for radiography is similar to that of any other companion animal. Two views at right angles to each other are desirable to obtain a three-dimensional image of the patient. Lateral and dorsoventral views for chest radiographs and lateral and ventrodorsal or dorsoventral views for abdominal radiographs are standard. When radiographing limbs the dorsopalmar, dorsoplantar or craniocaudal views are required in addition to lateral ones. Many species considered here are so small that, for standard cassette film, separating limb views from whole body radiographs may be difficult. This is where the use of non-screen films, such as dental films, can be very useful, as they allow specific targeting of small areas and the viewing of fine details. These include radiography of the distal limbs and dentition of many of the species discussed in this manual. A useful technique for examination of ferret teeth, which are particularly prone to tartar formation and periodontal disease, is to use the bisecting angle positioning used in human and companion animal practice. This technique involves positioning the beam of the radiographic unit at 90 degrees to a line bisecting the planes of the radiographic film and the axis of the tooth to be examined.

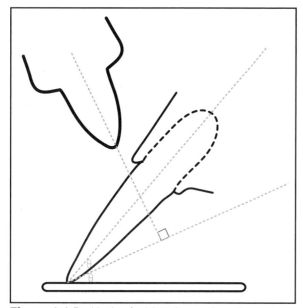

Figure 1.1 Positioning for bisecting angle radiographs.

This technique prevents distortion of the true length of the root of the tooth, which occurs with straightforward dorsoventral/lateral views, and allows assessment of the periodontal alveolar socket for early abscessation and periodontal disease (Figure 1.1).

Positioning for ultrasonography is again as for companion animal practice. The use of a table/bench with an area cut out to allow positioning of the transducer probe on the dependent side of the patient's body is extremely useful. Fur must be adequately shaved from the area to be examined and a coupling gel used to increase contact and enhance the image produced. Care should be taken not to cool the patient by excessive use of gel. Many more tractable species such as guinea pigs, rats and rabbits may be held consciously for this non-painful procedure, although patients may need chemical restraint if they show signs of struggling, especially when taking measurements of organs such as the heart.

Radiography

Equipment

Radiography unit

The basic requirements of a radiography unit are that it should be capable of producing a range of voltages from 40 to 70 kV, with a rapid exposure time of 0.008–0.016 seconds (Silverman, 1993). It is useful to have a radiographic unit that will allow variation of the focal film distance. This allows some magnification of areas being examined, which is particularly useful for smaller species. For some of the larger exotic species, a radiographic unit that is mobile and can be rotated to project the beam horizontally is useful. This is particularly so for examination of species such as the Vietnamese pot-bellied pig, as minimal chemical restraint can be employed and standing views taken of the limbs or torso. Horizontal X-ray beams are also useful when looking for fluid lines in body cavities.

Smaller radiography units, such as those used for human dental examinations, are also extremely useful for small species, as they offer a fixed voltage and amperage, the only variation being in exposure time, from 0.05 to 3 seconds. This means that some form of chemical restraint is often necessary, but the low power of the unit coupled with non-screen dental radiographic film makes fine detail possible.

Radiographic film and cassettes

Radiographic film used as mentioned is based on that utilized in companion animal practice. The Ultravision® series (DuPont®), the Kodak® series of non-screen dental films (DF50, DF75), and mammography films are extremely useful for enhancing fine skeletal detail.

To enhance the clarity of the image further, rare earth, detail or intensifying screens and cassettes should be used in conjunction with the respective radiographic film. The use of grids to reduce scatter effects should be restricted to the larger species, such as rabbits, where the thickness of the area to be imaged exceeds 10 cm (Stefanacci and Hoefer, 1997).

Contrast techniques

Contrast techniques are widely used in companion animal practice and may be performed in exotic small mammals.

Gastrointestinal tract: For gastrointestinal disease, such as screening for stomach ulcers in ferrets or trichobezoars in rabbits, barium sulphate may be administered orally or, in the case of rabbits, by nasogastric tube. The solution needs to be relatively dilute to pass through the 3–4 French diameter nasogastric tubes, with doses of 10–20 ml/kg bodyweight, and sequential radiographs should then be taken at time 0 and every 20 minutes thereafter. For detection of conditions such as megaoesophagus in ferrets, doses of 5–10 ml/kg should be given as barium swallows, and radiographs, or fluoroscopy if available, performed immediately. Examination of the intestinal lumen and walls by barium study is useful in carnivorous species such as ferrets, where some idea of lumen narrowing or wall thickening in conditions such as proliferative bowel disease or neoplasia can be gained. It is, however, a less useful technique for herbivorous species such as chinchillas, rabbits and guinea pigs, where the presence of large volumes of ingesta, fluid and gas are common and where caecotrophy and hence recycling of the barium occurs. Air gastrograms are also useful, especially for detecting trichobezoars in rabbits.

Urinary tract: Examinations of the urinary system can also be enhanced by the use of positive contrast studies. They allow the examination of the lining of the bladder, the highlighting of any uroliths and the separation of the urinary bladder shadow from other organs, such as the female reproductive system, which may act as an aid in the diagnosis of uterine enlargement and tumours. The techniques for this differ from procedures for dogs and cats, as the often small size of the patients involved makes urethral catheterization extremely difficult. Intravenous techniques are often employed, using radiopaque iodine-based substances (e.g. Conray®) at doses of 1–2 ml/kg bodyweight to gain an excretory urogram. Radiographs can be taken from 0–5 minutes after administration, as the substance is removed from the bloodstream by the kidneys and excreted into the bladder.

Many uroliths, particularly in small herbivores, are radiopaque as they are usually calcium carbonate based, or triple phosphate/struvite crystals in ferrets. However, less radiopaque oxalate crystals may be found. In ferrets, many males are large enough for the urethra to be catheterized with latex 23–25 gauge intravenous catheters, or in some larger males, a 3 French tomcat catheter. This allows the use of positive and negative, or even double, contrast techniques to be employed. Care should be taken with volumes of air/contrast media administered, with a maximum of 10 ml in an adult ferret.

Nasolacrimal duct: Other areas that benefit from the use of positive contrast techniques include the naso-lacrimal ducts of rabbits when investigating dental disease and oculonasal discharges. The solitary lacrimal punctum of the lower lid for either eye may be catheterized with a specialized tear duct cannula or with a 25–27 gauge latex intravenous catheter. Volumes of 0.5–1 ml of iodine-based contrast medium may then be flushed through the duct and lateral or oblique lateral radiographs taken immediately.

Interpretation of radiographs of small mammals

The radiographs in this chapter illustrate the normal anatomy of the most commonly examined small mammals. Some abnormal findings are highlighted for comparison. A few points of significance in individual species are mentioned.

Rats and mice

Right lateral and dorsoventral whole body radiographs of a male rat are shown in Figure 1.2.

The abdomen of the mouse, and particularly that of the rat, is disproportionately large in relation to the thorax. The caecum may be found as a dilated ingesta-filled organ in the left caudal abdomen. The stomach tends to be part buried in the liver mass on the left side and is an elongated organ. In cases of enteritis, the small intestinal loops often become gas-filled in the mid-abdomen, with the stomach becoming obviously enlarged with luminal gas. The liver contains no gallbladder in the rat and is a flattened organ tucked underneath the ribcage in the normal adult. The testes may be retracted into the abdomen but even when in the scrotal region a fat body projects from their cranial aspect into the caudoventral abdomen.

The heart fills the cranial and ventral aspect of the thorax and is often difficult to view clearly due to the

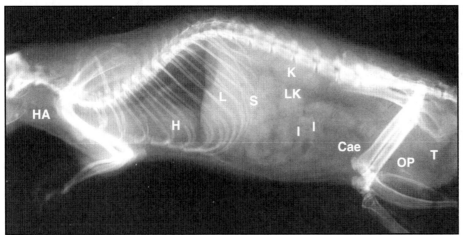
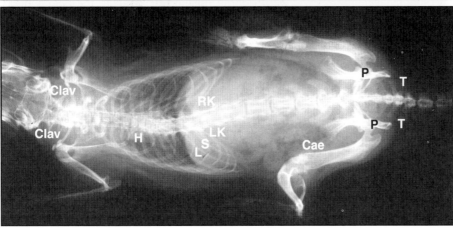

Figure 1.2 Right lateral and dorsoventral whole body radiographs of a male rat. Cae = caecum; Clav = clavicle; H = heart; HA = hyoid apparatus; I = intestine; K = kidney; L = liver; LK = left kidney; OP = os penis; P = pelvis; RK = right kidney; S = stomach; T = testis.

interference of the forelimb musculature in lateral radiographs. A bronchial pattern is a not uncommon finding in older rats and mice, and may reflect the high incidence of respiratory disease in these species.

An os penis is present in both rats and mice.

Hamsters

Left lateral abdominal and thoracic radiographs of a male hamster are shown in Figure 1.3.

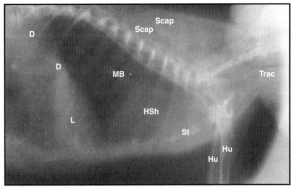

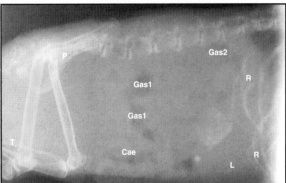

Figure 1.3 Left lateral thoracic and abdominal radiographs of a male hamster. Cae = caecum; D = diaphragm; Gas1 = gas in sacculated caecum; Gas 2 = gas in non-glandular portion of stomach; HSh = heart shadow; Hu = humerus; L = liver; MB = main bronchus; P = pelvis; R = calcified sternal portion of ribs; Scap = scapula; St = sternebrae; T = testis; Trac = trachea

The abdomen of the hamster is filled with a large intestinal mass, with a dilation of the caecum into a sacculated organ in the lower left abdomen. The small intestine is longer than in many other small mammals and is coiled. The large volume of the gastrointestinal tract results in poor abdominal detail for other organs such as the kidneys and spleen. The stomach has two portions, a non-glandular proximal section and a glandular distal section, which are noticeably distinct. The non-glandular portion often possesses a gas bubble.

The thorax is small in relation to the abdomen and filled cranioventrally by the heart, which can become globoid and much enlarged due to valvular damage from endocarditic lesions in later life. The sternal portion of the ribs commonly calcifies with age.

The skeletal structure is fine, and spondylosis lesions are a not uncommon finding in the lumbar region of the spine. Fractures of the tibia are very common in hamsters that fall from the bars of their cages.

Chipmunks

Radiographically chipmunks resemble the form of the ferret (see below). The skull, however, is similar to that of other rodents, and overgrowth or malocclusion of the incisors is a common finding (Figure 1.4). Other common radiographic abnormalities include fractures of the hindlimbs and the lumbar spine due to bullying or falls from the bars of aviary-style enclosures.

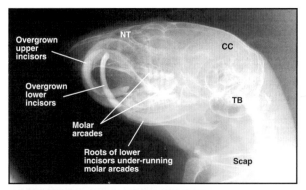

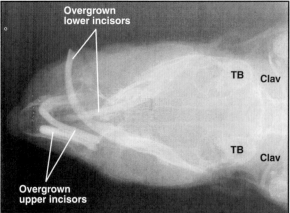

Figure 1.4 Right lateral and dorsoventral skull radiographs of a chipmunk with overgrown incisors. CC = cranial cavity; Clav = clavicle; NT = nasal turbinates; Scap = scapula; TB = tympanic bulla.

Guinea pigs

Right lateral and dorsoventral whole body radiographs of an entire male guinea pig are shown in Figure 1.5.

The abdomen of the guinea pig is much the same as that of the rabbit (see below), being mainly filled with the large intestine and caecum, the latter containing haustrae that give it a segmental appearance on radiographs. This large hindgut tends to produce an amorphous radiographic picture due to the gas and ingesta, making the clarity of abdominal radiographs poor. The stomach tends to be much smaller and to contain less ingesta on average in relation to the rest of the gastrointestinal tract than is the case in the rabbit. Urolithiasis is not uncommon; the uroliths tend to be calcium carbonate or calcium oxalate and so are radiopaque. A common presenting problem of older female guinea pigs is cystic ovarian disease (Figure 1.6). The ovaries can attain enormous sizes due to persistent rete ovarii cysts, which may well be accompanied by pathological changes or even tumours of the reproductive system.

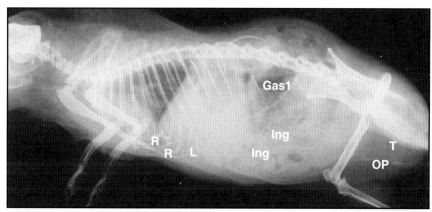

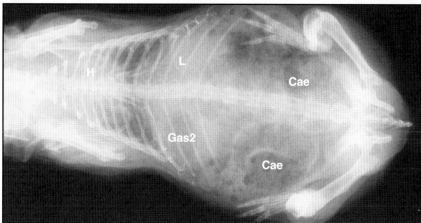

Figure 1.5 Right lateral and dorsoventral whole body radiographs of an entire male guinea pig. Cae = caecum; Gas1 = gas in caecum (haustrae); Gas2 = gas in fundus of stomach; H = heart; Ing = ingesta in caecum and large intestine; L= liver; OP = os penis; R = calcified sternal portion of ribs; T = testis.

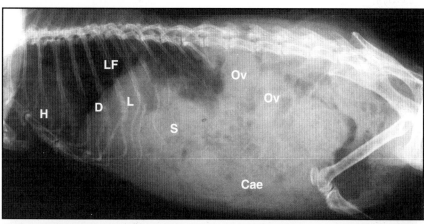

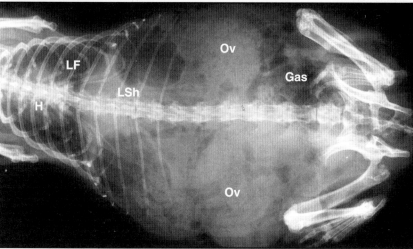

Figure 1.6 Right lateral and dorsoventral whole body radiographs of a 4-year-old entire female guinea pig with cystic ovarian disease. Cae = caecum; D = diaphragm; Gas = gas in caecum; H = heart; L = liver; LF = lung field; LSh= liver shadow; Ov = bilateral cystic ovaries; S = stomach.

The thorax of guinea pigs is small in relation to the abdomen. This is particularly the case for the cranial lung area, which appears much reduced on radiographs, the heart and thymus, which persist in the adult, appearing to fill the cranioventral thorax.

The skeletal structure of guinea pigs is similar to that of chinchillas and rabbits, being relatively fine boned compared with body size. This makes them susceptible to fractures of the lumbar spine and limbs, and if guinea pigs are housed with rabbits rib fractures are not uncommon. The characteristic three digits of the hindlimbs distinguish the radiographs of guinea pigs from those of other small mammals.

The male guinea pig possesses an os penis.

Chinchillas

Right lateral and dorsoventral whole body radiographs of a male chinchilla are shown in Figure 1.7.

The abdomen of the chinchilla is similar to that of the guinea pig. Like most of the small herbivores, the chinchilla is a hindgut fermenter with an extremely long large intestine. The proximal third of this large intestine is sacculated, giving a segmental appearance on radiographs. The distal two thirds of the large intestine is unsacculated and has a much smaller diameter, although it often has a beaded appearance due to the faecal pellets present in its lumen. The liver is a flattened organ in the most cranial portion of the abdomen. The testes in the male sit in the inguinal region, rather than

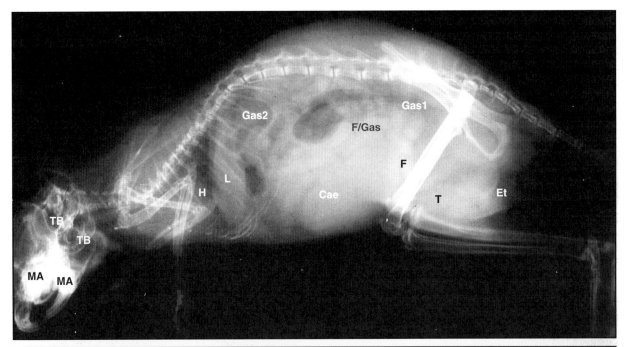

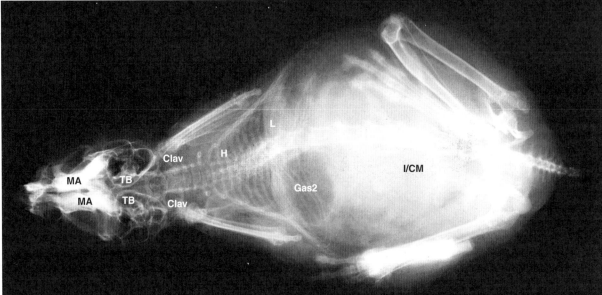

Figure 1.7 Right lateral and dorsoventral whole body radiographs of a male chinchilla. Cae = caecum; Clav = clavicle; Et = tail of epididymis; F = fat body of testes projecting into abdomen; F/Gas = fluid and gas in sacculated proximal large intestine leading from caecum; Gas 1 = gas in sacculated areas of proximal large intestine; Gas 2 = gas in fundus of stomach; H = heart; I/CM = intestinal/caecal mass; L = liver; MA = molar arcade; T = testis; TB = tympanic bulla.

a true scrotal position, although the tails of the epididymes do sit scrotally. A large fat body extends into the abdominal cavity from the cranial pole of each testicle.

The thorax of the chinchilla is small in relation to the abdomen. The heart fills most of the cranioventral thoracic space.

The skeletal structure, as with the rabbit and guinea pig, is relatively delicate radiographically. The most obvious aspect of skull radiographs in chinchillas are the large auditory/tympanic bullae housing the middle ear. Lateral head radiographs (Figures 1.8 and 1.9) are an important tool for detecting and assessing dental disease in chinchillas (see Chapter 7). Not only can the visible molar crowns overgrow orally, but the roots can protrude through the ventral aspect of the mandible

and into the nasal passages and the orbit of the eye in the maxilla. The latter problem can lead to persistently watery eyes and a nasal discharge as well as inappetence due to dental pain. A test to see if the molars are slightly over-long is to extend a line from the nasal bones and the ventral aspect of the mandible rostrally. These lines should converge; if they diverge or remain parallel, the molars are likely to be too long.

Chinchillas possess clavicles similar to rabbits and ferrets. Male chinchillas possess a small os penis in the distal portion of the penis.

Rabbits

Right lateral and dorsoventral views of the trunk of a male Netherland dwarf rabbit are shown in Figure 1.10.

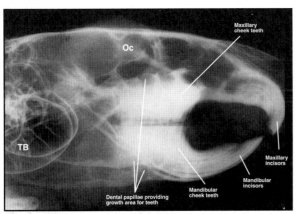

Figure 1.8 Left lateral radiograph of a chinchilla's head, showing the normal positions of molar and incisor. TB = tympanic bulla; Oc = ocular orbit.

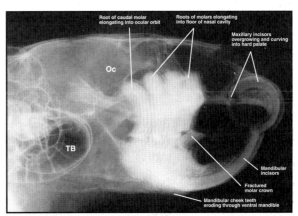

Figure 1.9 Left lateral radiograph of a chinchilla's head, showing overgrown incisors and molar roots. TB = tympanic bulla; Oc = ocular orbit.

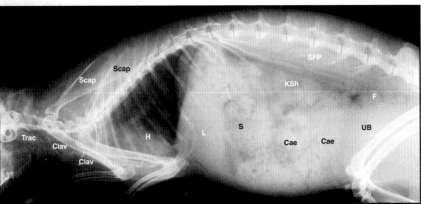

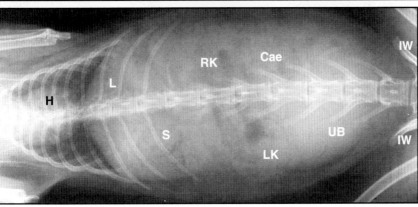

Figure 1.10 Right lateral and dorsoventral whole body radiographs of a male Netherland Dwarf rabbit. Cae = caecum; Clav = clavicle; F = faecal pellet in rectum; KSh = kidney shadow; H = heart; IW = ilial wing; L = liver; LK = left kidney; RK = right kidney; S = stomach; Scap = scapula; SFP = sublumbar fat pad; Trac = trachea; UB = urinary bladder.

The abdomen of the rabbit is largely occupied by the extensive caecum and large intestine. The caecum sits ventrally, predominantly on the right side, and is full of ingesta and some small volumes of gas in the healthy animal. In cases of bloat or advanced intestinal disease/mucoid enteropathy, excessive gas pockets and fluid build-up may be seen, indicative of colic and intestinal ileus. These signs often carry a grave prognosis as endotoxic shock is commonly the sequel. The dorsal aspect of the abdomen is occupied by the retroperitoneal/sublumbar fat pads, which are usually extensive in the house rabbit. These push the kidney silhouettes ventrally. Renal calculi are commonly found. The liver often appears as a relatively flattened organ, cranial to the stomach (which is always full). The stomach may become overfilled with ingesta or trichobezoars and project caudally beyond the extent of the ribcage. It may also develop a significant gas cap to the fundus. The bladder is commonly filled with small calcium carbonate crystals in adult rabbits (Figure 1.11), due to the rabbit's unique calcium metabolism, especially if dietary calcium levels are high. This appears as a radiodense amorphous mass in-filling the bladder lumen. In some cases individual spherical bladder calculi may be found.

The thorax of the rabbit is relatively small in relation to the abdomen, as is the case for most small herbivores. This makes the heart seem abnormally large, as it occupies most of the cranioventral part of the thoracic cavity. This is often further obscured by the presence of fat deposits in overweight rabbits, which occur around the heart itself, often smudging the cardiac silhouette and persistent remnants of the thymus. It also means that relatively little lung pathology needs to be present, such as that found in association with rabbit snuffles, for the rabbit's respiratory efficiency to be severely compromised. The lungs are also one of the main sites for secondary spread of the uterine adenocarcinomas seen in older entire does (Figure 1.12).

The skeletal structure of the rabbit is delicate. Only 6–7% of the total bodyweight is skeleton, compared with 12–13% in domestic cats. Rabbits possess clavicles similar to ferrets (see below). The scapula has a unique hooked suprahamate process of the acromion (compared with the shorter one of the domestic cat), as well as a triangular infraspinous fossa.

Dental disease is a common problem in rabbits and lateral skull radiographs are extremely useful to determine root elongation of cheek teeth, periodontal

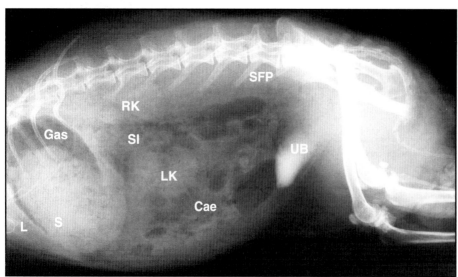

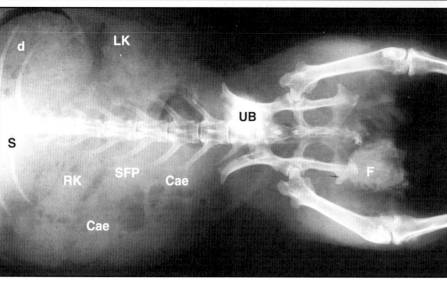

Figure 1.11 Right lateral and ventrodorsal abdominal radiographs of a neutered female rabbit with urolithiasis. Cae = caecum, full of digesta, found mainly on the right side; d = digesta in stomach; F = faecal material adhering to fur (external); Gas = gas cap in fundus; L = liver; LK = left kidney; RK = right kidney; S = stomach, with large volume of digesta; SFP = sublumbar fat pad; SI = small intestine; UB = urinary bladder with calcium carbonate crystals.

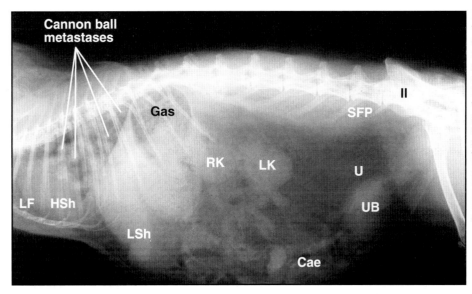

Figure 1.12 Right lateral whole body radiograph of entire 5-year-old female rabbit with uterine adenocarcinoma and secondary metastases to the lung field. Cae = caecum, with digesta and gas; Gas = gas cap in fundus of stomach; HSh = heart shadow; Il = ilium; LF = lung field; LK = left kidney; LSh = liver shadow; RK = right kidney; SFP = sublumbar fat pad; U = uterus; UB = urinary bladder, with calcium carbonate urolithiasis.

disease and abscess formation (Figures 1.13 and 1.14). Many of the problems associated with an oculonasal discharge in rabbits have their source in dental disease. This can be shown by plain and contrast lacrimal duct studies (Figure 1.15) to demonstrate

narrowing or blockage of the lacrimal duct as it passes over the cheek teeth roots or around the roots of the maxillary incisors.

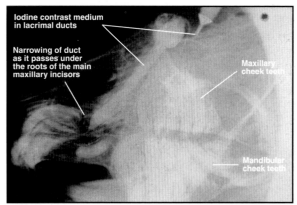

Figure 1.15 Oblique lateral radiograph of the head of a neutered female rabbit using positive contrast study of the lacrimal ducts.

Figure 1.13 Right lateral radiograph of normal dentition in a neutered female rabbit. There are six maxillary cheek teeth each side; the height of the roots should not project above the arch of the maxillary incisors. There are five mandibular cheek teeth each side; the roots should not distort the line of the mandible ventrally.

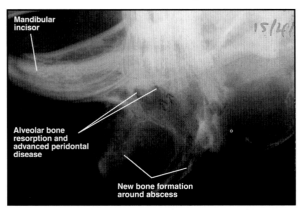

Figure 1.14 Right lateral radiograph of a mandibular abscess, periodontal disease and new bone formation in a rabbit.

Ferrets

Right lateral and dorsoventral whole body radiographs of a 3-year-old castrated male ferret are shown in Figure 1.16.

The abdomen of the ferret has a few notable features. Its form is very elongated but organs are often well delineated due to the retroperitoneal fat present. The spleen is often a relatively large organ in the adult ferret. There may be some small volumes of gas within the gastrointestinal tract, although excessive volumes are suggestive of inflammatory bowel disease or, if accompanied by gastric dilation, an intestinal foreign body, which is very common in ferrets. The male ferret possesses a prostate, and negative contrast techniques can be useful for detecting enlargement.

The thorax of the ferret is very elongated and narrow. The heart should cover 2–2.5 rib space widths. When cardiomyopathies are suspected, the heart often becomes globoid in shape, although ultrasonography is required to distinguish hypertrophic from dilated forms. The heart may be seen to be pushed caudally in cases of thymic lymphoma, with a precardiac shadow.

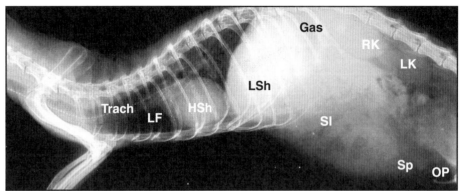

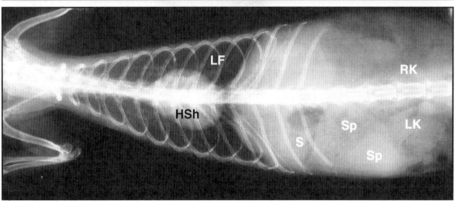

Figure 1.16 Right lateral and dorsoventral whole body radiographs of a 3-year-old castrated male ferret. Gas = gas pocket of fundus; HSh = heart shadow; LF = lung field; LK = left kidney; LSh = liver shadow; OP = os penis; RK = right kidney; S = stomach; SI = small intestine; Sp = spleen; Trach = trachea.

The skeletal structure follows the basic quadruped form. The male ferret possesses an os penis, and both sexes possess vestigal clavicles.

Dental disease is common (Figure 1.17).

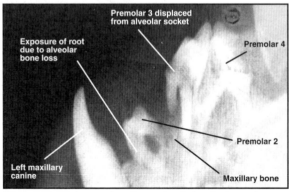

Figure 1.17 Intraoral radiograph of alveolar bone loss around premolar 2/premolar 3 of the left maxillary arcade of a 4-year-old castrated male ferret.

Fancy pigs

The Vietnamese pot-bellied pig is probably the most commonly encountered fancy pig. Radiography of an adult is extremely difficult for anything other than the extremities. In the case of lameness or limb pathology, a mobile large animal radiographic unit for craniocaudal and lateral extended and flexed radiographs can be employed. For thoracic or abdominal radiography, larger fixed units, such as those employed in large animal teaching hospitals and equine hospitals, should be considered in the case of adult pigs. Juveniles and piglets may be radiographed more routinely using small animal facilities, although use of grids to avoid scatter and voltages up to 80kV may still need to be employed for larger animals.

Primates

Most of the smaller pet primates may be radiographed using standard companion animal facilities. Radiographic surveys are particularly useful for the assessment of bone quality in cases of suspected nutritional secondary hyperparathyroidism and/or vitamin D deficiency (rickets). In addition, radiography can be essential in the detection of tuberculous lesions in the lymph nodes of the thorax and abdomen, the detection of foreign bodies and in assessing the extent of dental disease.

Ultrasonography

Equipment

Ultrasound unit

The standard units for companion animal practice are suitable for small mammal work. The important points are that a sector probe transducer should be used rather than the linear array form used in examinations of the reproductive system of farm animals. In addition probes of higher frequency are preferred. The 5 MHz sector probe is satisfactory for most small mammals such as rabbits, ferrets and the larger guinea pigs and chinchillas. For smaller species, such as the rodent family, a 7.5 MHz sector probe can give better detail, and the decreased depth penetration is not important with this size of patient. In general the most widely used and useful form of ultrasound for small mammals is the B-mode form, which provides a two-dimensional 'real-time' image. The M-mode form may also be used for measurement of the heart's contractility and wall thickness, useful for species prone to cardiomyopathy lesions, such as the ferret. Finally, Doppler technology can be used to assess turbulence within the heart itself, useful in species such as hamsters, which commonly have endocarditic lesions.

Additional equipment

Additional equipment for ultrasonography is relatively limited, but nonetheless vital. The main component is for a coupling mechanism to allow the ultrasound waves to reach the skin surface. Standard coupling gels as provided for companion and farm animals can be used. It is necessary to shave fur prior to the application of the gel and to apply the gel some minutes before examination begins to allow it to permeate the area. Care should be taken to ensure that these procedures do not lead to chilling.

The provision of a solid worktop surface with a hole cut into it to allow the sector probe to be applied to the dependent side of the recumbent patient can also be useful. In the case of many of the very small species, manual or chemical restraint may be needed to enable the animal to remain still enough for a meaningful examination.

Finally, the presence of video recording equipment or a printer may be helpful for post-examination interpretation and to allow a library of 'normal' organ examinations to be built up for comparison.

Interpretation of ultrasound images

In the interpretation of ultrasound images in small mammals, the same basic principles apply as for companion and farm animals. Fluids are anechoic and appear black, allowing clear examination of structures deeper to them. Gas and very dense substances such as bone appear hyperechoic and white on the screen, with a 'shadow' effect effectively blocking examination of deeper structures.

The chest is therefore not a good body cavity for ultrasound examination except for the heart or when there is a pleural effusion. The abdominal cavity makes a better subject, particularly in the ferret and rodents. The rabbit, guinea pig and chinchilla make relatively good ultrasound subjects, though the presence of large amounts of caecal and large intestinal gas often leads to hyperechoic interference. However, with patience and using the bladder as an 'acoustic window,' all of the major organs may be examined. This is particularly useful for the examination of the reproductive tract to determine early stage pregnancy, which in the case of rabbits may be determined from 10–14 days after conception.

Figures 1.18 to 1.21 give an idea of the structures that can be examined in some small mammals.

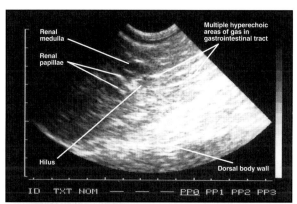

Figure 1.18 Ultrasound image in longitudinal section of a normal left kidney in a rabbit.

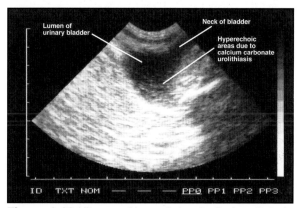

Figure 1.19 Ultrasound image in longitudinal section of the urinary bladder in a rabbit.

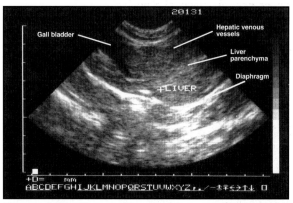

Figure 1.20 Ultrasound image of the normal liver and gallbladder of a neutered female rabbit.

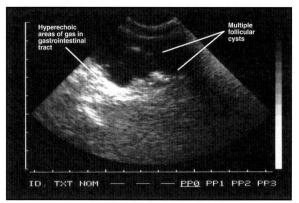

Figure 1.21 Ultrasound image of a cystic ovary in a guinea pig.

CT and MRI examinations

Computed tomography (CT) creates a cross-sectional image of the patient and is useful for examining skeletal structure and form, such as that described for the analysis of dental disease in chinchillas (Crossley *et al.*, 1998). Anaesthesia is required, as the animal must be totally stationary while a rotating X-ray beam images the patient in segments.

Magnetic resonance imaging (MRI) is a relatively new technique that relies on aligning protons within the patient inside a strong magnetic field. It is useful for soft tissue diagnostic imaging as soft tissues that appear of similar density on CT and conventional radiography can be easily differentiated with MRI. It is therefore of use in determining the presence of soft tissue changes such as tumours, polyps and haematomas. MRI also requires the patient to be totally immobilized.

Both techniques are in their infancy with application to exotic mammals but, as time progresses, more centres are gaining the expertise and equipment, making these techniques a feasible diagnostic tool for the future.

References and further reading

Aitken V (1983) Radiographic studies of exotic species. *Radiography* **49**, 179–202

Crossley DA, Jackson A, Yates J and Boydell IP (1998) Use of computed tomography to investigate cheek tooth abnormalities in chinchillas. *Journal of Small Animal Practice* **39**, 385–389

Rubel GA, Isenbugel E and Wolverkamp P (1991) *Atlas of Diagnostic Radiology of Exotic Pets.* WB Saunders, Philadelphia

Silverman S (1993) Diagnostic imaging of exotic pets. *Veterinary Clinics of North America: Small Animal Practice* **23**, 1287–1299

Stefanacci JD and Hoefer HL (1997) Small mammal radiology. In: *Ferrets, Rabbits and Rodents: Clinical Medicine and Surgery*, ed. EV Hillyer and KE Quesenberry, pp. 358–377. WB Saunders, Philadelphia

2

Rats and mice

Hannah E. Orr

Introduction

The common pet rat (*Rattus norvegicus*) and mouse (*Mus musculus*) are rodents (from the Latin word *rodere*, to gnaw) of the Family Muridae. These two species are the most likely to be kept as pets, and in many countries they are bred to show standards and exhibited. Fancy mice and rats have been bred for exhibition for at least 100 years in the UK. Because of the drive to breed and exhibit new varieties, there are many colours and markings.

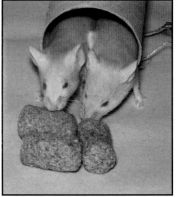

Figure 2.1 Two fancy mice.

The varieties of fancy mice (Figure 2.1) are classified in five sections:

- Self: solid coat colour (11 recognized self-colours)
- Tan: self upper body and tan belly
- Marked: e.g. Banded, Tri-colour, Himalayan
- Satin: self-coloured, with high-gloss fur
- Any Other Variety (AOV): all other recognized standards (e.g. Longhaired, Brindle, Seal Point).

Fancy rats (Figure 2.2) are also classified in five sections:

- Self: one solid colour (10 recognized self-colours)
- Marked (e.g. Irish, Berkshire, Hooded, Capped)
- Silver: recognized self-colour containing equal numbers of silver and non-silver guard hairs
- AOV (e.g. Siamese, Agouti)
- Rex: coat with as few guard hairs as possible and evenly curled (even the whiskers will sometimes be curly).

Advice to clients on buying rats and mice

Rats and mice can be very suitable pets for both adults and children.

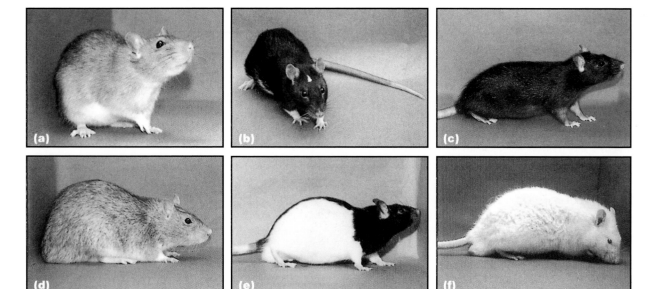

Figure 2.2 Examples of fancy rat varieties. (a) Agouti. (b) Berkshire. (c) Black. (d) Chinchilla. (e) Hooded. (f) Pink-eyed white rex. (Courtesy of Supreme Petfoods).

- Rats in particular make excellent pets as they rarely bite, especially if well socialized from an early age; they display more individual 'personality' than mice and they can also be trained
- Rats tend to be more nocturnal than mice and spend most of the day asleep, hence their suitability as pets for those who are out all day
- Mice tend to be more active and move faster than rats and sometimes leap out of a small child's hands. They cannot be trained to the same extent as rats
- For both species, the more enrichment that is provided in their environment and the more time an owner spends with them, the more an animal's 'personality' comes across
- Male rats tend to be more docile than females and if allowed out of their cages will often simply sleep on their owner's lap
- Males tend to smell stronger than females but neutering of males may reduce the smell to some extent
- A high percentage of female rats develop mammary tumours in later life (frequency up to 50% in many laboratory strains)
- A rat or mouse will benefit from being housed with a companion of the same species and demonstrate a wider range of behaviours when group housed
- A pair of rats or mice from the same litter will usually live together for their lifespan without fighting
- Introducing adult males to each other is not to be recommended (Figure 2.3); it is easier to introduce older females of both species.

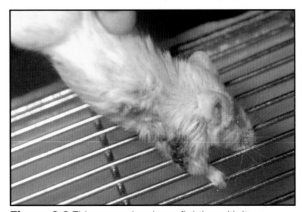

Figure 2.3 This mouse has been fighting with its companions.

Pet rats and mice are available from breeders, animal rescue centres and pet-shops. It is best to buy direct from a good breeder as this should ensure that the animal's parents are in good health and the young have been handled on a regular basis. In the UK the National Fancy Rat Society maintains a 'Kitten Register' listing breeders with baby rats that are suitable as pets (see 'Useful Contacts' at the end of this chapter).

The potential pitfalls of buying an animal from a pet shop are that it is of unknown health status, it has been mixed with animals from various sources and it is often difficult to determine the extent to which the animal has been handled and socialized. Early socialization with people plays an important part in the making of a friendly pet.

Biology

Biological data for rats and mice are summarized in Figure 2.4 and normal haematological and biochemical values in Figure 2.5.

	Rats	**Mice**
Life expectancy	$2^1/_2$–$3^1/_2$ years	$1^1/_2$–$2^1/_2$ years

Weight
  Male
  Female
	
	267–500 g
	225–325 g
		
		20–40 g
		22–63 g

Dentition	2 (I1/1 C0/0 P0/0 M3/3)	
Respiratory rate	70–150 breaths per minute	100–250 breaths per minute
Tidal volume	1.5–1.8 ml	0.3–0.5 ml
Heart rate	260–450 beats per minute	500–600 beats per minute
Blood volume	70 ml/kg	80 ml/kg
Rectal temperature[a]	38 °C	37.5 °C
Water intake (av. daily)	10 ml/100 g	15 ml/100 g
Urine production	13–23 ml/day	1–2 ml/day
Environmental temperature	21–24 °C	24–25 °C
Sexual maturity	6–8 weeks	6–7 weeks
Oestrous cycle	4–5 days	4–5 days
Duration of oestrus	14 hours	14 hours
Gestation	20–22 days	19–21 days
Litter size (average)	6–16 (10)	6–12 (8)
Birthweight	4–7 g	1–1.5 g
Eyes open	12–14 days	12–14 days
Weaning age, earliest	21 days	21 days

Figure 2.4 Biological data for rats and mice.

a There is large individual variation in normal rectal temperature with age, sex and strain of animal and with the environmental temperature.

Dentition

When rats and mice are gnawing, the cheeks are pulled into the diastema (the space between the incisors and molars) so that particles can be easily expelled from the mouth. The incisor teeth are constantly erupting and are worn down by the gnawing action. The front surface of the incisor teeth is covered in a layer of hard enamel but the back surface has only an outer layer of softer dentine; therefore the teeth wear unevenly, producing the characteristic 'chisel' shape. It is normal for the teeth to have a yellowish colour, caused by the presence of iron pigments.

	Reference range rats	Reference range mice
ALT (IU/l)	50–150	68–85
AP (IU/l)	100–250	100–200
AST (IU/l)	192–262	200–400
Total protein (g/dl)	5.9–8.4	5.6–6.25
Albumin (g/dl)	3.2–4.3	3.5–4.6
Globulin (g/dl)	2.9–4.8	–
Urea (mg/dl)	12–25.8	13.9–28.3
Creatinine (mg/dl)	0.39–2.29	0.3–1.0
Glucose (mg/dl)	89.5–183.3	62.8–176
Sodium (mEq/l)	129–150	128–145
Calcium (mg/dl)	9.6–11.0	3.2–8.5
Potassium (mEq/l)	4.6–6.0	4.85–5.85
Chloride (mEq/l)	97–110	105–110
Phosphorus (mg/dl)	6.0–8.0	2.3–9.2
Haematocrit/PCV (%)	36.0–52.0	40.4 ± 3.8
RBC (×10 power 12/l)	5.00–12.0	8.39 ± 1.2
Haemoglobin (g/dl)	11.1–18.0	13.1 ± 1.5
MCV	44.5–69.0	49.1 ± 3.4
MCH	12.0–24.5	15.9 ± 1.1
MCHC (%)	21.6–42.0	32.3 ± 1.4
Clotting time (minutes)	–	2–10
PTT (seconds)	–	55–110
Prothrombin time (seconds)	–	7–19
Reticulocytes	–	4.7 ± 3.3
Leucocyte count		
Total (×10 power 3/µl)	9.98 ± 2.68	8.4 (5.1–11.6)
Neutrophils (%)	4.00–50.0	17.9 (6.7–37.2)
Lymphocytes (%)	40.0–95.0	69 (63–75)
Monocytes (%)	0.00–8.00	1.2 (0.7–2.6)
Eosinophils (%)	0.00–4.00	2.1 (0.9–3.8)
Basophils (%)	0.00–2.00	0.5 (0–1.5)

Figure 2.5 Normal haematological and biochemical values in rats and mice. This table is provided as a rough guide only: it is compiled from data reported in the literature and gives values for animals of mixed sex, breed and age. It should be noted that, for chemistry in particular, values should come from the laboratory running the test, as methods of testing and test machines vary. This is not as crucial for haematology but breed, sex and age of the animals do have considerable effects on some parameters.

Sexing

Sexing of rats and mice is performed by contrasting the shorter anus-to-vulva distance of the female with the longer anus-to-penis distance in the male (Figure 2.6). Rats are easier to sex than mice since the testicles are visible even in juvenile animals. If this is not the case then the animal should be held vertically, which will cause the testes to pass through the inguinal canal into the scrotum. Neonatal rats and mice are harder to sex than the adults, as the testicles of the males are not yet visible and so the only guide is anogenital distance. If animals of both sexes are available, comparison will enable the distinction to be made.

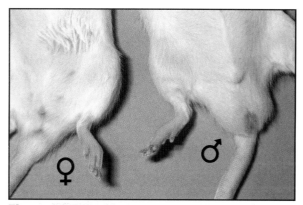

Figure 2.6 Female and male rats, illustrating the difference in anogenital distance.

Husbandry

Housing

Rats and mice like to gnaw and so a cage made of wire with a solid plastic bottom, or an aquarium with a mesh roof, is recommended. The former is preferable as it is better ventilated. Although a wire mesh lid will increase aquarium ventilation, the number of air changes per hour will be fewer than in a more traditional cage.

Ventilation and cage cleanliness are particularly important with respect to the build-up of ammonia, which is formed by the action of microbial urease on urea in the urine. Ammonia is a potent respiratory irritant: levels of 100 ppm cause excessive blinking in rats (the maximum level permitted for staff working with animals in the USA is 25 ppm) and between 25 and 250 ppm there is a positive correlation between rising NH_3 levels and prevalence of *Mycoplasma pulmonis* lung lesions. Limiting ammonia build-up will thus help to prevent respiratory disease and will palliate the clinical signs if the animal does have a respiratory problem.

Frequency of cage cleaning should be balanced against the stress that removal of scent marking and olfactory clues causes. It will also vary with the size of the cage and the number of animals in it.

Cages should supply sufficient space for the occupants to exercise and to allow environmental enrichment (Figure 2.7):

- A shelter to provide the animals with a 'bolt-hole' and a place to sleep should be included in the cage, such as a plastic house from a pet shop for mice or a piece of drain-pipe as a rat's sleeping quarters; these are easily cleaned
- The cage floor should be covered with an absorbent substrate (e.g. sawdust, wood-shavings)
- Nesting material (e.g. shredded newspaper, commercial rodent bedding) should be provided
- Some of the diet can be scattered in the sawdust (in clean areas) to allow foraging
- Other provisions for environmental enrichment include empty cardboard boxes, sheets of paper to tear up, drain-pipes suspended from the cage lid, exercise wheels (with a solid back to prevent long tails getting caught in the side supports as the wheel turns), cat 'treat balls' and ladders.

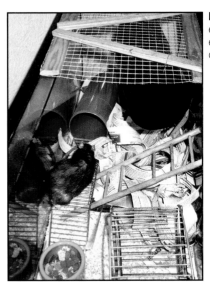

Figure 2.7 An environmentally enriched rat cage.

Many rat owners choose to give their pets 'out-of-cage' time, allowing them the run of a room or even the house, and will often carry them around inside clothing or on a shoulder. Supervised out-of-cage playtime can be rewarding for both rat and owner but careful 'rat proofing' of the area in question is essential.

Diet
Rodents are omnivorous or herbivorous. To avoid dietary imbalances it is best to feed rats and mice primarily on a commercial rodent diet, which can be supplemented with a wide variety of fresh food, fruit and vegetables – in moderation. Excessive supplementation can result in dietary imbalance, obesity or gastric upsets. 'Treats' such as chocolate and yoghurt drops or sticks consisting of dried grains, fruit and vegetables held together with molasses or honey are sold by pet shops and are readily consumed. They should be reserved for special occasions, or as training rewards, as overfeeding of these foods can easily result in obesity and dental caries.

Food bowls should be heavy enough to prevent them being tipped over. A source of water should always be available. A water bottle is probably better than a bowl, as the water is unlikely to become contaminated with cage debris, but it is possible to get an air lock in the sipper tube of a bottle. This is one of the first areas to check if a sick rat or mouse is presented with no significant clinical signs other than looking unwell and dehydrated.

Breeding
Rats and mice are polyoestrous, with no specific breeding season. The stage of the oestrous cycle may be determined by microscopic examination of vaginal smears. Following mating, a plug of ejaculate forms in the vagina. This vaginal plug confirms that mating has taken place, but it can fall out and so may not be observed. Normal reproductive and growth parameters are summarized in Figure 2.4.

To breeders, male rats and mice are known as bucks, females as does and the young as kittens or pups. There are three main breeding methods:

- In monogamous pairs (a male and a female permanently caged together)
- In harems (one male and several females caged together)
- In same-sex groups (if breeding is required a female is introduced to a male, on the male's territory, for a short time).

In the first two systems the male can be left with the female throughout the pregnancy and at birth, but it should be noted that a postpartum oestrus occurs and mating will often take place. Thus a 'population explosion' can be a major problem. The third system allows better control of population numbers.

Parturition occurs most commonly between midnight and 4 a.m. and it can be delayed if the mother is lactating. The pups are normally born within 1–2 hours and any born dead are usually consumed by the mother at birth. The pups receive maternal antibodies in the milk until they are weaned. Bedding material will be used to make a nest for the pups and hide them. It is best not to disturb the mother and pups (Figure 2.8) for 2–3 days after birth, as excessive handling may cause the mother to eat her young – a particular risk with rats. The more familiar the female is with people and being handled, the more tolerant she will be of disturbance.

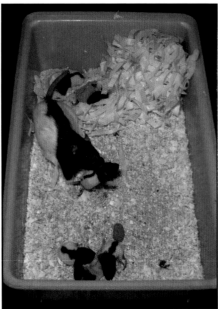

Figure 2.8 Female rat with young.

A female rat may bite those who disturb her and her young. If it is necessary to examine the mother or pups in the first weeks after birth, it is best to move the mother to a separate cage. Distress to the mother is minimized if latex gloves are worn when handling the pups, to stop the handler's scent covering the young.

Handling and restraint

The key to handling either of these species is to be gentle yet firm and decisive.

Mice

Mice in unfamiliar surroundings will often try to bite and so should be handled with care. If the animal is brought to the practice in its cage, the owner should be asked to remove it to a smaller container. From this, the mouse can be picked up by the base of the tail and placed on a rough surface: it will instinctively pull away (Figure 2.9a). With the tail held with one hand, the skin of the scruff can be grasped with the other hand (Figure 2.9b). Ensure that sufficient scruff is grasped to prevent the mouse from turning its head and biting. The mouse can then be lifted and the grip on the tail transferred to the third and fourth fingers (Figure 2.9c).

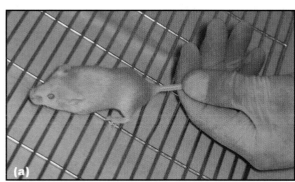

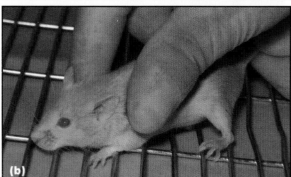

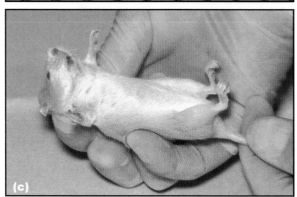

Figure 2.9 Handling techniques for mice.

Rats

Unlike mice, rats rarely bite, even when startled, and this is especially true if they are used to human contact and have been socialized from an early age. If a rat does bite when handled, it is often because it is in pain or very fearful. Remember to wash hands between handling carnivores and these rodents.

Rats, being more nocturnal, will often be asleep when brought into the practice. It is wise to ensure that a rat is awake and aware of the veterinary surgeon's presence before it is picked up.

The rat should be grasped around the shoulders, supporting the hindfeet with the other hand if necessary. To restrain it for a painful procedure (such as injection), place a thumb under the mandible to prevent biting. Hold the animal firmly, but take care not to impair respiration (Figure 2.10). If a rat seems aggressive (such as a doe with young), it can be picked up by the base of its tail. Picking up by the scruff will often cause considerable distress and should be avoided.

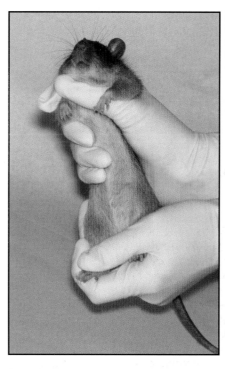

Figure 2.10 Restraint technique for a rat.

Diagnostic approach

Physical examination
Monitoring the weight of rats and mice can be a useful prognosticator.

History
The following questions should be asked:

- What age is the animal?
- When and where was it acquired?
- Does it have companions of the same species? If so, where did they come from and when were they introduced?
- Do animals of other species live in the household?
- What is the diet (including basic ration and treats)?
- Has the diet been changed recently? How was this implemented and what was the animal fed previously?
- Does the animal drink from a bowl or a sipper bottle? How much does it drink each day and has this increased or decreased recently?

Species	Average adult bodyweight	Approximate blood volume	Sample volume	Recommended routes
Rat	300–500 g	70 ml/kg = 21–35 ml	2.4–4 ml	Lateral tail vein Saphenous vein
Mouse	25–40 g	80 ml/kg = 2–3.2 ml	0.2–0.32 ml	Lateral tail vein Saphenous vein

Figure 2.11 Sample volumes and routes for blood sampling in rats and mice. (The address of a web page site showing a saphenous vein bleeding technique in mice is given in the 'Useful contacts' section.)

- What type of housing is used and of what dimensions? What bedding is used? How often is the cage cleaned out?
- Have there been any changes in the amount or consistency of the faeces or the wetness of the cage contents?
- Is the animal handled regularly? If so, how often and by whom?
- Does the animal have out-of-cage playtime? Is this always supervised and, if so, by whom?
- What problem is the animal being presented for? When was this first noticed and what caused the owner to notice the problem?

Sample collection

Blood
It is assumed rats and mice have approximately 70 and 80 ml of blood per kilogram of bodyweight, respectively. No more than 10% of that volume should be removed from any healthy animal in a period of 3–4 weeks and volumes should be reduced appropriately in sick rats or mice. Figure 2.11 gives sample volumes and routes for rats and mice.

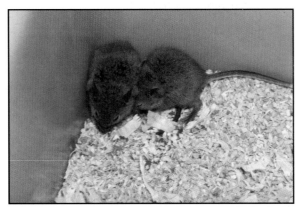

Figure 2.12 Sick mice exhibiting typical clinical signs.

Urine
Rats and mice that are not accustomed to being handled will often urinate when restrained as an alarm reflex. Otherwise a sample can be obtained by placing the animal on a non-absorbent surface. Cystocentesis and urethral catheterization are generally not practicable in these animals.

Common conditions

Healthy rats and mice spend a large proportion of their waking hours grooming, which keeps their coats well kempt, clean and shiny. Signs of ill health are frequently reflected in their external appearance: the coat becomes ruffled and 'staring'. They also eat and drink less and lose weight; their activity decreases and they finally display a characteristic clinical picture: hunched up with an unkempt coat, isolated from cage mates, disinterested in surroundings and reluctant to move (Figure 2.12).

Pet rats and mice develop a range of clinical conditions (Figure 2.13). Extrapolation from techniques for the more familiar species will often enable diagnosis and treatment of conditions. A drug formulary for rats and mice is summarized at the end of this chapter (see Figure 2.25).

Dental disease
In contrast to the molars, the incisors are open rooted and can overgrow. Incisor malocclusion (Figure 2.14) can be inherited or may be acquired due to trauma. Gnawing on cage bars and loosening tooth roots can be the cause. The resulting anorexia or reduced food intake is often the reason that these animals are presented by the owners to the veterinary surgeon. Treatment is by regular trimming every 4–5 weeks. Clipping with nail clippers may shatter the teeth, causing pain and loosening them, and so burring them with a dental burr is best. Removal can be performed but is difficult because of the incisors' long roots.

Organ system	Rats	Mice
Respiratory	Chronic respiratory disease	Chronic respiratory disease
Ocular	Red tears (porphyrin staining)	
Digestive	Incisor malocclusion, enteritis	Incisor malocclusion, enteritis, endoparasites
Integumentary	Ectoparasites	Ectoparasites, bite wounds, abscesses, barbering
Reproductive	Mammary neoplasms (often benign)	Mammary neoplasms (often malignant)
Urinary	Chronic renal disease	
Neurological	Head tilt (often associated with agents causing chronic respiratory disease)	

Figure 2.13 Summary of the most common conditions and clinical signs in rats and mice.

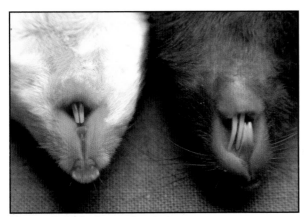

Figure 2.14 Incisor malocclusion.

Ocular system disease

'Red tears' (chromodacryorrhoea)

In rodents, a red occulonasal discharge may be observed as a non-specific response to stress and disease (Figure 2.15). This material consists of various porphyrins secreted from the Harderian gland located behind the eyes and should not be mistaken for crusts of blood. The underlying cause should be investigated and addressed.

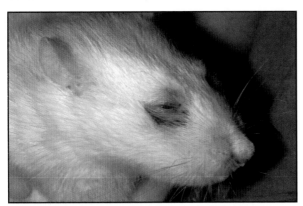

Figure 2.15 Rat with periocular porphyrin staining.

Retinal atrophy

This age-related change is seen in some albino rats, exacerbated by the levels of lighting intensity that occur in most households. It is reported that some of these animals are seen to 'head weave'. It is not known whether this is a behavioural or a neurological problem.

Gastrointestinal disease

Enteritis and diarrhoea are common signs of ill health in rats and mice and can be caused by a wide range of agents. General supportive therapy should be employed in addition to specific therapies (see section on emergency cases). A sudden change of diet can result in diarrhoea; this should be treated by reintroducing the normal diet, plus supportive therapy.

Bacterial enteritis

Salmonella: *Salmonella typhimurium* or *S. enteritidis* can cause acute or chronic diarrhoea. Because of the zoonotic aspect, euthanasia of the animal is recommended if this agent is involved; treated animals become carriers. It is important to remember that an animal infected with salmonella can present with clinical signs other than diarrhoea.

Tyzzer's disease: Caused by *Clostridium piliforme* (previously know as *Bacillus piliformis*), this disease is important in mice and rats as well as gerbils and hamsters. It produces diarrhoea, generalized signs of illness, dehydration and death. Environmental stress caused by factors such as overcrowding, poor husbandry, high environmental temperatures and concurrent disease may trigger the disease. The source of infection is usually spore-contaminated food or bedding. The organism exists in spore and vegetative forms and cannot be cultured. Diagnosis is on postmortem findings and by silver, Geimsa or PAS staining of tissues for the organism. Treatment of affected individuals is invariably unsuccessful, but supportive therapy and oral tetracycline for 30 days may decrease morbidity in group situations.

If other bacterial agents are thought to be involved in episodes of diarrhoea, treatment consists of antibiotics (neomycin for 5–7 days may be effective) and supportive care.

Viral enteritis

This is rarely seen in pet rats and mice. Mouse hepatitis virus (MHV) is a coronavirus of mice and can manifest as severe enteritis in neonates.

Parasitic enteritis

Faeces can be examined for the presence of endoparasites. Although relatively common in rats and mice, many are coincidental findings and considered non-pathogenic unless heavy worm burdens are observed (Figure 2.16).

Respiratory disease

Respiratory disease is one of the most common problems of rats and mice. Typical clinical signs include dyspnoea (but not mouth breathing), 'rattling' respiratory sounds, sneezing and rhinitis. As the disease progresses these signs may be accompanied by weight loss, 'red tears' (see Ocular disease, above) and adoption of the typical 'sick rodent' posture, interspersed with periods of laboured breathing where the rodent may be observed extending its neck to make breathing easier.

The aetiology of these conditions tends to be mixed. In mice the most common causal agents are *Mycoplasma pulmonis* (chronic disease) and Sendai virus (acute disease); in rats the agent most commonly involved is *M. pulmonis*, though synergistic interaction with other agents such as *Streptococcus pneumoniae*, *Corynebacterium kutscheri*, Sendai virus and cilia-associated respiratory (CAR) bacillus is likely.

	Parasite	Disease	Diagosis	Treatment
Protozoa	*Giardia muris, Spironucleus muris*	May cause mild enteritis in large numbers	Detection of large numbers of oocytes in faeces	Metronidazole or dimetridazole in drinking water. May need to sweeten water to increase palatability
Pinworms (Nematodes)	*Syphacia obvelata* and *Aspicularis* species	May cause mild enteritis in young animals; large worm burdens can result in rectal prolapse caused by straining	Diagnosis by adhesive tape impression of anal area to observe *Syphacia* eggs; faecal flotation for *Aspicularis*	Ivermectin given orally has proved effective, three doses at 2-week intervals. Proper sanitation controls egg dispersion until problem is eliminated
Tapeworms (Cestodes)	*Hymenolepis nana* and *Hymenolepis diminuta*	Heavy infections may cause weight loss and diarrhoea	Identification of egg in faecal floats	Praziquantel. Proper sanitation controls egg dispersion until problem is eliminated

Figure 2.16 Gastrointestinal parasites that can infect rats and mice.

Treatment of affected individuals rarely resolves the disease but rodents can live for some time with chronic disease whilst undergoing periods of palliative treatment and supportive therapy. Treat with appropriate antibiotics: enrofloxacin is often administered for at least 7 days. High-dose tetracyclines, tylosin, cephalosporins and potentiated sulphonamides have also been reported to be occasionally effective. Adjunctive therapy with mucolytics (e.g. bromhexine) and bronchodilators (e.g. clenbuterol) may be of use. Environmental stressors may exacerbate clinical disease and proper cage sanitation to control levels of ammonia, which is a potent respiratory irritant, should also be employed.

Urinary system disease

Chronic progressive nephropathy

This is a significant disease in aged rats. Glomerulosclerosis and interstitial fibrosis are histological features. Dietary factors seem to have a role to play in the development of the disease, and preventive measures include caloric restriction and feeding a reduced-protein ration (4–7%), which will also limit the severity of the disease if it does occur. Clinical signs are polydipsia and marked proteinuria (> 10 mg/l). Treatment, in addition to basic supportive therapy, involves feeding a reduced protein intake and administration of anabolic steroids.

Ejaculatory plugs

These are often seen in the bladder of male mice and rats on postmortem examination. They are formed from epithelial cells and spermatozoa and should not be mistaken for uroliths causing a urinary tract obstruction.

Fractures

Fractures may be seen in rats and mice that have been dropped or trapped in a cage lid or door. Limb or tail amputation is well tolerated and may be the most humane method of treatment in some cases.

Neurological disease

Torticollis

Torticollis (Figure 2.17) and circling are seen more commonly in rats than mice and can be caused by central lesions in the brain, but are more often secondary to otitis interna (often associated with *M. pulmonis* infection). Medical treatment is frequently unrewarding but in acute cases steroids and antibiotics may be effective.

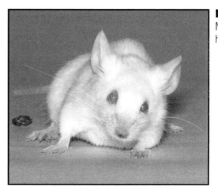

Figure 2.17 Mouse with a head tilt.

Skin disease

Parasites

Ectoparasites are the most common cause of dermatoses in rats and mice. Diagnosis is by identification of the parasite (adult, nymph or egg) by examining the animal's coat with a hand lens (×20), or in pelt brushings or skin scrapings.

Mites: The most commonly occurring mouse and rat fur mites are *Myobia musculi* (Figure 2.18), *Radfordia affinis* and *Mycoptes musculinus* (mouse only). Affected animals are often pruritic, with areas of alopecia or generalized thinning of the hair over the head, abdomen and thorax, and miliary lesions over the head and neck, induced by self-trauma. Treatment is with ivermectin given orally, topically or subcutaneously three times at intervals of 7–10 days.

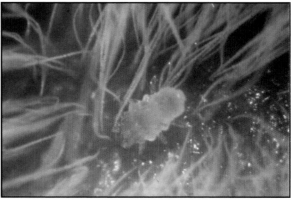

Figure 2.18 *Myobia musculi*, a mouse fur mite.

Lice and fleas: These can occur on rats and mice but are unlikely to be encountered.

Fungal diseases

Dermatophytosis occurs rarely in rats and mice, but *Microsporum* and *Trichophyton* species can cause alopecia, scaling and sometimes mild pruritus. Diagnosis is by Wood's lamp examination, microscopic hair examination and fungal culture. Treatment for individuals consists of enilconazole wash twice weekly until two cultures are negative; for groups, enilconazole spray can be made up and used to treat the environment twice weekly for 20 weeks. Alternatively oral griseofulvin can be administered.

Bacterial diseases

Skin abscessation often occurs secondarily to bite wounds or some other trauma. If possible, abscesses should be excised and the wound flushed. If this is not possible, then the abscess should be opened, drained and flushed under anaesthesia and managed as an open wound. Culture and sensitivity of the contents of the abscess are recommended; in the meantime a broad-spectrum antibiotic may be administered presumptively for 5–7 days. Advice should be given on husbandry and housing if the primary cause is fighting between cagemates.

Neoplasms

Mammary tumours are the most common tumour to occur in rats and mice (Figure 2.19). In mice, they are likely to be malignant carcinomas and adenocarcinomas; in rats, they are usually benign fibroadenomas. Rat mammary gland tumours (carcinomas and fibroadenomas) are known to respond to hormone stimuli. The incidence of carcinomas increases with the administration of oestrogen; prolonged administration of growth hormone will increase the incidence of fibroadenomas. In addition, spontaneously occurring pituitary tumours (which result in increased levels of circulating growth hormone) are often found in animals that have mammary fibroadenomas, further suggesting that these tumours may be related. Tumours must be removed surgically or, if surgery is not opted for in the case of fibrosarcomas in rats, the animal should be euthanased before the tumour inhibits movement or becomes ulcerated. In the rat, a good prognosis may be given if the lesions are successfully removed.

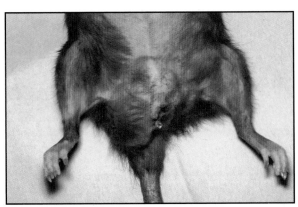

Figure 2.19 Rat with mammary tumours.

Environmental and behavioural problems

Aggression

Sustained aggressive behaviour in male rats can sometimes be controlled by castration, depending on the age of onset of the aggression and how soon castration is performed.

Barbering

If housed in groups, rats and mice will establish a dominance hierarchy and this may be especially obvious in a group of mice. The dominant male or female in the group may chew off sharply delineated patches of facial or body hair from the less dominant group members (Figure 2.20). This is known as 'barbering', as the areas of skin look clean-shaven. Often the dominant group member will be the only one without hair-loss. The skin has a normal appearance and the condition does not cause any problems, aside from unsightly bald patches.

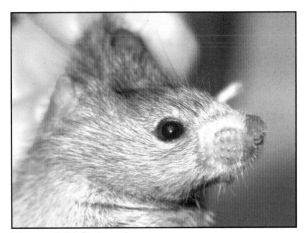

Figure 2.20 Barbered mouse.

Bites

The dominance hierarchy described above can also manifest as repeated bites to the subordinate group members by the dominant animal. These may progress to abscesses, or alternatively areas of alopecia and dermal ulceration that may become extensive. The problem may be alleviated to some extent by adding environmental enrichment to the cage but the situation can only be resolved by removing the dominant group member.

Supportive care

Drug administration

Injection

Injection sites, volumes and needle gauges are given in Figure 2.21. Intravenous administration (via the tail vein) is difficult to carry out but can be mastered with practice. It is much easier if the animal, or simply the tail, has been pre-warmed, using either a 60 watt lightbulb for 10–15 minutes, an incubator at 35°C, or a bowl of warm water (30–35°C) into which the tail is immersed.

The dilated veins of the tail will then be clearly visible in mice and young rats. Older rats have thicker skin on their tails but careful cleaning can help to make the vessels more visible. Disposable insulin syringes with a pre-attached 25-gauge needle are a convenient size for venepuncture and injection in rats and mice.

Medication

Medication can be administered orally via the drinking water, by mixing with small amounts of food (e.g. mixing with gelatine made up in ice-cube trays for rats, by administration directly into the mouth with a syringe or dropper, or by gavage using a polyethylene catheter or commercial gavage needle. Administration via the drinking water carries the risk of under- or overdosing; underdosing is more of a risk if the drug has an unpleasant taste.

Emergency cases

* Give oxygen therapy if the mucous membranes are blue tinged or there are respiratory difficulties. The prognosis is guarded. Take care not to chill the animal inadvertently whilst it is receiving oxygen
* Administer warmed parenteral fluids (e.g. lactated Ringer's). The intraperitoneal route is preferable: subcutaneous takes longer to be absorbed. Volumes for administration: 10–15 ml i.p., 5–10 ml s.c. in rats; 1–3 ml i.p., 1–2 ml s.c. in mice
* Warm the animal's environment, whether at home or hospitalized (approximately 23–26°C); take care not to overheat, as these animals cannot pant or sweat
* Hospitalize away from cats and dogs
* Offer enticing foods in addition to the animal's basic ration (e.g. warmed fruit/vegetable baby food); also offer some of the usual diet soaked in warm water to increase fluid intake and make consumption easier. Syringe feeding of small quantities of warmed foods is an option
* Provide additional nesting material
* Only isolate the animal from its companions if absolutely necessary.

Anaesthesia and analgesia

Rats and mice can be anaesthetized safely and effectively. An awareness of the potential problems that must be overcome will lead to greater success.

Risk factors

Risk factors that may be overcome by pre-anaesthetic preparation include:

* Obesity
* Pre-existing illness (careful preoperative clinical examination is required)
* Animals in poor condition because they are presented late in the course of disease
* Old age (this risk factor may be countered to some extent by pre-anaesthetic preparation).

Risk factors that arise primarily because of the small size of the animals include:

* Rapid heat loss due to high ratio of surface area to volume and disturbance of normal thermoregulatory mechanisms
* Difficulty in accessing the airway (for intubation) or veins (for intravenous drug or fluid administration)
* Small muscle mass for intramuscular drug administration, often resulting in pain and muscle necrosis
* Prolonged recovery times as routes other than the intravenous route are used for injectables and relatively large doses have to be given. It is not possible to administer drugs 'to effect' by intraperitoneal, intramuscular or subcutaneous routes, because of the slow rate of onset in action compared with the intravenous route
* A very wide range of variation in response to injectable anaesthetics. Use drugs that have a wide safety margin if possible, especially agents with a specific antagonist
* Failure of monitoring devices to detect small signals; the monitoring device fails, or fails to display correct reading.

Pre-anaesthetic preparations

* Rats and mice cannot vomit and so do not require preoperative fasting
* Evaluate and stabilize the patient if required
* Weigh the animal, in order to dose accurately with anaesthetic agent (dilute where necessary)
* Select the anaesthetic regime. It is often preferable to use a volatile anaesthetic, since this allows better control of anaesthetic depth and frequently more rapid recoveries in comparison with injectable agents.

Species	Subcutaneous	Intramuscular[a]	Intraperitoneal	Intravenous
Rat	Scruff or flank 25–23 gauge 5–10 ml	Quadriceps 25–23 gauge 0.3 ml	23 gauge or less 10–15 ml	Lateral tail vein 25 gauge 0.5 ml
Mouse	Scruff or flank 25–23 gauge 2–3 ml	Quadriceps 25–23 gauge 0.05 ml	23 gauge or less 1–3 ml	Lateral tail vein 25 gauge 0.2 ml

Figure 2.21 Sites of injection, needle gauges and maximum volumes for injection in rats and mice.

[a] Note that intramuscular administration of any substance often causes pain and muscle damage, due to the small muscle mass available; this route should be avoided if possible.

Recommended concentrations of inhalational anaesthetics, sedative and tranquillizer dose rates, injectable anaesthetic dose rates and analgesic dose rates are given in Figures 2.22–2.25. It should be noted that these rates are provided as a guide only: many of the drugs listed are not licensed for use in rats and mice and considerable individual variation in response can occur.

Perioperative care

- To prevent heat loss during surgical site preparation, clip the minimum area required, use warmed skin disinfectants and avoid alcohol-based sprays
- Provide patient warming at all times
- Oxygen should be provided even when solely injectable agents are being used

Anaesthetic	Halothane	Isoflurane
Induction concentration %	3–4	3–4
Maintainance concentration %	1–2	1.5–3

Figure 2.22 Recommended concentrations of inhalational anaesthetics.

- If respiration becomes depressed, assistance can be given by manually compressing the thorax
- Be aware that seemingly small amounts of blood and fluid loss can be a significant proportion of the patient's circulating volume: replace losses (with warmed fluids) accordingly
- Take care not to rest hands or instruments on the patient's chest, thus inhibiting respiration.

Postoperative care

- Keep the animal warm, using a fleece blanket and a heat lamp. Monitor environmental temperature: keep at 32°C at first and then lower to 26–28°C. Give some nesting material once the animal is recovered. Overheating must be avoided – rats and mice cannot sweat or pant but rely on radiant heat loss and peripheral vasodilation
- Provide the patient with a quiet environment whilst it is recovering, away from dogs and cats
- Check the animal at frequent intervals until it is able to rise

Species	Acepromazine	Diazepam	Medetomidine	Midazolam	Xylazine
Rat	2.5 mg/kg i.p.	2.5 mg/kg i.p.	30–100 µg/kg s.c.	2.5 mg/kg i.p.	10 mg/kg i.p.
Mouse	5 mg/kg i.p.	5 mg/kg i.p.	30–100 µg/kg s.c.	5 mg/kg i.p.	10 mg/kg i.p.

Figure 2.23 Recommended sedative and tranquillizer dose rates.

Drug	Dose rate	Effect	Duration of anaesthesia (min)	Sleep time (min)
Alphaxalone/alphadolone	Rat: 10–12 mg/kg i.v. Mouse: 10–15 mg/kg i.v.	Surgical anaesthesia	5	10
Fentanyl/fluanisone and diazepam	Rat: 0.6 + 2.5 mg/kg i.p. Mouse: 0.4 + 5 mg/kg i.p.	Surgical anaesthesia	45–60	120–240
Fentanyl/fluanisone and midazolam[a]	Rat: 2.7 ml/kg i.p. Mouse: 10 ml/kg i.p.	Surgical anaesthesia	45–60	120–240
Ketamine/medetomidine	Rat: 75 + 0.5 mg/kg i.p. Mouse: 75 + 1.0 mg/kg i.p.	Rat: Surgical anaesthesia Mouse: Immobilization/anaesthesia	20–30	Rat: 120–240 Mouse: 60–100
Ketamine/xylazine	Rat: 75–100 mg/kg + 10 mg/kg i.p. Mouse: 80–100 mg/kg + 10 mg/kg i.p.	Rat: Surgical anaesthesia Mouse: Immobilization/anaesthesia	20–30	Rat: 120–240 Mouse: 60–120
Pentobarbitone	40–50 mg/kg i.p.	Immobilization/anaesthesia **Narrow safety margin!**	Rat: 5 Mouse: 20–40	Rat: 10 Mouse: 120–180
Propofol	Rat: 10 mg/kg i.v. Mouse: 26 mg/kg i.v.	Surgical anaesthesia	5	10

Figure 2.24 Recommended injectable anaesthetic dose rates (adapted from Flecknell, 1996a).

a This dose is in ml/kg and consists of a mixture of one part fentanyl/fluanasone plus two parts water for injection and one part midazolam (5 mg/ml initial concentration).

Species	Buprenorphine	Butorphanol	Carprofen	Meloxicam	Ketofen	Flunixin	Nalbuphine
Rat	0.05 mg/kg s.c.	2 mg/kg s.c.	5 mg/kg s.c. bid	2 mg/kg s.c. or 4 mg/kg orally	5 mg/kg s.c.	2.5 mg/kg s.c.	1–2 mg/kg i.v.
Mouse	0.1 mg/kg s.c.	1–5 mg/kg s.c.	Unknown	Unknown	Unknown	2.5 mg/kg s.c.	4–8 mg/kg s.c.

Figure 2.25 Suggested analgesic dose rates.

- Ensure that food and water are available once the patient has recovered sufficiently to eat and drink
- Ensure that the animal receives adequate analgesia. If it is losing weight or is anorexic the day following surgery, consider administering further pain relief.

Common surgical procedures

Rats and mice have a very similar anatomy (see Chapter 1). Rodents frequently remove skin sutures with their teeth and so wound closure with subcuticular sutures using 4-0 to 5-0 absorbable suture material is recommended. Tissue glue or skin staples can also be used.

Ovariohysterectomy

Using a ventral midline approach, enter the abdominal cavity and identify the bicornate uterus and ovaries. Ligate the ovarian pedicles and the uterine body with 4-0 or 5-0 monofilament absorbable suture and remove them. Close the abdominal incision in two layers, using an interrupted suture pattern for the muscle layer and a subcuticular suture pattern for the skin closure.

Castration

In mice and rats, the testicles do descend into the scrotal sac but the inguinal canals remain open and the testicles are easily retracted into the abdomen. The surgical approach for castration can be scrotal, prescrotal or midline intra-abdominal. If the scrotal or prescrotal approach is used, and the testes have been retracted into the abdomen, it is possible to move them back into the scrotum by applying gentle pressure to the caudal abdomen, using a rolling motion.

In an open technique the testes are removed from the scrotum by incising the tunic to expose the testicle and spermatic cord; the vas deferens and the spermatic blood vessels are then ligated. In the rat, the wall of the scrotum and the skin should be closed in separate layers. In the mouse, this is not possible and they have to be closed as a single layer. If an open technique is chosen, it possible to close the inguinal rings if the prescrotal or midline intra-abdominal techniques are used. Use of an open technique does not seem to be associated with herniation of the abdominal contents into the inguinal canal and scrotum in these species, perhaps because of effective closure of the canal by the remaining adipose tissue.

Mammary tumour removal

Mammary tissue extends from the axillae to the inguinal region. The general principles of tumour removal apply to the removal of mammary tumours in rats and mice. Haemostasis is especially important when performing these procedures: a seemingly small volume of blood loss can comprise a significant percentage of the animal's circulating volume and many mammary tumours are highly vascular.

Drug formulary

Drug	Dose/comments
Antibacterials	
Amoxycillin	Rat: 150 mg/kg i.m. Mouse: 100 mg/kg s.c.
Ampicillin Injection, 15% w/v Oral preparations	50–150 mg/kg s.c. 200 mg/kg orally
Cephalosporins Cephalexin	60 mg/kg orally Rat: 15 mg/kg s.c. Mouse: 30 mg/kg s.c.
Chloramphenicol Injectable Oral preparations	Rat: 10 mg/kg i.m. bid Mouse: 50 mg/kg i.m., s.c. bid Rat: 20–50 mg/kg bid Mouse: 200 mg/kg tid
Clavulanate-potentiated amoxycillin	2 ml/kg orally (Synulox)
Enrofloxacin	10 mg/kg s.c., orally sid
Neomycin Oral preparations	Rat: 50 mg/kg s.c. Mouse: 2.5 g/l in drinking water Rat: 2.0 g/l in drinking water
Oxytetracycline, long-acting injection	60 mg/kg s.c., i.m. every 3 days (Curl, 1988)
Potentiated sulphonamides (e.g. trimethoprim/ sulphadiazine)	120 mg/kg s.c., i.m. 24% solution = 240 mg/ml = 0.5 ml/kg
Sulphamerazine	0.02% in drinking water
Tetracycline Injectable tetracyclines Oral tetracycline	100 mg/kg s.c. (high dose used in respiratory disease) 5 mg/kg orally in drinking water
Tylosin	10 mg/kg s.c.
Miscellaneous	
Dimetridazole	2.5 mg/ml drinking water
Enilconazole Wash Environmental spray treatment	Twice weekly washing of individuals 50 mg/m^2 twice weekly for 20 weeks
Frusemide	2.5 mg/kg i.p., s.c.
Griseofulvin	25 mg/kg orally sid or 0.75 mg/kg feed for 28–42 days
Ivermectin Oral dose Topical Subcutaneous	200–400 µg/kg (in oil or propylene glycol), three doses at weekly interval (rats), two doses 10-day intervals (mice) Dilute to 1:100 in equal parts with water and propylene glycol and place a few drops on neck/head (Donnelly, 1997) 200–400 µg/kg s.c. (three injections 7–10 days apart in treatment of fur mites)
Metronidazole Oral preparation	20 mg/kg s.c. sid or 2.5 mg/ml in drinking water, for 7–10 days 1 ml in 150 ml drinking water (Flagyl)
Oxytocin	3 IU/kg s.c.
Praziquantel	5 mg/kg s.c. or 10 mg/kg orally
Steroids Betamethasone (anti-inflammatory dose)	0.1 mg/kg s.c.

Figure 2.26 Formulary for rats and mice. Note that streptomycin and procaine penicillin are toxic to rats and mice.

References and further reading

Altman NH and Goodman DG (1979) Neoplastic diseases. In: *The Laboratory Rat, Volume One, Biology and Diseases*, ed. HJ Baker *et al.*, pp. 333–376. ACLAM Medicine Series, Academic Press, New York

Curl JL, Curl JS and Harrison JK (1988) Pharmacokinetics of long acting oxytetracycline in the laboratory rat. *Laboratory Animal Science* **38**, 430

Donnelly TM (1997) Disease problems of small rodents. In: *Ferrets, Rabbits and Rodents: Clinical Medicine and Surgery*, ed. EV Hillyer and KE Quesenberry, pp. 307–327. WB Saunders, Philadelphia

Flecknell PA (1996a) Anaesthesia and analgesia for rodents and rabbits. In: *Handbook of Rodent and Rabbit Medicine*, ed. K Laber-Laird *et al.*, pp. 219–237 Elsevier, Oxford

Flecknell PA (1996b) *Laboratory Animal Anaesthesia, 2nd edn.* Academic Press, London

Flecknell PA (1998) Placement of a subcuticular suture and use of an Aberdeen knot for anchoring the suture. *In Practice* **20**, 294–295

Flecknell PA (2000) *BSAVA Manual of Rabbit Medicine and Surgery.* BSAVA, Cheltenham

Flecknell PA and Waterman-Pearson A (2000) *Pain Management in Animals.* WB Saunders, Philadelphia

Harkness JE and Wagner JE (1983) *The Biology and Medicine of Rabbits and Rodents*, 3rd edn. Lea and Febiger, Philadelphia

Hawk CT and Leary SL (1995) *Formulary for Laboratory Animals.* Iowa State University Press, Ames, Iowa

Hillyer EV and Quesenberry KE (1997) *Ferrets, Rabbits and Rodents: Clinical Medicine and Surgery.* WB Saunders, Philadelphia

Inglis JK (1980) *Introduction to Laboratory Animal Science and Technology.* Pergamon Press, Oxford

Jacoby RO and Fox JG (1984) Biology and diseases of Mice. In: *Laboratory Animal Medicine*, ed. JG Fox *et al.*, pp. 31–89. ACLAM Medicine Series, Academic Press, New York

Jain MC (1994) *Essentials of Veterinary Haematology.* Lea and Febiger, Philadelphia

Kaneky JJ and Harvey JW (1997) *Clinical Biochemistry of Domestic Animals, 5th edn.* Academic Press, New York

Kelly PJ, Millican KG and Organ PJ (eds) (1992) *The Principles of Animal Technology, I.* The Institute of Animal Technology

Krinke GJ (ed.) (2000) Immunology and haematology. In: *The Handbook of Experimental Animals – The Laboratory Rat*, pp. 441–442. Academic Press, New York

Laber-Laird K, Swindle MM and Flecknell PA (1996) *Handbook of Rodent and Rabbit Medicine.* Elsevier, Oxford

Lee KP (1986) Ultrastructure of proteinaceous bladder pugs in male rats. *Laboratory Animal Science* **36**(6), 671–677

Loeb WF and Quimby FW (1989) *The Clinical Chemistry of Laboratory Animals.* Pergamon Press, New York

Meredith A (1996) Aspects of rodent, lagomorph and ferret medicine. Lecture handout, RDSVS, University of Edinburgh

Mitruka BM and Rawnsley HM (1977) *Clinical Biochemical and Haematological Reference Values in Normal Experimental Animals.* Masson Publishing, New York

Percy DH and Barthold SW (2001) *Pathology of Laboratory Rodents and Rabbits, 2nd edition.* Iowa State University Press, Ames, Iowa

Robinson R (1979) Taxonomy and genetics. In: *The Laboratory Rat, Volume One, Biology and Diseases*, ed. HJ Baker *et al.*, pp. 37–54. ACLAM Medicine Series, Academic Press, New York

Ringler DH and Dabich L (1979) Haematology and clinical biochemistry. In: *The Laboratory Rat, Volume One, Biology and Diseases*, ed. HJ Baker *et al.*, pp. 105–121 Academic Press, New York

Seymour C and Gleed R (1999) *Manual of Small Animal Anaesthesia and Analgesia.* BSAVA Publications, Cheltenham

Tennant B (1999) *BSAVA Small Animal Formulary, 3rd edn.* BSAVA Publications, Cheltenham

Useful contacts

- **National Rat Fancy Society**, PO Box 24207, London SE9 5ZF. *http://www.nfrs.org/*
  Society for pet keepers as well as breeders and exhibitors. Include a stamped addressed envelope for joining details or to obtain a copy of the 'Kitten Register' (a list of young rats that are suitable as pets)
- **London & Southern Counties Mouse and Rat Club** (LSCMRC), 153 Kenilworth Crescent, Enfield, Middlesex EN1 3RG. *http://www.miceandrats.com/index.htm*
- **Pet Rat Information Sheet** (information sheet produced by A. Swierzy and A. Horn for owners of pet rats) available on the internet at *http://www.quite.co.uk/rats/*
- **The Rat and Mouse Club of America** (RMCA), *http://www.rmca.org*
- The web site illustrating the technique for carrying out saphenous vein bleeds in mice can be found at: *http://www.uib.no/vivariet/mou_blood/Blood_coll_mice_.html*
- The National Fancy Rat Society (address above) and Supreme Petfoods (The Briars, Waterberry Drive, Waterlooville, Hants PO7 7YH) produce a range of posters illustrating rodent and rabbit varieties, including a poster of popular fancy rat varieties.

3

Hamsters

Gidona Goodman

Introduction

Hamsters are rodents in the family Cricetidae. Several species of hamster are kept as pets or for research purposes. The Syrian hamster (*Mesocricetus auratus*; Figure 3.1) originates from hamsters bred in 1930 at the Hebrew University of Jerusalem. Syrian hamsters are indigenous to northwest Syria. They are also referred to as 'golden hamsters,' as this was the original coat colour. Today different colour variations exist (e.g. grey, black and cinnamon) as well as different coat types (short-haired, long-haired or Rex). Syrian hamsters are the most common pet hamsters. They are nocturnal solitary animals and will hibernate if room temperatures remain below 10°C.

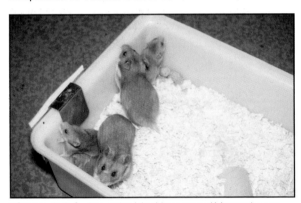

Figure 3.1 Syrian or 'golden' hamsters (*Mesocricetus auratus*). Courtesy of Paul Flecknell.

The Russian dwarf hamster (*Phodopus sungorus sungorus*; Figure 3.2) is also nocturnal and is housed in pairs or groups (one male with several females or two males together). Other species of dwarf hamster are Roborovski (*Phodopus roborovskii*), Campbelli (*Phodopus sungoris campbelli*) and Chinese or striped hamster (*Cricetulus griseus*; Figure 3.3). The Chinese hamster has a longer tail than the other dwarf hamsters. It is also more aggressive to fellow cagemates and is better housed alone.

Biology

Hamsters are characterized by large cheek pouches, short tails and thick bodies. The cheek pouch is an evagination of the lateral buccal wall. It can be everted with forceps for examination. The cheek pouches are

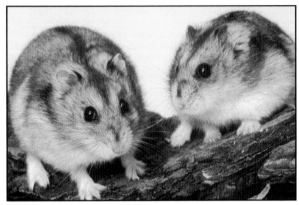

Figure 3.2 Russian dwarf hamsters (*Phodopus sungorus sungorus*).

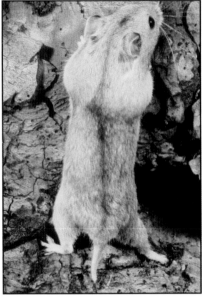

Figure 3.3 Chinese hamster (*Cricetulus griseus*).

used to transport and store food and to conceal a newly born litter when danger is present.

Hamsters are born with their incisor teeth erupted. The incisors are open rooted and grow continuously. Hamsters lack canine and premolar teeth. The dental formula is $2(I_1C_0P_0M_3)$. The dental enamel is yellow/orange in colour.

The hamster has a distinctly compartmentalized stomach consisting of two parts: the forestomach (*pars cardiaca*) and the glandular stomach (*pars pylorica*). The parts are divided by a muscular sphincter.

	Syrian hamster	Chinese hamster	Russian hamster
Adult weight	Male: 85–130 g Female: 95–150 g	Male: 30–35 g Female: 27–32 g	Male: 40–50 g Female: 30 g
Life expectancy	1½–2 years	2½–3 years	1–2 years
Heart rate	280–412 beats per minute		
Respiratory rate	33–127 breaths per minute		
Sexual maturity	6–8 weeks	7–14 weeks	6–8 weeks
Gestation	15–18 days	21 days	18 days
Litter size	5–9	4–5	4
Weaned	21–28 days	21 days	16–18 days

Figure 3.4 Biological data.

Hamsters generally urinate in one corner of the cage, and their urine is cream in colour.

Figure 3.4 summarizes the biological data for the different hamster species.

Sexing

Male and female hamsters can be distinguished by measuring the anogenital distance, which is greater in males (Figure 3.5). In females there are three openings: the anus, vagina and urethra. The female generally has 12 or 14 nipples. Hamsters are seasonally polyoestrous, with oestrus every 5–7 days, and they secrete a copious whitish vaginal discharge that can be mistaken for pyometra. If disturbed when nursing their litter, they may eat their young. The young should not be touched or handled until they are at least 5 days old.

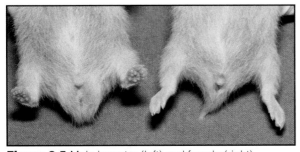

Figure 3.5 Male hamster (left) and female (right). Courtesy of Paul Flecknell.

Adult male hamsters have prominent testicles, and the inguinal canal remains open. Males also have prominent bilateral scent or flank glands (Figure 3.6). The glands are poorly developed in females. With age the glands become darkly pigmented and covered with coarse fur. Secretions from these sebaceous glands play a part in territorial marking and mating behaviour.

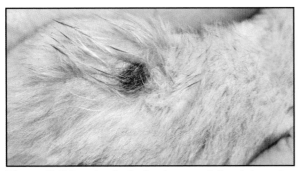

Figure 3.6 Scent or flank gland on an adult male hamster.

Husbandry

Housing

Hamsters are constantly trying to find ways to escape, and cages need to be resistant to gnawing. In the wild hamsters will travel long distances at night and thus require plenty of exercise in captivity. They enjoy using exercise wheels and other 'toys.' The hair of long-haired hamsters should be trimmed to avoid it getting caught in the wheel.

Aquaria with screen tops, conventional cages (wire with plastic base) with several floors, or solid plastic caging with plastic connecting tunnels can be used to house hamsters. A nest box should be available for the animal to retreat into, with paper or hay as nesting material. It should be cleaned regularly as hamsters tend to hoard food. Hamsters are burrowing animals by nature and like a deep layer of bedding. A variety of bedding is available (wood shavings, beet pulp or ground corncob).

Diet

Hamsters in the wild are omnivorous, hoard food and are coprophagic. Pet hamsters are usually fed a commercial hamster mix, which can be supplemented with fruit, vegetables and nuts. Hamsters begin eating solid foods at 7–10 days of age. Adult hamsters consume about 5–10 g of food a day. The daily calorie requirement is as estimated for rats and mice:

Maintenance = $110W^{0.75}$ kcal/day

where W = bodyweight in kg.

Protein requirements range from 16% for maintenance up to 20% for reproduction. Requirements for carbohydrate are 60–65% and for fat 5–7%.

Hamsters drink 10 ml/100 g bodyweight of water daily, usually provided in a water bottle with sipper tube.

Handling and restraint

Hamsters have a reputation for being biters, but if handled correctly and not startled they can be examined without injury. They can be lifted in the palm of cupped hands (Figure 3.7) or by grasping the excess skin at the back of the neck. To restrain them for examination, grip the skin over the neck and dorsum between thumb and fingers. An aggressive hamster may turn and bite if the skin is held too loosely. If startled, hamsters will exhibit threatening behaviour by rolling on their backs and vocalizing, and they may bite.

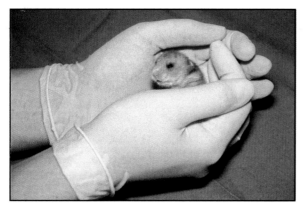

Figure 3.7 Lifting a hamster in cupped hands.

Diagnostic approach

Sample collection

Blood

The circulating blood volume of a hamster is 78 ml/kg. Up to 10% of this volume can be withdrawn at one time from a healthy hamster. Usually it is necessary to sedate or anaesthetize the animal to obtain a blood sample.

To obtain blood samples from a hamster, a tourniquet is applied to the foreleg and blood collected from the cephalic vein with a 27 gauge needle and a capillary tube. For larger volumes, blood can be obtained from the anterior vena cava. Blood can be taken from the lateral saphenous vein, which runs dorsally and then laterally over the tarsal joint, by using a 25 gauge needle, and collected in a heparinized syringe or haematocrit tube. In the author's experience, obtaining blood samples from hamsters can be difficult, especially if a large volume is needed for blood biochemistry. Figure 3.8 gives the blood values for normal hamsters.

Haematology	Syrian hamster	Chinese hamster
Red blood cells (10^{12}/l)	7.5	
Packed cell volume (%)	44.1–53.9	
Haemoglobin (g/dl)	14.5–18	12.4
White blood cells (10^9/l)	7.62	
Neutrophils (%)	18.6–32.1	17–21
Eosinophils (%)	0.46–1.22	1.0–2.4
Basophils (%)	0–3	0.11–0.19
Lymphocytes (%)	59.4–81.9	75
Monocytes (%)	1.4–2.4	1.8–2.4
Biochemistry: mean values		
Calcium (mmol/l)	2.75	
Phosphorus (mmol/l)	2.29	
Glucose (mmol/l)	7	
Blood urea nitrogen (mmol/l)	13.5	
Creatinine (µmol/l)	51.27	
Total protein (g/l)	61	
Albumin (g/l)	42	
Globulin (g/l)	34	
Alkaline phosphatase (IU/l)	131	
Lactate dehydrogenase (IU/l)	224	
Aspartate aminotransferase (IU/l)	57	

Figure 3.8 Normal blood values for hamsters.

Common conditions

Ill hamsters become irritable and often bite. They may move reluctantly, with a stiff gait. Their eyes may look dull and sunken and often produce a conjunctival discharge. Most of the diseases described in this chapter relate to Syrian hamsters. Figure 3.9 summarizes the common diseases that may cause certain clinical signs.

Clinical problem	Differential diagnosis
Diarrhoea	Proliferative ileitis Tyzzer's disease *Escherichia coli* infection *Salmonella* infection Antibiotic-associated toxicity
Alopecia	*Demodex* infestation Hyperadrenocorticism Dermatophytes Epitheliotropic lymphoma
Polyuria/polydipsia	Hyperadrenocorticism Diabetes mellitus Arteriolar nephrosclerosis Amyloidosis
Ocular discharge	Respiratory infection General malaise
Dyspnoea	Bacterial pneumonia Cardiac thrombosis

Figure 3.9 Differential diagnosis of common clinical problems in hamsters.

Dental disease

Incisors grow continuously throughout a hamster's life. Owners often want their hamsters' teeth clipped because they think they are too long. In general the crown to length ratio for the upper to lower incisors is around 1:3. Anorexia, weight loss, swelling and ptyalism can result from overgrown incisors or incisor/molar malocclusion due to trauma. Maloccluded incisors need to be trimmed periodically. Teeth can be cut with dental burrs. Nail clippers should be avoided.

Cheek pouch impaction

Impaction is usually presented as large persistent swellings on one or both sides of the face. Under general anaesthesia the pouches can be everted, carefully emptied with forceps and flushed with water. Abrasion can be treated with topical antibiotic ointment. Any dental malocclusion should be ascertained.

Gastrointestinal disease

Bacterial enteritis

In some references 'wet tail' is synonymous with all forms of enteritis, whereas in others it refers only to proliferative ileitis. Enteritis is considered the most common disease in hamsters.

Proliferative ileitis: This mainly affects weanlings aged 3–8 weeks. The bacterium *Lawsonia intracellularis* is currently considered the aetiological agent of proliferative ileitis in hamsters (Cooper *et al.*, 1997). Previously, *Campylobacter jejuni* and *Desulfovibrio* spp. (Fox *et al.*, 1994) were thought to be involved in proliferative ileitis.

Other factors involved in the development of clinical disease are stress, weaning and dietary change. Early clinical signs include lethargy, anorexia and ruffled coat, followed by diarrhoea. Signs associated with diarrhoea include dehydration and hunched back. On abdominal palpation thickened bowels can be felt. If the individual survives the acute stage of the disease, ileal obstruction, impaction, intussusception and peritonitis may follow. A prolapsed rectum is usually accompanied by an intussusception of the colon. Prognosis is guarded. Treatment includes supportive care and antibiotics such as chloramphenicol, tetracycline, neomycin or erythromycin (see Figure 3.13 for doses).

Tyzzer's disease: The causative agent of Tyzzer's disease is the unusual Gram-negative spore-forming bacterium *Clostridium piliforme* (previously named *Bacillus piliformis*) that multiplies only within hepatic, intestinal epithelial or myocardial cells. Clinical signs include sudden onset of pale yellow watery diarrhoea, dehydration, lethargy and death. Tetracycline can be used in a group outbreak.

Other bacteria isolated from hamsters with enteritis are *Escherichia coli* (β-haemolytic) and *Salmonella*. Salmonellosis is rarely observed; clinical signs resemble enteric disease (faeces may be soft or normal) but the bacteria may cause an acute septicaemic disease with high mortality, abortion or chronic wasting. Salmonellosis is a zoonotic disease, and an asymptomatic carrier state may occur after treatment.

Antibiotic-associated toxicity or colitis
The predominant bacteria in the flora of a hamster's intestine are *Lactobacillus* and *Bacteroides*. Even antibiotics routinely recommended for use in hamsters can potentially induce toxicity. The disease generally develops 4–10 days after administration. Proliferation of *Clostridium difficile*, with production of lethal toxins, results in diarrhoea and death. Penicillin, ampicillin, erythromycin, vancomycin, gentamicin, cephalosporins (first generation) and lincomycin have been reported to induce diarrhoea and death in hamsters. Dihydrostreptomycin is lethal to hamsters, causing an ascending paralysis. Treatment should include fluid therapy and supportive care. Vancomycin has been used but may have to be given indefinitely because no normal flora will be able to re-establish to compete with *C. difficile*.

Parasitic disease
Hymenolepis nana, the dwarf tapeworm, has a direct and indirect life cycle, with fleas or beetles as an intermediate host. It is zoonotic. Most hamsters fail to show clinical signs. Diagnosis is on the basis of finding eggs in the faeces. Treatment is with niclosamide at 100 mg/kg bodyweight given at 7-day intervals or at 0.3% of the active ingredient in feed for 7 days.

The mouse pinworm (*Syphacia obvelata*) and the rat pinworm (*Syphacia muris*) may infect hamsters.

Protozoans are abundant in the hamster. Most are commensal organisms or at best opportunistic. *Trichomonas* spp. are relatively non-pathogenic. *Giardia* spp. and *Spironucleus* may contribute to enteric disease.

Neoplasia
Neoplasms occurring in the hamster stomach are usually benign and are primarily gastric squamous papillomas in the glandular portion of the stomach. Intestinal adenomas are the other most commonly reported benign neoplasm.

Respiratory disease

Bacterial pneumonia
Bacterial respiratory infections are reported to be the second most common disease in hamsters. However hamsters seem more resistant to infectious respiratory disease than other rodents. *Mycoplasma* has been isolated from hamsters but its pathogenic potential is not known. The bacteria most often isolated are *Pasteurella* and *Streptococcus*. *Pasteurella* can be present in carriers without clinical signs. Other bacteria include *Staphylococcus*, *Klebsiella* and *Bordetella*. Common clinical signs are dyspnoea, head tilt and ocular and nasal discharge. Some organisms reside as normal flora in the respiratory and gastrointestinal tracts and cause opportunistic infection.

Treatment with antibiotics should be on the basis of bacterial culture and sensitivity.

Urogenital disease
Arteriolar nephrosclerosis seems to be related to the level of dietary protein. Affected hamsters develop uraemia, proteinuria and polyuria and progress to end-stage renal disease. Amyloid deposition often occurs concurrently (see Amyloidosis, below).

Endometritis
Female hamsters have a 4-day oestrous cycle, with a copious white discharge at the end of the cycle. Pyometra has been observed clinically, and a definite diagnosis can be made by ultrasonography and cytological examination of the discharge. Ovariohysterectomy is the treatment of choice.

Neoplasia
Tumours of the ovary are usually unilateral and metastasis is uncommon. Uterine endometrial adenocarcinoma is reported in Chinese hamsters with vaginal haemorrhage.

Endocrine disease

Hyperadrenocorticism
Hyperplasia, adenomas and carcinomas of the adrenal cortex are more common in male than in female hamsters and generally occur in aged animals. Clinical signs include bilateral and symmetrical alopecia, hyperpigmentation and thinning of the skin, polydipsia, polyuria and polyphagia. Plasma cortisol levels are increased (normal range 13.8–27.6 nmol/l). Treatment with metyrapone (8 mg orally sid for 1 month) was effective in one hamster (Bauck *et al.,* 1984).

Diabetes mellitus
Genetically determined spontaneous diabetes mellitus has been reported in Chinese hamsters (single or two recessive genes, with the onset of glucosuria regulated by a multiple-gene system). Glucose blood levels

increase above 16.65 mmol/l (non-fasting), with glucosuria, ketonuria, polydipsia, polyuria and hyperphagia. Onset of symptoms can be delayed by restricting food quantities as for a non-diabetic hamster, reducing fat content and replacing animal fat with vegetable fat. As hamsters are an insulin-deficient model, they should be treated with NPH insulin.

Skin disease

Dermatophytosis is rare in hamsters and is caused by *Trichophyton mentagrophytes*. Infection may be asymptomatic, or dry circular skin lesions can develop. Treatment is with griseofulvin. Staphylococcal pyoderma is relatively common and treated with enrofloxacin. Allergic dermatitis attributed to cedar or pine shavings has been reported (Burgmann, 1991).

Demodicosis

Demodex is the most common ectoparasite of the hamster and is found in skin scrapings from healthy hamsters. Transmission occurs from mother to young during suckling. *Demodex criceti* inhabits the keratin and pits of the epidermal surface, and *D. aurati* inhabits the hair follicles. Predisposing factors for the development of overt disease are concurrent disease, immunosuppression and ageing. Clinical signs include alopecia and dry scaly skin on the dorsal thorax and lumbar area. Pruritus does not usually occur. Diagnosis is made on the basis of skin scrapes. Treatment is with amitraz (diluted to 100 ppm, once weekly until 4 weeks after skin scrapings give negative results) or ivermectin. It is important to know that the condition is indicative of an underlying problem.

Other mites include the hamster ear mite (*Notoedres notoedres*) and the cat mange mite (*N. cati*). *N. notoedres* produces scabby lesions around the ears, nose, feet and perianal area. Both infestations can be treated with ivermectin.

Neoplasia

Melanomas and melanocytomas are the most commonly reported cutaneous neoplasms. A higher incidence occurs in males. Epitheliotropic lymphoma (mycosis fungoides; Figure 3.10) is the next most common cutaneous neoplasm in hamsters. This can manifest from alopecia, pruritus and flaky skin to cutaneous plaques and nodules, which may become ulcerated and crusted. Diagnosis is by biopsy, and euthanasia is recommended.

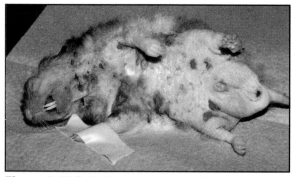

Figure 3.10 Epitheliotropic lymphoma (mycosis fungoides) in an adult hamster.

Hamster papovavirus is thought to be the cause of transmissible lymphoma, and it has been identified as a cause of cutaneous epitheliomas in hamsters. The virus is host-specific, and lesions are found in hamsters aged from 3 months to 1 year. The lesions are wart-like and occur most often around the eyes, mouth (Figure 3.11) or perianal area. The virus is highly contagious (passed through urine), has a long incubation period and is very resistant. There is no spontaneous resolution.

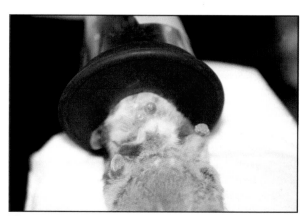

Figure 3.11 A 3-month-old hamster infected with hamster papovavirus.

Systemic conditions

Lymphocytic choriomeningitis

Lymphocytic choriomeningitis is caused by an arenavirus (LCMV). Its manifestation depends on the age and immune status of the host and virus strain. A chronic fatal wasting disease occurs in young hamsters that do not eliminate the virus or subclinical infection. Diagnosis is on the basis of serology. A common reservoir of infection, through direct or indirect contact, is wild mice. The virus is shed in urine and saliva of infected carriers. Congenital infection also occurs. Because of its zoonotic potential, animals positive for the virus should be euthanased. In humans LCMV produces influenza-like symptoms that can progress to choriomeningitis.

Neoplasia

Malignant lymphomas are the most common neoplasm in Syrian hamsters and consist predominantly of lymphosarcomas of the lymph gland and small intestine and reticulum cell sarcomas of the lymph nodes.

Polycystic disease

Polycystic disease in hamsters is a benign congenital disease, generally observed incidentally. Cysts are grossly visible and most often seen in liver. The condition has not been associated with clinical signs.

Geriatric diseases

Two of the most common geriatric diseases are amyloidosis and thrombosis. Amyloidosis is often associated with thrombosis.

Amyloidosis: This usually involves the kidney, spleen, adrenal gland or liver. Females have a higher incidence. Clinical signs are associated with organ failure, and a nephrotic syndrome is often associated.

Anorexia, oedema, ascites, proteinuria, hypercholesterolaemia, decreased serum albumin and increased total globulin are usually present. Polyuria, polydipsia and haematuria are seen occasionally. Treatment is largely palliative through decreased protein in the diet and adequate hydration.

Cardiac thrombosis: The left atrium is the most common location of cardiac thrombosis in hamsters. Cardiomyopathy, vascular disease, coagulopathy and amyloidosis have been suggested as contributors to thrombus formation. Clinical signs include hyperpnoea, tachycardia and cyanosis. Reported treatments include digoxin, diuretics, angiotensin converting enzyme inhibitors, anticoagulants and verapamil (0.25–0.5 mg s.c. bid over 4 weeks; Bauck and Bihun, 1997).

Supportive care

Drug administration

Injection
Hamsters may be injected subcutaneously, intramuscularly or intraperitoneally. Intravenous injections are difficult to perform in hamsters. Subcutaneous injections are preferred. Figure 3.12 summarizes the injection routes and recommended volumes for hamsters.

Fluid therapy
A hamster's daily fluid intake is 10 ml per 100 g bodyweight. Up to 5 ml of fluid can be given subcutaneously. Fluids should be warmed before injection.

Environmental temperature
Providing a warm environment is particularly important after surgery. Initially a temperature of 35–37°C is recommended. A hospitalized animal benefits from environmental temperatures between 20 and 25°C.

Supplementary feeding
Hospitalized animals should be weighed daily. If bodyweight is not maintained or the animal is anorexic, the hamster should be syringe-fed. Semi-liquid baby foods can be fed by syringe several times a day until weight is maintained or the animal resumes eating.

Anaesthesia and analgesia

Hamsters have a relative high metabolic rate and lose body heat and fluids rapidly. Maintaining body temperature during and after surgery is essential. Blood loss should be kept to a minimum, and warmed preoperative fluids should be given. Analgesia should be provided after surgery.

Isoflurane is the recommended inhalant anaesthetic agent. Anaesthesia can be induced in a gas chamber and maintained by mask.

Common surgical procedures

Common surgical procedures include castration, ovariohysterectomy, rectal prolapse and repair of limb fractures.

Castration
Castration should be performed with a closed technique. If an open technique is used, the tunics should be closed to avoid herniation. Recently castrated rodents should be kept away from intact females until at least 3 weeks after surgery.

Ovariohysterectomy
Rodents have a bicornate uterus with a short uterine body and one cervix. The broad ligament is a site of fat storage. Ovariohysterectomy is performed through a midline incision. Ovarian ligaments are easily stretched, and the ovarian vessels and uterine body ligated with 4-0 or 5-0 absorbable monofilament.

Rectal prolapse
It is important to ascertain which part of the bowel is prolapsed and to address and treat the underlying cause. A non-necrotic rectal prolapse can be replaced and a purse-string suture placed in the anus with 5-0 non-absorbable suture material. A 5 French catheter should be placed centrally when positioning the suture. If the prolapsed rectum is necrotic it should be amputated at the junction with healthy tissue. Healthy rectum should be sutured to healthy anus with 6-0 absorbable synthetic suture material.

Fracture repair
Fracture healing is rapid, with callus formation after 7–10 days. Most fractures in rodents can be treated by external coaptation with splints and slings. To discourage chewing, the tape can be hardened with glue, bitter sprays applied or Elizabethan collars used. Small mammals generally adapt to the loss of a limb; the same principles should be applied as for amputations in dogs and cats.

Euthanasia

The author prefers to anaesthetize hamsters before injecting a lethal dose of intracardiac barbiturate.

Route	Site	Volume
Subcutaneous	Skinfold along the back or flank	3–5 ml
Intramuscular	Gluteal or quadricep muscles	0.1 ml per site with a 23 gauge needle or smaller
Intraperitoneal	Lower right quadrant of abdomen (restraining animal head down)	3–4 ml

Figure 3.12 Injection routes and injection volumes in hamsters.

Drug formulary

Agent	Dosage	Comments
Amitraz	1.4 ml/l topically every 14 days for 3–6 treatments	Apply with cotton bud, not recommended in young
Aspirin	100–150 mg/kg orally every 4 hours 240 mg/kg orally sid	
Atropine	0.004–0.01 mg/100 g s.c. or i.m.	
Buprenorphine	0.05–0.1 mg/kg s.c. tid	
Butorphanol	1–5 mg/kg s.c. every 2–4 hours	
Chloramphenicol	50 mg/kg orally bid	
Chlortetracycline	20 mg/kg s.c. or i.m. bid	
Dexamethasone	0.1–0.6 mg/kg s.c. or i.m.	
Diazepam	3–5 mg/kg i.m.	
Enrofloxacin	10 mg/kg i.m., s.c. or orally bid	
Erythromycin	0.13 mg/ml drinking water	Control of proliferative ileitis, can cause enterotoxaemia
Fenbendazole	20 mg/kg orally sid for 5 days	
Flunixin meglumine	2.5 mg/kg s.c. sid–bid	
Griseofulvin	25 mg/kg orally sid for 14–60 days	Not to be used in pregnant animals. Can cause diarrhoea, leucopenia and anorexia
Insulin	2 IU s.c.	Used in glucose tolerance study
Ivermectin	0.2–0.5 mg/kg orally or s.c. every 14 days for 3 treatments	
Metyrapone	8 mg per hamster orally sid for 1 month	
Neomycin	50–100 mg/kg orally sid 0.5 mg/ml drinking water	
Niclosamide	100 mg/kg orally then repeat after 7 days	
Oxytetracycline	0.25–1.0 mg/ml drinking water 16 mg/kg s.c. sid	
Tetracycline	0.4 mg/ml drinking water 10–20 mg/kg orally tid–bid	Control of proliferative ileitis for 10 days
Trimethoprim/sulphonamide	30 mg/kg orally, s.c. or i.m. sid–bid	
Verapamil	0.25–0.5 mg/kg s.c. bid	

Figure 3.13 Drug formulary for hamsters.

References and further reading

Battles AH (1985) The biology, care and disease of the Syrian hamster. *Continuing Education* **7**, 815–825

Bauck L and Bihun C (1997) Basic anatomy, physiology, husbandry and clinical techniques. In: *Ferrets, Rabbits and Rodents: Clinical Medicine and Surgery*, ed. EV Hillyer and KE Quesenberry, pp. 291–306. WB Saunders, Philadelphia

Bauck L, Orr JP and Lawrence KH (1984) Hyperadrenocorticism in three teddy bear hamsters. *Canadian Veterinary Journal* **25**, 247–250

Biggar JR, Schmidt TJ and Woodall JP (1977) Lymphocytic choriomeningitis in laboratory personnel exposed to hamsters inadvertently infected with LCM virus. *Journal of the American Veterinary Medical Association* **171**, 829–832

Brown SA (2000) Neutering of rabbits and rodents. In: *Kirk's Current Veterinary Therapy XIII: Small Animal Practice*, ed. JD Bonagura, pp. 1337–1340. WB Saunders, Philadelphia

Burgmann P (1991) Dermatology of rabbits, rodents and ferrets. In: *Practical Exotic Animal Medicine: The Compendium Collection*, ed. KL Rosenthal, pp. 174–194. Veterinary Learning Systems, Trenton

Burke TJ (1995) Wet tail in hamsters and other diarrhoeas of small rodents. In: *Kirk's Current Veterinary Therapy XII: Small Animal Practice*, ed. JD Bonagura and RW Kirk, pp. 1336–1339. WB Saunders, Philadelphia

Carpenter JW, Mashima TY and Rupiper DJ (1996) *Exotic Animal Formulary*. Greystone, Kansas

Cooper DM, Swanson DL, Barns SM and Gebhart CJ (1997) Comparison of the 16S ribosomal DNA sequences from the intracellular agents of proliferative enteritis in a hamster, deer, and ostrich with the sequence of a porcine isolate of *Lawsonia intracellularis*. *International Journal of Systematic Bacteriology* **47**, 635–639

Diani A and Gerritsen G (1987) Use in research. In: *Laboratory Hamsters*, ed. GL Van Hoosier and CW McPherson, pp. 329–347. Academic Press, London

Donnelly TM (1997) Disease problems of small rodents. In: *Ferrets, Rabbits and Rodents: Clinical Medicine and Surgery*, ed. EV Hillyer and KE Quesenberry, pp. 307–327. WB Saunders, Philadelphia

Dulisch ML (1976) A castration procedure for the rabbit, rat, hamster and guinea pig. *Journal of Zoo Animal Medicine* **7**, 8–11

Fox JG, Dewhirst FE, Fraser GJ, Paster BJ, Shames B and Murphy JC (1994) Intracellular *Campylobacter*-like organism from ferrets and hamsters with proliferative bowel disease is a *Desulfovibrio* sp. *Journal of Clinical Microbiology* **32**, 1229–1237

Frisk CS (1987) Bacterial and mycotic diseases. In: *Laboratory Hamsters*, ed. GL Van Hoosier and CW McPherson, pp. 112–134. Academic Press, London

Harkness JE (1994) Small rodents. *Veterinary Clinics of North America: Small Animal Practice* **24**, 89–102

Hem A, Smith AJ and Solberg P (1998) Saphenous vein puncture for blood sampling of the mouse, rat, hamster, gerbil, guineapig, ferret and mink. *Laboratory animals* **32**, 364–368

Hubbard GB and Schmidt RE (1987) Non-infectious diseases. In: *Laboratory Hamsters*, ed. GL Van Hoosier and CW McPherson, pp. 169–178. Academic Press, London

Huerkamp MJ (1995) Anaesthesia and postoperative management of rabbits and pocket pets. In: *Kirk's Current Veterinary Therapy XII: Small Animal Practice*, ed. JD Bonagura and RW Kirk, pp. 1322–1327. WB Saunders, Philadelphia

Johnson-Delaney CA (1998) Disease of the urinary system of commonly kept rodents: diagnosis and treatment. *Seminars in Avian and Exotic Pet Medicine* **7**, 81–88

Kirkman H and Algard FT (1968) Spontaneous and nonviral-induced neoplasms. In: *The Golden Hamster: Its Biology and Use in Medical Research*, pp. 227–240. Iowa State University Press, Ames.

Kupersmith DS (1998) A practical overview of small mammal nutrition. *Seminars in Avian and Exotic Pet Medicine* **7** (3) 141–147.

Ladiges WC (1987) Diseases. In: *Laboratory Hamsters*, ed. GL Van Hoosier and CW McPherson, pp. 321–328. Academic Press, London

Lipman NS and Foltz C (1996) Hamsters. In: *Handbook of Rodent and Rabbit Medicine,* ed. K Laber-Laird *et al.,* pp. 59–89. Pergamon, Oxford

Mitruka BM and Rawnsley HM (1981) *Clinical Biochemical and Haematological Reference Values in Normal Experimental Animals and Normal Humans.* Masson Publishing USA, New York

Morris TH (1995) Antibiotic therapeutics in laboratory animals. *Laboratory Animals* **29,** 16–36

Mullen H (1997) Soft tissue surgery. In: *Ferrets, Rabbits, and Rodents: Clinical Medicine and Surgery,* ed. EV Hillyer and KV Quesenberry, pp. 329–336. WB Saunders, Philadelphia

Muller and Kirk (1995) Dermatoses of pet rodents, rabbits and ferrets. In: *Muller and Kirk's Small Animal Dermatology, 5ᵗʰ edn,* ed. DW Scott *et al.,* pp. 1127–1173. WB Saunders, Philadelphia

Murphy JC, Fox JG and Niemi SM (1984) Nephrotic syndrome associated with renal amyloidosis in a colony of Syrian hamsters. *Journal of the American Veterinary Medical Association* **185,** 1359–1984

Parker JC, Ganaway JR and Gillet CS (1987) Viral diseases. In: *Laboratory Hamsters*, ed. GL Van Hoosier and CW McPherson, pp. 95–111. Academic Press, London

Perey DH and Barthold SW (1993) Hamsters. In: *Pathology of Laboratory Rodents and Rabbits,* ed. DH Perey and SW Barthold, pp. 115–136. Iowa State University Press, Ames

Rehg JE and Lu YS (1982) *Clostridium difficile* typhlitis in hamsters not associated with antibiotic therapy. *Journal of the American Veterinary Medical Association* **181,** 1422–1423

Schuchman SM (1989) Individual care and treatment of rabbits, mice, rats, guineapigs, hamsters and gerbils. In: *Current Veterinary Therapy X: Small Animal Practice,* ed. RW Kirk, pp. 738–764. WB Saunders, Philadelphia

Strandberg JD (1987) Neoplastic disease. In: *Laboratory Hamsters*, ed. GL Van Hoosier and CW McPherson, pp. 157–168. Academic Press, London

Swindle MM and Shealy PM (1996) Common surgical procedures in rodents and rabbits. In: *Handbook of Rodent and Rabbit Medicine,* ed. K Laber-Laird *et al.,* pp. 239–254. Pergamon, Oxford

Toft JD (1992) Commonly observed spontaneous neoplasms in rabbits, rats, guinea pigs, hamsters and gerbils. *Seminars in Avian and Exotic Pet Medicine* **1,** 80–92

Verhoef-Verhallen E (1997) Hamsters. In: *Konijnen and Knaagdieren Encyclopedie,* pp. 111–144. Rebo, Lisse

Wagner JE and Farrar PL (1987) Husbandry and medicine of small rodents. *Veterinary Clinics of North America: Small Animal Practice* **17,** 1061–1087

Wagner JE (1987) Parasitic disease. In: *Laboratory Hamsters*, ed. GL Van Hoosier and CW McPherson, pp. 135–156. Academic Press, London

Whittaker D (1999) Hamsters. In: *The UFAW Handbook on the Care and Management of Laboratory Animals, 7ᵗʰ edn,* ed. T Poole, pp. 356–366. Blackwell Science, Oxford

Zook BC, Huang K and Rhorer RG (1977) Tyzzer's disease in Syrian hamsters. *Journal of the Veterinary Medical Association* **171,** 833–836

4

Gerbils

Emma Keeble

Introduction

Gerbils are small desert rodents with a wide geographical distribution, originating from Central Asia, India, the Middle East and Africa. They belong to the suborder Myomorpha (rats, mice, gerbils and hamsters) and family Cricetidae (hamsters and gerbils). Gerbils (also known as jirds) belong to a separate subfamily, the Gerbillinae. The most common pet species is known as the Mongolian gerbil or clawed jird (*Meriones unguiculatus*). Other gerbil species that may now be encountered in veterinary practice include the Libyan gerbil *M. libycus*, the duprasi or fat-tailed gerbil *Pachyuromys duprasi* (see Chapter 10) and Shaw's jird *M. shawii*. This chapter refers to the Mongolian gerbil.

Mongolian gerbils originate from the semi-desert regions of Mongolia and northeastern China. In the wild, gerbils live in large family groups of around 20 animals, with one dominant male and female. They dig deep burrows consisting of several chambers for nesting and food storage, with multiple entrances. Environmental temperatures can vary from –40°C in winter to >50°C in the summer. Gerbils do not hibernate.

Gerbils are specially adapted to this desert lifestyle, with low water requirements and the production of scant, concentrated urine. They have an acute sense of hearing and smell, and communicate via a series of foot drummings. Both sexes have a prominent ventral scent gland, used for marking territorial boundaries.

Gerbils make good children's pets because:

- They are relatively long lived (average lifespan 3–4 years), generally hardy, and diurnal
- They are odourless (to humans) and their housing does not need cleaning out as often as that of other rodents
- They are highly sociable, create extensive burrow systems and are fun to watch
- They rarely bite and are docile.

Common problems when keeping gerbils are that they:

- Can be difficult to handle, resulting in degloving injuries to the tail
- Are destructive and may chew wires and carpets.

Many colour varieties of gerbil exist. The most common is agouti (Figure 4.1), the natural colour in the wild. Variations on agouti include cinnamon (lacks

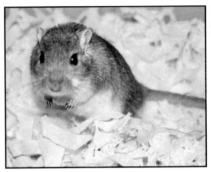

Figure 4.1
Agouti or 'wild type' coloration.

black guard hairs) and argente (silvery sheen). Self-varieties (albino, black, grey, lilac, dove) are all one body colour. Marked and variegated colour varieties also exist.

Foot stomping is a normal communicative behaviour in gerbils and is used as an alarm call.

Biology

Biological data are summarized in Figure 4.2.

Life expectancy	3–4 years
Adult weight	70–120 g
Heart rate	300–400 beats per minute
Respiratory rate	90–140 breaths per minute
Body temperature	37–38.5°C
Food consumption	5–8 g/day
Water consumption	4–7 ml/day
Sexual maturity	10–12 weeks
Duration of oestrus	4–6 days
Gestation	24–26 days non-lactating; 27–48 days lactating
Litter size	3–7 (average 5)
Birth weight	2.5–3.5 g
Number of litters per year	4–10 (average 7)
Weaned	2–26 days

Figure 4.2 Biological data.

Sexing

The distance between the anus and genitals in male gerbils is twice the length of that in females (Figure 4.3). Young male gerbils have dark coloured skin over the scrotum and a more pronounced ventral abdominal scent gland.

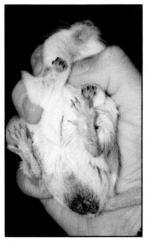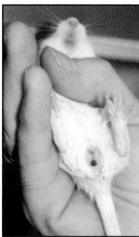

Figure 4.3 External genitalia of adult male (left) and female (right) gerbils.

Husbandry

Housing

Gerbils are highly social animals and should be kept as single sex groups (introduced before sexual maturity, ideally at 6–8 weeks), breeding pairs or harems. Adult females are more likely to fight than males, even if kept together since birth.

Gerbils should be housed in a 'gerbilarium' (Figure 4.4), a large glass or plastic tank (minimum 75 cm in length, 40 cm wide and 40 cm high). A wire mesh or plastic tight-fitting lid with ventilation holes should be fitted. Wire cages are not suitable, as gerbils are unable to burrow in them. Deep substrate (15 cm) should be used, such as sawdust, wood shavings or a mixture of peat and hay. Sand should be avoided as it may lead to rostral abrasions during burrowing. A separate sand bath should be provided to maintain the coat.

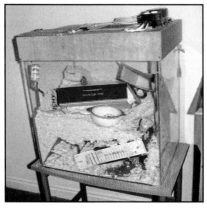

Figure 4.4 A 'gerbilarium' as recommended for housing gerbils.

Nesting material should be provided (shredded paper, toilet tissue). Synthetic bedding may cause impactions if ingested or may wrap around the legs.

Playthings alleviate boredom and prevent stereotypical behaviours. Wood and cardboard should be provided for chewing (e.g. fruit tree branches, wooden cotton reels, cardboard tubes, egg boxes). Ceramic flower pots and old mugs provide good areas to hide in. New items should be added weekly.

The tank should be kept away from direct sunlight and radiators to prevent overheating. Humidity should be kept low (below 30%), or the coat will become roughened and starey.

Gerbils create their own system of tunnels, which changes constantly. They produce scant urine so the tank needs cleaning only three or four times a year. Sawdust and shaving substrates are associated with higher levels of ammonia, which reduces air quality and predisposes to respiratory disease. If used, these substrates should be changed every 4–6 weeks.

Diet

In the wild gerbils feed on coarse grasses, roots, seeds and occasional invertebrates (Agren *et al.*, 1989). They store food over winter in burrows. In captivity they may be fed commercial rodent mixes (one tablespoon per day) with added fresh fruit and vegetables, such as lettuce, apple and carrot (Brain, 1999). Hay may also be provided. For occasional treats, raisins, melon seeds and sunflower seeds should be given.

Gerbils eat over a 24-hour period and are coprophagic. Sunflower seeds are high in cholesterol and low in amino acids, vitamins and minerals, particularly calcium. Gerbils often eat sunflower seeds to the exclusion of other foods. This may lead to obesity, reduced growth and nutritional osteodystrophies.

Water should be changed daily and provided via a water bottle.

Captive breeding

Gerbils form monogamous pairs in captivity and share parental responsibilities. Harems may be kept, although fighting is more likely. The female is polyoestrous and cycles throughout the year. Pseudopregnancy is possible following infertile mating, lasting 14–16 days. If lactating, delayed implantation may occur, resulting in a prolonged gestation period (see Figure 4.2). The male may remain with the female after birth; however, a postpartum oestrus does occur. Caesarean section is reportedly rare.

The young, or pups, are altricial, with ears opening at 5 days and eyes at 16–17 days. Incisors erupt at 12–14 days. Cannibalization or litter abandonment occurs only rarely and may be secondary to small litter size, excessive handling, mastitis, agalactia or lack of a nesting area. Fostering and hand rearing of young is rarely successful, although in the author's experience hand rearing can be achieved, particularly in older pups. Potential milk substitutes include goats' milk or high fat milk substitutes. Pups are fed via an intravenous catheter sleeve and 1 ml syringe, initially every 2 hours. At 3 weeks of age the young start to eat small amounts of seed, fruit and vegetables. It is important to ensure water and food sources are within reach of the pups at this stage or deaths may occur at weaning.

Handling and restraint

Gerbils should always be handled over a table or flat surface in case they are dropped. Limb fractures are common from improper handling. Gerbils rarely bite, except when unused to handling. They should never be picked up by the tail as the skin may strip away to expose the underlying bone. Correct handling is either by scruffing the skin over the neck and supporting the body with the other hand or by holding the body, with the thumb under the gerbil's mandible (Figure 4.5). Grasping the scruff stimulates an immobility response (Cruz and Junquera, 1993). Gerbils may also be picked up by cupping both hands over the animal.

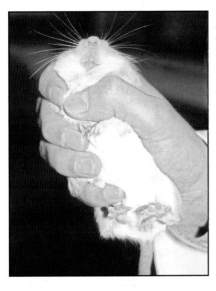

Figure 4.5 Correct technique for handling a gerbil.

Diagnostic approach

Physical examination
Clinical examination, initially at a distance, allows observation of the respiratory rate and character. Evidence of blood, porphyrin staining, droppings and urine can also be evaluated in the cage. Direct examination should follow this.

An accurate weight is essential as a guide to health status and for calculation of therapeutic doses. Body temperature should be recorded before the gerbil becomes too distressed. Clinical examination should be carried out as for any other animal species, starting with the head and working caudally. Important examinations include assessment of the oral cavity, thoracic auscultation and abdominal palpation.

Sample collection

Blood
Sampling sites include the lateral tail vein and the saphenous vein (Hem *et al.*, 1998). A gerbil's total blood volume is around 7% of total bodyweight (70 ml/kg). Of this circulating volume only 10% can be safely withdrawn at any one time (7 ml/kg). Thus, 0.5–0.8 ml of blood may be taken from a gerbil weighing 70–120 g (Hem *et al.*, 1998). A safe resampling period is 3–4 weeks.

The red blood cells of gerbils have a rapid turnover (average life span 10 days) and typically show pronounced basophilic stippling. The blood has high circulating cholesterol levels, possibly a reflection of

Parameter (units)	Normal range *(McClure, 1999)*
Red blood cells (×10^{12}/l)	8–9
PCV (%)	43–49
Haemoglobin (g/dl)	12.6–16.2
White blood cells (×10^9/l)	7–15
Neutrophils (%)	5–34
Lymphocytes (%)	60–95
Monocytes (%)	0–3
Eosinophils (%)	0–4
Basophils (%)	0–1
Platelets (×10^9/l)	400–600
Glucose (mmol/l)	2.8–7.5
Blood urea nitrogen (mmol/l)	6.1–9.6
Creatinine (μmol/l)	53–124
Total protein (g/l)	43–125
Albumin (g/l)	18–55
Globulin (g/l)	12–60
Total bilirubin (μmol/l)	21–103
Calcium (mmol/l)	0.90–1.50
Inorganic phosphorus (mmol/l)	1.20–2.00
Alkaline phosphatase (IU/l)	3.7–7.0
Cholesterol (mmol/l)	2.33–3.91

Figure 4.6 Normal haematological and biochemical values in gerbils.

a gerbil's high fat diet in captivity and preference for sunflower seeds (Bauck and Bihun, 1997). Normal haematological and biochemical ranges are shown in Figure 4.6.

Diagnostic tests and techniques

Urinalysis
A urine sample may be collected from voluntary urination during handling or from the cage. Gerbil urine is alkaline and normally contains small amounts of protein, glucose, bilirubin and acetone.

Faecal analysis
Gerbils often pass droppings while being handled, and these may be screened for parasitology, bacteriology and fungal culture. The anal tape test may be used to identify some species of pinworm (*Syphacia muris* and *S. obvelata*).

Radiography
Gerbils should be sedated or anaesthetized for radiography. The thorax is not easily visualized due to its small size relative to the abdominal cavity and the superimposition of the triceps muscle over the cranial thoracic cavity. The liver and gastrointestinal tract occupy the cranial abdomen. In the male, large scrotal fat pads occupy the caudal abdomen from the level of the os penis to the umbilicus.

Ultrasonography
In the author's experience ultrasonography may be rewarding for diagnosis of pyometra and abdominal masses. A stand off and 7.5 MHz sector scanner may be used successfully.

Common conditions

General signs of disease include a rough hair coat, porphyrin-stained ocular secretions, lethargy, dehydration, anorexia and small scant droppings.

Dental disease

Incisor malocclusion
As with other rodents the incisors of gerbils are open rooted and constantly erupting. Malocclusion may be congenital or acquired. Treatment with regular corrective burring and provision of substances to gnaw may help. The long-term prognosis is poor. Incisor removal has been described but this is not a practical option because of the length of the tooth roots.

Gastrointestinal disease

Figure 4.7 lists the common gastrointestinal disorders of gerbils.

Enteritis
Enteritis results in diarrhoea, starey coat, hunched posture and skin tenting associated with dehydration. General supportive treatment should be initiated. There are many causes of diarrhoea in gerbils (see Figure 4.7), and a full clinical history is essential, including diet, recent changes in husbandry, the environment and the introduction of new animals.

Gastric dilation
In the author's experience gastric dilation is common in gerbils. Gaseous distension of the stomach may occur secondary to feeding inappropriate or stale diets. Gerbils have a well developed ridge at the junction between the oesophagus and the stomach, so they are unable to eructate or vomit. Bloat may also occur as a sequel to intestinal ileus and anorexia. Clinical signs include abdominal tympany, tooth grinding, dyspnoea and cardiovascular compromise. Treatment is essential. Gas may be reduced by using a wide-bore stomach tube or by direct aspiration with a needle and syringe. Fluid therapy and non-steroidal anti-inflammatories are indicated.

Ileus
Ileus is common after anaesthesia, malocclusion or periods of anorexia. Scant dry droppings or lack of droppings are seen clinically. Increased gas is present in the small intestine on radiography. Supportive treatment with oral fluids, probiotics and intestinal stimulants such as cisapride and metoclopramide is indicated.

Bacterial enteritis

Tyzzer's disease: Gerbils are particularly susceptible to infection with *Clostridium piliforme*. This organism is an obligate intracellular Gram-negative bacterium, which survives as spores for over a year in bedding, soil or contaminated feed. Spores are resistant to most disinfectants but are killed by 0.5% sodium hypochlorite, peracetic acid or prolonged heat treatment. Predisposing factors include poor hygiene, overcrowding, concurrent disease or recent transportation. Infection is via the faecal–oral route, with weanlings being most

Disease	Aetiology	Clinical signs	Differential diagnosis	Diagnostic options	Treatment options
Incisor malocclusion	Congenital or acquired	Overgrowth of incisors			Regular burring; removal difficult due to long roots and fragile skull
Gastric dilation (bloat)	Stale or inappropriate diet, anorexia, malocclusion	Tympany, tooth grinding, dyspnoea, cardiovascular compromise	Respiratory, cardiovascular or underlying systemic disease	Clinical signs, abdominal palpation, radiography	Reduce gas by stomach tube or needle aspiration Fluid therapy, metoclopramide, cisapride, carprofen
Ileus	Post-anaesthesia, abdominal surgery, malocclusion, anorexia	Scant small droppings, lack of droppings	Intestinal impaction or foreign body, gastric dilation, underlying systemic disease	Clinical signs, abdominal palpation, radiography	Parenteral/oral fluid therapy, probiotics, metoclopramide, cisapride, high fibre diet
Bacterial enteritis					
Tyzzer's disease	*Clostridium piliforme*	Acute: lethargy, death Chronic: weight loss, diarrhoea, head tilt, incoordination, death	Bacterial, parasitic enteritis	Gross postmortem, histopathology and special stains (PAS, silver, Giemsa), ELISA on serum sample	Improve husbandry and hygiene, disinfect environment, fluid therapy Oxytetracycline, chloramphenicol, probiotics
Parasitic enteritis					
Protozoal	*Giardia, Trichomonas, Entamoeba,* coccidians	Ranging from no clinical signs to diarrhoea	Bacterial, parasitic enteritis, Tyzzer's disease	Faecal parasitology	Coccidiosis: Sulphadimidine, sulfamethazine, sulfadimethoxine Others: Metronidazole, dimetronidazole, fenbendazole
Helminths	*Syphacia, Aspicularis,* Oxyurids, *Hymenolepis, Taenia*	Weight loss, starey coat, diarrhoea, rectal prolapse	Bacterial, parasitic enteritis, Tyzzer's disease	Faecal parasitology, adhesive tape for pinworm	Ivermectin, fenbendazole Niclosamide (tapeworm infection)

Figure 4.7 Common gastrointestinal disorders of gerbils.

susceptible. Acute infection causes lethargy and death (within 24–48 hours). Chronic infection causes weight loss, watery diarrhoea, head tilt, incoordination and death. The initial enteric infection spreads rapidly to the liver, heart and central nervous system. Deaths are common in animals aged 3–7 weeks. Diagnosis can be made on postmortem examination, where ulceration of the ileocaecocolic junction, hepatomegaly with necrotic white foci, and necrotizing myocarditis are common. Bacterial culture is difficult. An ELISA is available and may aid diagnosis. Treatment is rarely successful but has been described with oxytetracycline 0.1 mg/ml in the drinking water daily for 30 days to decrease morbidity. Chloramphenicol at 50 mg/kg by mouth every 8 hours or 30 mg/kg i.m. every 8 hours may also be effective. Carrier status may develop after treatment. Prevention should be aimed at improving husbandry and hygiene.

Other causes of bacterial enteritis in gerbils include infections with *Salmonella*, *Escherichia coli* and *Citrobacter rodentium* (Puente-Redondo *et al.*, 1999). Diagnosis is based on culture of the organism. Animals diagnosed with salmonellosis should be euthanased because this is a zoonosis and asymptomatic carrier status may develop after infection.

Parasitic enteritis
Endoparasitic infections in gerbils are rare and often have no associated clinical signs.

Protozoal infections reported include coccidiosis (*Eimeria* sp.), *Trichomonas*, *Entamoeba muris* and *Giardia* (FELASA, 1996). Diagnosis is based on faecal parasitology.

Helminth infections include those caused by pinworms (*Syphacia muris*, *S. obvelata*, *Aspicularis tetraptera*), oxyurids (*Dentostomella translucida*), the dwarf tapeworm *Hymenolepis nana* and the tapeworm *Taenia crassicollis*. Pinworm infections have been associated with rectal prolapse and are easily diagnosed by placing adhesive tape over the perineum and examining it under a microscope for ova. Oxyurid infection may be detected on faecal parasitology. Although tapeworm infections are rare, it should be noted that *Hymenolepis nana* is zoonotic.

Neoplasia
Intestinal adenocarcinoma has been reported in the gerbil.

Respiratory disease
Respiratory diseases are reportedly rare in gerbils, although the author has seen several cases in practice. Clinical signs are cyanosis, weight loss, dyspnoea, anorexia, porphyrin staining around the eyes and, occasionally, sneezing. Bacterial sinusitis has been described, and lower respiratory tract infections with *Mycoplasma pulmonis*, *Pasteurella pneumotropica*, *Streptococcus pneumoniae* and *Bordetella bronchiseptica* have been recorded. Gerbils can also be carriers of Sendai virus and pneumonia virus of mice. Diagnostic aids include radiography and bacterial culture from nasal swabs. Initial stabilization in an oxygen chamber may help alleviate clinical signs. Antibiotics, non-steroidal anti-inflammatories, mucolytics, bronchodilators and diuretics may be useful.

Cardiovascular disease
Arteriosclerosis and focal myocardial degeneration have been reported in ageing gerbils.

Urogenital disease

Renal failure
Chronic interstitial nephritis is common in ageing gerbils and may be associated with weight loss, reduced appetite, polydipsia/polyuria, and cystitis. Renal fibrosis, glomerulosis and amyloidosis have also been reported. Diagnosis is based on urinalysis (presence of protein, blood, casts and cells) and biochemistry. Supportive care with fluid diuresis and anabolic steroids may slow the progression of renal failure. Clients should be encouraged to provide fresh water and food at all times and to avoid stressful situations that could predispose to acute renal failure.

Reproductive tract
Cystic ovaries are extremely common in older female gerbils. Cysts can grow to 5 cm in diameter and are often bilateral. Reproductive performance is reduced. Abdominal distension and dyspnoea occur in severe cases. Drainage may be attempted, but ovariohysterectomy is the treatment of choice.

Pyometra can occur in gerbils. Ovariohysterectomy is recommended.

Neoplasia of the reproductive tract may present with a vulval discharge similar to pyometra. This is often associated with secondary bacterial infections. Tumours of the reproductive tract include granulosa and thecal cell tumours, leiomyoma and adenocarcinoma of the uterus. Testicular teratomas and seminomas have been reported in the male.

Endocrine disease
Diabetes mellitus may be a sequel to obesity in gerbils because obese individuals are predisposed to hyperglycaemia and glucose intolerance (Laber-Laird, 1996). A reduction in weight may alleviate clinical signs, but care should be taken because hepatic lipidosis may occur after rapid dietary changes.

Hyperadrenocorticism has rarely been reported in ageing gerbils.

Cortical adenomas and carcinomas of the adrenal gland have also been reported in ageing gerbils, although these were findings at postmortem examination.

Neurological disease

Epilepsy
Spontaneous epileptiform seizures are common in certain genetic lines of gerbil. It is thought this behaviour may have developed as a survival mechanism to deter predators (Laber-Laird, 1996). Evidence suggests that these gerbils lack the enzyme glutamine synthetase, which is necessary for conversion of glutamate to glutamine, one of the excitatory amino acids of the central nervous system. Seizures occur from 2–3 months and may become more severe up to 6 months of age. They are usually stimulated by a change in environment or handling. Episodes last for a few minutes only and

range from mild hypnotic episodes to generalized grand mal seizures. If gerbils are handled frequently within the first 3 weeks of life, epilepsy may be less likely to develop. Treatment is rarely indicated, although phenytoin and primidone may be used.

Head tilt

Head tilt is common in ageing gerbils and may be associated with bacterial infection, secondary to respiratory infections (otitis media, otitis interna), aural cholesteatoma, papilloma or polyp formation. Cholesteatoma formation occurs as an accumulation of keratinized epithelium. Affected gerbils may become deaf. There is no treatment. Bacterial infections are rare because the external auditory canal in gerbils is vertical, allowing pus to drain easily. Treatment for bacterial infections with appropriate antibiotics may prevent worsening of clinical signs but rarely provides resolution. Papilloma or polyps in the external ear canal may be removed surgically, although regrowth is possible after incomplete removal.

Viral infections

Gerbils can act as carriers of lymphocytic choriomeningitis virus, which is zoonotic. In some cases infection can cause meningitis and convulsions.

Fractures

Fractures are common in gerbils, and management is as for other species. Cage rest may be sufficient in some cases. Amputation of the affected limb may be necessary, and in the author's experience both hind- and forelimb amputations are well tolerated, provided the animal is monitored closely. Occasionally an underlying calcium deficiency may cause metabolic bone disease and pathological fractures. This is seen in gerbils fed primarily on sunflower seeds.

Skin disease

Figure 4.8 lists the common skin disorders of gerbils. Occasional litters may be born with abnormal hair pigmentation and stunted growth. The aetiology is unknown (Laber-Laird, 1996).

Disease	Aetiology	Clinical signs	Differential diagnosis	Diagnostic options	Treatment options
Parasitic					
Demodicosis	*Demodex meroni*	Alopecia, scaling, dermatitis	Fungal, bacterial	Microscopy of hair pluck/skin scrape	Topical amitraz every 2 weeks, 3–6 treatments Ivermectin injection every 7–10 days, 3 treatments
Fungal					
Dermatophytosis	*Microsporum gypseum, Trichophyton mentagrophytes*	Focal alopecia, hyperkeratosis	Parasitic, bacterial	Microscopy of hair pluck, fungal culture, Wood's lamp (*Microsporum*)	Disinfect environment, clip hair Oral griseofulvin for 3 weeks Enilconazole baths twice weekly until 2 negative cultures
Bacterial					
Nasal dermatitis	Hypersecretion of Harderian gland, secondary staphylococcal infection	Alopecia, crusting, dermatitis surrounding nares, spreading to paws, abdomen	Bald nose, barbering	Clinical signs, bacterial culture, cytology of impression smears	Identify underlying stressors Provide sand Topical antibiotic (fusidic acid, chloramphenicol), topical iodine, systemic chloramphenicol, potentiated sulphonamides, penicillins, cephalosporins
Sebaceous gland dermatitis	*Staphylococcus Streptococcus*	Reddened, ulcerated ventral scent gland	Adenoma, adenocarcinoma	Histopathology	Topical (fusidic acid, chloramphenicol) or systemic antibiotics (potentiated sulphonamides, chloramphenicol, penicillins, cephalosporins) Surgical removal
Neoplasia					
Ventral scent gland neoplasia	Adenoma, adenocarcinoma, squamous cell carcinoma, basal cell carcinoma	Ulceration, proliferation of scent gland	Bacterial infections	Histopathology	Total surgical excision
Environmental/behavioural					
Barbering	Fur chewed by others	Hair loss tail base and top of head	Fungal	Observation, chewed hairs microscopically	Reduce stocking density, remove dominant animal
Bald nose	Nose rubbed by bars	Hair loss around nose	Nasal dermatitis, barbering	Observation	Feed inside cage, house in 'gerbilarium'
Tail slip	Incorrect handling	Degloving of skin from tail	N/A	Clinical signs	Amputate proximal to injury
Fight injuries	Staph. Infection	Bite marks on head, tail, perineum, abscesses	Bacterial dermatitis, trauma	Observation	Remove dominant animal, topical and systemic antibiotics
High humidity	Humidity >50%	Starey coat	General ill health and disease	High humidity recorded	Regular cleaning, check water bottle, underlying disease needs to be investigated

Figure 4.8 Common skin disorders of gerbils.

Bacterial infections

Nasal dermatitis ('sore nose', 'facial dermatitis'):

Nasal dermatitis (Figure 4.9) is extremely common in gerbils, particularly in sexually mature animals housed in groups that may be stressed by overcrowding and high humidity. Lesions start as small focal areas of alopecia and crusting around the external nares and may progress to involve the face, medial paws and abdomen, with associated alopecia and dermatitis. Severe infection may be associated with debility and mortality. Hypersecretion of the Harderian gland results in accumulation of porphyrin pigment around the nares. This is irritant and may lead to self-trauma and secondary staphylococcal infection. Digging through abrasive bedding could be a predisposing factor. Diagnosis is based on clinical signs, bacterial culture and cytology of impression smears. Harderian gland secretions may increase with stress. Improving husbandry, environmental temperature and humidity (below 50%) helps resolve this problem. Provision of a sand bath helps to improve fur quality and encourage grooming. Removal of the Harderian gland has been described, although the long-term effects of this surgery are not known (Thiessen and Pendergrass, 1982; Farrar et al., 1988). Topical or systemic antibiotic treatment is indicated.

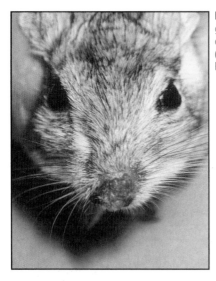

Figure 4.9 A gerbil with nasal dermatitis. (Courtesy of Paul Flecknell.)

Fungal infections

Microsporum gypseum or Trichophyton mentagrophytes infections rarely occur but are associated with focal alopecia and hyperkeratosis. Diagnosis is based on hair examination and fungal culture. Infections are zoonotic. Treatment involves disinfection of the environment, clipping of the surrounding hair and oral griseofulvin at 30 mg/kg daily for 3 weeks. For large groups, griseofulvin may be added to the food (0.75 mg/kg of feed, 10 g/kg of 7.5% powder in dry feed), although this is expensive. Washes with enilconazole twice weekly, until two cultures give negative results, have also been described.

Parasites

Compared with other small rodent species, ectoparasites are not common in gerbils.

Infestation with Demodex meroni has been reported (Burgmann, 1997). This species is specific to gerbils and causes alopecia, scaling and focal ulcerative dermatitis with secondary bacterial infections. Diagnosis is based on microscopic examination of plucked hair and deep skin scrapes. Treatment consists of topical amitraz, 0.66 ml per pint of water, three to six times at 2-week intervals. In the author's experience demodicosis may respond to three treatments of injectible ivermectin at 200 µg/kg, 7–10 days apart. Generalized Demodex infestation is often associated with immunosuppression and underlying disease due to old age, poor nutrition or husbandry-related problems such as overcrowding and poor ventilation.

Other ectoparasites include Liponyssoides sanguineous, the mouse fur mite, although this has not been associated with any adverse clinical signs. The fur mite Acarus farris has been associated with clinical signs in gerbils. Diagnosis is based on microscope examination of plucked hairs (Jacklin, 1997).

Sebaceous gland dermatitis

Gerbils have a large ventral abdominal sebaceous gland, which is used in territorial marking and scent identification of pups. Size is androgen-dependent, so the gland is larger in the male. The gland may become inflamed and infected with staphylococci and streptococci, appearing reddened and ulcerated. Early neoplastic changes may have a similar appearance and should be considered as differentials, particularly in older animals. Treatment is with topical or systemic antibiotics. If the condition does not respond, total gland excision is recommended because neoplasia is common.

Neoplasia

Skin neoplasms are relatively common in gerbils, particularly in older animals. Adenoma of the ventral scent gland (Figure 4.10) is most common; however, squamous cell carcinomas and basal cell carcinomas have been reported. These develop as raised ulcerated masses. Treatment is early total gland excision. Some advocate castration at the same time because growth is androgen-dependent (Jackson et al., 1996). Early excision is often curative, although the author has seen local spread to inguinal lymph nodes in advanced cases.

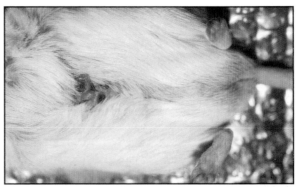

Figure 4.10 Ventral scent gland adenoma in a gerbil. (Courtesy of Anna Meredith.)

Other common skin neoplasms include melanomas, melanocytomas and squamous cell carcinoma of the feet and pinnae and, less commonly, papilloma, subcutaneous fibrosarcoma and mammary gland adenocarcinoma. Diagnosis is based on cytology and treatment is by wide surgical excision.

'Tail slip'

This is common after incorrect handling. If the tail is grasped, the skin may deglove, leaving exposed muscle and bone. Amputation proximal to the injury site is indicated.

Environmental and behavioural problems

High humidity

If the relative humidity exceeds 50% gerbils become starey coated. The rise in humidity can be caused by damp bedding, polyuria, diarrhoea or leakage of the water bottle. Starey coat is also a general sign of ill health.

Fighting

Boxing and play fighting is part of normal gerbil behaviour. Fighting, however, is a common problem, particularly between females. Gerbils are highly territorial and will fight to the death. Gerbils older than 10 weeks should preferably not be introduced to others; however, introduction may be possible using a temporary division, so that the individuals can smell each other but are not in direct contact. Each gerbil should be given a period on either side of the partition to become accustomed to the other animal's scent and to deposit its own. On introduction into neutral territory they should be closely monitored for at least 3 hours and separated at any sign of fighting. Fighting occurs when animals lack the space they would have in the wild to leave the group and establish their own colony. It is commonly seen in young gerbils trying to establish themselves in the hierarchy. Overcrowding or large tanks that allow separate territories to be set up are common underlying causes.

Fight wounds commonly occur on the head, tail base, gluteals and perineum and are often associated with abscesses. Clipping and lavage of the affected area, followed by treatment with topical and systemic antibiotics and addressing the underlying cause, are indicated.

Stereotypy

Stereotypical burrowing can occur when gerbils are not given access to suitable burrowing substrates (Weidenmayer, 1997). This results in repetitive burrowing in the corners of the cage. It can be avoided by housing in a 'gerbilarium' (see Figure 4.4).

Barbering

Barbering may occur in large groups, appearing as alopecia of the dorsal head and tail base. Stocking density should be reduced and the individual responsible for the hair loss removed.

Bald nose

This is associated with feeding through wire cages. Hair loss occurs when the nose is rubbed through the cage bars. This may be prevented by feeding inside the cage or housing in a glass tank.

Toxicities

Antibiotics

Streptomycin is toxic to gerbils and should be avoided. It inhibits acetylcholine release, resulting in neuromuscular block and paralysis.

Lead

Lead toxicity is common in gerbils as they gnaw at metal structures, such as cage wire and metal bowls. They also produce highly concentrated urine, leading to chronic lead accumulation. Clinical signs include weight loss, anorexia, starey coat, anaemia and neurological signs (ataxia and seizures). Chronic intoxication leads to hepatic and renal failure and microcytic hypochromic anaemia with basophilic stippling. Diagnosis is by history, radiography and measurement of lead levels in blood. Treatment with chelating agents (EDTA or D-penicillamine) and removal of the lead source is indicated.

Nutritional problems

Obesity

Obesity (Figure 4.11) is very common in gerbils fed large quantities of sunflower seeds. Dietary protein levels should be 22% and fat <4% to avoid problems with obesity and hypercholesterolaemia.

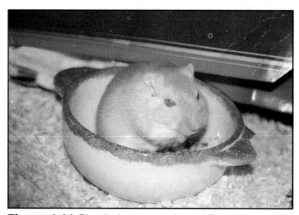

Figure 4.11 Obesity is common in gerbils.

Hypercholesterolaemia

Gerbils rapidly develop increased serum and liver cholesterol levels, even when fed a diet relatively low in fat. This increase in levels and increased liver storage is related to differences in hepatic enzymes involved in cholesterol metabolism.

Ocular disease

Figure 4.12 lists the common ophthalmological disorders of gerbils.

Disease	Aetiology	Clinical signs	Differential diagnosis	Diagnostic options	Treatment options
Cataracts	Old age, diabetes, post-anaesthesia	Opacity lens	See aetiology	Clinical history, urinalysis	None if transient post-anaesthetic Reduce weight (diabetes)
Corneal ulcers	Trauma, irritants	Blepharospasm, epiphora	Anterior uveitis	Fluorescein dye	Topical antibiotics
Proptosis	Trauma, improper handling, molar abscess	Prolapse of globe	See aetiology		Replacement or enucleation under anaesthesia

Figure 4.12 Common ophthalmological disorders of gerbils.

Cataracts

Cataracts may occur associated with old age, diabetes or general anaesthesia. Those associated with anaesthesia are transient and are thought to be caused by changes in composition of the aqueous humour.

Corneal ulcers may occur secondary to trauma or irritation. Calcification of the cornea is an ageing change, resulting in white plaques developing centrally (Kirschner, 1997).

Ocular emergencies

Proptosis can occur secondary to trauma, handling or molar abscess. In aged gerbils it is associated with protrusion of the nictitating membrane and conjunctiva, although the exact aetiology is not known. Proptosis, corneal abrasions and anterior uveitis should be treated as for other domestic species.

Miscellaneous diseases

Neoplasia

The incidence of neoplasia is high in gerbils older than 2 years. Sites most commonly affected are the reproductive tract, adrenal gland and skin (see above). Lymphoma, thymoma and osteosarcoma have also been seen. Clinical signs may be non-specific. Early surgical intervention is the treatment of choice.

Supportive care

Drug administration

Injection

Figure 4.13 lists the injection routes and volumes for gerbils. In general, for any injection the smallest needle size should always be used (25–27 gauge). Figure 4.14 shows an intraperitoneal injection into a gerbil.

Route	Site	Volume
Subcutaneous	Scruff of neck	2–3 ml
Intramuscular	Quadricep muscle	0.05–0.1 ml
Intravenous	Lateral tail vein or saphenous vein[a]	0.2 ml
Intraperitoneal (see Figure 4.14)	Right caudal quadrant, abdomen	3–4 ml

Figure 4.13 Injection routes and volumes for gerbils.
[a]From Hem et al., 1998.

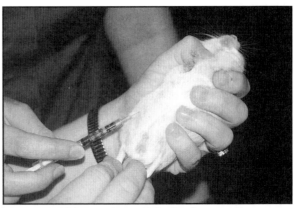

Figure 4.14 Intraperitoneal injection in a gerbil.

Nutritional support

Nutritional support is essential for long-term critical care and oral routes help prevent development of gastric stasis and intestinal ileus. Assisted feeding, either by syringe or gastric gavage, using sweet flavours, is well tolerated. A metal blunt-ended gavage needle can be introduced into the stomach to give a volume of 1–2 ml of a simple, non-sterile solution such as baby food, a commercial oral rehydration product or soaked and ground-up food pellets. Care must be taken not to damage the oesophagus or to intubate the trachea.

Probiotics, multivitamins (particularly vitamin B complex), gut transfaunation, motility modifiers and kaolin-based products may all be useful as supportive therapy in sick gerbils.

Fluid therapy

Daily maintenance fluid requirements are 40–60 ml/kg/day. Dehydration deficits are added to this as a percentage of bodyweight, based on clinical signs of dehydration. Shock fluid volumes of 10 ml/kg may be administered to gerbils over 20 minutes, with no detectable signs of volume overload. As a general rule, assume 10% dehydration for debilitated gerbils, replace 50% of the fluid deficit in 12 hours and the remainder (plus maintenance and concurrent losses) in 48–72 hours. Figure 4.15 shows volumes for fluid therapy.

Emergency cases

An oxygen cage may be created by piping oxygen into a small container in which gerbils can be placed. Gerbils are nasal breathers.

Route	Volume (ml)	Advantages	Disadvantages	Suggested Fluids
Subcutaneous injection	2–3	Large volume Simple technique	Slow absorption Sterile solution required	Isotonic crystalloids
Intraperitoneal injection	3–4	Rapid absorption Simple technique	Aseptic technique Risk of peritonitis and adhesions	Isotonic crystalloids
Intravenous injection	1 ml/100g as bolus[a]	Rapid rehydration	Skill required May need general anaesthesia	Crystalloids and colloids
Intraosseus catheter (femur, tibia)	1 ml/100g as bolus[a]	Rapid rehydration Large volumes Easy access if vascular collapse	Aseptic procedure Requires anaesthesia (local, general)	Crystalloids and colloids

Figure 4.15 Fluid therapy in gerbils.

[a] (Oglesbee, 1995)

Anaesthesia and analgesia

Preoperative considerations

Fasting is not required before anaesthesia in gerbils because vomiting does not occur. Fasting could lead to hypoglycaemia and dehydration due to the gerbil's high metabolic rate. Assessment of health status should be routine practice prior to anaesthesia. Fluid therapy may be indicated.

General anaesthesia may be monitored with normal reflexes, as described for other animals. The pedal withdrawal reflex is the most useful response in gerbils. Subclinical respiratory disease is common, and oxygen should be given routinely via a face mask or a nasal catheter. Tracheal intubation is difficult, requiring either tracheotomy or specialized endotracheal tubes and laryngoscopes (Huerkamp, 1995). Small intravenous catheter sleeves may be used as endotracheal tubes, although these are easily occluded by mucous secretions (Antinoff, 1999).

Gerbils have a large surface area for heat loss relative to body mass, and under anaesthesia normal thermoregulatory functions are affected. Hypothermia may be prevented by using bubble wrap and additional heat sources, such as heat lamps, heat pads and heated operating tables. Incubators are useful for postoperative recovery and administration of oxygen.

Inhalational anaesthesia

Induction using an anaesthetic induction chamber is preferred. Oxygen should be given for several minutes prior to induction. The gerbil may then be transferred to an Ayre's T-piece circuit with face mask. Figure 4.16 gives gas concentrations.

Injectable anaesthesia

A wide variety of injectable anaesthetic agents are available for use in the gerbil. These are primarily used in laboratory situations, but they may be of use for sedation or induction in practice. Individual variations are common, and overdoses are possible. The animal should be weighed prior to induction. Injectable agents may be used as total anaesthesia, or for induction to be followed by maintenance with a gaseous anaesthetic (Figures 4.17–4.19).

Anaesthetic Agent	Induction concentration (%)	Maintenance concentration (%)
Halothane	3–4	1–3
Isoflurane	3.5–4.5	1.5–3

Figure 4.16 Concentrations of inhalant general anaesthesia used in the gerbil.

Sedative	Dose rate	Sedative effect	Analgesia	Comments
Acepromazine	3 mg/kg i.m.	Light sedation	None	Not commonly used; may induce epileptic fit
Atropine	0.04 mg/kg s.c.	Anticholinergic	None	Reduces secretions
Diazepam	5 mg/kg i.m., i.p.	Light sedation	None	Anxiolytic
Fentanyl/fluanisone	0.5–1.0 ml/kg i.m., i.p.	Moderate sedation	Moderate	Commonly used for minor procedures, reversible
Ketamine	100–200 mg/kg i.m.	Heavy sedation	Mild	Dissociative, poor muscle relaxation, not commonly used
Medetomidine	100–200 µg/kg i.p.	Light to heavy sedation	Mild	Minor procedures, reversible, hypothermia, cyanosis and reduced blood pressure common
Midazolam	5 mg/kg i.m., i.p.	Light to moderate sedation	None	Anxiolytic
Xylazine	2 mg/kg i.m., i.p.	Light sedation	Mild	Not commonly used, reversible, hypothermia, cyanosis and reduced blood pressure common

Figure 4.17 Dose rates for sedatives and tranquillizers used in the gerbil.

Reversal agent	Dose rate	Drug reversed
Atipamezole	1 mg/kg i.m., i.p., s.c., i.v.	Medetomidine, xylazine
Buprenorphine	0.01–0.05 mg/kg s.c., i.p.	Fentanyl
Butorphanol	2mg/kg i.m., i.p., s.c.	Fentanyl
Doxapram (respiratory stimulant)	5–10 mg/kg i.m., i.p., i.v.	All anaesthetics
Nalbuphine	1–2 mg/kg i.m.	Fentanyl
Naloxone	0.01–0.1 mg/kg i.m., i.p., i.v.	Fentanyl
Yohimbine	0.2 mg/kg i.v., 0.5 mg/kg i.m.	Xylazine, medetomidine

Figure 4.18 Dose rates of reversal agents used in the gerbil.

Drug	Dose rate	Effect	Duration	Comments
Fentanyl/fluanisone/midazolam ([a])	8 ml/kg i.p.	Light – Surgical anaesthesia	20 mins	Partially reversible, commonly used
Fentanyl/fluanisone plus diazepam	0.3 ml/kg i.m., i.p. + 5 mg/kg i.p.	Light – Surgical anaesthesia	20 mins	Partially reversible, commonly used
Ketamine/medetomidine	75 mg/kg + 0.5 mg/kg i.p., s.c., i.m.	Medium depth anaesthesia	20–30	Partially reversible, commonly used
Ketamine/xylazine	50 mg/kg + 2 mg/kg i.p., s.c., i.m.	Immobilization		Partially reversible
Ketamine/diazepam	50 mg/kg + 5 mg/kg	Immobilization		
Alphaxalone/alphadalone	80–120 mg/kg i.p.	Immobilization		

Figure 4.19 Dose rates of injectable general anaesthetics used in the gerbil.

[a] Dose as mixture of 1 part fentanyl/fluanisone + 2 parts water for injection + 1 part midazolam (5 mg/ml solution)

Analgesia

Figure 4.20 lists the dose rates for analgesic agents used in the gerbil.

Drug	Dose rate	Frequency of dosing
Aspirin	100–150 mg/kg orally	4 hourly
Buprenorphine	0.01–0.05 mg/kg s.c., i.m., i.p.	8 hourly
Butorphanol	1–5 mg/kg s.c., i.m., i.p.	2–4 hourly
Carprofen	5 mg/kg s.c.	8–12 hourly (anecdotal)
Flunixin	2.5 mg/kg s.c., i.m.	12–24 hourly
Pethidine	10 mg/kg s.c., i.m.	2–3 hourly

Figure 4.20 Dose rates of analgesics used in the gerbil.

Common surgical procedures

Removal of the ventral scent gland

This is a simple procedure. The entire gland should be excised, using a circumferential incision with a wide margin into normal skin. Haemostasis is important to prevent excessive blood loss. Closure with continuous subcuticular absorbable monofilament sutures (5-0, 6-0) is the preferred method.

Tail amputation

This is carried out with the gerbil in ventral recumbency. The skin is debrided to healthy tissue and the tail amputated through the most cranial coccygeal vertebra visible in the wound. Haemorrhage is minimal and can be controlled by cauterization. The subcutis and skin are closed with simple interrupted absorbable suture material (5-0, 6-0). Injection of local anaesthetic into the tail tip and careful atraumatic handling should prevent self-trauma to the tail after surgery.

Other surgical procedures described in gerbils include ovariohysterectomy, caesarean section, routine castration (closed technique), limb amputation and fracture repair.

Euthanasia

Euthanasia is defined as the 'killing of an animal with the minimum of physical and mental suffering'. Intraperitoneal injection of barbiturate may be slow in onset of action and cause painful irritation of the peritoneum. The author's preferred method of euthanasia is general anaesthesia (using inhalant gaseous induction) followed by intracardiac injection with barbiturate.

Drug formulary

Drug	Dose	Licence category
Antibacterials		
Ampicillin	2–10 mg/100 g s.c. tid	Veterinary
Chloramphenicol palmitate	50 mg/kg orally bid	Veterinary
Chloramphenicol succinate	30 mg/kg i.m., s.c. bid, 50 mg/60 ml water for 2 weeks	Veterinary
Ciprofloxacin	10 mg/kg orally bid	Human
Dimetronidazole	0.25–1% in water for 5–7 days	Human
Enrofloxacin	10 mg/kg i.m., s.c., orally, bid	Licensed for gerbils
Gentamicin	5 mg/kg i.m., s.c. sid	Veterinary
Neomycin	100 mg/kg orally sid for 7 days, 10 g/gallon water for 5 days, then 5 g/gal for 5 days	Veterinary
Oxytetracycline	800 mg/l water, 20 mg/kg s.c. sid, 0.1 mg/ml water daily for 30 days (Tyzzer's disease)	Veterinary
Tetracycline	250 mg/100 ml water for 14 days, 20 mg/kg orally, i.m. bid	Veterinary
Trimethoprim sulfadiazine	30 mg/kg s.c. sid	Veterinary
Trimethoprim sulfamethoxazole	15 mg/kg orally bid	Veterinary
Trimethoprim/Sulphonamide (240mg/ml)	120 mg/kg orally bid	Veterinary
Tylosin	10 mg/kg orally sid for 21 days, 10 mg/kg i.m., s.c. sid 5–7 days	Veterinary
Antifungals		
Enilconazole	Twice-weekly washes	Veterinary
Griseofulvin	25–30 mg/kg orally sid for 3 weeks, in feed 0.75 mg/kg (10 g/kg of 7.5% powder in dry feed)	Veterinary
Antiparasitic drugs		
Amitraz	0.66 ml per pint water, 3–6 topical treatments, 14 days apart	Veterinary
Dimetronidazole	0.25–1% in water for 5–7 days, 0.1% in water for 14 days	Human
Fenbendazole	50 mg/kg orally sid for 5 days	Veterinary
Ivermectin	200 μg/kg s.c., orally, topically every 7–10 days, 3 treatments 4 ml/l water for 7 days on, 7 days off, 3 treatments (pinworm)	Veterinary
Mebendazole	2.2 mg/ml water per animal sid for 5 days orally	Veterinary
Metronidazole	1 ml/150ml water daily for 10 days, 7.5 mg/ 70–90 g animal orally every 8 hours	Veterinary
Niclosamide	100 mg/kg orally, repeat in 7 days **or** 7 days on, 7 days off, 7 days on	Human
Piperazine	3–5 mg/ml water treat for 7 days on, 7 days off, repeat once, 0.5 g/l water for 3 days	Veterinary
Praziquantel	30 mg/kg orally every 14 days, 3 treatments	Veterinary
Sulphadimadine	0.2% in water daily for 7–10 days	Veterinary
Sulphadimethoxine	75 mg/kg orally sid for 7–14 days	USA
Sulfaquinoxaline	0.1% in water daily for 14 days	USA
Miscellaneous drugs		
Cisapride	0.5 mg/kg orally bid	Human
Dexamethasone	0.6 mg/kg s.c., i.m., i.p.	Veterinary
Diphenylhydantoin	25–50 mg/kg orally bid	USA
D-Penicillamine	50 mg/kg orally bid	Human
EDTA	30 mg/kg i.m., s.c. bid	Veterinary
Frusemide	2.5 mg/kg s.c., i.p.	Veterinary
Metoclopramide	0.5 mg/kg s.c. tid	Veterinary
Oxytocin	0.2–3 units/kg s.c., i.m.	Veterinary
Phenobarbitone	10–20 mg/kg	Veterinary
Primidone	0.05–0.1 ml of 50 mg/ml solution orally bid	Veterinary

Figure 4.21 Drug dosages and therapeutic regimens in the gerbil. Data from Carpenter *et al.* (1996), Laber-Laird *et al.* (1996), Marx and Roston (1996), Hawk and Leary (1999) and Tennant (1999).

References and further reading

Agren G, Zhou Q and Zhong W (1989) Ecology and social behaviour of Mongolian gerbils, *Meriones unguiculatus,* at Xilinhot, Inner Mongolia, China. *Animal Behaviour* **37**, 11–27

Allen KL, Bruggen van N and Cooper JE (1993) Detection of bacterial sinusitis in the Mongolian gerbil (*Meriones unguiculatus*) using magnetic resonance imaging. *Veterinary Record* **132,** 633–635

Anderson N (1995) Intraosseous fluid therapy in small exotic animals. In: Kirk's *Current Veterinary Therapy XII: Small Animal Practice,* ed. JD Bonagura, pp. 1331–1335. WB Saunders, Philadelphia

Antinoff N (1999) Critical care. In: *Veterinary Clinics of North America: Exotic Animal Practice*, ed. AE Rupley, vol 2, no 2, pp. 153–175. WB Saunders, Philadelphia

Bauck L and Bihun C (1997) Small rodents; basic anatomy, physiology, husbandry and clinical techniques. In: *Ferrets, Rabbits and Rodents: Clinical Medicine and Surgery*, ed. E Hillyer and K Quesenberry, pp. 291–306. WB Saunders, Philadelphia

Brain PF (1999) The laboratory gerbil. In: *The UFAW Handbook on the Care and Management of Laboratory Animals*, 7th edn, vol 1, Terrestrial Vertebrates, ed. T Poole, pp. 345–355. Blackwell Science, Oxford

Burgmann P (1997) Dermatology of rabbits, rodents and ferrets. In: *Practical Exotic Animal Medicine: The Compendium Collection*, ed. K Rosenthal, pp. 175–179, 184–185. Veterinary Learning Systems, New Jersey

Carpenter JW, Mashima TY and Rupiper DJ (1996) *Exotic Animal Formulary*, pp 189–208. Greystone Publications, Kansas

Collins BR (1988) Common diseases and medical management of rodents and lagomorphs. In: *Contemporary Issues in Small Animal Practice, vol 9, Exotic Animals*, ed. ER Jacobson and GV Kollias, pp. 261–271. Churchill Livingstone, New York

Cruz F and Junquera J (1993) The immobility response elicited by clamping, bandaging and grasping in the Mongolian gerbil (*Meriones unguiculatus*). *Behavioural Brain Research* **54**, 165–169

Daviau J (1999) Physical examination and preventative medicine. In: *The Veterinary Clinics of North America: Exotic Animal Practice*, vol 2, no 2, ed. CJ Orcutt, pp. 429–445. WB Saunders, Philadelphia

Donnelly T (1997) Disease problems of small rodents. In: *Ferrets, Rabbits and Rodents: Clinical Medicine and Surgery*, ed. E Hillyer and K Quesenberry, pp. 322–324. WB Saunders, Philadelphia

Farrar P, Opsomer M, Kocen J and Wagner J (1988) Experimental nasal dermatitis in the Mongolian gerbil: effect of bilateral Harderian gland adenectomy on the development of facial lesions. *Laboratory Animal Science* **38**, 72–76

FELASA (1996) FELASA recommendations for the health monitoring of mouse, rat, hamster, gerbil, guinea pig and rabbit experimental units. *Laboratory Animals* **30**, 193–208

Flecknell P (1996) *Laboratory Animal Anaesthesia, 2nd edn*, pp.160–182. Academic Press, London

Flecknell P (1996) Anaesthesia and analgesia for rodents and rabbits. In: *Handbook of Rodent and Rabbit Medicine*, ed. K Laber-Laird, *et al.*, pp. 219–238. Pergamon, Oxford

Flecknell P, Laber-Laird K and Swindle M (1996) Appendix 1, drug dosages for rodents and rabbits. In: *Handbook of Rodent and Rabbit Medicine*, ed. K Laber-Laird, *et al.*, pp. 255–263. Pergamon, Oxford

Harkness JE and Wagner JE (1989) *The Biology and Medicine of Rabbits and Rodents*, 3rd edn, pp. 34–40, 95–100, 139–140, 148–149, 198–201. Lea and Febiger, Philadelphia

Harkness J (1994) Small rodents in exotic pet medicine. In: *The Veterinary Clinics of North America: Small Animal Practice*, vol 24, pp. 89–102. WB Saunders, Philadelphia

Hawk CT and Leary SL (1999) *Formulary for Laboratory Animals, 2nd edn*. Iowa State University Press, Ames

Hem A, Smith A and Solberg P (1998) Saphenous vein puncture for blood sampling of the mouse, rat, hamster, gerbil, guinea pig, ferret and mink. *Laboratory Animals* **32**, 364–368

Huerkamp MJ (1995) Anesthesia and postoperative management of rabbits and pocket pets. In: *Kirk's Current Veterinary Therapy XII: Small Animal Practice*, ed. JD Bonagura, pp. 1322–1327. WB Saunders, Philadelphia

Jacklin MR (1997) Dermatosis associated with *Acarus farris* in gerbils. *Journal of Small Animal Practice* **38**, 410–411

Jackson TA, Heath LA, Hulin MS, Medina CL, Scarlett LM, Rogers KL, Chrisp CE and Dysko RC (1996) Squamous cell carcinoma of the midventral abdominal pad in three gerbils. *Journal of the American Veterinary Association* **209**, 789–791

Kirschner S (1997) Ophthalmological diseases in small mammals. In: *Ferrets, Rabbits and Rodents, Clinical Medicine and Surgery*, ed. E Hillyer and K Quesenberry, pp. 339–345. WB Saunders, Philadelphia

Knapka J (1998) Husbandry and nutrition. In: *Veterinary Clinics of North America: Exotic Animal Practice*, vol 1, no 1, ed. JR Jenkins, pp. 153–167. WB Saunders, Philadelphia

Laber-Laird K (1996) Gerbils. In: *Handbook of Rodent and Rabbit Medicine*, ed. K Laber-Laird, *et al.*, pp. 39–58. Pergamon, Oxford

Laming P, Cosby S and O'Neill J (1989) Seizures in Mongolian gerbils are related to differences in glutamine synthetase. *Comparative Biochemistry and Physiology* **94**, 399–404

Levine JF and Lage AL (1985) House mouse mites infecting laboratory rodents. *Laboratory Animal Science* **34**, 393–394

Marx KL and Roston MA (1996) *The Exotic Animal Drug Compendium, an International Formulary*. Veterinary Learning Systems, New Jersey

McClure DE (1999) Clinical pathology and sample collection. In: *Veterinary Clinics of North America: Exotic Animal Practice*, vol 2, no 3, ed. DR Reavill, pp. 565–590. WB Saunders, Philadelphia

Mighell J S and Baker A E (1990) Caesarian section in a gerbil. *Veterinary Record* **126**, 441

Motzel SL and Gibson SV (1990) Tyzzer's disease in hamsters and gerbils from a pet store supplier. *Journal of the American Veterinary Association* **197**, 1176–1178

Oglesbee BL (1995) Emergency medicine for pocket pets. In: *Kirk's Current Veterinary Therapy XII: Small Animal Practice*, ed. JD Bonagura, p. 1330. WB Saunders, Philadelphia

Olson GA, Shields RP and Gaskin JM (1977) Salmonellosis in a gerbil colony. *Journal of the American Veterinary Medical Association* **171**, 970–972

Percy DH and Barthold SW (1993) Gerbil. In: *Pathology of Laboratory Rodents and Rabbits*, pp. 137–144. Iowa State University Press, Ames

Potgieter FJ and Wile PI (1996) The dust content, dust generation, ammonia production, and absorption properties of three different rodent beddings. *Laboratory Animals* **30**, 79–87

Puente-Redondo VA, Gutierrez-Martin CB, Perez-Martinez C, del Blanco NG, Garcia-Iglesias MJ, Perez-Garcia CC and Rodriguez-Ferri EF (1999) Epidemic infection caused by *Citrobacter rodentium* in a gerbil colony. *Veterinary Record* **145**, 400–403

Richardson VCG (1997) *Diseases of Small Rodents*, pp. 72–105. Blackwell Science, Oxford

Ringler DH, Lay DM and Abrams GD (1972) Spontaneous neoplasms in ageing Gerbillinae. *Laboratory Animal Science* **22**, 407–414

Tennant B (1999) Drug doses for exotic pets. In: *BSAVA Small Animal Formulary*, 3rd edn, pp. 289–291. BSAVA Publications, Cheltenham

Thiessen DD and Pendergrass M (1982) Harderian gland involvement in facial lesions in the Mongolian gerbil. *Journal of the American Veterinary Association* **181**, 1375–1377

Toft JD (1992) Commonly observed spontaneous neoplasms in rabbits, rats, guinea pigs, hamsters and gerbils. *Seminars in Avian and Exotic Pet Medicine*, vol 1, no 2, pp. 80–92

Wiedenmayer C (1997) Causation of the ontogenetic development of stereotypic digging in gerbils. *Animal Behaviour* **53**, 461–470

Wolvekamp P and Oschwald CH (1991) Small mammals, gerbil. In: *Atlas of Diagnostic Radiology of Exotic Pets*, ed. GA Rubel, *et al.*, pp. 66–67. Wolfe Publishing

5

Chipmunks

Anna Meredith

Introduction

Chipmunks are rodents of the family Sciuridae. The chipmunk genus *Tamias* (or *Eutamius)* is made up of 24 species, inhabiting North America and Asia. Despite the many species occurring naturally in North America, pet chipmunks in the USA and Europe are almost exclusively the species *T. (E.) sibericus,* the Siberian chipmunk, also known as the Korean or Japanese squirrel. This chapter refers to this species, although the information is largely applicable to others.

Chipmunks are diurnal burrowing rodents, although they will also nest in tree hollows. They inhabit mainly forests and open woodland, but are largely ground dwelling, although they will climb trees if necessary to obtain food. Wild-type chipmunks have brown–grey fur with characteristic white stripes along the back, white fur around the eyes and a whitish yellow underbelly (Figure 5.1). The tail is long and bushy with white-tipped hairs. Cream and albino variants (see Figure 5.5) are now available.

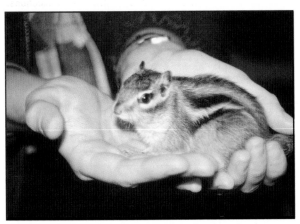

Figure 5.1 Wild-type pet chipmunk *Tamias sibericus.*

Like squirrels, chipmunks are hoarders of food and possess large cheek pouches. They exhibit coprophagy, which allows uptake of vitamins B and K.

Biology

Figure 5.2 summarizes the biological data of chipmunks.

Life expectancy	Variable: male up to 8 years, female up to 12 years in captivity. Generally 4–6 years
Respiratory rate	75 breaths per minute
Body temperature	38.0°C (A few degrees above environmental temperature when hibernating)
Bodyweight of adult	72–120 g
Bodyweight of newborn kit	3 g
Food consumption	25–30 g/day

Figure 5.2 Physiological data for the chipmunk.

Sexing

The anogenital distance is greater in male chipmunks than it is in females. The prepuce is obvious in males. During the breeding season (January to September in the northern hemisphere) the testes are obvious in mature males.

Husbandry

Chipmunks have very different husbandry requirements from other rodents of similar size, and in many ways do not make ideal pets. They remain essentially wild in captivity, and their welfare can be severely compromised if their behavioural needs are not met.

The advantages of chipmunks as pets are that they are:

* Attractive
* Diurnal and constantly active.

The disadvantages of chipmunks as pets are that they are:

* Best kept outdoors in large enclosures
* Usually difficult to handle
* Easily stressed and exhibit stereotypical behaviour.

Housing

In the wild chipmunks live in loose colonies but have individual burrows. They are extremely active, and therefore rodent cages sold for other small rodents are not suitable for chipmunks. Cages should be as large as possible, which can make housing indoors difficult. Minimum sizes of 1.2 m high or base plus length plus height of 3.5–4.5 m are quoted, but no cage can be large enough. An outdoor shed or outdoor aviary-type enclosure is more suitable. If kept indoors, cages should be situated out of direct sunlight and away from television sets (see Behavioural problems) and cigarette smoke.

Chipmunks are good at escaping and will gnaw wood or plastic to achieve that goal, though escapees generally return to the home cage. Strong metal mesh (2.5 cm) should be used with metal supports, or the wire should be fixed inside wood supports. Double doors are recommended on outdoor enclosures. Chipmunks burrow avidly, so the base of the cage or enclosure should be solid. A layer of substrate should be provided to permit normal burrowing behaviour – peat or wood chips are ideal for this purpose.

Cage furniture such as branches (fruit trees are safe), thick ropes and drainpipes on the ground provide interest and activity.

Chipmunks can be housed singly, in pairs or in harems with one male to two or three females. Single-sex groups can work if there is sufficient space, but adult males do tend to fight (Figure 5.3).

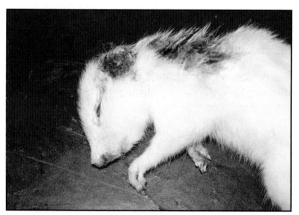

Figure 5.3 Fight wounds on a male chipmunk.

Chipmunks use one area of the cage as a latrine, and this should be cleaned as often as necessary. To minimize disturbance, cleaning can be undertaken at night or when the animals are secured within nest boxes.

One nest box per animal must be provided, to mimic the wild situation where they live individually in burrows. Nest material should be paper-based, hay or straw, as synthetic fibres can become impacted in the cheek pouches. It is useful to be able to close the nest box to contain the animal while cleaning the cage or for capture. Nest boxes should be cleaned about once a month, except in winter when they should be left undisturbed.

Hibernation
Chipmunks do not enter prolonged periods of hibernation in cold weather but will 'hibernate' in their burrows or nest boxes in a torpid state, waking every few days to eat and excrete. Extra nest material should be provided over this period. Prior to hibernation, hoarding of food occurs and so plentiful supplies must be available in the autumn. Food stores in nest boxes should not be removed over the winter. Increased aggression is often seen at this time. In captivity, individuals often become torpid and stay in their nest boxes on cold days rather than entering true hibernation. Survival rate and life expectancy is greater when chipmunks do not hibernate.

Diet
Chipmunks are omnivorous, although in the wild the diet is made up largely of seeds, buds, leaves and flowers. Commercial dry mixes specifically for chipmunks are available or other rodent mixes can be used, supplemented with fresh and dried fruit, vegetables and nuts. Sunflower seeds and nuts, although greatly enjoyed, are high in fat and low in calcium and should be fed in moderation. Dog biscuits and animal protein such as mealworms, cooked meat, hard-boiled eggs and day-old chicks from a reputable source are also enjoyed. Extra protein is important for pregnant and lactating females.

Fresh food should be regularly removed from food hoards to prevent mould.

Water is best provided from a sipper bottle.

Captive breeding
In the spring the male's testes descend into the scrotum. Females are in oestrus for 3 days, during which they chirp repeatedly to the male. Mating generally occurs on the second day. Females should be taken to the male for mating unless they are housed as a pair, as she will be aggressive if not in oestrus. Although rising temperature and increasing day length stimulate reproductive activity, artificially long days indoors can lead to infertility. Female chipmunks generally have one litter per breeding season, although if the kits are weaned by 7 weeks a second smaller litter may be produced.

The young are altricial (naked and blind) and remain in the nest for about 35 days (Figure 5.4). Females have four pairs of mammary glands and benefit from supplementary protein during pregnancy and lactation. Any stress, such as television or proximity of predators, may result in abandonment of the young. Chipmunks do not have a post-partum oestrus.

Oestrous cycle length	13–14 days (range 11–21 days)
Gestation	31–32 days (range 28–35 days)
Breeding season	March–September
Emergence of young from nest	Approx. 35 days
Weaning	Approx. 42 days
Litter size	3–5 (range 1–10)
Mammary glands	4 pairs

Figure 5.4 Reproductive parameters for the chipmunk.

Hand rearing can be successful if the young are over a week old. Diluted evaporated milk (1:2 with water) fed from a small syringe can be provided every 4 hours for the first week, after which baby cereal can be added and fed every 6–8 hours as age increases. Probiotics may be added. Urination and defecation should be stimulated after each feed by rubbing the anogenital area with moist cotton wool.

Handling and restraint

Most pet chipmunks are not tame and resent being handled, inflicting a powerful bite. Although many learn to take food from the hand, it is still not possible to grasp and pick them up. Some hand-reared animals may allow handling by cupping in the hands (see Figure 5.1) or grasping the scruff. In the veterinary consulting room escapes can easily happen. Chases are stressful to the chipmunk and should be avoided. Leather gloves are generally not advisable, as the lack of sensitivity can result in damage to the animal. A lightweight net is useful – once caught the animal can be carefully grasped around the shoulders (Figure 5.5) or scruffed as for a mouse (see Chapter 2). The tail must not be grasped, as degloving injuries can occur. For any useful clinical examination to take place it is recommended that the animal is sedated or anaesthetized (see below).

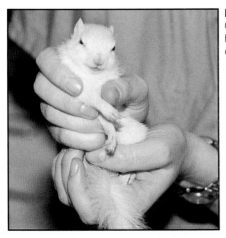

Figure 5.5 Correct handling of a chipmunk.

Diagnostic approach

Physical examination
Clinical examination of the conscious chipmunk is often difficult. Observation while the animal is in its cage or in a small transparent plastic container can allow some information to be gained. In the author's experience, a full clinical examination is best carried out under gaseous anaesthesia.

Sample collection

Blood
Blood samples are obtainable from the jugular vein under anaesthesia.

Common conditions

Diseases
Chipmunks are generally hardy and have relatively few disease problems (Figure 5.6). There is little published literature on diseases and veterinary care of this species and much is anecdotal or extrapolated from other rodent species. When presented with a sick chipmunk, first principles often need to be relied upon. Reference to chapters on other rodents in this manual may help. Veterinary surgeons making definitive diagnoses of disease in chipmunks, whether as clinical cases or at postmortem examination, are encouraged to publish their findings to increase knowledge of this species.

Wild chipmunk species in the USA and Asia are known to be asymptomatic hosts for various infectious diseases and parasites, including *Borrelia burgdorferi* (Lyme disease), rabies, *Cryptosporidium parvum*, ticks (*Ixodes* spp.) and fleas. Wild chipmunk fleas have been associated with *Yersinia pestis* (plague).

If chipmunks are brought in as wildlife casualties or if members of the public rescue and domesticate wild chipmunks, their potential as vectors of serious zoonotic disease should be seriously considered. Wild chipmunks are known to carry many species of *Eimeria* and other gastrointestinal parasites, but their clinical significance is not known.

General signs of illness, pain or distress are as for other rodent species – immobility, hunched posture, piloerection and anorexia. Sick animals are often attacked and may be killed by cagemates.

Behavioural problems
Chipmunks are extremely susceptible to stress. Important stressors are:

- Small cage, resulting in inability to exhibit normal foraging and exploratory behaviour
- Overcrowding and insufficient nest boxes
- Aggression from cagemates – dominant animals of either sex will be aggressive to subordinates. Aggression often increases in autumn as food-hoarding activity increases
- Proximity of predators, e.g. cats and dogs
- Television – prolonged exposure can result in death; this is thought to be due to electromagnetic and ultrasonic radiation from the 15.6 kHz time-based oscillator
- Catching and handling
- Transportation and trips to a veterinary surgery.

After a stressful event, many chipmunks remain quiescent for about 24 hours. Hyperactivity is a sign of stress, and in small cages chipmunks often show stereotypic behaviour, such as continually repeated horizontal or vertical circling of the cage walls.

Supportive care

Daily fluid requirements are estimated at 75–100 ml/kg. Figure 5.7 gives information on fluid and nutritional therapy.

Disease	Aetiology	Clinical signs	Diagnosis	Treatment
Bacterial cystitis/urethritis	May be associated with struvite urolithiasis	Haematuria, dysuria (often vocalize), penile swelling and protrusion, anorexia	Urinalysis	Antibiosis, analgesia, anti-inflammatories
Bacterial enteritis	e.g. *Salmonella*. Wild rodents can act as source	Diarrhoea, weight loss, death	Faecal culture	Appropriate antibiosis, fluid therapy Euthanasia if zoonosis (e.g. *Salmonella*)
Cage paralysis	Thought to be due to vitamin E deficiency	Weakness, paresis, paralysis	Clinical signs, elevated CPK and cholesterol, radiography to eliminate spinal fracture	Dietary supplementation with Vitamin E
Cataracts	Unknown aetiology. Reported in older chipmunks, especially males	Partial/complete blindness	Ocular examination	None
Ectoparasites	Fleas, burrowing mites and harvest mites reported. Species not reported	Alopecia, pruritus	Visual identification of parasite	Pyrethrin powder, fipronil, ivermectin
Seizures	Epilepsy RARE – unknown aetiology; bacterial or viral meningitis	Repetitive running followed by quivering and loss of consciousness; death can occur	Clinical signs, postmortem examination	None reported
Fracture	Limbs or spine, following a fall or mishandling	Lameness, paresis, paralysis	Radiography	Cage rest (confined space), analgesia, amputation if severe (dressings not tolerated) Euthanasia if paralysed
Hypocalcaemia	Generally following parturition though can occur in males	Posterior paresis/paralysis, incoordination, semi-consciousness	History and clinical signs, serum calcium levels	0.5 ml 10% calcium borogluconate s/c Prevent by calcium supplementation or calcium-rich foods, e.g. cheese, milk powder
Incisor overgrowth	Insufficient wear (poorly abrasive diet), trauma causing misalignment	Anorexia, salivation, facial soft tissue penetration and infection, pawing at mouth. May cause a rhinitis	Dental examination, skull radiography	Burr teeth under sedation/anaesthesia (do not clip) Correct the diet to include more abrasive items, e.g. nuts in shell, dog biscuits; provide branches to gnaw
Mammary tumours	Usually benign fibroadenomas	Mammary mass	Clinical signs, fine needle aspiration, biopsy	Surgical removal
Metritis/pyometra	Metritis: usually due to retained fetus. Often progresses to peritonitis and toxaemia Pyometra: as for other species	Vaginal discharge, abdominal enlargement, anorexia	Clinical signs, bacterial culture of discharge	Antibiosis, supportive care, ovariohysterectomy
Pneumonia	Predisposing stressors: overcrowding, poor ventilation, damp conditions. Bacteria involved not reported. Can contract human influenza viruses	Dyspnoea, tachypnoea, anorexia. Often fatal	Clinical signs, radiography	Antibiosis – systemic or by nebulization Supportive care – warmth, fluids, oxygen, assisted feeding, mucolytics
Rhinitis	May occur in association with incisor overgrowth and chronic suppurative periodontal disease	Nasal discharge, upper respiratory tract stridor, epistaxis, face rubbing	Clinical signs, skull radiography	Antibiosis, supportive care, analgesia Euthanasia if severe disease

Figure 5.6 Diseases of chipmunks.

Route	Volume	Suggested Fluids
Oral (gavage, syringe feeding)	2–5 ml	Oral rehydration solutions, baby foods
Subcutaneous	3–5 ml	Crystalloids
Intraperitoneal	5–10 ml	Crystalloids (warm)
Intravenous	50–70 ml/kg for shock	Crystalloids and colloids
Intraosseous catheter (femur, tibia)	50–70 ml/kg for shock	Crystalloids and colloids

Figure 5.7 Fluid and nutritional therapy for chipmunks.

Anaesthesia and analgesia

Anaesthesia

An inhalational method is the simplest way of anaesthetizing chipmunks. This is the least stressful method, as anaesthesia can be achieved without handling the chipmunk. Isoflurane or halothane can be administered into a scavenged anaesthetic chamber. Once anaesthetized the chipmunk can be removed and anaesthesia maintained with a small facemask (see Figure 5.8). Coaxial scavenged masks designed for laboratory rodents are useful.

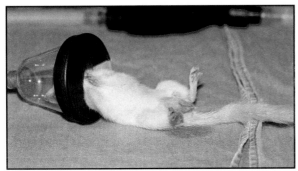

Figure 5.8 The chipmunk can be maintained under anaesthesia with a facemask after gaseous induction in a chamber.

Injectable agents can probably be used as for other rodents. Alphaxalone with alphadalone (Saffan®) 40 mg/kg is the only agent reported. Dose rates are unavailable for other agents.

See Chapter 2 on rats and mice for information on perioperative care.

Analgesia

Buprenorphine 0.1 mg/kg s.c. every 6–12 hours can be used for analgesia. Dose rates are not available for other agents, but doses used in the mouse and rat are probably safe and effective.

Common surgical procedures

Castration

Castration is a simple procedure, and a closed technique should be used to prevent herniation of abdominal contents.

Ovariohysterectomy

Ovariohysterectomy is not usually carried out routinely but is used as a treatment for pyometra. The technique is as for other rodents.

Drug formulary

There are no published drug doses for chipmunks. The reader is referred to Chapter 2; as chipmunks are of similar size to rats, the author uses the doses for rats.

References and further reading

Childs JE, Colby L, Krebs JW *et al.* (1997) Surveillance and spatiotemporal associations of rabies in rodents and lagomorphs in the United States 1985–1994. *Journal of Wildlife Diseases* **33(1)**, 20–27

Henwood C (1989) *Chipmunks.* TFH Publications, Neptune City, New Jersey

Gillett KE and Temple JD (1991) Chipmunks. In: *BSAVA Manual of Exotic Pets*, pp. 23–30. BSAVA Publications, Cheltenham

Gillett KE (1988) *Chipmunks, the Siberian Chipmunk in Captivity.* Bassett Publications

Mannelli A, Kitron U, Jones CJ *et al.* (1993) Role of the eastern chipmunk as a host for immature *Ixodes dammini* in northwestern Illinois. *Journal of Medical Entomology* **30(1)**, 87–93

Matsui T, Fujino T, Kajima J *et al.* (2000) Infectivity to experimental rodents of *Cryptosporidium parvum* oocysts from Siberian chipmunks (*Tamias sibiricus*) originated in the People's Republic of China. *Journal of Veterinary Medicine and Science* **62(5)**, 487–489

Perz JF and Le Blancq SM (2001) *Cryptosporidium parvum* infection involving novel genotypes in wildlife from Lower New York State. *Applied Environmental Microbiology* **67(3)**, 1154–1162

Richardson VCG (1997) *Diseases of Small Domestic Rodents.* pp. 53–72. Blackwell Science, Oxford

Seville RS and Patrick MJ (2001) *Eimeria* spp from the eastern chipmunk (*Tamias striatus*) in Pennsylvania with a description of one new species. *Journal of Parasitology* **87(1)**, 165–168

Slacherjt T, Kitron UD, Jones CJ *et al.* (1997) Role of the eastern chipmunk (*Tamias striatus*) in the epizootiology of Lyme borreliosis in northwestern Illinois, USA. *Journal of Wildlife Diseases* **33(1)**, 40–46

6

Guinea pigs

Paul Flecknell

Introduction

Guinea pigs (cavies) originated from the mountains and grasslands of South America, where both domesticated and wild strains are kept as food animals. In the wild, they live in small social groups of five to ten animals. They are hystricomorph rodents – a group characterized by having long gestation periods, precocious offspring, and a membrane that covers the vaginal opening except at oestrus and during parturition. They are generally non-aggressive and make suitable pets for children. They are highly vocal animals: as well as the squeals of alarm noted during clinical examination and handling, they emit a wide range of other calls.

Guinea pigs are bred by enthusiasts as show animals and a number of different hair types and colour varieties have been produced. Hair types include smooth-coated varieties (English, or American Shorthair), wiry coats that form rosettes (Abyssinians) and very long fine hair (Peruvians). Coat colouring can be solid single colours ('selfs') or blocks and bands of colours (Figure 6.1). Descriptions of different breeds and varieties can be found in Robinson (1978).

Biology

Biological data for guinea pigs are summarized in Figure 6.2 and normal haematological and biochemical values in Figure 6.3.

Guinea pigs are social animals and are best housed in pairs or small groups – either single-sex or mixed-sex groups with the males neutered. Hospitalized animals often benefit from the presence of their normal cagemate.

Provided the animals have been reared together from a young age, they form stable groups and fighting is rare. Entire females and males may fight but neutering will often resolve such problems. In any group, dominant animals may occasionally bully subordinates, and this may become apparent as 'barbering', when the dominant animal chews the coat of subordinates, producing patches of hair loss.

It is possible to introduce animals into an established group but plenty of hiding places should be provided, so that the newly introduced guinea pig can escape from aggression. It is best not to keep guinea pigs with rabbits, as cross-infection with agents such

Variety	Coat colour
Self	Solid single colour including black, white, cream, golden beige, lilac, red and chocolate
Dutch	White cheeks, white blaze and white forequarters, thorax and abdomen, with hindquarters and remainder of head being coloured
Tortoiseshell	Red and black blocks of hair
Bicolours	Blocks of two different colours
Tortoiseshell and white	Red, black and white blocks of hair
Tricolours	Blocks of two different colours and white
Himalayans	White body and black or chocolate nose, feet and ears
Roans	Even mixture of black and red hairs
Brindles	Even mixture of black and white hairs

Figure 6.1 Coat colours of guinea pigs.

Lifespan	4–8 years
Weight	Male 1000–1200 g Female 750–1000 g
Dentition	2(I1/1 C0/0 P1/1 M3/3)
Respiratory rate	90–150 breaths per minute
Tidal volume	5–10 ml/kg
Heart rate	190–300 beats per minute
Blood volume	70 ml/kg
Rectal temperature	38.6°C (37.2–39.5°C)
Water intake (average daily)	10 ml/100 g bodyweight
Urine pH	9
Sexual maturity	Male: 9–10 weeks Female: 4–6 weeks
Oestrous cycle	15–17 days
Duration of oestrus	1–16 hours
Length of gestation	59–72 days (depending on litter size)
Litter size	1–6 (average 3–4)
Birthweight	60–100 g
Weaning age	3 weeks

Figure 6.2 Biological data for the guinea pig.

Haematocrit (l/l)	0.4 (0.35–0.45)
Haemoglobin (g/dl)	14.3
Red blood cell count (per litre)	5.0×10^{12}
White blood cell count (per litre)	11.2×10^9
Neutrophils	37%
Lymphocytes	56%
Alkaline phosphatase (IU/l)	55–108
Bilirubin (mg/dl)	0.3–0.9
BUN (mg/dl)	9–32
Calcium (mg/dl)	5.3–12
Cholesterol (mg/dl)	16–43
Chloride (mEq/l)	90–115
Creatinine (mg/dl)	0.6–2.2
Glucose (mg/dl)	60–180
Phosphorus (mg/dl)	3.0–7.6
Potassium (mg/dl)	3.8–7.9
SGOT (IU/l)	27–68
SGPT (IU/l)	25–59
Sodium (mEq/l)	120–152
Total protein (g/dl)	4.7–6.4
Albumin (g/dl)	2.1–3.9
Globulin (g/dl)	1.7–2.6

Figure 6.3 Normal ranges of haematological and biochemical parameters (data from Harkness and Wagner, 1995; Manning *et al.*, 1984; Mitruka and Rawnsley, 1981). Note that these values are only a general guide, and the laboratory that analyses the samples should be asked to provide its opinion on expected normal ranges.

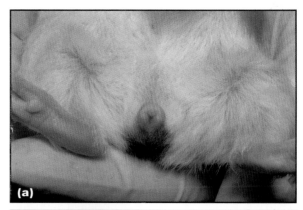

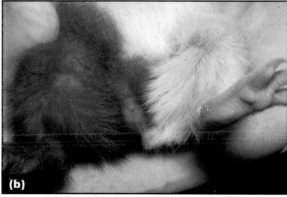

Figure 6.4 Appearance of external genitalia in male (a) and female (b) guinea pigs.

as *Bordetella bronchiseptica* (which can be carried asymptomatically by rabbits) can occur. In addition, there may be bullying by either species.

Sexing

Determination of the sex of guinea pigs is reasonably simple, though both males and females have an obvious pair of nipples in the inguinal region and the external genitalia are superficially similar. There is no obvious scrotum but the penis can be protruded by pressing gently on either side of the genital opening. In very young animals, the penis can be palpated in the midline, just cranial to the genital opening. The female has a shallow vaginal groove between the urethral orifice and the anus (Figure 6.4). The vagina is covered by a membrane except during oestrus and parturition.

Husbandry

Housing

Guinea pigs are best kept in a hutch, with either a large run connected to it or a separate pen for exercise and grazing. The minimum size for a hutch should be 0.9 m² per adult guinea pig. The hutch should have an enclosed solid-sided nesting area for shelter, and a mesh-fronted section.

Since they are a prey species, guinea pigs can become apprehensive in large open spaces and so hiding places and shelter, such as a section of plastic drain-pipe, should be provided in the run. Guinea pigs make greatest use of the edges of their enclosure: upturned boxes and other objects in a run can increase the space utilized by the animals, as well as providing environmental enrichment.

The pen or run can be outdoors in summer, but in countries such as the UK guinea pigs are best brought indoors to a garage or outbuilding in the winter, and provided with a well insulated hutch and plenty of bedding. If possible, an indoor run should be provided. In milder climates, they can be housed outdoors for the whole year. The preferred temperature range is 16–24°C. Temperatures above 27–30°C can cause heat stroke.

Enclosures must be strong enough to exclude cats and other predators. Ideally, they should also prevent the entry of wild birds, which may be sources of infection with *Yersinia* and *Salmonella* spp. (see below).

Hutches and runs are usually constructed from wood but guinea pigs may eventually gnaw through wood panels, unless they are protected by wire-mesh. Flooring in a hutch should be smooth. Sawdust, wood shavings, shredded paper or hay should be provided as bedding. Use of sawdust as the basic bedding with the addition of hay is recommended as the latter provides a dietary supplement and also some variety in the environment. Hutches must be cleaned frequently, typically two or three times a week, as guinea pigs are rather messy animals.

Diet

A variety of commercial diets is available, including complete pelleted diets and mixtures of pellets, grains and other vegetable material. Since guinea pigs can be highly selective feeders, complete pelleted diets are often preferable as they help to ensure that the animal receives a balanced diet. Variety should be provided by supplementing with hay and fresh vegetables. Hay or grass must be available *ad libitum*; the fibre content is very important, as it ensures normal dental wear.

It is essential that guinea pigs receive an adequate intake of vitamin C, as they are unable to synthesize this vitamin. If there is doubt about the adequacy of the vitamin C content of a diet, a supplement should be added (for example, in liquid form in the drinking water). Guinea pigs require a daily intake of approximately 10 mg/kg and this is increased to 30 mg/kg/day during pregnancy.

Some forms of vitamin C supplement are unstable and oxidize readily, and so the amount of vitamin in the diet reduces rapidly. Typically, relatively high quantities of vitamin C (800 mg/kg) are added to try to offset this. Stabilized forms of the vitamin are now used in several of the leading brands of commercial diets in the UK, and these often have lower quantities of vitamin C (200–300 mg/kg) as less vitamin is lost during storage.

Irrespective of the type of supplement added, it is important to observe the manufacturer's recommendations for shelf-life and storage conditions of the diet.

Water should be provided *ad libitum* in bowls or water bottles. Any change in the watering system should be introduced gradually, as guinea pigs may not use the new source of water initially. If water bottles with metal drinking tubes are used, these will oxidize any vitamin C added as a supplement fairly rapidly and daily changing of the supplemented water will be required.

Breeding

Mating of females is best delayed until the animals are 12–14 weeks old. The female is polyoestrous, with oestrus every 15–17 days. Oestrus can be detected by behavioural changes, including arching of the back when the back and rump are stroked, and mounting by other females. Following mating, a plug of ejaculate ('vaginal plug') usually forms in the vagina. This plug usually drops out after 24–48 hours.

Pregnancy can be diagnosed by gentle abdominal palpation at about 4–5 weeks, or by use of ultrasonography. Females increase markedly in size in the second half of pregnancy, often doubling their bodyweight by the end of gestation. The duration of pregnancy is variable (see Figure 6.2): the larger the litter, the shorter is the gestation period. The approach of parturition can be detected by palpation of the pubic symphysis. In the last weeks of pregnancy there is a gradual relaxation of the pubic ligaments and separation of the symphysis. Just before parturition the gap is about 2–3 cm (finger-width). Parturition normally takes around 30 minutes, with an interval of 3–10 minutes between deliveries. If breeding of a female has been delayed such that she is over 9–12 months of age, separation may not occur and dystocia will result, with caesarian section being required.

As a postpartum oestrus occurs 24–48 hours after parturition, the male should be separated from the female in late pregnancy if immediate breeding is not intended. Pregnant females should be separated from other animals in late gestation, and housed together with their young until weaning.

Small groups of breeding females can be housed together with their young but they may inadvertently injure the young if startled. Females housed together will cross-suckle offspring from others in the group, and this can help the survival of young from sows who have an inadequate milk supply. It can also cause problems, however, if older offspring deprive younger animals of their milk supply.

At birth, guinea pigs are relatively mature, with open eyes and fur. Although their teeth have erupted, they eat only small quantities of solid food in the first few weeks of life.

Handling and restraint

Guinea pigs are relatively easy to handle and restrain but may run at high speed to escape capture. Any objects or other obstructions should be removed. The animal should be grasped rapidly and firmly around the shoulders and lifted clear of its pen or cage. As it is lifted from its pen, the hindquarters should be supported (Figure 6.5). Avoid grasping around the abdomen, as excessive force can result in liver rupture. The guinea pig can then be placed on an examination table but should be restrained at all times as it may try to escape and, if it falls from the table, it may injure itself.

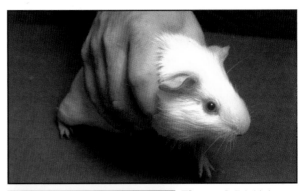

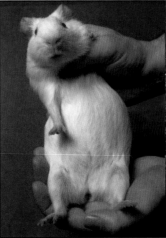

Figure 6.5 Initial restraint of the guinea pig is by grasping around the shoulders. The animal is then lifted and the hindquarters are supported.

Diagnostic approach

History

It is especially important to obtain a detailed case history. In particular, the adequacy of the vitamin C content of the diet should be checked, as subclinical hypovitaminosis C can predispose to the development of other clinical disease. An accurate description of the husbandry regimen should be obtained, as irregular feeding and watering can lead to the development of gastrointestinal disorders.

Physical examination

As with other species, a general clinical examination should be carried out.

- Guinea pigs will often be apprehensive, resulting in tachycardia and tachypnoea
- Vocalization is also common but usually subsides. Repeated vocalization associated with handling a particular area may indicate pain
- It is easiest to examine the animal with an assistant providing restraint. This also enables procedures such as clipping overgrown nails and injection of drugs.

Animals in ill health often show a series of non-specific clinical signs:

- Their body posture is altered, so that they appear hunched, rather than 'sausage-shaped'
- The fur is ruffled
- The eyes may appear sunken
- There may be discharges around the eyes and nose.

Common conditions

Figure 6.6 summarizes the common clinical conditions seen in the guinea pig. A drug formulary for the guinea pigs is summarized at the end of this chapter (see Figure 6.18).

Dental disease

The incisors, molars and premolars of guinea pigs grow continuously, and overgrowth and malocclusion are relatively common (see chinchilla dental disease in Chapter 7). The underlying cause may be congenital or inherited defects, or a result of lack of fibre in the diet. Chronic hypervitaminosis C has also been associated

Body system	Clinical signs	Common causes	Diagnostic procedure	Treatment
Skin/integument	Alopecia	Barbering	Abdominal palpation, ultrasonography, ? genital enlargement	Address husbandry problems, enrich environment
		Cystic ovarian disease		Ovariohysterectomy
	Pruritis	*Trixacarus caviae*	Skin scrapings, response to treatment (mites not always found)	Ivermectin (200–400 µg/kg), repeat every 2 weeks. Treat in-contact animals, clean environment
	Ruffled fur coat	General sign of ill-health	If no other clinical signs, consider metabolic disorders and pain	Address underlying cause
	Subcutaneous swellings	Abscess (usually secondary to trauma)	Exploratory surgery	Drain or excise, antibiotic therapy
Respiratory system	Dyspnoea, ocular and nasal discharge	*Bordetella bronchiseptica*	Physical examination, culture of nasal/ocular discharge if present	Antibiotic therapy and supportive care, may require oxygen, give vitamin C supplement
Gastrointestinal system	Diarrhoea	Clostridial infection (often secondary to antibiotic therapy)	History, faecal examination	Fluid therapy, probiotics, address potential underlying cause (e.g. poor husbandry)
		Coccidiosis (in group-housed animals)		As above plus sulphonamides
	Anorexia	Non-specific sign of disease, but always examine teeth (often see ptyalism)	Examine teeth, general physical examination	Treat tooth overgrowth, check for possible underlying causes, give vitamin C supplement
Musculoskeletal system	Reluctance to move, lameness	Hypovitaminosis C	History, clinical examination, response to therapy	Vitamin C (100 mg/kg daily)

Figure 6.6 Common clinical conditions in the guinea pig.

with malocclusions, as has periodontal disease. The molars and premolars are angled, so that the lower teeth are directed slightly inwards, towards the tongue. As a consequence, small spurs on these teeth will rapidly cause pain on eating, and the animal will quickly become inappetent. The lack of chewing will then exacerbate the condition, as normal wearing of the teeth will not occur. Affected animals typically show weight loss, ptyalism, and anorexia.

A thorough oral examination should be carried out, including radiography if underlying dental abnormalities are suspected. If malocclusion is noted, it is essential to carry out the dental examination under sedation or general anaesthesia. The teeth should be trimmed using a dental burr, analgesia provided, and the diet and any other predisposing causes corrected.

Gastrointestinal disease

Bacterial enteritis
Diarrhoea associated with infection with *Escherichia coli*, and more rarely *Clostridium piliforme* and *Campylobacter* spp., may occur in guinea pigs. Often the cause is uncertain and disease develops after some form of stress (e.g. elective surgery) or dietary changes. Fluid therapy and other supportive treatment, together with antibiotics, may be successful.

Antibiotic-induced enterotoxaemia
Guinea pigs are particularly susceptible to disruption of their normal gut flora by administration of antibiotics. The disturbance in the balance of organisms can allow enterotoxin-producing clostridia to multiply, and result in diarrhoea or more acute illness and death associated with enterotoxaemia. A wide range of antibiotics has been associated with this syndrome, including ampicillin, bacitracin, cephalosporins, clindamycin, erythromycin, gentamicin, lincomycin, penicillins, spiromycin and tetracyclines.

The effects of antibiotic administration vary considerably and in some animals no ill-effects are observed. This leads to considerable confusion regarding which antibiotics can be considered 'safe' in guinea pigs. In general, broad-spectrum antibiotics seem less likely to induce this condition than narrow-spectrum agents, and oral administration seems more likely to result in problems than subcutaneous or intramuscular administration. Chloramphenicol, trimethoprim/sulphonamides and enrofloxacin appear least likely to cause gastrointestinal disturbances. Those agents associated with enterotoxaemia should only be administered when results of bacteriological culture and sensitivity indicate that they are the only suitable agents.

Pseudotuberculosis (yersiniosis)
Infection with *Yersinia pseudotuberculosis* usually results in gradual weight loss, diarrhoea, loss of condition and death after several weeks of illness. Some animals can die rapidly with septicaemia, or develop non-fatal infection restricted to the cervical lymph nodes. At postmortem examination, animals may have enlarged mesenteric lymph nodes, and necrotic foci in the liver and spleen. The organism can be cultured from the lymph nodes, or from blood in the septicaemic form of the condition. The source of infection in many instances is believed to be contamination of feed by wild rodents or birds. The condition is zoonotic and so treatment is not advised.

Coccidiosis
Coccidiosis in guinea pigs, caused by *Eimeria caviae*, is uncommon but may cause watery diarrhoea, particularly in groups of younger animals. As with other species, overcrowding, poor husbandry and other intercurrent infections predispose to the development of disease. A diagnosis can be confirmed by examination of a faecal smear. Treatment with sulphadimidine or sulphamethazine (2% in drinking water for 7–10 days) is usually effective, especially when combined with general improvements in housing and husbandry.

Salmonellosis
In contrast to other species, salmonellosis in guinea pigs often results in septicaemia and sudden death, rather than enteritis. Pregnant animals may abort and chronic infections may occur, characterized by progressive weight loss and poor general condition. Since *Salmonella* is zoonotic, affected animals should be euthanased.

Candidiasis
Although *Candida albicans* is part of the normal gut flora of guinea pigs, diarrhoea associated with an overgrowth of *Candida* has been seen, especially in animals receiving long-term antibiotic therapy (pers. comm., Meredith and Redrobe).

Respiratory disease

Bacterial pneumonias
The commonest cause of respiratory disease is infection with *Bordetella bronchiseptica*, though disease can also be caused by *Streptococcus pneumoniae*. Typically, animals develop an ocular and nasal discharge, which may progress to signs of dyspnoea. There may be abnormal respiratory sounds and sneezing. Affected animals are often anorexic, depressed and lethargic. If the disease progresses, weight loss may occur, and animals frequently die.

Animals may respond well if antibiotic therapy is started early in the course of the condition, especially when combined with general supportive therapy (fluids, vitamin C supplementation, assisted feeding, and use of oxygen for dyspnoeic animals).

Animals that recover from the infection may continue to carry the organism. Outbreaks of these diseases in groups of guinea pigs are often associated with overcrowding, poor husbandry and inadequate diet, especially vitamin C deficiency. Porcine and canine vaccines have been used to reduce clinical disease in guinea pig colonies, but vaccination does not prevent the development of a carrier state.

Viral pneumonia
Outbreaks of respiratory disease caused by adenovirus have been reported in laboratory colonies but the incidence in pet and show animals is unknown.

Chlamydiosis

Conjunctivitis can be caused by infection with *Chlamydia psittaci*. Examination of conjunctival scrapings can confirm the diagnosis. Treatment with enrofloxacin is usually effective but the condition is often self-limiting.

Urinary system disease

Urolithiasis and cystitis

Cystitis appears relatively common in guinea pigs but often results in relatively minor clinical signs. Owners may notice haematuria, and occasional straining, but severely affected animals can show signs of abdominal pain and general ill-health. Treatment with antibiotics (e.g. trimethoprim/sulphonamide) may resolve the condition, but recurrence is common.

It is important to establish that urolithiasis is not present. Uroliths are relatively uncommon in guinea pigs and even when present they may not be associated with clinical signs of cystitis or urethral obstruction. Large single and multiple small calculi occur. They are usually formed of calcium oxalate, and so are radio-opaque. Clinical signs include dysuria, haematuria and generalized depression and collapse if complete obstruction occurs and goes undetected. Large stones, or a large accumulation of small calculi, may be palpable through the body wall, and examination of urine may show the presence of a few small calculi. Cystotomy is indicated to remove the calculi, and antibiotics may be required to control the cystitis. The cause of calculi formation is uncertain and no specific measures to prevent recurrence can be given. Acidification of the urine is not possible.

Urethral obstruction may also occur in males due to plugging of the urethra with material from the accessory sexual glands. These plugs are sometimes visible at the end of the penis and can be removed by gentle traction.

Reproductive disease

Pregnancy toxaemia

Pregnancy toxaemia may occur in pregnant females and in non-pregnant obese animals. In pregnant animals it occurs in late pregnancy or shortly after parturition. Animals become depressed and anorexic (Figure 6.7); if untreated, this progresses to collapse and coma. Occasionally convulsions may be seen, and pneumonia with associated dyspnoea can occur in the later stages of the condition. Animals are ketoacidotic and urinanalysis will usually show ketonuria, proteinuria and acidurea. Treatment with fluids (warmed dextrose/saline i.p. and s.c.), oral glucose and corticosteroids is often successful early in the course of the condition, but animals presented for treatment in a collapsed state often die despite aggressive therapy.

Obesity and fasting, especially in late pregnancy, can trigger the condition, as can other stress. Owners should therefore be advised to avoid overfeeding breeding females, and to ensure a regular supply of food and water during pregnancy.

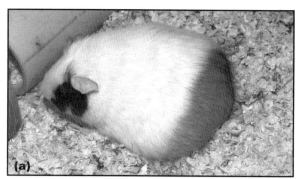

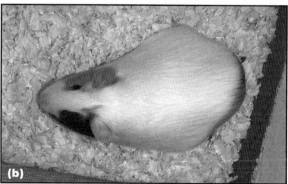

Figure 6.7 Guinea pig with pregnancy toxaemia. (a) Note the ruffled fur coat, sunken eyes and pale ears that are relatively non-specific signs of severe ill health. (b) Appearance 24 hours after treatment with intraperitoneal glucose–saline and glucose by mouth.

Musculoskeletal disease

Hypovitaminosis C ('scurvy')

Guinea pigs have an absolute requirement for vitamin C and an inadequate dietary intake can result in clinical signs of deficiency developing in 2–3 weeks. The clinical signs are due to defects in collagen synthesis and include lameness, an altered, shuffling gait, swelling of the joints and costochondral junctions, petechiation of mucous membranes and a variety of non-specific signs including depression, rough hair coat, ptyalism due to malocclusion and poor wound healing. As mentioned earlier, affected animals also show an increased susceptibility to infection. They gradually deteriorate and die unless treated.

Response to oral supplementation (100 mg/kg/day) is often rapid, even in severely affected animals. To prevent a recurrence of the condition, ensure a commercial supplemented guinea pig diet forms the bulk of the diet, check its vitamin content and method of storage, advise feeding of greens, and consider adding ascorbic acid to the animal's drinking water (daily, 200–400 mg/l) – especially in winter, when fewer green vegetables may be available for feeding.

Skin disease

Parasites

Mites: Dermatitis caused by *Trixacarus caviae*, a sarcoptid mite, is a common problem in guinea pigs. Infection can result from direct or indirect contact.

Active infections cause severe pruritis and the severity of lesions may be exacerbated by self-trauma (Figure 6.8). The severity of the pruritis can be such that handling of the guinea pig results in apparent seizures. These normally subside if the animal is returned to its transport box but can also be controlled with diazepam. The diagnosis can be confirmed by demonstration of mites in skin scrapings but these can be difficult to find, especially in traumatized lesions.

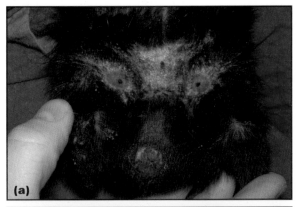
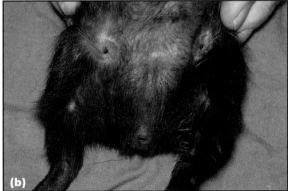

Figure 6.8 (a) Severely pruritic lesions caused by *Trixacarus caviae* infection. (b) Two weeks after treatment.

Recommended treatment is with ivermectin (200–400 µg/kg s.c., three doses 12–14 days apart). If the animal is severely pruritic, a low dose of corticosteroid or an NSAID can be administered. Response to ivermectin is usually rapid, with a marked improvement in the condition in 3–7 days. It is important also to treat unaffected animals that are in contact, as the mite can remain as a subclinical infection (singly housed individuals can develop clinical signs after several years of isolation from other guinea pigs). Poor planes of nutrition, poor husbandry and intercurrent infections all appear able to trigger clinical disease. In addition to treating all animals, the cage environment should be thoroughly cleaned.

Lice: Louse infestation with *Gliricola porcelli* or *Gyropus ovalis* rarely causes pruritis unless infestation is severe. Lice can be seen relatively easily on the coat, and can be detected in skin and hair samples or by applying adhesive cellophane tape to the coat, followed by microscopic examination. Transmission of the parasites is by direct contact, but since infestations are often subclinical, it is important to treat all in-contact

animals and to clean the pens and hutches. Treatment with ivermectin is normally effective. As with *Trixacarus* infestations, clinical signs can be triggered by stress, intercurrent disease or inadequate husbandry.

Abscesses and fight wounds

Localized abscesses are often seen in guinea pigs and can be caused by bites in group-housed animals, or trauma from sharp objects in the cage. The abscess material is often thick and paste-like, so that simple lancing is ineffective and surgery to establish drainage is required (see below).

Cervical lymphadenitis

Infection with *Streptococcus zooepidemicus* can result in abscess formation but this is usually restricted to the cervical lymph nodes. The organism is found in the oropharynx of healthy animals and infection is thought to follow abrasions of the mucosa secondary to eating coarse feeds. Bite wounds may be a source of infection, and spread by aerosol or sexual contact is also possible. The infected nodes may burst and discharge pus. Some animals may die of acute septicaemia and the condition can cause high mortality in large groups of guinea pigs, especially if the animals' overall state of health has been compromised. The diagnosis can be confirmed by cytology or bacteriology of infective material.

Individual animals can be treated by surgical excision of the node, or incision to establish drainage, and use of systemic antibiotics to eliminate the infection. Cephalosporins have been recommended for treatment but use of these antibiotics can cause enterotoxaemia.

Pododermatitis

Ulceration of the plantar surfaces of the feet, particularly of the hindlimbs, can occur – often as a result of poor husbandry. The condition is usually associated with rough cage flooring or inadequate cleaning and is more common in older, obese animals. Inadequate dietary vitamin C can also predispose to development of the condition. Lesions can be mildly erythematous, with some hyperkeratosis, but can progress to severe ulcerative lesions (Figure 6.9) and eventually to osteomyelitis.

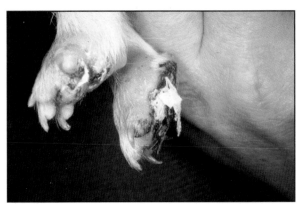

Figure 6.9 Severe pododermatitis in a guinea pig. (Courtesy of S. Wolfensohn.)

Treatment of established severe lesions is difficult but milder lesions often respond to changing the caging to provide a smoother floor, softer bedding and increased cleanliness, and increasing dietary vitamin C. Established lesions should be treated with topical antibiotic therapy, with systemic drugs if osteomyelitis has been demonstrated. Surgical debridement and bandaging can be attempted but the prognosis for such severe lesions should remain guarded. Analgesics should be given if the animal is lame, or if debridement is carried out.

'Barbering'

Chewing of the fur, either by other guinea pigs as an expression of dominance, or as self-mutilation, is relatively common. If self-inflicted, the head and neck will not be affected. Adding complexity to the animals' environment, particularly increasing the number of shelters and hiding places, can help to reduce the problem. Female guinea pigs may occasionally barber their offspring, but this usually resolves after weaning.

Alopecia

The term 'hormonal alopecia' has been used to describe the hair loss seen in females in late pregnancy and shortly after parturition. It is particularly common in females who have been bred repeatedly and are in poor condition. Improving the animal's general health and delaying subsequent mating usually resolves the problem.

Alopecia caused by development of ovarian cysts produces a similar non-pruritic hair loss, but the loss is often bilaterally symmetrical and may also be associated with enlargement of the external genitalia and abdominal distension (Figure 6.10). Cysts can be detected by ultrasonography or radiography, and large cysts by abdominal palpation. Affected sows may show persistent oestrous behaviour. Temporary remission of clinical signs can occur after administration of HCG (100 IU i.m. weekly for 3 weeks) but ovariohysterectomy is recommended.

Cheilitis

This condition is characterized by ulcerative scabbing lesions around the lips (Figure 6.11). Animals may be anorexic, or in otherwise apparently good health. The cause of the condition is uncertain; some cases may be due to pox-virus infection and it has been suggested that others may be due to eating acidic or abrasive food.

Treatment is non-specific, with cleaning and (if needed) debriding of the lesions. If severe, they can be packed with 'Orabase' (Squibb). Steroids should be avoided because of the involvement of pox-virus in some cases. Changing the diet to avoid acidic or abrasive foods may be of value. The condition may resolve spontaneously but this can take several months.

Dermatophytosis

Ringworm can produce typical scaly lesions with hair loss but can also cause inflamed pruritic lesions. Combined infections with mange mites can occur. As *Trichophyton mentagrophytes* is most frequently isolated, ultraviolet fluorescence is not often helpful for confirming a diagnosis. Direct microscopic examination of hair samples or culture can confirm the diagnosis.

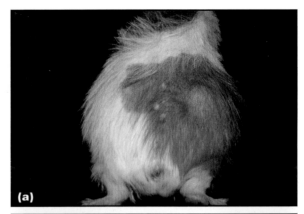
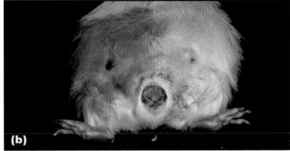

Figure 6.10 (a) Bilateral alopecia associated with cystic ovarian disease. (b) Enlargement of the external genitalia associated with cystic ovarian disease. (Courtesy of A. Meredith.)

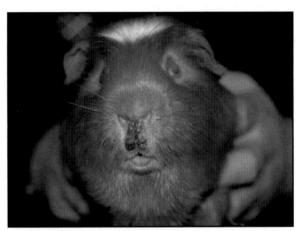

Figure 6.11 Cheilitis in a guinea pig. (Courtesy of A. Meredith.)

Treatment with griseofulvin (15–25 mg/kg for 14–28 days) is usually successful, and the condition will also respond to treatment with topical fungicidal treatment (e.g. enilconazole).

Mastitis

Mastitis is seen occasionally in guinea pigs, with a variety of organisms being isolated. It is likely that poor husbandry and overcrowding predispose to the development of the condition. Treatment with antibiotics, coupled with an improvement in hygiene and husbandry, is often successful. NSAIDs should be given to reduce pain and inflammation in the early stages of therapy. If the glands are severely affected and ulceration has occurred, treatment should include use of a topical wound-cleaning cream.

Ear disease

Otitis media is relatively common in guinea pigs but purulent exudate in the tympanic bulla may be an incidental finding at postmortem. Clinically affected animals show typical signs of head tilting and circling or loss of balance. A number of different organisms, including *Bordetella bronchiseptica*, *Streptococcus zooepidemicus* and *Pasteurella* spp., have been isolated from affected animals. Treatment with antibiotics is occassionally successful but a guarded prognosis should be given. Successful treatment by surgical drainage of the bulla has not been reported.

Endocrine disease

Diabetes mellitus

Affected animals have glycosuria and occasionally become ketotic but are often in apparent good health. Some animals may develop chronic weight loss, polydipsia, polyuria and diabetic cataracts. The majority of animals do not require treatment, and spontaneous remission (judged by absence of glycosuria) appears common. Successful management of severely affected animals with insulin has not been reported.

Supportive care

Drug administration

Injections

Restraint and the site for subcutaneous injection is shown in Figure 6.12. For intramuscular and intraperitoneal injections, the animal is restrained by an assis-

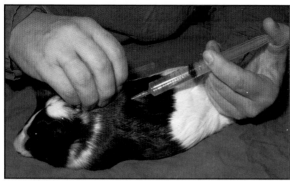

Figure 6.12 Subcutaneous injection is given into the scruff.

tant as in Figure 6.5. Intraperitoneal injection is made into a posterior quadrant of the abdomen, along the line of the extended hindlimb. Intramuscular injection is made into the quadriceps muscle. Intravenous injection is difficult, though the ear veins in adults may be sufficiently large for venepuncture using a 24–25-gauge needle. Application of local anaesthetic approximately 30 minutes prior to attempting venepuncture will prevent the animal from moving in response to the injection, thus minimizing the risk of damage to the small and delicate blood vessels. Alternative sites for venepuncture are the medial and lateral tarsal veins, on either side of the hindfeet, or the brachiocephalic veins on the forelimbs.

Oral administration

Drugs can be administered orally using a syringe placed in the diastema, though the animal may not swallow the material. In this case it may be preferable to insert a small mouth gag (made by drilling a hole through the barrel of a 1 ml syringe) into the diastema. A 2 mm catheter or stomach tube can then be threaded through the gag and into the oesophagus or stomach.

Postoperative care

Environmental temperature

Guinea pigs should be provided with warm, comfortable bedding after surgery. Drybed® (William Daniels, UK) is ideal for the initial recovery period, and once the animal has regained activity it can be transferred to a cage or pen with good quality hay or straw.

In the initial recovery period, supplemental heat should be provided: a temperature of 35–36°C should be maintained while the animal is unconscious but this can be reduced to 23–24°C when the animal has regained its righting reflex.

Fluid therapy

Water should be provided, and it is advisable to administer warmed (37°C) subcutaneous or intraperitoneal dextrose/saline at the end of surgery to provide some fluid supplementation in the immediate postoperative period (Figure 6.13).

To minimize the risks of stress-induced gastrointestinal disorders, it is important for guinea pigs to eat as soon as possible after surgery.

Treatment	Indication	Administration
Normal saline, dextrose (4%)/ saline (0.18%) Lactated Ringer's (Hartmann's solution)	Fluid deficits – use lactated Ringers when fluid and electrolyte deficit present Dextrose/saline for primary water deficit	If loss severe (> 5–10%, skin tenting) give i.v. if possible (24G catheter in peripheral vein, see text). Replace at 7–15 ml/kg/h. Alternatively, give i.p. (up to 30 ml/kg) or s.c. (up to 20 ml/kg). Repeat every 5–6 hours. Always warm fluid to 38°C
Glucose, 5% and 20–50%	Pregnancy toxaemia	Give 5% dextrose i.v. or i.p. (as above) and 20–50% by mouth (5 ml/adult every hour)
Liquidized diet (use liquidized pellets, liquidized vegetables, or proprietary nutritional support products)	Nutritional support	By hand-feeding or via oro/oesophageal tube using mouth gag, 5–10 ml/adult/feed. Add 10–30 mg vitamin C/kg to diet

Figure 6.13 Guidance on fluid and supportive therapy for guinea pigs.

Anaesthesia and analgesia

Guinea pigs, like many small mammals, are considered to be at higher risk of anaesthetic-related morbidity and mortality. This apparent increased risk of complications can be reduced significantly by adoption of best anaesthetic practice, coupled with careful perioperative care. Careful clinical examination is required to identify problems associated with pre-existing illness; for example, guinea pigs may have chronic bronchopneumonia or chronic renal disease.

Guinea pigs presented for treatment late in the course of an illness may be in generally poor clinical condition. For example, animals requiring dental procedures may have had reduced fluid and food consumption for several weeks, and so be at risk of circulatory failure during anaesthesia and also more prone to develop stress-related gastrointestinal tract disturbances in the postsurgical period.

If the animal is dehydrated, anaesthesia should be postponed and fluid therapy administered. This is easily achieved by intraperitoneal or subcutaneous injection of an appropriate fluid (e.g. 0.18% saline, 4% dextrose to correct dehydration, 10–20 ml/kg). In cases with severe dehydration, subcutaneous administration of fluids may be ineffective until peripheral circulatory function is improved. Intravenous injection is difficult in guinea pigs (see above) but it is possible to place a 24-gauge over-the-needle catheter in the medial or lateral tarsal vein. If time allows, oral rehydration therapy should also be commenced, using a syringe to deliver small mouthfuls of fluid (see above).

It is not necessary to withhold food and water for prolonged periods preoperatively in guinea pigs, as these animals do not vomit. They often retain food material at the back of the pharynx and removing food and water 1 hour prior to induction of anaesthesia is sufficient to minimize this.

Selection of method of anaesthesia

Because of the difficulty of intravenous administration, injectable anaesthetics are generally given by the intramuscular, intraperitoneal or subcutaneous routes. It is therefore not possible to adjust the dose to provide the desired effect in a particular individual. Since large variations in response can occur, it is advisable to select an anaesthetic regimen with a wide safety margin and, if possible, one that is completely or partially reversible.

Difficulties of physical restraint limit the use of local anaesthetics as the sole means of providing analgesia, but use of local anaesthetic techniques to provide additional analgesia in conjunction with low doses of injectable anaesthetics or low concentrations of inhalants can be valuable.

Many of these problems can be overcome by using an inhalational anaesthetic regimen and in many instances these are the agents of choice in guinea pigs. Anaesthetics, dosages and routes are set out in Figure 6.14.

Drug	Doseage
Acepromazine	0.5–1.0 mg/kg i.m.
Alphaxalone/alphadolone	40 mg/kg i.p.
Atipamezole	1 mg/kg s.c., i.m., i.p., i.v.
Atropine	50 µg/kg s.c., i.m.
Buprenorphine	50 µg/kg s.c.
Butorphanol	1 mg/kg s.c.
Carprofen	5 mg/kg s.c. uid
Diazepam	2.5 mg/kg i.m., i.p.
Diclofenac	2 mg/kg orally uid
Doxapram	5–10 mg/kg i.v.
Fentanyl citrate/fluanisone	0.5 ml/kg i.m.
Fentanyl citrate/fluanisone + diazepam	1 ml/kg i.m. + 2.5 mg/kg i.p.
Fentanyl citrate/fluanisone + midazolam	8 ml/kg i.p.[a]
Frusemide	5–10 mg/kg bid
Ketamine	100 mg/kg i.m., i.p.
Ketamine + acepromazine	100 mg/kg + 5 mg/kg i.p.
Ketamine + medetomidine	40 mg/kg + 500 µg/kg i.p.
Ketamine + midazolam	1.0 mg/kg + 5 mg/kg i.p.
Ketamine + xylazine	40 mg/kg + 5 mg/kg i.p.
Methohexital	30 mg/kg i.p.
Morphine	5 mg/kg s.c.
Naloxone	10–100 µg/kg i.m., i.p., i.v.
Oxytocin	1 IU total dose i.m., s.c.
Pentobarbital	25 mg/kg i.v.
Pethidine	5–10 mg/kg s.c., i.m.

a Dose is in ml/kg of a mixture made up of 2 ml Hypnorm™ (Janssen) plus 4 ml water for injection plus 2 ml Hypnovel™ (Roche).

Figure 6.14 Anaesthetics and analgesics.

Injectable anaesthetic regimens

Neuroleptanalgesic combinations: Fentanyl/fluanisone, when administered alone, produces sedation and sufficient analgesia for superficial surgery in most guinea pigs. Muscle relaxation is generally poor and marked respiratory depression can occurs with high dose rates. If fentanyl/fluanisone is administered in combination with a benzodiazepine (e.g. midazolam), surgical anaesthesia with good muscle relaxation and only moderate respiratory depression is produced. It is possible partially to reverse the effects of the combination by administering butorphanol, or other mixed agonist/antagonists. The benzodiazepine antagonist flumazenil can be used to speed recovery further but repeated doses are needed to avoid re-sedation. Even when reversal agents are used, recovery can be prolonged, especially if the animal's body temperature is not maintained by supplemental heating.

Ketamine combinations: Ketamine, when used alone, immobilizes guinea pigs but has little analgesic effect.

- Light anaesthesia is produced when combined with midazolam, diazepam or acepromazine
- If combined with infiltration of local anaesthetic, or low concentrations of volatile agents, these combinations can be sufficient for major surgery
- Administration of ketamine with xylazine or medetomidine produces deeper levels of anaesthesia, but this combination is not as reliable as it is in other rodents and in rabbits
- If anaesthesia is not sufficient to allow the required surgical procedure to be undertaken, it is preferable to deepen anaesthesia using an inhalational agent, or to provide additional analgesia using local anaesthetic
- As in other species, medetomidine and xylazine produce glycosuria and polyuria.

A significant advantage of the technique is that reversal of medetomidine or xylazine with atipamezole greatly speeds recovery. Note that if atipamezole is used following surgery, an analgesic should be administered to provide postoperative pain relief (see below).

Pentobarbitone: Although it has a veterinary product licence for use in guinea pigs in the UK, pentobarbitone has a very narrow margin of safety and very variable effects. If it is to be used, a relatively low dose (25 mg/kg i.p.) should be used to immobilize and sedate the animal. Anaesthesia should be deepened using a low concentration of a volatile agent (e.g. 0.5–1% isoflurane).

Inhalational anaesthetics

Halothane and isoflurane can be used to produce safe and effective anaesthesia in guinea pigs but it can be more difficult to maintain a stable plane of anaesthesia in this species than in other small mammals. Guinea pigs may become apnoeic even when given normally safe concentrations of anaesthetic and should be monitored carefully throughout the period of anaesthesia.

- Halothane can cause marked hypotension and has been associated with hepatic damage
- Isoflurane also has some disadvantages: guinea pigs may lacrimate and salivate during induction, presumably due to irritation of the mucous membranes
- On balance, isoflurane probably has a greater margin of safety and thus is to be preferred.

Induction can be via a face mask, but it is often easier and may be less stressful to use an anaesthetic induction chamber, filled from an anaesthetic machine. Suitable chambers can be purchased commercially or constructed from clear plastic containers. It is important to fill the chamber from the bottom and remove waste anaesthetic gas from the top, as the anaesthetic vapour is denser than air. Removal of gas from the bottom of the chamber can significantly increase the time taken to achieve an appropriate concentration for induction of anaesthesia (4% halothane, 5% isoflurane). After induction of anaesthesia, the guinea pig can be removed from the chamber and very brief procedures (< 1 minute) may be carried out. Anaesthesia can easily be maintained using a face mask (1.5–2.5% halothane,

1.5–2.5% isoflurane). Induction of anaesthesia is rapid (2–3 minutes) and recovery, even after relatively prolonged periods of anaesthesia (e.g. 30 minutes), is short (< 10 minutes).

Intraoperative care and anaesthetic monitoring

The risks of complications during anaesthesia are greatly reduced by monitoring the patient and by adopting high standards of intraoperative care. Monitoring of respiratory and cardiovascular function is important but the relatively small size of guinea pigs makes maintenance of body temperature particularly important. The small size can also complicate routine surgical procedures. It is important to remain aware that traction during surgery, placing instruments across the animal's chest or steadying the surgeon's hand on the animal can seriously compromise respiratory movements and must be avoided.

Body temperature

Rectal temperature should be monitored throughout anaesthesia and in the early stages of recovery, using an electronic thermometer.

- Body temperature should be maintained by placing the guinea pig on a heating pad (at 38°C) and, if necessary, by covering it with insulating material (e.g. 'space blanket' or bubblewrap)
- Shaving and preparation of the surgical site should be kept to the minimum compatible with maintaining asepsis
- Any fluids administered should first be warmed to body temperature.

Measures to maintain body temperature must be continued in the postoperative period.

Respiratory monitoring

Respiratory rate can be monitored either by direct observation or by use of a respiratory monitor. Detection of gradual changes can often alert the anaesthetist to impending problems but sudden apnoea can occur in guinea pigs. Adequacy of respiration can also be monitored by means of a pulse oximeter, with the probe placed on the foot (Figure 6.15). It is important to note that the rapid heart rate of guinea pigs (> 300) may exceed the upper limits of some instruments. Whichever anaesthetic regimen is used, it is advisable to deliver oxygen by face mask throughout anaesthesia and in the early stages of recovery.

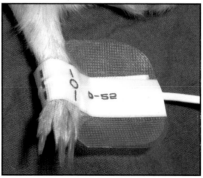

Figure 6.15
Pulse oximeter probe placed on the hindfoot of a guinea pig.

If respiratory depression occurs, respiration can be assisted by manual compression of the chest and by administration of respiratory stimulants such as doxapram. Endotracheal intubation is very difficult in guinea pigs and is not routinely carried out.

Cardiovascular monitoring

Assessment of circulatory function by clinical monitoring is difficult in guinea pigs, though capillary refill time can be assessed in larger animals by using the mucous membranes of the mouth. Some indication of cardiovascular function can be obtained by use of a pulse oximeter, and cardiac function can be monitored using a suitable ECG (as with pulse oximetry, an instrument capable of detecting low signal strengths and high frequencies is needed).

Techniques for supporting the circulation or treating cardiac arrest are similar to those for larger species, but one practical problem is the difficulty of venous access. Preventive measures are therefore particularly important:

- Avoid overdose with injectable anaesthetics by carefully weighing the animal
- Maintain body temperature and respiratory function
- Administer oxygen
- Minimize haemorrhage by careful surgical technique.

Analgesia

Pain is one of the major causes of postoperative inappetence. Suggested dosages and routes for the administration of analgesics in guinea pigs are given in Figure 6.14.

- When major surgery is undertaken the opioid analgesic, buprenorphine, should be given, either alone or in combination with an NSAID such as carprofen or ketoprofen, since this may provide more effective pain relief
- Gut motility modifiers (metoclopramide, cisapride) may be used to prevent postoperative ileus
- Infiltration of the surgical site with a long-acting local anaesthetic such as bupivacaine can be a useful adjunct to the use of systemic analgesics
- Less extensive procedures (e.g. uncomplicated ovarohysterectomy or castration) may require only administration of a potent NSAID. Following an initial dose at the time of surgery, an additional dose of an NSAID can be given by mouth 16–24 hours later.

In most circumstances, provision of analgesia for 24–48 hours appears sufficient. There is little detailed information regarding the clinical efficacy of many of these analgesics in guinea pigs, but the agents have been shown to be safe and effective in laboratory studies. There can be few indications, then, for withholding analgesics.

Common surgical procedures

Orchidectomy

Because guinea pigs have an open inguinal canal, a closed approach is preferred. Although the scrotum is not readily visible, the testes can be palpated lateral to the penis.

- An incision is made over the testis (Figure 6.16a), through the skin and subcutis, and the testis and its surrounding tunics are gently dissected free from the scrotum (Figure 6.16b)
- Gentle traction is applied and the cord and tunics are double-clamped
- A transfixing ligature is placed proximal to the clamps
- The cord is then transected between the two clamps and gently released
- The procedure is then repeated with the other testis.

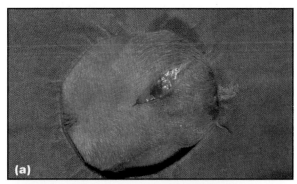

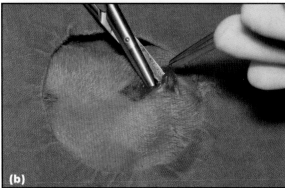

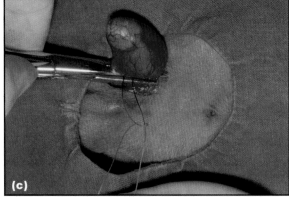

Figure 6.16 Castration. (a) An incision is made over the testis. (b) Blunt dissection is used to mobilize the testis in the scrotum, and it is then exteriorized. (c) The testis is clamped and ligated, and then removed.

If the tunic is damaged and the tear extends up into the incision, the incision should be lengthened so that the tunic can be repaired, or the inguinal canal closed. The skin should be closed with a subcuticular technique.

Caesarian section

If females are mated for the first time when they are over 9–12 months of age, separation of the pubic symphysis at parturition may be inadequate. Dystocia can also occur because of fetal oversize, and in obese females (who may also develop pregnancy toxaemia).

Females should be observed closely in late gestation and owners advised to contact their veterinary surgeon if the animal becomes depressed or inappetent, or shows other signs of ill-health. If the animal develops a bloody or olive-green vaginal discharge, it should be seen urgently unless pups are produced within about an hour.

The surgical technique is via a midline approach, in a similar manner to that used in the cat and dog. The skin is best closed using a subcuticular technique. High standards of perioperative care are required and fluid therapy is often essential to a successful outcome.

Unfortunately the young are often dead when delivered and maternal mortality can also be high. Orphaned guinea pigs can be fed on a mash of commercial pelleted diet and on diluted cow's milk, using a dropper or syringe. If several females are kept and another has recently given birth, the young can be cross-fostered.

Ovariohysterectomy

The surgical approach is via a midline incision, and the ovaries and uterus are normally easily identifiable. The ovarian pedicles, uterine body and associated vessels are ligated, as in other species, and removed. In obese guinea pigs, the ovarian and uterine vessels may be embedded in adipose tissue, and care must be taken to identify them so that they can be incorporated when ligating the tissues.

Treatment of superficial abscesses

Localized abscesses are common and are usually filled with thick, paste-like pus.

- The skin should be shaved and disinfected and the abscess opened with a large cruciform incision (Figure 6.17)
- The contents can then be removed, the cavity flushed with saline or a wound cleansing fluid and the cavity filled with a wound-cleaning cream

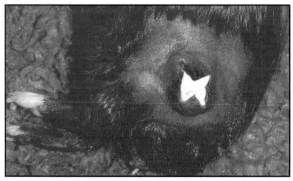

Figure 6.17 Drainage of a superficial abscess.

- Systemic antibiotic therapy is not usually required, unless the animal appears to have signs of systemic infection
- Check that the wound remains open for 2–3 days, and repack with wound-cleaning cream if necessary.

Euthanasia

Guinea pigs can be humanely killed by intraperitoneal administration of pentobarbitone (200 mg/kg). Animals can also be killed by cervical dislocation but as this technique requires considerable skill it is not recommended.

Drug formulary

Drug	Dose
Antibiotics	
Cephalexin[a]	15 mg/kg i.m. twice daily
Chloramphenicol	50 mg/kg orally 3 times daily, 20 mg/kg i.m. twice daily
Enrofloxacin	50–100 mg/l drinking water 5 mg/kg orally, s.c. twice daily
Gentamicin[a]	5–8 mg/kg s.c. once daily
Griseofulvin	25 mg/kg orally once daily for 2 weeks 800 µg/kg feed
Neomycin	5 mg/kg orally twice daily
Sulphadiazine with trimethoprim	120 mg/kg s.c. once daily
Sulphadimidine	20 g/l drinking water
a Note that adverse reactions are possible with these antibiotics (see text).	
Endoparasiticides	
Fenbendazole	20 mg/kg orally daily for 5 days
Ivermectin	200–400 µg/kg s.c. 500 µg orally
Piperazine	3 g/l drinking water for 7 days
Thiabendazole	100 mg/kg orally daily for 5 days
Ectoparasiticides	
Ivermectin	As above
Permethrin	Dusting powder

Figure 6.18 Drug formulary for the guinea pig.

References and further reading

Harkness JE and Wagner JE (1995) *The Biology and Medicine of Rabbits and Rodents, 4th edn.* Williams and Williams, Baltimore

Manning PJ, Wagner JE and Harkness JE (1984) Biology and diseases of guinea pigs. In: *Laboratory Animal Medicine*, ed. JG Fox *et al.*, pp. 149–177. Academic Press, New York

Mitruka BM and Rawnsley HM (1981) *Clinical Biochemical and Haematological Reference Values in Normal Experimental Animals and Normal Humans, 2nd edn.* Year Book Medical Publishers, Chicago

Popesco P, Rajtova V and Horak J (1992) *A Colour Atlas of Small Laboratory Animals. Vol. 1, Rabbit and Guinea Pig.* Wolfe, London

Robinson R (1978) *Coat Colour Genetics in Small Mammals.* Watmoughs Ltd, Bradford

7

Chinchillas

Heidi L. Hoefer and David A. Crossley

Introduction

The chinchilla is a medium-sized rodent that originates from the Andes. There are two species, *Chinchilla laniger* and *C. brevicaudata.* The latter is much larger, with a shorter tail and smaller ears (Walker, 1975) but is now considered rare, possibly extinct (Jimenez, 1996). Known for their luxurious pelts, chinchillas have been trapped to near extinction in their native countries of Peru, Bolivia, Chile and Argentina. By the early 1900s the wild population was sparse. With government assistance, an American man trapped 11 wild chinchillas in 1923 (*C. laniger*) and transported them to California in an attempt to establish ranch breeding for the fur industry. This small group of captive-bred chinchillas has formed the basis of the national population; over 3000 ranchers have been estimated to have a growing population of pet chinchillas.

Chinchillas are non-burrowing animals that live in groups in rock crevices or burrows at elevations above 4000 m (15,000 ft). They are adapted to a barren mountainous terrain; the thick fur protects them from cold temperatures and the footpads allow agility on rocky surfaces. Chinchillas are social animals that rarely fight. They are generally nocturnal and prefer a quiet environment during the day, although some individuals can be active in the daytime. Chinchillas do not hibernate.

Chinchillas are known for their soft and dense fur. There are about 60 hairs per follicle, and the hairs are loosely attached. The tail is long and covered with short coarse hairs. Chinchillas have long vibrissae, about 110 mm long, on either side of the upper lip, and these are used as sensory organs to assist in nocturnal navigation.

The natural colour is a smoky blue–grey, but several colour mutations have been developed, including white, silver, beige and black (Figure 7.1). They are clean, odourless to humans and inquisitive, and are relatively easy to care for. Chinchillas can be shy, jumpy and reluctant to sit still for long, making them more appropriate as pets for older children and adults.

Biology

Biological data for chinchillas are summarized in Figure 7.2.

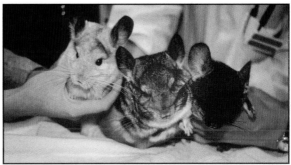

Figure 7.1 Coat colours in juvenile chinchillas: (from left) silver, natural grey and black velvet.

Life expectancy	Average 8–10, maximum 18 years
Adult weight	400–600 g (females larger)
Rectal temperature	37–38°C
Heart rate	100–150 beats per minute
Sexual maturity	6–8 months
Gestation	111 days
Litter size	1–6, average 2
Weaning age	6 weeks

Figure 7.2 Biological data for chinchillas.

Sexing and reproductive biology

The female has a cone-shaped urogenital papilla that, at a quick glance, may resemble a prepuce (Figure 7.3a). The urethral opening is seen within this papilla. There is a vaginal closure membrane that is only open during oestrus (3–5 days) and parturition. The female has two uterine horns that open separately into the cervix. There are three pairs of mammary glands.

In the male, the testes are located in the inguinal canal without a true scrotal sac. The urogenital distance is greater than in the female (Figure 7.3b). Males have open inguinal rings that require surgical closure during castration.

Female chinchillas are seasonally polyoestrous from November to May, with an oestrous cycle of about 40 days. The female in oestrus is easy to identify by the loss of the vaginal membrane, making the opening slightly moist and easy to visualize (see Figure 7.3a). During oestrus the female expels a waxy plug from the vaginal opening. She also expels a plug after a successful mating (Figure 7.4).

Females do not usually use a nest. The young are typically born early in the morning, They are

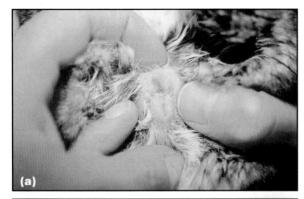

Figure 7.3 (a) Female chinchilla in oestrus. The vaginal membrane is open and lies between the urethral papilla and anus. (b) Male chinchilla.

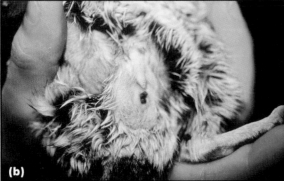

Figure 7.4 Vaginal plugs found in cage after successful mating.

precocious: fully furred, open-eyed and active at birth. Although they can eat solids from birth, weaning takes place at about 6 weeks.

Dentition

Chinchillas have four prominent, strongly curved, incisor teeth, one in each quadrant of the mouth. There is a single premolar and three molar teeth in each quadrant (Figure 7.5). All teeth grow continuously. The part of the teeth embedded in the alveolus is frequently referred to as the 'root', although continuously growing teeth do not form true anatomical roots, a more accurate term being 'reserve crown' with the visible part being the 'exposed crown'.

Dental Formula : 2 × I 1/1 C 0/0 P 1/1 M 3/3

The facial surfaces of the incisors are covered by enamel with superficial yellow to orange pigmentation. The exposed incisor crowns should appear short, with the oral surfaces being worn to a chisel-like pattern that

finishes flush with the gingiva (Figure 7.6). The abrasive effect of the substrate is responsible for the bulk of the tooth wear, an additional component coming from an active tooth-on-tooth grinding action used for 'self-maintenance' of the teeth. Self-maintenance of the occlusal pattern requires a normal jaw movement range and so is inhibited by tooth elongation and oral dysfunction.

The premolars and molars ('cheek teeth') of each quadrant are arranged in a straight line, the arcades converging mesially, i.e. towards the front of the mouth. The cheek teeth all have a similar form, composed of multiple folded parts which produce transverse ridges at the occlusal surface of maxillary and oblique ridges on the mandibular teeth. The difference in angulation of the ridging at the mandibular and maxillary occlusal surfaces allows them to slide smoothly over each other without risk of interlocking during the propalineal chewing action, one cheek tooth arcade being drawn along the opposing one (i.e. diagonally). Differential wear of

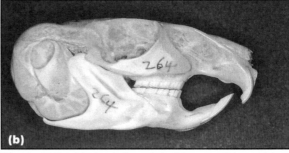

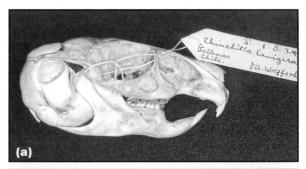

Figure 7.5 (a) Lateral view of skull from a wild-caught chinchilla. Note that all tooth crowns are short and bone outlines smooth. Courtesy of the Natural History Museum collection. (b) Lateral view of skull from a clinically healthy captive-bred chinchilla. Captive-bred chinchillas tend to be larger than their wild counterparts, with disproportionately longer teeth.

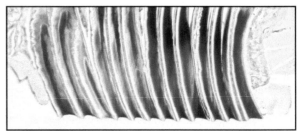

Figure 7.6 Ground section of maxillary dental arcade showing pattern of occlusal surface wear. Dentine and cementum (dark stained areas) are worn preferentially compared with harder enamel (unstained), forming a highly efficient grinding surface.

the exposed enamel, dentine and cementum produces a highly effective surface for grinding thin fibrous plant material (see Figure 7.6). The cheek teeth in each quadrant abut closely and wear to form a continuous horizontal occlusal surface that should be flush with the gingiva except at the mesial surface of the mandibular premolar. As with the incisor teeth, the occlusal surface requires continual maintenance. When eating a natural diet of tough fibrous plants with a high phytolith (plant silicate) content, tooth wear is rapid, new teeth being formed and erupting to replace those lost by attrition.

Gastrointestinal tract

Chinchillas are hindgut fermenters. The gastrointestinal tract is long, averaging 2.5 to 3.0 m. The stomach and caecum are relatively large, and the jejunum is very long. The colon is highly sacculated.

Ears and eyes

Chinchillas have very large ears with thin-walled pinnae and well developed auditory bullae. They are common subjects of auditory research and are especially useful in investigations of acoustic trauma (Bettcher, 1990).

Chinchillas have a shallow orbit, a large cornea and a densely pigmented iris with a vertical pupil. The mean intraocular pressure in one study of 14 animals was 18.5 (SD 5.75) mm Hg (Peiffer and Johnson, 1980).

Husbandry

Housing

Chinchillas can be housed in pairs, single-sex groups or polygamous groups of one male per five females. Chinchillas are active and require a fair amount of space. They like to jump and climb, and a large multilevel cage is recommended. A wire mesh cage is better than wood because they like to gnaw. The mesh must be small enough to prevent foot and limb injury (15 mm ×15 mm) and part of the floor should be solid. A wooden nest box is recommended for hiding or sleeping.

Chinchillas are fastidious groomers and require dust baths as part of their weekly bathing. There are commercial dust products available; beach-type sand should not be used. Volcanic ash can be used when available, or a fine mixture of Fuller's earth (a type of kaolin) and silver sand (1:9). A small amount (2–3 cm deep) should be placed in a container large enough for the chinchilla to roll around in (Figures 7.7). These baths need to be kept clean and free of faeces and should be removed when not in use. The dust bath can be used 3–4 times weekly; overuse can lead to an irritative conjunctivitis in some individuals.

The chinchilla's native habitat provides low humidity and sharp variations between daytime and evening temperatures. High temperatures and high humidity must be avoided all year round. Chinchillas are comfortable at cooler temperatures, as low as 0°C if dry and free of drafts. They are prone to heat stroke if the environmental temperature rises above 28°C, especially when coupled with high humidity.

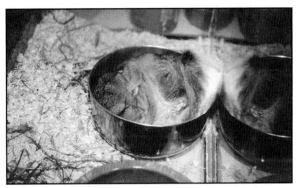

Figure 7.7 Dust bathing. Chinchillas spin rapidly in shallow bowls of dust.

Diet

The chinchilla is a hindgut fermenting herbivore. Free-ranging chinchillas survive on a diet of grasses, cactus fruit, leaves and the bark of small shrubs and bushes. The chinchilla originates from an area of the Andes where vegetation is tough and fibrous and low in energy content. This requires a high intake and prolonged mastication for extraction of nutrients. Chinchillas need this high-fibre diet to prevent enteric problems and to maintain the integrity of their open-rooted teeth. Although it is difficult to reproduce the natural diet in captivity, the recommended chinchilla diet consists of a good quality grass hay (e.g. Timothy) and a small amount of chinchilla pellets. Because the diet must be high in fibre, the sole feeding of pellets must be avoided. Pellets should be limited to 1–2 tablespoons per day. Fruit and small amounts of greens can be offered as treats. Any change in diet should be made gradually over several days and faecal output monitored periodically.

Handling and restraint

Chinchillas are usually easy to handle and rarely bite. However, they can be shy and nervous and reluctant to stay still for prolonged periods. They can move quickly and are best caught right from the carrying case to prevent problems on the examining table. The best approach is to hold the animal gently around the thorax (Figure 7.8). Alternatively, the tail can be held at the base

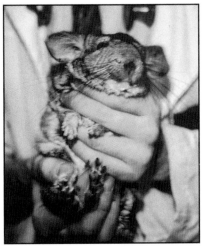

Figure 7.8 Restraining a chinchilla during examination.

as long as the body is supported. Chinchilla fur, although dense, is not tightly attached and this serves as a defence mechanism to predator attack. The fur should not be grasped roughly during handling; it may result in a dropped patch of fur in a frightened animal ('fur slip').

Diagnostic approach

Sample collection

Blood

Small volumes of blood for quick assessment tests can be collected from peripheral veins. For larger volumes of blood, the jugular vein can be used. It lies superficially in the jugular furrow and can be palpated or visualized in some chinchillas. In laboratory settings, the orbital sinus and transverse sinus are used for blood collection but these are not recommended for routine use in pet chinchillas (Bettcher, 1990).

Reference blood values may change with the laboratory performing the tests, but the values in Figure 7.9 may serve as a reference point. As with the guinea pig, the chinchilla is a 'lymphocytic species' and the lymphocyte percentage of the total white cell count may be as high as 75%, with an average white cell count of 8000–12,000/mm³.

Red blood cell count ($\times 10^{12}$/l)	7 (.16)
Packed cell volume (%)	43 (1.9)
White blood cell count ($\times 10^9$/l)	4.5 (1.6)
Neutrophil count ($\times 10^9$/l)	2.6 (.82)
Lymphocyte count ($\times 10^9$/l)	1.9 (1.2)
Platelet count ($\times 10^9$/l)	350 (92)
Total protein (g/l)	47 (2.8)
Urea (mmol/l)	8 (1.4)
Creatinine (μmol/l)	42 (13)
Alanine aminotransferase (IU/l)	27 (19)
Alkaline phosphatase (IU/l)	72 (49)
Calcium (mmol/l)	2.3 (.24)

Figure 7.9 References values (SD) for blood tests in chinchillas. Data from an unpublished study by DA Crossley.

Urinalysis

Chinchilla urine is alkaline, with a pH of about 8.5 and contains calcium crystals. The specific gravity can be high, with values above 1.045 (Merry, 1990).

Common conditions

There is a paucity of information available in the literature on diseases of pet chinchillas. Much of what we know is based on personal experiences and anecdotal information from veterinary surgeons and breeders. Most conditions in chinchillas are outlined below. Neoplasia is not mentioned; there are no contemporary reports of neoplasia in pet chinchillas and only rare mention in the older literature of farm ranchers. Medicine and surgery in the chinchilla should be considered an open field, and any disease process is possible. Thorough investigations are recommended whenever appropriate.

Dental disease

Dental disease is very common in captive chinchillas. When attrition is within the natural range, the rate of tooth growth and eruption vary to match the rate of attrition. A reduction in attrition rate results in elongation of the exposed crown, increased occlusal contact increasing the occlusal stress, which impedes further eruption. Tooth growth is reduced to compensate for reduced eruption, but below about half the normal rate the reduction in growth is less than the reduction in eruption. Tooth growth continues at a slow rate, even when there is no eruption. Continued apical growth stimulates remodelling of the surrounding tissues, allowing root elongation. This results in palpable changes on the ventrolateral border of the mandible. In the maxilla, premolar and first molar root elongation tends to obliterate the lacrimal ducts, resulting in impaired drainage from the eye. Elongation of the second and third maxillary molar roots initially prevents retraction of the eyes into their sockets and in extreme cases may lead to proptosis. Changes in the apical tissues lead to dysplasia of the newly formed tooth due to physical distortion or disruption of the germinal tissues. Slower growth leads to increased curvature of the teeth.

The basic eruption and growth control mechanisms are also influenced by other factors such as extreme nutritional deficiencies, stress, inflammation, injury and other disease.

A recent study identified early changes in about one third of chinchillas examined in the United Kingdom (Crossley, 2001). These animals had signs (altered head profile, visibly elongated incisors and palpable mandibular changes) indicative of tooth elongation. Many chinchillas cope well with simple tooth elongation but the problem is progressive if not corrected by provision of a more abrasive low energy diet at an early stage. Continued elongation with altered tooth curvature predisposes to reduced chewing efficiency, interproximal food packing, periodontal pocketing and spike formation on the edges of the occlusal surfaces (causing soft tissue damage). Clinically affected animals show a range of signs (Figure 7.10), the most significant being weight loss. Many lesions are difficult to find on examination of the conscious animal, so anaesthesia and radiography are required for a thorough assessment (Figure 7.11). Even with this approach a high proportion of lesions will not be recognized, 50% more lesions generally being detected on postmortem examination.

As the teeth elongate and prevent closure of the mouth (Figure 7.12) there is a progressive decrease

Weight loss
Difficulty eating
General loss of condition
Change in faecal droppings
Altered chewing pattern
Palpable deformity of ventral mandible
Palpably abnormal cheek tooth occlusion
Visible elongation of incisors or wear abnormality
Discomfort on facial palpation
Restricted jaw movement range
Excessive salivation
Ocular discharge

Figure 7.10 Clinical signs associated with dental lesions.

in the efficiency of swallowing (try swallowing with your mouth open!) with a tendency for chewed food material to be retained in the mouth. In the past this has often been misdiagnosed as paralysis of the pharyngeal muscles.

> Irregular cheek tooth wear
> Spikes on cheek teeth
> Mucosal ulceration
> Periodontal pocketing
> Food impaction between cheek teeth
> Coronal elongation
> Root elongation
> Root deformity
> Resorptive lesions
> Caries lesions
> Missing teeth
> Jaw deformity

Figure 7.11 Additional findings on intraoral examination and radiography of anaesthetized animals with dental disease.

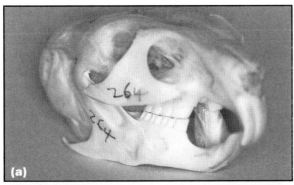

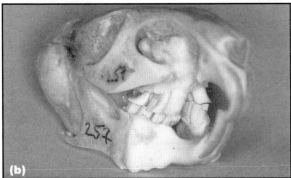

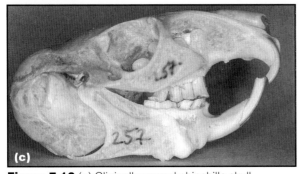

Figure 7.12 (a) Clinically normal chinchilla skull. (b,c) Skull with grossly elongated teeth holding mouth open. There is also ventral mandibular distortion, increased curvature and 'spike' formation on buccal occlusal surfaces of maxillary cheek teeth, the 'roots' of which have elongated into the infraorbital foramen and orbit.

Treatment

Prevention of dental diseases is desirable, through provision of a diet and environment which promote normal rapid attrition. Inclusion of fresh leafy vegetation, particularly from monocotyledonous plants, ensures a normal chewing pattern and provides adequate vitamin A intake. If dental problems are recognized in the early stages, they can usually be arrested, though rarely cured, by the same approach.

As most animals do not show any clinical signs until there is serious dysfunction, most chinchillas presented with dental problems have advanced disease. In cases of uncomplicated tooth elongation, with or without 'spike' formation, attempts may be made to restore the occlusal surfaces to a normal height by use of fine dental burrs, provided the tooth roots have not already penetrated the surrounding bone and there are no gross tooth deformities. Rasping and tooth clipping are contraindicated as they cause significant periodontal trauma and do not restore the teeth to a normal shape. Fine diamond-coated files can be used but are very slow and best reserved for final finishing. When a significant length is removed from the cheek teeth there will be additional oral dysfunction as the jaw muscles require several weeks to adapt back to a normal length. During this time supportive feeding is required and the teeth tend to elongate again, so treatment usually needs to be repeated several times at intervals of 6–8 weeks.

When there is caries of the occlusal surfaces, a combination of coronal reduction, as above, with elimination from the diet of items containing sugars and starch may prove successful. Treatment of periodontal disease is unlikely to prove successful. Lateral and interproximal food and hair impaction into periodontal pockets frequently leads to lateral abscessation and may extend to the root apices. Correction of occlusal problems, cleaning of the pockets and packing them with a (non-toxic) antibiotic or antiseptic gel may help, but recurrence should be expected in the short term. Systemic use of an antibiotic effective against periodontal pathogens (but unlikely to upset the caecal flora) is also beneficial in the short term.

It is important to advise owners of the poor prognosis in most dental cases. Assessment of the patient's quality of life can be difficult. If it cannot be assured then euthanasia is preferable to continued disease that is likely to result in prolonged suffering.

Gastrointestinal disease

Lower gastrointestinal disease is a common problem in chinchillas. High fibre low-energy diets are essential for the chinchilla's digestive physiology. Disruption to the system results in anorexia, colic, diarrhoea, hair and faecal impaction, intussusception, mucoid enteritis, ileus, bloat and rectal prolapse. Hepatic lipidosis is a common sequel to prolonged anorexia.

Predisposing factors include an abrupt change in diet, inappropriate antibiotic use, overcrowding and stress, and diets too low in fibre and too high in fat and protein. Changes in enteric pH or normal gut flora results in bacterial overgrowth and can lead to enterotoxaemia. *Clostridium, Escherichia coli, Proteus* and *Pseudomonas* are common isolates. Clostridial enterotoxaemia (*C. perfringens*) causes severe diarrhoea, shock and acute death. Diagnosis is based on clinical signs and history. Anorexia and decreased faecal output are early warning signs. Whole body radiographs should be taken to assess both body cavities. Varying amounts of gas and ingesta may be seen normally in hindgut fermenters. With gastroenteritis, there is an increase in gas production and usually evidence of ingesta, despite persistent anorexia (Figure 7.13). It can be difficult to determine simple gas production from an obstructive ileus; barium can be given orally by syringe if necessary to aid in visualization and the determination of motility.

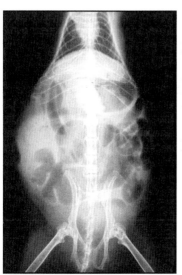

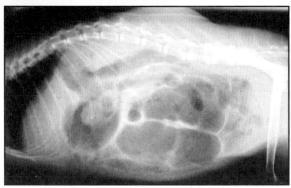

Figure 7.13
Radiographs of an anorexic chinchilla with generalized ileus. The stomach contains small amounts of ingesta and there is increased gas production throughout the gut. This chinchilla had an impacted gut loop.

Treatment for the acute abdomen includes supportive care (fluids, temperature regulation), anti-inflammatories (flunixin hydrochloride) or analgesics (buprenorphine or butorphanol), antibiotics, and surgery if obstructed. Human paediatric anti-gas preparations containing simethicon may be helpful to decrease gas production. Motility modifiers (metoclopromide or cisapride) can be useful in cases of non-obstructive ileus, which is not always easy to determine. A sick chinchilla is a poor surgical candidate, and medical management is usually indicated prior to abdominal surgery. Blood testing is recommended in anorexic individuals (complete blood counts and plasma chemistry).

Other reported causes of gastroenteritis in chinchillas include *Salmonella, Listeria monocytogenes* and *Yersinia pseudotuberculosis*. Intestinal parasitism is uncommon but nematodes, coccidians, *Giardia* and *Cryptosporidium* can sometimes be found in chinchillas. Low numbers of *Giardia* are thought to be normal in chinchillas but an overgrowth can lead to diarrhoea. Faecal examinations should be performed in any animal with diarrhoea. There are anecdotal reports of hepatotoxicity to metronidazole in some chinchillas, although this author (HH) has not seen it.

Respiratory system

Overcrowding, high humidity, poor ventilation and other stress-inducing factors may result in pneumonia in chinchillas. Affected animals are typically emaciated, have poor hair coats and show abdominal breathing. Some animals become septicaemic and develop anorexia, depression, dyspnoea, nasal discharge and lymphadenitis. Chronic respiratory disease can be caused by *Bordetella, Streptococcus* or *Pasteurella*, often in combination. Antibiotics should be targeted at the common bacterial isolates. Combination antibiotics, e.g. trimethoprim–sulphonamide and enrofloxacin, may be indicated in individuals with moderate respiratory disease. Prognosis is poor once respiratory distress is evident.

Heart disease with subsequent heart failure can also be seen in chinchillas. These animals are acutely dyspnoeic, and the condition may be difficult to distinguish from a primary respiratory condition. Thoracic radiographs and echocardiography are important to distinguish heart disease from lung disease.

Cardiovascular system

Most reports of cardiac disease in chinchillas are anecdotal. At the author's (HH) previous practice (the Animal Medical Center in New York), several chinchillas were found to have heart conditions on postmortem examination. Cardiomyopathy and valvular disease were seen. Unfortunately, most chinchillas with cardiac disease present in heart failure. These animals are acutely dyspnoeic but often in good body condition. Pleural effusion, pulmonary oedema and cardiomegaly can be seen radiographically. Prognosis is poor with fulminant cardiac failure.

Heart murmurs are occasionally auscultated in otherwise normal chinchillas. What part this plays, if any, in signalling a cardiovascular problem is unknown. Two young chinchillas with significant murmurs picked up during routine examination had echocardiograms performed at the Animal Medical Center. Results were considered to be within normal limits. Another young chinchilla with a murmur survived neutering but died suddenly several years later, with cardiac abnormalities seen at postmortem examination.

Reproductive system

Fur ring

Adult male chinchillas may present with paraphimosis, caused by a ring of matted fur caught around the penis inside the prepuce. This is called 'fur ring' (Figure 7.14). It is more commonly seen in breeding males, although it can develop in other males. Treatment includes lubrication of the penis

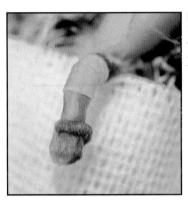

Figure 7.14
Paraphimosis in a chinchilla caused by a ring of fur encircling the exposed penis.

and the gentle removal of the fur ring. The penis of all male breeding chinchillas should be checked several times during the breeding season.

Dystocia

Dystocias can occasionally be found in chinchillas. Malpositioned fetuses, uterine inertia and uterine torsion are possible causes. Affected females are restless and may bleed. Caesarean section should be considered after 4 hours of unproductive labour, using routine techniques as in other small animals. Pyometras are uncommonly diagnosed in chinchillas.

Neurological disease

Listeriosis

Chinchillas are highly susceptible to infection with *Listeria monocytogenes*, and there are several reports in animals raised on farms (Finley and Long, 1977). Encephalitic and enteric forms of the disease are seen. Although listeriosis tends to be peracute in chinchillas, clinical signs observed prior to death may include ataxia, circling and convulsions. Poor sanitation and contaminated feed are often implicated in outbreaks of listeriosis. Oral chloramphenicol (50 mg/kg bid) or injectable oxytetracycline (10 mg/kg i.m. bid) are recommended; however, treatment is unlikely to be effective once clinical signs appear.

Cerebrospinal nematodiasis

Cerebrospinal nematodiasis caused by *Baylisascaris procyonis* has been reported in chinchillas housed outdoors in the USA (Sanford, 1991). Affected animals developed an acute progressive disease of the CNS, characterized by ataxia, torticollis and paralysis. Diagnosis was confirmed with sections of brain tissue taken at postmortem examination. The most likely source of nematodiasis is raccoon faeces. Raccoons infected with *B. procyonis* are most common in northern temperate regions of North America, especially in the midwestern and northeastern parts of the USA. Hay, straw or feed contaminated by raccoon faeces must be avoided. Owners need to be warned of the zoonotic potential of this indiscriminate parasite.

Torticollis

Torticollis can be caused by otitis media or otitis interna. Infections with *Streptococcus* spp. can progress to otitis media, and affected chinchillas may also present with subcutaneous abscesses, septic arthritis and chronic respiratory disease. Bulla disease can be identified radiographically and may require an osteotomy to allow flushing and drainage.

Dietary deficiencies

Dietary deficiencies may play a part in the development of neurological symptoms. Deficiencies of thiamine (vitamin B) can result in circling and convulsions. A minimum of 1 mg of vitamin B per kilo of feed should be available in the diet (Wallach and Boever, 1983). Calcium deficiencies can also result in convulsions, especially in young rapidly growing animals or pregnant adults.

Lymphocytic choriomeningitis

Lymphocytic choriomeningitis is a naturally occurring viral disease of mice that has been reported to affect the chinchilla (Wallach and Boever, 1983). Clinical signs include conjunctivitis, tremors and convulsions. The virus has zoonotic potential, and although it is uncommon, it can cause meningoencephalitis in humans. There is no treatment.

Lead poisoning

Lead poisoning has been seen by the author (HH) as a cause of acute convulsions and blindness in an apartment-dwelling chinchilla. Diagnosis was based on an increased level of lead in the blood (34 mg/dl in one case) and a positive response to chelation therapy using calcium disodium versenate (EDTA at 30 mg/kg s.c. bid).

Skin disease

Dermatophytosis

The most important infectious disease of the skin in chinchillas is dermatophytosis. Infection with *Trichophyton mentagrophytes* is most common but *Microsporum canis* and *M. gypseum* can occur. Subclinical infections are also possible. Dermatophytosis resembles the disease in other species: small scaly patches of alopecia on the nose, ears and feet are typical. Oral griseofulvin can be given for 3 or 4 weeks. Dips containing lime sulphur can be beneficial.

Ectoparasites

Ectoparasites are uncommon in the chinchilla because of its dense fur. Fur mites (*Cheyletiella*) have been reported anecdotally and can be treated with ivermectin and dips containing lime sulphur.

Abscesses

Bite wounds with subsequent abscess formation occur in chinchillas kept in groups. *Streptococcus* and *Staphylococcus* are common isolates. Inspissated abscesses are typical in chinchillas, and so surgical excision is recommended.

Fur loss

Barbering and fur chewing are thought to be behavioural and may be related to overcrowding, stress or possibly nutritional deficiencies. Chinchillas that are handled roughly or fight release a patch of fur, leaving the skin clean and smooth ('fur slip'). Fur regrowth may take several months.

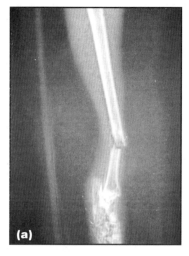

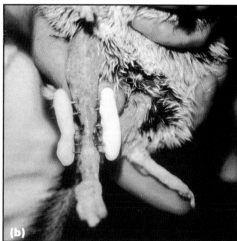

Figure 7.15 (a) Traumatic fracture of the tibia in a caged chinchilla. Note the long bone with thin cortices. (b) Type II Kirschner–Ehmer external fixator used to repair the transverse fracture. Small non-threaded K wires were used and connected using hand-rolled polymethylmethacrylate bars.

Heat stroke

Because chinchillas are adapted to low environmental temperatures, prolonged exposure to temperatures above 28°C (80°F) can result in heat prostration. Affected animals become recumbent and hyperthermic and they pant. Treatment consists of cool water baths, intravenous fluids and corticosteroids in advanced cases. Owners should be reminded to place chinchilla cages away from radiators or sunny windows.

Fractures

In the author's (HH) practice, the most common traumatic fracture in chinchillas is of the tibia, which is a long straight bone with little soft tissue covering. Tibial fractures tend to be short spiral or transverse (Figure 7.15a). Soft padded bandages and lateral splints can be applied but may not provide adequate stabilization for the active chinchilla. Surgical repair can be difficult due to the long thin nature of the bone. External fixators (type II Kirschner–Ehmer apparatus) can be applied and have been used with success by the author (Figure 7.15b). Soft padded bandages may have a better success rate for forelimb fractures (radius and ulna and distal). Care must be taken when applying tape 'stirrups' to the skin when dressing a bandage; irritation can be substantial in some chinchillas. Because chinchillas can be active, non-unions are possible. Strict cage rest without climbing or jumping room for a minimum of 4 weeks is essential.

Supportive care

Fluid therapy and nutritional support plus other supportive therapy is detailed in Figure 7.16.

Drug administration

Injections

Subcutaneous injections can be given dorsally behind the neck or in the flank area. The thick fur can make it easy to miss the skin; parting the fur and wetting it down with an alcohol swab aids in correct needle placement. Intramuscular injections can be given in the rear leg (semitendinosis or quadriceps femoris muscle). Only small gauge needles (23 or 25) should be used for intramuscular injections, and no more than 0.3 ml of a solution should be given in one site in an adult.

Maintenance fluids	75–100 ml/kg/day i.v.; s.c. (lactated Ringer's solution)
Anti-inflammatories	Flunixin 2.5 mg/kg i.m. bid
Antibiotics	Enrofloxacin 10–15 mg/kg i.m., s.c. or i.v. slow and dilute, chloramphenicol 50 mg/kg i.m. or s.c.
Analgesics	Butorphanol 0.5–1 mg/kg s.c. bid to tid, buprenorphine 0.05–0.1 mg/ s.c. bid, carprofen 2–4 mg/kg orally sid
Anticholinergics	Atropine 0.05–0.10 mg/kg s.c. or i.m.
Corticosteroids	Dexamethasone sodium phosphate 2 mg/kg i.m.; i.v. (short-term use only)
Motility modifiers	Metoclopramide 0.5–1.0 mg/kg s.c. tid
Nutritional support	Strained vegetable baby food; human enteral lactose-free formulas; soaked and pulverized pellets; by syringe orally tid

Figure 7.16 Emergency and supportive therapy for chinchillas.

Intravenous injections are difficult but are possible with 25 gauge needles or insulin syringes (28 gauge). Peripheral veins are small, but the lateral saphenous or cephalic veins may be accessible.

Antibiotics

Chinchillas rely on a complex balance of microorganisms in the digestive tract to ferment non-digestible fibre. Any disruption in this system can change pH, interfere with gut motility and promote bacterial overgrowth. Gram-negative bacteria and clostridial overgrowths can lead to diarrhoea, enterotoxaemia and death. Antibiotics that have a selective Gram-positive spectrum should be avoided. This includes the β-lactams (penicillins and cephalosporins), clindamycin, lincomycin and the erythromycins. Safe antibiotics include those listed in Figure 7.20 at the end of the chapter. Commonly used antibiotics include chloramphenicol, enrofloxacin, trimethoprim–sulphonamide and the aminoglycosides.

Anaesthesia and analgesia

Chemical restraint can be used if prolonged sedation is needed (Figure 7.17). The anxiolytic drug midazolam can be used as an intramuscular agent, either alone for mild sedation and stress reduction (0.5–1 mg/kg i.m.) or in combination with ketamine 20–40 mg/kg i.m.

Drug	Dosage and route	Comments
Acepromazine	0.5–1.0 mg/kg i.m.	Preanaesthetic and light sedation
Atropine	0.05–0.10 mg/kg s.c. or i.m.	Anticholinergic
Buprenorphine	0.05–0.10 mg/kg s.c. bid	As needed
Butorphanol	0.5–2 mg/kg i.m. tid	Analgesic
Carprofen	1–4 mg/kg	Analgesic
Diazepam	1–5 mg/kg i.m., 0.5–1.0 mg/kg i.v.	Sedation; preanaesthetic
Flunixin meglumine	1–2.5 mg/kg i.m.	Non-steroidal anti-inflammatory, analgesia
Glycopyrrolate	0.01–0.02 mg/kg s.c. or i.m.	Anticholinergic
Halothane	2–5% induction; 2–3% maintenance	
Isoflurane	2–5% induction; 2–4% maintenance	
Ketamine	20–40 mg/kg i.m.	Preanaesthetic, moderate sedation, works best in combination (see below)
	10–20 mg/kg i.v.	For short procedures; use with diazepam
Meperidine	20 mg/kg s.c. or i.m.	Analgesic
Midazolam	1–2 mg/kg s.c. or i.m.	Mild sedation; anxiolytic drug
Morphine	2–5 mg/kg i.m.	Analgesic
Oxymorphone	0.2–0.5 mg/kg s.c. or i.m. bid or tid	Analgesic
Paracetamol	1–2 mg/ml in drinking water	Analgesic
Xylazine	2–10 mg/kg i.m.	Lower dose when used in combination
Yohimbine	2.0 mg/kg i.m.	Reversal of xylazine

Figure 7.17 Anaesthetic and analgesic agents for chinchillas. Doses are based on review of the literature and author's experience.

Combination	Commments
Acepromazine 0.5 mg/kg i.m. and ketamine 40 mg/kg i.m.	5 minutes to induction, 45–60 minutes surgical anaesthesia, 2–5 hours recovery (Morgan *et al.*, 1981)
Acepromazine 0.5 mg/kg i.m., ketamine 10 mg/kg i.m. and atropine 0.05 mg/kg i.m.	Preanaesthetic sedation for use with isoflurane inhalation
Ketamine 40 mg/kg i.m. and xylazine 2 mg/kg i.m.	2 hours surgical anaesthesia; reversal with yohimbine 2 mg/kg i.m. (Hargett *et al.*, 1989)
Ketamine 20–40 mg/kg i.m. and diazepam 3–5 mg/kg i.m.	Diazepam can irritate muscle. Midazolam better absorbed intramuscularly
Ketamine 10–15 mg/kg i.m., midazolam 0.5 mg/kg i.m. and atropine 0.05 mg/kg i.m.	Author's preferred combination as a preanaesthetic to isoflurane
Tiletamine and zolazepam combination 20–40 mg/kg i.m.	Recovery can be prolonged

Figure 7.18 Combination pre-anaesthetic and anaesthetic protocols. Doses are based on review of the literature and author's experience.

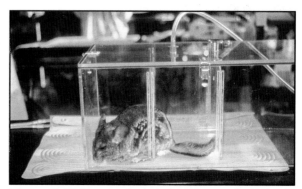

Figure 7.19 Chamber for inducing gaseous anaesthesia.

for stronger sedation and as a pre-anaesthetic (Figure 7.18). Ketamine (40 mg/kg) with acepromazine (0.5 mg/kg) given intramuscularly provides about 40–60 minutes of anaesthesia time (Morgan *et al.*, 1981). Ketamine (40 mg/kg i.m.) with xylazine (2 mg/kg) provides up to 2 hours anaesthesia time but can be reversed with yohimbine 2.1 mg/kg i.p. (Hargett *et al.*, 1989). Combinations of injectable ketamine and valium also work well. A small intravenous bolus of ketamine and diazepam (a quarter to half the intramuscular dose) can be given for quick procedures like oral examinations, radiography and tooth trimming. The preferred method of inhalant anaesthesia is isoflurane. Anaesthesia is usually delivered through a small face mask, and isoflurane is the agent of choice, although halothane has been used successfully in chinchillas. It has a rapid induction and recovery time and high margin of safety. Gas delivery is through an induction chamber (Figure 7.19) or a face mask. Chinchillas are difficult to intubate; respirations and anaesthetic depth must be carefully monitored during prolonged procedures.

Analgesics are essential for painful procedures (see Figure 7.17).

Common surgical procedures

Operations are uncommonly performed in the chinchilla. Chinchillas of both sexes are neutered for population control only, as there is no evidence to support neutering for health reasons.

Castration

Males are presented more commonly than females for elective neutering. Because males have open inguinal rings, a closed castration technique should be used and scrotal incisions can be made. The scrotal skin can then be closed with tissue glue or subcuticular absorbable sutures.

Euthanasia

Euthanasia is best accomplished by inducing anaesthesia with isoflurane or halothane in a chamber, followed by an intraperitoneal injection of pentobarbitone.

Drug formulary

Drug	Dosage and route	Comments
Antibacterials		
Amikacin	2–5 mg/kg s.c. or i.m. bid or tid	
Chloramphenicol	50 mg/kg s.c. or orally bid	Veterinary drug, oral suspension not available in USA
Chlortetracycline	50 mg/kg orally bid	
Ciprofloxacin	10–15 mg/kg orally bid	Human formulation
Doxycycline	2.5 mg/kg orally bid	Paediatric syrup available in USA
Enrofloxacin	10–15 mg/kg s.c., i.m. or orally bid	Not for repeated subcutaneous injections as it can cause skin sloughs
Gentamicin	2–4 mg/kg s.c. or i.m. bid or tid, 5 mg/kg s.c. or i.m. sid	
Metronidazole	10–40 mg/kg orally bid	Anecdotal reports of hepatotoxicity
Oxytetracycline	50 mg/kg orally bid, 1 mg/ml in drinking water	
Tetracycline	50 mg/kg orally bid, 0.3–2.0 mg/ml in drinking water	
Trimethoprim–sulphonamide	30 mg/kg s.c. or orally bid	Oral paediatric suspension; injectable must be compounded in USA
Antifungals		
Griseofulvin	25 mg/kg orally sid, 1.5% in DMSO topically	Long-term use; 4–6 weeks. 5–7 days usage
Captan powder	1 tsp/2 cups dust	Fungicide for use in bathing dust
Lime–Sulphur dip	Once or weekly for 6 weeks	Dilute 1:40 with water before use
Antiparasiticides		
Carbaryl 5% powder	Dust lightly once weekly	Veterinary ectoparasiticide
Fenbendazole	20 mg/kg orally sid for 5 days	Nematocide
Ivermectin	0.2–0.4 mg/kg s.c. weekly for 3 weeks	
Metronidazole	30–50 mg/kg orally bid	Treats giardiasis
Piperazine citrate	100 mg/kg orally sid for 2 days	
Sulphamerazine	1 mg/ml in drinking water	Coccidiostat
Sulphadimethoxine	10–15 mg/kg orally bid	Coccidiostat
Thiabendazole	50–100 mg/kg orally sid for 5 days	Nematocide
Miscellaneous		
Calcium EDTA	30 mg/kg s.c. bid	Heavy metal chelation. Dilute with saline
Cimetidine	5–10 mg/kg bid or tid	Gastrointestinal ulcers, reflux oesophagitis, choke
Dexamethasone (SP)	0.5 mg–2 mg/kg bid or tid	Use tapering dose; short term only
Frusemide	2–4 mg/kg bid or tid	Diuretic
Oxytocin	0.2–3.0 IU/kg	Delayed parturition
Prednisone	0.5–2.0 mg/kg	Anti-inflammatory

Figure 7.20 Drug formulary for chinchillas. Doses are based on review of the literature and author's experience. There are no pharmocokinetic studies of drugs in chinchillas.

References and further reading

Boettcher FA, Bancroft BR and Salvi RJ (1990) Blood collection from the transverse sinus in the chinchilla. *Laboratory Animal Science* **40**, 223–224

Bryer LW (1957) An experimental evaluation of the physiology of tooth eruption. *International Dental Journal* **7**, 432–478

Crossley DA (2001) Dental disease in chinchillas in the United Kingdom. *Journal of Small Animal Practice* (in press)

Crossley DA, Dubielzig RR and Benson KG (1997) Caries and odontoclastic resorptive lesions in a chinchilla (*Chinchilla laniger*). *Veterinary Record* **141**, 337–339

Crossley DA, Jackson A, Yates J and Boydell IP (1998) The use of computed tomography to investigate cheek tooth abnormalities in *Chinchilla laniger*. *Journal of Small Animal Practice* **39**, 385–389

Donnelly TM and Schaeffer DO (1997) Disease problems of guinea pigs and chinchillas. In: Ferrets, Rabbits, and Rodents, Clinical Medicine and Surgery, ed. EV Hillyer and KQ Quesenberry, pp. 270–281. WB Saunders, Philadelphia

Finley GG and Long JR (1977) An epizootic of listeriosis in chinchillas. *Canadian Veterinary Journal* **18**, 164–167

Hagen KW and Gorham JR (1972) Dermatomycoses in fur animals: chinchilla, ferret, mink and rabbit. *Veterinary Medicine/Small Animal Clinician* **38**, 43

Hargett CE, Record JW, Carrier M, Bordwell KC and Patterson JH (1989) Reversal of ketamine-xylazine anesthesia in the chinchilla by yohimbine. *Laboratory Animal* Oct, pp. 41–43

Hoefer HL (1994) Chinchillas. *Veterinary Clinics of North America: Small Animal Practice* **24**, 103–111

Jenkins JR (1992) Husbandry and common diseases of the chinchilla (*Chinchilla laniger*). *Journal of Small Exotic Animal Medicine* **2**, 15–17

Jimenez J (1996) The extirpation and current status of wild chinchillas, *Chinchilla laniger* and *C. brevicaudata*. *Biological Conservation* **77**, 1–6

Kennedy AH (1952) Diseases affecting the mouth, teeth and oesophagus. In: *Chinchilla Diseases and Ailments*. Clay Publishing, Bewdley, Ontario

Kertesz P (1993) Dental diseases and their treatments in captive wild animals. In: *A Colour Atlas of Veterinary Dentistry and Oral Surgery*. Wolfe Publishing, London

Kraft I (1987) Diseases of chinchillas. TFH Publications, Neptune City, New Jersey

Merry CJ (1990) An introduction to chinchillas. *Veterinary Technician* **11,** 315–331

Moore RW and Greenlee HH (1975) Enterotoxaemia in chinchillas. *Laboratory Animals* **9,** 153–154

Morgan RJ, Eddy LB, Solie TN and Turbes CC (1981) Ketamine-acepromazine as an anesthetic agent for chinchillas (*Chinchilla laniger*). *Laboratory Animals* **15,** 281–283

Peiffer RL and Johnson PT (1980) Clinical ocular findings in a colony of chinchillas (*Chinchilla laniger*). *Laboratory Animals* **14,** 331–335

Sanford SE (1991) Cerebrospinal nematodiasis caused by *Baylisascaris procyonis* in chinchillas. *Journal of Veterinary Diagnostic Investigation* **3,** 77–79

Schour I and Medak H (1951) Experimental increase in rate of eruption and growth of rat incisor by eliminating attrition. *Journal of Dental Research* **30(4),** 521

Taylor AC and Butcher EO (1951) The regulation of eruption rate in the incisor teeth of the white rat. *Journal of Experimental Zoology* **117,** 168–188

Walker EP (1975) *Mammals of the World, 3rd edn*, vol 2. Johns Hopkins Press, Baltimore

Wallach JD and Boever WJ (1983) *Diseases of Exotic Animals*, pp. 135–195. WB Saunders, Philadelphia

Webb RF (1991) Chinchillas. In: *Manual of Exotic Pets*, ed. PH Beynon PH and JE Cooper JE, pp. 15–21. BSAVA Publications, Cheltenham

Wiggs RB and Lobprise HB (1990) Dental disease in rodents. *Journal of Veterinary Dentistry* **7(3),** 6–8

Wiggs RB and Lobprise HB (1995) Dentistry in pet lagomorphs and rodents. In: *BSAVA Manual of Small Animal Dentistry, 2nd edn*, ed. DA Crossley and S Penman. BSAVA Publications, Cheltenham

Wiggs RB and Lobprise HB (1997) Diseases in rodents and lagomorphs. In: *Veterinary Dentistry, Principles and Practice*. Lippincott-Raven, Philadelphia

Williams CSF (1976) *Practical Guide to Laboratory Animals*, pp. 3–11. CV Mosby, St Louis

Yamini B and Raju NR (1986) Gastroenteritis associated with *Cryptosporidium* sp. in a chinchilla. *Journal of the American Veterinary Medical Association* **189,** 1158–1159

8

Rabbits

Anna Meredith and David A. Crossley

Introduction

Over the centuries, the rabbit has been used for food, sport and clothing, as a scientific model, and as a hobby (the rabbit 'fancy'). In the UK, the keeping of rabbits as pets developed in Victorian times, since when their popularity has grown enormously: rabbits are now the UK's third most popular mammalian pet. Many are kept as house pets and true companion animals. They are relatively long-lived in captivity (up to 10 years) and this should be borne in mind when acquiring a young animal.

All domestic rabbits are the same species as the wild European rabbit (*Oryctolagus cuniculus*). There are many other species of rabbit and these, along with cottontails, pikas and hares, make up the order Lagomorpha. There are many recognized rabbit breeds and varieties (Figure 8.1) and more are constantly evolving by selective breeding and mutation. Many pet rabbits are cross-breeds.

Advantages of rabbits as pets include:

* Generally docile and responsive
* Good house pets
* Can be house-trained to use litter-tray.

Disadvantages include:

* Can become aggressive, or nervous and difficult to handle
* Can be destructive in the house, and unneutered animals can exhibit territorial marking
* Can be easily damaged by incorrect handling
* Larger breeds are difficult for young children to handle.

Biology

Rabbits are highly social, burrowing herbivores that are natural prey for a large number of carnivores. In the wild they live in warrens of 70 or more individuals, broken down into small groups of two to eight. They spend a lot of time engaged in mutual grooming and lying together but their displays of greeting behaviour, pain and fear are poor. Scent is much more important than sight and each animal has an individual scent profile. They can distinguish between familiar and unfamiliar humans, and between human genders. Thumping with the hindleg is an alarm call. Fear elicits either complete immobility or a flight response, often with frantic attempts to escape and screaming. As a prey species they have evolved to be constantly vigilant, lightweight and fast-moving, with a highly efficient digestive system that enables them to spend the minimum time possible above ground and in danger of capture. Biological data for the rabbit are summarized in Figure 8.2.

Digestive tract anatomy

Rabbits are hindgut fermenters, adapted to digest a low quality, high-fibre diet consisting mainly of grass. Gut transit time is rapid and fibre is eliminated from the digestive tract as soon as possible. This permits body size and weight to remain low, which is advantageous in a prey species. In the wild, feeding takes place mainly in the early morning and evening and at night. Indigestible fibre (lignocellulose) stimulates gastrointestinal motility and has a protective effect against enteritis.

The stomach is thin-walled and poorly distensible. Vomiting is not possible. Food, hair and caecal pellets are always present in the stomach. Bacterial fermentation takes place in the caecum, which is very large,

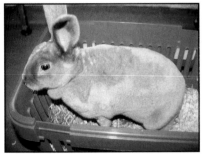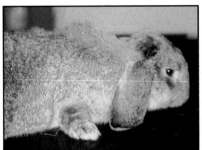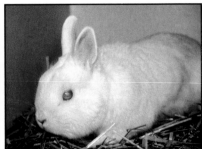

Figure 8.1 Examples of rabbit breeds: Rex, Dwarf Lop, Netherland Dwarf.

Lifespan	5–10 years
Weight	1–10 kg (breed dependent)
Dentition	I 2/1 C 0/0 P 3/2 M 3/3
Respiratory rate	30–60 breaths per minute
Heart rate	180–300 beats per minute
Blood volume	60 ml/kg
Rectal temperature	38.5–40°C
Water intake (daily)	50–150 ml/kg
Food intake (daily)	50 g/kg
Urine production (daily)	10–35 ml/kg
Sexual maturity	4–8 months (does earlier than bucks)
Oestrous cycle	Reflex ovulation; oestrus Jan–Oct
Length of gestation	28–32 days
Litter size	4–12
Birthweight	30–80 g
Weaning age	6 weeks

Figure 8.2 Biological data for the rabbit.

thin-walled and coiled and has many sacculations (or haustrae). It terminates in the vermiform appendix, which is rich in lymphatic tissue. The caecum lies on the right side of the abdomen. Caecal contents are normally semi-fluid. The colon is sacculated and banded. Colonic contractions separate fibrous from non-fibrous particles, and fibre moves rapidly through for excretion as hard faecal pellets. Antiperistaltic waves move fluid and non-fibrous particles back into the caecum. Three to eight hours after eating, mainly at night, soft, mucus-covered caecal pellets are expelled and eaten directly from the anus (a process known as caecotrophy, coprophagy, refection or pseudorumination). Arrival of the caecotrophs at the anus triggers a reflex licking of the anus and ingestion of the caecotrophs, which are swallowed whole and not chewed. A muscular band of richly innervated tissue with a thickened mucosa, the fusis coli, lies at the end of the transverse colon and acts to regulate colonic contractions and controls production of the two types of pellet.

The mucous covering protects the caecal pellet bacteria from the low pH of the stomach. Caecotrophs remain in the stomach for up to 6 hours, with continued bacterial synthesis, and eventually the mucous layer dissolves and the bacteria are killed. This process of caecotrophy allows absorption of nutrients and bacterial fermentation products (amino acids, volatile fatty acids and vitamins B and K) and the redigestion of previously undigested food.

Dentition

Rabbits have six unpigmented incisor teeth: one in each mandible and two each side of the premaxilla. The second upper incisor is much smaller than the rest (it is commonly referred to as a 'peg tooth') and is palatal to the first incisor. There is a long diastema between the incisor and premolar teeth. The premolar teeth are similar in form to the molar teeth and are frequently described together as the 'cheek teeth'.

All the teeth grow continuously and never form anatomical roots. The part of the tooth embedded in the alveolus should therefore be described as 'reserve crown', though it is more commonly referred to as the 'root'. The visible part of the tooth is correctly described as the 'exposed crown'.

The first incisor teeth are normally kept very short, with the occlusal surfaces taking on a chisel-like shape (Figure 8.3) the lingual profile of which is flush with the gingiva. Incisor wear, growth and eruption are generally balanced over time, at a rate of about 3 mm per week.

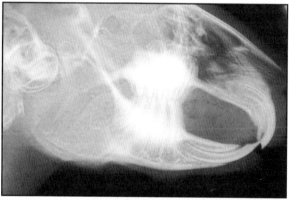

Figure 8.3 Lateral radiograph showing the features of healthy rabbit dentition: chisel-shaped first incisor wear pattern, approximately 45 degrees upper, 30 degrees lower; smooth incisor tooth surface, longitudinally grooved in maxillary first incisor teeth; tips of the mandibular incisors rest between the maxillary first and second incisors; transversely ridged cheek tooth occlusal surfaces angled at about 10 degrees to horizontal; tooth wear patterns bilaterally symmetrical; short teeth with very short exposed crown; distinct radiographic dental and periodontal outlines with large apical radiolucencies and no distortion of adjacent bone; oral cavity profile narrowing rostrally; and smooth ventrolateral border to the mandible.

The mandible is narrower than the maxilla, with the temporomandibular articulation positioned dorsal to the occlusal line. Functionally the incisor teeth are used with a largely vertical scissor-like slicing action. Cut vegetation is then moved to the back of the mouth by the tongue and ground between the cheek teeth. When grinding fibrous natural foods, the mandible has a wide lateral chewing action, concentrating on one side at a time. This wears the whole cheek tooth occlusal surface. Grass is highly abrasive, as it has a high content of silicate phytoliths, so there is rapid wear of the teeth (around 3 mm per month) with equally rapid tooth growth and eruption to compensate for this. Mandibular teeth, incisors and cheek teeth, grow and erupt faster than their maxillary counterparts.

Sexing

The anogenital distance is greater in the male (buck), which has a round preputial opening. The female (doe) has an elliptical vulval opening (Figure 8.4). Within a breed, does tend to be slightly larger than bucks, but bucks have broader heads.

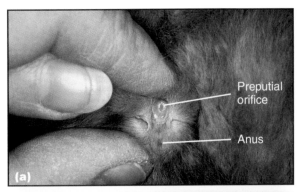

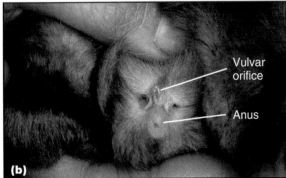

Figure 8.4 Sexing may be difficult in immature animals (before testicular descent in the male). (a) The preputial orifice is always circular. (b) The vulvar orifice is elliptical. The anogenital distance is longer in males than in females. Courtesy of D. Malley.

Husbandry

Housing

Rabbits are social animals and should be provided with a companion wherever possible.

- Litter mates can be kept together but should be neutered if of different sexes
- Unrelated females will usually tolerate each other if sufficient space is provided, but they can fight
- Intact bucks will fight and inflict severe injuries
- All introductions should be supervised
- Neutering minimizes the risk of conflicts
- The most stable pairing is a neutered buck and neutered doe.

It is not recommended that rabbits are kept with guinea pigs, as bullying by both species can occur – especially by the rabbit. Rabbits can also harbour *Bordetella bronchiseptica*, which is pathogenic to guinea pigs.

Outdoor housing

- Rabbits are generally hardy but need protection from extremes of weather
- Avoid direct sunlight, as heat stress and heat stroke occur easily
- The hutch should be raised off the ground
- A waterproof roof and louvred panel to cover the mesh-fronted area in bad weather should be provided

- The hutch should at least be big enough for the rabbit to stretch out fully, stand upright on its hindlegs and, if confined to the hutch for long periods, be able to perform at least three 'hops' from one end to the other
- A solid-fronted nesting area and a mesh-fronted living area should be provided, bedded with wood shavings and hay or straw
- Good ventilation is essential, to prevent respiratory disease
- Rabbits need daily exercise and need to graze: the hutch should be placed within an enclosure, or a separate ark or run should be provided (Figure 8.5); alternatively, a shed or garage can be used to provide a floor-pen. Raised shelves or platforms are readily used
- Rabbits will burrow, so precautions should be taken to prevent escape
- Rabbits can jump well and covering the run or pen with a mesh top will prevent escape, as well as providing protection from predators
- Rabbits should always be provided with appropriate 'bolt-holes', such as empty cardboard boxes or drain-pipes, to use if alarmed
- Contact with wild rabbits should be prevented, to minimize the risk of disease transmission by direct contact (e.g. viral haemorrhagic disease) or by vectors such as the rabbit flea (myxomatosis)
- Fly and mosquito control should be considered in summer months.

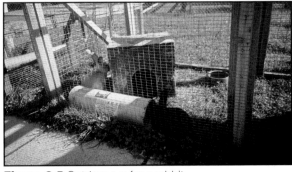

Figure 8.5 Outdoor run for a rabbit.

House rabbits

- House rabbits should have a secure cage area where they can be restrained when the owner is not present. Wire cages with plastic bases are suitable
- Exercise around the house and garden should be encouraged
- Rabbits will readily learn to use cat-flaps to gain indoor/outdoor access
- Rabbits are easily trained to use a litter tray, by repeatedly placing them in it (it may be necessary initially to place some droppings in the tray). Wood or paper-based litter should be used, as Fuller's earth products can be harmful if ingested

- Electrical cables must be protected from chewing, and poisonous house plants such as *Dieffenbachia* (dumb cane) avoided
- Chewable toys are enjoyed, such as cardboard boxes, telephone directories, or commercial bird toys.

Diet

The best diet for a rabbit is grass and good quality grass hay (e.g. Timothy) with a small amount of a high-fibre (18–24%) commercial diet with protein levels around 15%. Wild plants can be given if available (e.g. bramble, groundsel, chickweed, dandelion). Alfalfa hay can be given, especially to growing animals, but care should be taken as alfalfa is high in calcium and large amounts could predispose to urolithiasis. Hay should always be available and can be fed from racks or nets to increase time spent feeding. Fresh vegetables such as kale, cabbage, watercress, root vegetables and their leaves, should also be provided; carrots or other root vegetables can be suspended from the cage roof to act as edible toys and increase time spent eating.

Grass is approximately 20–25% crude fibre, 15% crude protein and 2–3% fat. Commercial rabbit diets are often too low in fibre and too high in protein, fat and carbohydrate. These cause caecocolic hypomotility, prolonged retention of digesta, increased volatile fatty acid production and adverse alterations in caecal pH and microflora, leading to diarrhoea, ileus and death, especially around the time of weaning.

The energy requirements of a rabbit can be met rapidly on a concentrate diet, but this can lead to dental disease due to lack of wear (Crossley, 1995), obesity, and boredom-associated problems such as stereotypic behaviour and aggression. Many rabbits are selective eaters and leave the pellet and biscuit component of a commercial mix, favouring grains and pulses, which are low in calcium. It is thought that this can lead to osteoporosis and dental disease (Harcourt-Brown, 1995). Commercial mixes, consisting of pulses, grains, grass pellets and biscuits, should not be fed *ad libitum*, as this can encourage selective feeding and obesity.

Sudden changes in diet, frosted or mouldy food, and lawnmower clippings should be avoided. Rabbits enjoy sweet foods but sugar-rich treats should not be fed, though they may be of use if tempting an anorexic animal to feed.

Water intake is approximately 10% of bodyweight daily. Drinking bottles are easier to keep clean than water bowls and they avoid wetting the dewlap, which can lead to a moist dermatitis.

Breeding

Onset of puberty depends on breed, but is at approximately 4–5 months in the female and 5–8 months in the male. Smaller breeds mature earlier than larger ones.

Rabbits are reflex ovulators. There is no definitive oestrous cycle: receptive periods usually occur for 12–14 days, followed by 2–4 days of non-receptivity, but this can vary, and some does become receptive every 4–6 days during the breeding season (January to October in the UK).

A receptive doe is very active, rubbing her chin on objects and exhibiting lordosis. The vulva becomes congested and reddish-purple. Does may mount each other and this, or an infertile mating, can induce ovulation, leading to a pseudopregnancy of approximately 18 days.

Does tend to be more territorial than bucks and the doe should be taken to the buck or to neutral territory for breeding, to avoid aggression. Sexually mature bucks will mate at any time.

Nest-building behaviour involves burrowing and pulling of fur from the dewlap, flanks and belly to line the nest and expose the nipples. Pregnancy can be detected by palpation at 14 days; gestation is 30–32 days. Parturition usually occurs in the early morning. The kits are altricial (hairless, with ears and eyes closed). Passive immunity is acquired by placental transfer before birth. Rabbit milk is exceptionally nutritious and nursing is for a few minutes once (occasionally twice) a day.

Kits emerge from the nest at about 2–3 weeks of age, when they start to show interest in solid food. Coprophagy starts at about 3 weeks and weaning can take place at 4–6 weeks.

Hand-rearing can be achieved using cat milk substitute 3–5 times a day, to which probiotics can be added. Hay should be introduced at 2–3 weeks. Concentrates should only be introduced once the young are established on hay.

Handling

Rabbits should be held by the scruff and with the weight of the body supported (Figure 8.6). Twisting and kicking out by the powerful hindlegs must be deterred, as serious back injury can result.

Turning the rabbit on to its back results in a trance-like state ('hypnotization' or tonic immobility). This behaviour is a defence mechanism, i.e. 'playing dead' if caught by a predator. This useful technique can be employed single-handed with the rabbit cradled in one arm, but it should be remembered that it is stressful for the rabbit and should be used for the minimum time possible. Under no circumstances should painful procedures be carried out using this technique as restraint.

> Rabbits should *never* be picked up by the ears!

Diagnostic approach

Physical examination

Most of the clinical techniques employed in dogs and cats can be applied to the rabbit. As with any animal, a systematic clinical examination, carried out in a consistent fashion, is important.

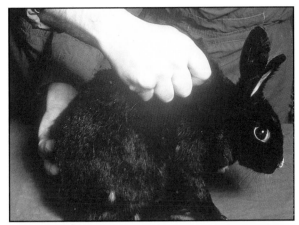

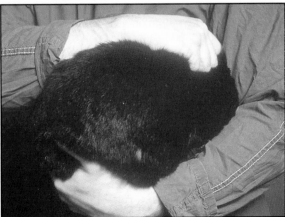

Figure 8.6 Handling techniques.

A non-slip surface should be used when carrying out a physical examination, and an assistant should hold the rabbit to prevent it jumping off the table. Placing one hand over the eyes and the other on the rump provides good restraint. The incisor teeth, ventrum, feet and nails are best examined with the rabbit held on its back. Special attention should be paid to the plantar metatarsal surface (plantar pododermatitis), and perineum (accumulation of caecotrophs, myiasis). The rectal temperature can also be taken in this position.

A rabbit in pain is immobile, with a hunched posture, and may grind its teeth and show increased aggression.

Oral examination
Sedation or anaesthesia is required to examine the mouth properly. An otoscope can be used for a cursory inspection but lesions such as tooth spurs can easily be overlooked.

Ocular examination
Purulent discharge from the nasolacrimal duct punctum is often present (see Dacryocystitis). Pressure over the medial canthus often causes expulsion of pus from the lacrimal sac. The optic nerve is above the horizontal midline of the eye, and retinal vessels spread outwards from the optic disc. Rabbits have no tapetum lucidum.

Abdominal examination
Palpation of the thin-walled abdomen is easily achieved. Vertical restraint, with the back of the rabbit held against the handler's chest, is useful for auscultation and ballotment of the abdomen. The caecum lies on the right side.

Diagnostic tests and techniques

Blood sampling
Blood collection sites are the marginal ear vein, jugular vein (Figure 8.7), cephalic vein or saphenous vein. The use of local anaesthetic cream is recommended. Blood volume is approximately 65 ml/kg and it is safe to remove 10% in a normal animal, or up to 1% of bodyweight (i.e. 6.5–10 ml/kg). Normal haematological and biochemical values are summarized in Figure 8.8.

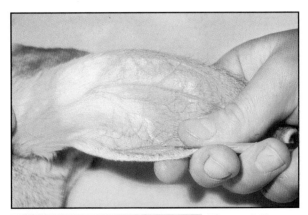

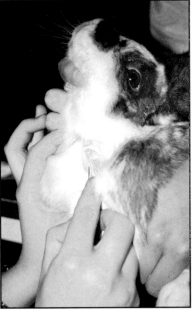

Figure 8.7 Blood collection from the marginal ear vein and jugular vein.

Cystocentesis
Cystocentesis can be achieved in a conscious rabbit, using a method similar to that for the cat. Rabbit urine is alkaline (Figure 8.9), contains albumin, calcium carbonate and ammonium magnesium phosphate crystals, and is often pigmented.

Parameter	Average	Range
Total WBC (x 10⁹/l)	8.55 6	5–12 5.0–8.0
Neutrophils (x 10⁹/l)		3–20 1.5–4.0
Neutrophils (%)	48	34–60 40–70
Band neutrophils (x 10⁹/l)	0.2	0–0.2
Lymphocytes (x 10⁹/l)	5.4	2–20
Lymphocytes (%)	53 47	43–62 20–80
Monocytes (x 10⁹/l)	0.41	0–1.8
Monocytes (%)	3	0–4 0–7.0
Eosinophils (x 10⁹/l)	0.26	0–0.8
Eosinophils (%)	1	0–2 0–5
Basophils (x 10⁹/l)		0–0.84
Basophils (%)	2.5	0–1 0–7
Haemoglobin (mg/dl)	12	10–17.5 12–15
PCV (%)	40 39	34–50 33–47
RBC (x 10⁶/mm³)	6	5–8 5.1–7.9
MCV (fl)	69	50–75 59–79
MCH (pg)	21	18–24 16–23
MCHC (%)	33	27–34 28–36
Reticulocytes (%)		0–3
Platelets (x 10³/mm³)	290	240–600
In vivo coagulation time (minutes)	4	2–8
Protein (g/l)	61	49–71 50–71
Albumin (g/l)	31	27–36 33–50

Parameter	Average	Range
Globulin (g/l)	28	24–33 15–27
A/G ratio	1.09	0.7–1.89
Glucose (mmol/l)	7.5	6–8.9 4.2–8.3
Urea (mmol/l)	17	9.1–22.7 9.3–25.5
Creatinine (mmol/l)	88	53–124 70–150
Total bilirubin (mmol/l)		4.3–12.8
Triglycerides (mmol/l)		1.4–1.76
Bile acids (μmol/l)	11.6	3–20
Cholesterol (mmol/l)	1.1	0.62–1.68 0.1–2.0
Sodium (mmol/l)		134–150 130–155
Chloride (mmol/l)		92–120
Bicarbonate (mmol/l)		16–32
Potassium (mmol/l)		3.3–5.7 3.5–5.6
Phosphate (mmol/l)		1.0–2.2
Calcium (mmol/l)	3.55	2.17–4.59 5.5–7.8
Magnesium (mmol/l)		0.8–1.2
Iron (mmol/l)		33–40
Aspartate aminotransferase (IU/l)	57 < 50	33–99 5–50
Alanine aminotransferase (IU/l)	124 < 50	55–260 5–50
Alkaline phosphatase (IU/l)	51	12–96 100–400
Lactate dehydrogenase (IU/l)	187	132–252 50–500
Creatine phosphokinase (IU/l)	263	140–372 50–250
Gamma GT (IU/l)		0–5
Cortisol (resting) (μg/dl)		1.0–2.04
Cortisol (30 mins after stimulation with ACTH 6μg/kg i.m.) (μg/dl)		12.0–27.8

Figure 8.8 Haematology and biochemical values for the 'normal average rabbit'. This table gives an overview of the data published and should be treated as a guide rather than a definitive source of reference values. Reproduced from the *BSAVA Manual of Rabbit Medicine and Surgery*.

Parameter	Normal findings
Urine specific gravity	1.003 – 1.036
Urine average pH	8.2
Urine crystals normally present	Ammonium magnesium phosphate, calcium carbonate
Casts, epithelial cells, bacteria	Absent to rare
Leucocytes, erythrocytes	Occasional
Albumin	Occasional (young rabbits)

Figure 8.9 Normal composition of rabbit urine.

Catheterization

Bladder catheterization is possible in bucks but extremely difficult in does. Sedation is usually required.

Collection of cerebrospinal fluid

CSF can be collected under anaesthesia in lateral recumbency by flexing the head and inserting a needle in the midline halfway between the cranial edges of the wings of the atlas and the occipital protruberance.

Common conditions

Diseases of the rabbit are summarized in Figure 8.10. Differential diagnoses based on clinical signs are summarized in Figure 8.11. A drug formulary for the rabbit is presented at the end of this chapter (see Figure 8.18).

Disease	Aetiology	Clinical signs	Diagnosis	Treatment
Aberrant conjunctival overgrowth. Unique to rabbit	Unknown	Fold of non-adherent conjunctival tissue arising from limbus and covering variable area of cornea	Clinical signs	Surgical removal results in recurrence. Suturing fold to sclera allows vision
Abscess	*Pasteurella multocida, Staphylococcus aureus, Pseudomonas, Proteus, Streptococcus, Corynebacterium, Bacteroides* and other anaerobes. Local entry (wound) or haematogenous spread	Subcutaneous or facial swelling, draining tracts. May be dull, anorexic, pyrexic if bacteraemic. Also dyspnoea (pulmonary abscess). Neurological signs (cerebral/spinal abscess)	Aspirate. Bacterial culture. CBC and biochemistry. Radiography. Ultrasonography	Surgical removal – treatment of choice. Lance, drain and flush. Systemic antibiosis. Injection of gentamicin into capsule (0.5–1ml per rabbit empirically). Antibiotic-impregnated methylmethacrylate beads
Accumulation of caecotrophs	Excess caecotroph production (low fibre/high protein and carbohydrate diet) or reduced caecotrophy (overfeeding, physical problems, obesity, pain)	Caking of caecotrophs around perineum. Secondary myiasis. Often mistaken for diarrhoea, but faecal pellets normal	Clinical signs	Address underlying cause. Dietary reform to high fibre, low or no concentrate diet. May take several months on hay alone to resolve
Allergic/irritant rhinitis/bronchitis	Environmental allergens or irritants	Sneezing, dyspnoea, nasal discharge	Exclusion of other causes. Response to: elimination of suspected allergen; antihistamines/corticosteroids	Avoidance of allergen. Antihistamines. Corticosteroids (do not use if concurrent *Pasteurella* or other bacterial infection)
Antibiotic toxicity/enterotoxaemia (clostridial overgrowth)	Reported with all antibiotics except fluoroquinolones and potentiated sulphonamides. Especially ampicillin, amoxycillin, clindamycin, lincomycin, cephalosporins, erythromycin. Will occur only if clostridia already present in gut	Diarrhoea (brown, watery, foetid, bloody). Depression. Dehydration. Hypothermia. Abdominal distension. Collapse. Death	History of antibiotic usage. Faecal culture and toxin isolation (rarely performed)	Fluid therapy. Cholestyramine. Metoclopramide. Cisapride. Metronidazole. High fibre diet (assisted feeding). Probiotics
Bacterial dermatitis (*see also* pododermatitis). Primary bacterial dermatitis rare	Usually *Staphylococcus aureus* but also other bacteria	Alopecia. Erythema. Ulceration. Pruritus	Bacterial culture	Antibiosis (topical/systemic). Address underlying cause
Bacterial enteritis	*Escherichia coli, Salmonella,* Tyzzer's disease (*Clostridium piliforme*)	Diarrhoea. Depression. Weight loss. Hypothermia. Abdominal distension. Collapse. Death. High morbidity and mortality in young rabbits	Faecal culture. Postmortem histopathology for Tyzzer's	Fluid therapy. Appropriate antibiosis. Metoclopramide. Cisapride. High fibre diet. Probiotics
'Blue fur' disease	Secondary *Pseudomonas aeruginosa* infection	Moist dermatitis. Blue coloration of fur in moist areas (dewlap, skin folds)	Blue coloration pathognomonic. Culture of *P. aeruginosa*	Clip fur. Keep dry. Topical antiseptic. Address underlying cause
Clostridial overgrowth (see Antibiotic toxicity, above)				
Coccidiosis	*Eimeria* spp. *Eimeria stiedae* (hepatic coccidiosis)	Diarrhoea. Weight loss. Anorexia. Jaundice. Dehydration. Ascites. Death. Can cause high morbidity and mortality in young rabbits	Faecal oocysts. Postmortem examination	Sulpha drugs. Disinfection/good hygiene
Cystitis	Primary or secondary bacterial. Urolithiasis/hypercalciuria from high dietary calcium intake predisposes	Urinary incontinence. Urine scald. Dysuria. Haematuria	Urinalysis, culture and cytology. Radiography	Antibiosis. Analgesia. Fluid therapy. Reduce calcium content of diet
Conjunctivitis	Usually *Pasteurella multocida*. Also irritants – ammonia, dust	Photophobia. Blepharospasm. Chemosis	Bacterial culture	Topical and subconjunctival antibiosis. Topical corticosteroids if irritant and no corneal ulceration

Figure 8.10 Diseases of the rabbit. (continues) ▶

Disease	Aetiology	Clinical signs	Diagnosis	Treatment
Dacryocystitis (infection of nasolacrimal duct)	*P. multocida* and other bacteria	Lacrimation. Purulent ocular discharge	Bacterial culture	Flushing of nasolacrimal ducts until clear – may be necessary over several days. Topical antibiotic instillation. Investigate for underlying tooth root elongation
Dental disease/malocclusion	Primary congenital incisor malocclusion/mandibular prognathism (esp. dwarf breeds). Acquired dental disease due to insufficient dental wear. Cheek teeth malocclusion and overgrowth can lead to secondary incisor malocclusion. Low dietary calcium intake in some rabbits	Weight loss. Ptyalism. Dehydration. Lack of grooming. Lack of caecotrophy. Facial/retrobulbar abscesses. Ocular discharge. Dacryocystitis. Incisor wear abnormalities. Palpable swellings on ventral border of mandible. Ulceration of oral mucosa, tongue, cheek, palate, lip. Deep laceration to or scarring of the tongue or cheek. Spikes on the edges of cheek tooth occlusal surfaces. Pain on palpation of maxillary zygomatic process or mandibular manipulation. Food impaction between or around the cheek teeth. Missing teeth	Dental examination. Skull radiography	Burr sharp edges/spikes. Burr crowns to correct form. Tooth extraction. Incisor removal if primary malocclusion or uncorrectable secondary malocclusion. Antibiosis. Analgesia – may be required long term. Oral meloxicam recommended. Euthanasia if severe disease
Dermatophytosis	*Trichophyton mentagrophytes. Microsporum* (rare)	Alopecia. Scaling crusting, with or without pruritus	Fungal culture	Clip surrounding hair. Topical antifungal agents, e.g. miconazole, clotrimazole for small areas. Systemic griseofulvin for widespread lesions (25 mg/kg orally sid)
Dysautonomia (degeneration of autonomic ganglia leading to gut stasis; similar to equine grass sickness)	Cause and incidence unknown	Mucoid diarrhoea. Gut stasis. Caecal impaction. Dehydration. Anorexia. Weight loss. Abdominal pain and distension. Death	Histology of mesenteric autonomic ganglia	Fluid therapy. Metoclopramide. Cisapride. Analgesia. High fibre diet. Treatment usually ineffective
Ear mites	*Psoroptes cuniculi* (non-burrowing). 3-week life cycle on host	Pruritus. Head-shaking. Self-trauma. Thick crusts in external ear canal. Lesions can spread to face and neck	Identification of mite	Ivermectin, selamectin. Acaricidal ear drops for mild infections. Soften and remove debris – care not to damage ear canal. Analgesia in severe cases
Encephalitozoonosis (very common; antibodies not protective)	*Encephalitozoon cuniculi* (intracellular microsporidian parasite). Spores shed in urine and ingested or inhaled	Target organs kidney and CNS. Infection often asymptomatic but can cause neurological signs: ataxia; torticollis; posterior paresis/paralysis (floppy rabbit syndrome); urinary incontinence; tremors; convulsions. Chronic weight loss and polyuria/polydipsia	Clinical signs. Serology. Postmortem examination	Fenbendazole may be effective in eliminating or preventing infection. Albendazole can limit sporogeny. Supportive care. Treatment often ineffective if severe neurological signs. Cleaning and disinfection of environment; quaternary ammonium compounds inactivate spores
Endometrial hyperplasia (common in unmated does)	Ageing: continuum of changes from hyperplasia to adenocarcinoma	Haematuria. Bloody vaginal discharge. Palpably enlarged uterus	Radiography. Ultrasonography. Exploratory surgery and histology	Ovariohysterectomy
Endometrial venous aneurysm (rare)		Haematuria. Blood from vulva	Exclusion of other causes of haematuria. Ultrasonography. Examination of removed uterus	Blood transfusion if severe haemorrhage. Ovariohysterectomy
Entropion	Genetic factors	Keratoconjunctivitis. Corneal ulceration	Ocular examination	Corrective surgery
Eosinophilic granuloma	Usually secondary to parasitic or other skin disease	Skin ulceration. Self-trauma. Moist dermatitis	Direct smear. Histology of skin biopsy	Address underlying cause. Corticosteroids

Figure 8.10 continued Diseases of the rabbit. (continues)   ▶

Disease	Aetiology	Clinical signs	Diagnosis	Treatment
Fleas	Rabbit flea *Spillopsylla cuniculi* (important vector for myxomatosis). *Cediopsylla simplex* and *Odontopsyllus multispinosus* in USA. Also cat flea *Ctenocephalides felis*	Often none. Pruritus	Identification of flea or flea faeces	Feline/canine pyrethrum products. AVOID fipronil spray – adverse reactions reported
Fur mites	*Cheyletiella parasitovorax*: 5-week life cycle on host but can survive off host; ZOONOSIS. *Listorophorus gibbus* not pathogenic or zoonotic. *Demodex cuniculi* rarely reported	Alopecia. Scaling. Crusting. Minimal/no pruritus	Identification of mite	Ivermectin. Treat all in-contacts and environment (can use feline/canine environmental flea products)
Glaucoma/buphthalmia	Inherited in New Zealand white: recessive *bu* gene	Enlarged globe. Corneal opacity. Non-painful	Clinical signs. Tonometry	None
Leptospirosis	*Leptospira* spp. ZOONOSIS. Rabbits can acquire disease via contact with wild rodent hosts	Polyuria/polydipsia. Depression. Anorexia. Renal failure	Serology	Penicillin – but be wary of enterotoxaemia. Fluid therapy
Lice	*Haemodipsus ventricosis*	Pruritus. Anaemia	Identification of louse/eggs	Feline/canine louse powders or ectoparasitic shampoos
Listeriosis (rare)	Listeria monocytogenes.	Head tilt/torticollis from meningoencephalitis	CSF culture. Postmortem examination	Penicillin. Tetracycline (rarely effective)
Mastitis. Bacterial: infection of mammary glands (in lactation or in pseudopregnant does). Aseptic: in intact does over 3 years old	Often *P. multocida*, *S. aureus*, *Streptococcus*	Bacterial: Depression. Pyrexia. Anorexia. Polydipsia. Swollen painful abcessated mammary glands. Septicaemia. Death. Aseptic: Non-painful. May exude brown fluid	Bacterial: Clinical signs. Bacterial culture. Aseptic: Clinical signs. Biopsy	Bacterial: Antibiosis. Supportive care. Analgesia. Drainage of abscesses. Surgical excision for severe infections. Wean young Aseptic: Benign condition. Ovariohysterectomy will resolve
Myiasis (fly strike)	Primary or secondary myiasis occurs rapidly in warm weather. Flies often attracted to accumulated caecotrophs in perineal area	Depression. Collapse. Death	Presence of fly larvae	Fluid therapy and supportive care. Sedate and remove maggots. Clip fur. Flush wounds with antiseptic solution. Systemic antibiosis. Ivermectin. Address underlying cause. Fly control for outdoor rabbits
Myxomatosis	Poxvirus spread by the rabbit flea or other biting insects	Facial and genital oedema/swelling. Blepharitis. Conjunctivitis. Ocular and nasal discharge. Pyrexia. Subcutaneous masses. Nasal scabbing only in some cases. Depression. Death	Clinical signs	Supportive care in mild cases. Euthanasia. Prevention by vaccination
Otitis externa	*Psoroptes cuniculi* (see Ear mites, above)			
Otitis media/interna	Usually ascending bacterial infection via Eustachian tube from nasopharynx. *Pasteurella multocida* common	Head tilt/torticollis	Skull radiography. Bacterial culture	Antibiosis. Bulla osteotomy usually unrewarding
Pasteurellosis	*P. multocida* extremely common inhabitant of nasal cavity and tympanic bullae. Overt disease usually follows injury or stressor, e.g. overcrowding, intercurrent disease. Spread by direct and venereal contact, aerosol (slow), fomites, vertical/perinatal	Nasal discharge. Sneezing. Conjunctivitis. Dacrocystitis. Bronchopneumonia. Head tilt/torticollis. Abscesses. Pyometra. Mastitis. Orchitis. Epidydimitis. Depression. Anorexia. Pyrexia. Death	Bacterial isolation. (Serology.) Radiography (turbinate atrophy, pneumonia, pulmonary abscesses)	Antibiosis. Fluid therapy and supportive care. Nebulization with mucolytics (e.g. bromhexine, *N*-acetylcysteine) to break up nasal secretions. *See treatment for abscesses, pyometra, mastitis, metritis, orchitis, epidydimitis*

Figure 8.10 continued Diseases of the rabbit. (continues) ▶

Disease	Aetiology	Clinical signs	Diagnosis	Treatment
Pinworm	*Passalurus ambiguus*	Usually non-pathogenic even in large numbers	Identification of adult worm/ova in faeces or tape test from perineum. Can be seen within gut during abdominal surgery	Fenbendazole 10–20 mg/kg orally repeated in 14 days
Pododermatitis	Bacterial infection (often *S. aureus*, *Streptococcus*). Secondary to poor husbandry (wet soiled bedding), obesity, inactivity, genetic factors (Rex rabbits lack guard hairs on plantar surface)	Alopecia. Erythema. Skin thickening. Lameness. Ulceration. Abscessation. Osteomyelitis	Clinical signs. Bacterial culture	Antibiosis – topical and systemic. Analgesia/NSAIDs. Bandaging. Improve husbandry. Weight reduction
Pregnancy toxaemia/hepatic lipidosis	Affects pregnant, postpartum and pseudopregnant does or obese rabbits if for any reason anorexia occurs	Depression. Incoordination. Collapse. Dyspnoea. Convulsions. Coma. Death	Clinical signs. Ketonuria. Proteinuria. Aciduria	Intravenous lactated Ringer's and 5% glucose. Corticosteroids. Assisted feeding
Rabbit syphilis/venereal spirochaetosis	*Treponema cuniculi*. Direct contact/veneral spread. Kits can be infected at birth	Ulcerative, crusting lesions around genitalia and in face and legs from autoinoculation. Secondary bacterial infection and eosinophilic granuloma formation. Symptomless carrier state	Detection of organism in direct smear (dark field background) or biopsy (silver stain)	Penicillin – but be wary of enterotoxaemia
Splayleg	Inherited disease, several genes involved	1–4 legs held adducted. Subluxation of hip in some cases	Clinical signs. Radiography	None
Spondylosis/spondylitis ankylosis/osteomyelitis of a vertebral joint	Degenerative change. Infection, usually by haematogenous spread, e.g. *Pasteurella*	Reluctance to move. Paresis. Lack of caecotrophy	Radiography	Antibiosis. Analgesia. Euthanasia
Toxoplasmosis (rare)	*Toxoplasma gondii*	Ataxia. Tremors. Paresis/paralysis	Serology	Trimethoprim/sulphonamides. AVOID clindamycin – enterotoxaemia. Prevent contact with cat faeces
Tyzzer's disease	*Clostridium piliforme*	Watery diarrhoea. Depression. Death. Can cause high morbidity and mortality in young rabbits. Chronic weight loss in older rabbits	Postmortem examination	Poor response to antibiosis. Treatment only palliative once clinical signs observed – try supportive care and tetracyclines. Prevention by good husbandry. 0.3% sodium hypochlorite kills spores
Urolithiasis/hypercalciuria	Associated with high dietary calcium intake	Haematuria. Dysuria. Abdominal pain	Radiography. Ultrasonography. Urinalysis. Uroliths (usually calcium carbonate) can occur in kidney, ureter, bladder or urethra. Common to see radiodense 'sludge' in bladder, with or without clinical signs	Bladder lavage. Cystotomy and urolith removal. Antibiosis. Lower dietary calcium content. Not possible to acidify urine
Uterine adenocarcinoma (extremely common in older unmated does; progressive uterine changes from hyperplasia to adenocarcinoma; rapidly metastasize locally and to lungs)		Haematuria. Vulval discharge. Weight loss	Abdominal palpation. Radiography. Exploratory surgery	Ovariohysterectomy. Always radiograph thorax for pulmonary metastases
Viral enteritis	Rotavirus. Coronavirus (rare)	Diarrhoea. Depression. Anorexia. Death. High morbidity/mortality in young rabbits	Viral isolation	None
Viral haemorrhagic disease	Calicivirus. Spread by direct or indirect contact (fomites)	Usually sudden death. Pyrexia. Depression. Haemorrhagic discharge from nose and mouth	Postmortem examination	None. Prevention by vaccination

Figure 8.10 continued Diseases of the rabbit.

Clinical sign	Differential diagnoses	Further investigations
Abdominal distension	Ileus and gaseous distension of bowel. Ascites. Abdominal mass. Pregnancy. Obesity	Radiography, contrast studies. Ultrasonography. Peritoneal tap. Exploratory surgery
Abdominal mass	Trichobezoars. Foreign body (esp. at sacculus rotundus). Impaction (usually caecal – right hemiabdomen). Neoplasia. Uterine hyperplasia. Pyometra. Metritis. Hydrometra. Abdominal fat. Fetus(es)	Radiography, contrast studies. Ultrasonography. Exploratory surgery
Alopecia	Cheyletiellosis. *Listrophorus* (rare). Barbering. Normal moult. Dermatophytosis	Tape test. Skin scrape. Microscopic examination of hair. Fungal culture
Anaemia	Renal disease. Any chronic disease. Lead toxicity. Uterine hyperplasia/adenocarcinoma. Uterine venous aneurysm	CBC and blood biochemistry. Radiography. Ultrasonography. Exploratory surgery
Anorexia	Dental disease. Any systemic disease, especially gastrointestinal. Pain	CBC and blood biochemistry. Dental examination. Radiography – skull and body. Ultrasonography
Ascites	Abdominal neoplasia. Hepatic coccidiosis. Liver disease. Cardiac disease. Pleural effusion disease (coronavirus – rare)	CBC and blood biochemistry. Peritoneal tap. Radiography. Ultrasonography. Liver biopsy. Faecal analysis (coccidiosis). Virology
Dermatitis	Ectoparasites. Bacterial dermatitis/'blue fur disease'. Eosinophilic granuloma. Dermatophytosis. Self-trauma. Venereal spirochaetosis. Urine scald. Viral infection. Injection site reaction	Tape test. Skin scrape. Bacterial culture. Fungal culture. Skin biopsy. Investigate urinary tract disease (see below)
Diarrhoea	Bacterial enteritis. Viral enteritis. Coccidiosis (young rabbits). Clostridial enterotoxaemia. Low fibre, high carbohydrate diet. Gastric stasis/ileus. Dysautonomia	Dietary history. Faecal analysis – culture, parasitology. Radiography/contrast studies. Postmortem examination
Dyspnoea/collapse	Any respiratory disease. Cardiac disease. Pregnancy toxaemia/hepatic lipidosis. Severe pain	Radiography. Echocardiography. ECG. Urinalysis (ketones). CBC and blood biochemistry
Facial swelling	Myxomatosis. Facial/dental abscess. Cellulitis	Vaccination/contact history. Skull radiography. Dental examination
Haematuria	False haematuria – red/brown porphyrin pigments in urine. Cystitis. Urolithiasis/hypercalciuria. Uterine hyperplasia. Uterine adenocarcinoma. Uterine venous aneurysm. Bladder polyps. Renal infarcts. Disseminated intravascular coagulopathy	Urinalysis – dipstick, culture, cytology. CBC and biochemistry. Radiography/contrast studies. Ultrasonography
Lower respiratory signs	Bacterial pneumonia (esp. pasteurellosis). Pulmonary abscess. Pleural effusion disease (rare). Pulmonary neoplasia (esp. metastases from uterine adenocarcinoma). Thymoma. Cardiac disease	Radiography. Pleural fluid analysis. Bronchoalveolar lavage. Ultrasound-guided biopsy. Echocardiography
Neurological signs	Encephalitozoonosis. Otitis media/interna. Heat stroke. Trauma. Toxoplasmosis. Listeriosis. Baylisascariasis (USA). Epilepsy (rare). Pregnancy toxaemia. Splayleg. Hypovitaminosis A, E (rare)	Radiography (skull, spine). CBC and blood biochemistry. Serology
Paresis/paralysis	Spinal trauma (fracture/luxation). Spondylosis/spondylitis. Spinal abscess. Intervertebral disc disease. Encephalitozoonosis. Toxoplasmosis	Spinal radiography. Serology
Subcutaneous mass	Abscess. Lipoma. Other neoplasia. Myxomatosis. Injection reaction	Fine needle aspiration. Biopsy. Vaccination/contact history
Testicular swelling	Orchitis. Epididymitis. Myxomatosis. Venereal spirochaetosis. Testicular neoplasia	Fine needle aspiration. Bacterial culture. Histology
Torticollis	Encephalitozoonosis. Otitis media/interna. Meningitis. Listeriosis. Toxoplasmosis. Cerebral abscess. Baylisascariasis (USA). Hypovitaminosis A (rare)	Aural examination. Skull radiography. Bacterial culture. Serology. CBC and blood biochemistry
Upper respiratory signs	Pasteurellosis. Other bacterial URT disease. High environmental ammonia. Myxomatosis. Allergic/irritant rhinitis	Bacterial culture. Skull radiography. Environmental history
Urinary incontinence/ urine scald	Cystitis. Urolithiasis/hypercalciuria. Posterior paralysis/paresis. Obesity. Renal failure. Hormone-responsive incontinence (spayed does)	Urinalysis. Radiography. Serology. CBC and blood biochemistry. Response to stilboestrol
Vaginal discharge	Pyometra. Metritis. Uterine hyperplasia/adenocarcinoma. Dystocia	Culture and cytology of discharge. Radiography. Ultrasonography. Exploratory surgery
Weight loss	Dental disease. Any infectious or metabolic disease. Neoplasia. Bullying	Dental examination. Radiography. Ultrasonography. CBC and biochemistry. Serology. Faecal sample

Figure 8.11 Differential diagnoses based on clinical signs in the rabbit.

Dental disease

The incidence of dental disease is low in rabbits with conformation similar to those in the wild. If they are permitted to behave normally, feeding on fresh and dried grasses and other herbage, dental disease is rare. Unfortunately the incidence in some rabbits, particularly extreme dwarf and lop breeds, approaches 100% whatever their diet.

Rabbits that do not spend prolonged periods chewing typically show poor jaw bone development, or atrophy at muscle insertions. This is most prominent in the area of insertion of the pterygoid (medial) and masseter (lateral) muscles into the ramus; the bone in this area may be so thin that it is transparent, or there may even be a perforation where the bone has atrophied completely.

Dentistry techniques, including grinding and extraction, are dealt with under Common surgical procedures.

Spikes

There is reduced tooth wear when rabbits eat a higher energy or poorly abrasive diet. The teeth tend to continue growing more rapidly than necessary, with elongation of the exposed and embedded parts. The natural curvature of the cheek teeth, combined with elongation and incomplete surface wear, results in the formation of 'spikes' on the lingual occlusal surface of the mandibular cheek teeth and the buccal surface of the maxillary cheek teeth (Figure 8.12). The higher growth rate of mandibular teeth accounts for the more prominent spikes seen on these.

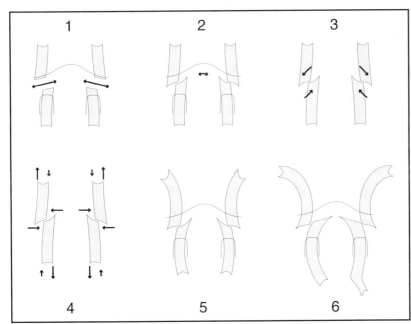

Figure 8.12 The process of cheek tooth 'spike' formation and development of apical deformities in rabbits. (1) Normal cheek teeth: chewing wears the whole occlusal surface evenly and rapidly, this being matched by tooth growth and eruption. (2) Early elongation of the exposed crown: reduced attrition and uneven wear with continued growth and eruption elongate one side of the exposed crowns. (3) Altered occlusal contact: the chewing action changes, altering the forces applied to the teeth. (4) Forces affecting the teeth: increased lateral and occlusally directed forces impede eruption affecting the apical germinal tissues, resulting in increased tooth curvature, and in extreme cases tipping of the teeth. (5) 'Root' elongation: spikes form at the occlusal surfaces interfering with chewing and further reducing attrition; increased occlusal contact reduces eruption but tooth growth continues, resulting in apical elongation and intrusion.

Tooth elongation

The most common dental disease in rabbits is that related to tooth elongation (Figure 8.13). Elongation of the cheek teeth prevents the mouth from closing fully. This separates the incisor teeth, reducing their wear until they have elongated sufficiently to compensate. Beyond a certain level of elongation, the incisors no longer function adequately and occlusal wear abnormalities become apparent.

Changes in incisor wear are also seen associated with jaw length discrepancies in some extreme dwarf and lop breeds. In these cases the problem can be detected at a very early age. When they no longer occlude, it is common for the mandibular incisors to become straighter (reduced occlusal pressure leads to a reduction in tooth curvature), preventing future correction of the problem. The maxillary incisors are not worn, but contact with the mandible maintains occlusal pressure so the tight spiral curvature of growth continues, the teeth eventually penetrating the palate or cheek if left untreated.

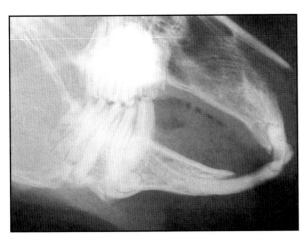

Figure 8.13 If not corrected at an early stage (before detectable apical changes have occurred) the process becomes self-perpetuating. Apical intrusion affects the germinal tissues, resulting in microscopic or, in extreme cases, gross dental dysplasia.

When detected in its earliest stages, uncomplicated tooth elongation can be corrected simply by dietary change, i.e. reduction then elimination of concentrate and processed rations and replacement with fresh and dried natural herbage.

Trauma

Traumatic injury (both accidental and iatrogenic) is a common presentation. Separation of the mandibular symphysis is more frequent than a true jaw fracture or dislocation of the temporomandibular joint. Incisor tooth fracture is quite common. In many cases this can be managed by smoothing any sharp edges and repeated trimming of occluding teeth until the fractured tooth has erupted back into function. Pulp exposure may occur associated with both dental fractures and professional trimming. If the exposure is small and the blood supply to the pulp is undamaged, it may heal unaided; however, pulpitis and pulp necrosis are common, with the formation of abscesses around the premolar tooth roots days to months later.

Abscesses

Mandibular and facial abscesses may also result from periodontal infection or mucosal damage caused by 'spikes'. Abscesses will not resolve without elimination of the cause. Unfortunately most dental abscesses result in gross changes in the surrounding tissues, including the jaw bone, so that there are residual problems even if the abscess is successfully treated. If not treated early, abscesses tend to behave as expansile masses. They can displace teeth over time and tooth roots may adapt, growing to follow the capsule (Figure 8.14).

Caries

High-carbohydrate diets, reduced attrition and arrested eruption predispose to development of caries, which may totally destroy the exposed crown and progress subgingivally, stimulating inflammatory 'root' resorption.

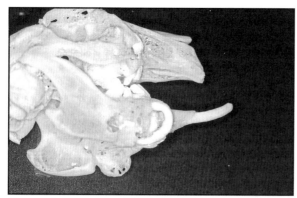

Figure 8.14 Slow expansion of a mandibular abscess has displaced the teeth, affecting the apical tissues and causing formation of an increasingly curved tooth structure which encircles the abscess.

Resorptive lesions

Resorptive lesions are also seen associated with periodontal disease and endodontic abscesses. If affected animals survive long enough, replacement resorption may eventually result in the disappearance of most of the cheek teeth. Affected rabbits often do well on a suitably processed diet, though there are continuing problems with progressive eruption of remaining non-occluding teeth.

Calcium deficiency

Once formed, the teeth are protected from resorption for systemic calcium homeostasis. Tooth formation is little affected by fluctuations in dietary calcium levels, a prolonged period of extreme deficiency being required before tooth growth and development are significantly affected. However, insufficient dietary calcium intake does appear to enhance the progression of concurrent dental resorptive lesions.

Behavioural problems

Rabbits have not been bred for positive behaviour traits and behavioural problems are common. Individual rabbits have distinct 'personalities', from timid to aggressive. In general, smaller breeds tend to be more highly strung.

Aggression is generally learned (the owner leaves the rabbit alone if it behaves aggressively). Other causes are territorial behaviour, boredom, pain, improper socialization and negative association (a previous aversive or traumatic situation). Behavioural aggression can be treated successfully in many cases with techniques similar to those used in dogs.

Does are more territorial than bucks, and as they reach sexual maturity may become aggressive towards other animals (and to their owners). Does may also bite, dig and chew flooring and household items, spray urine and mount other rabbits. If outdoors on soil, the doe may excavate deep tunnels.

Socialization of young rabbits is often overlooked. A well socialized pet rabbit will beg for treats, 'hum' and circle the owner, stand on its hindlegs and licking the owner's hands and arms. Rabbits are inquisitive and enjoy exploring. Picking up objects with the teeth and throwing them is common, as is exploratory chewing.

Supportive care

Injections

Injection sites and maximum volumes are shown in Figure 8.15.

Route	Sites	Amount
Subcutaneous	Scruff, flank	30–50 ml
Intramuscular	Quadriceps, lumbar muscles	0.5–1 ml
Intraperitoneal	Lateral to midline, lower third of abdomen	50–100 ml
Intravenous	Marginal ear vein, cephalic vein, jugular vein	
Intraosseous	Greater trochanter of femur	20 g, 1.5 inch spinal needle

Figure 8.15 Injection sites and maximum volumes in the rabbit.

Nutritional support

Assisted feeding is often necessary and should be instituted as soon as possible if the rabbit is anorexic, preferably within 24 hours. Fluid and electrolyte disturbances should be corrected before nutritional support is given (Figure 8.16).

- Daily maintenance requirements are 75–100 ml/kg/day
- Calculate dehydration as a percentage of bodyweight based on skin tenting and sunken eyes as for other mammalian species
- Use intravenous colloids if very hypotensive or hypoproteinaemic (normal serum protein is 50–71 g/l)
- Routes for fluid therapy are oral (syringe or via nasogastric tube), subcutaneous, intravenous, intraperitoneal or intraosseous (see Figure 8.15)
- If profoundly hypovolaemic, an i.v bolus of 100 ml/kg (preferably colloid) can be given over one hour
- If PCV <12% a blood transfusion can be given. Donors can give 10–15% blood volume of 65 ml/kg into acid citrate dextrose (1 part to 3.5 parts blood). Blood types are not established in the rabbit.

Figure 8.16 Fluid therapy for the rabbit.

Anorexia for 2–3 days or more has serious consequences, including gastrointestinal hypomotility and stasis, mucosal atrophy and hepatic lipidosis. Commercial enteral diets for rabbits are now available. A high fibre intake is necessary, and ground rabbit/alfalfa pellets made into a slurry can be fed via syringe. Probiotics can be added. Fresh hay, greens and the rabbit's normal diet should always be offered. Metoclopramide and cisapride are useful to stimulate gut motility.

High-fibre slurries may not pass down a nasogastric tube. In this case vegetable-based baby foods and vegetable juices are useful in the short term.

Amounts to feed vary with the type of diet selected. As a rough guide, the rabbit should be fed two or three times a day at a rate of 10–20 ml/kg bodyweight. If the calorific value of the food is known, the basal metabolic rate (BMR) can be approximated using the following equation:

$$\text{BMR (kcal/day)} = 70 \times \text{bodyweight (kg)}^{0.75} \text{ kcal/day}$$

To calculate the daily requirement, the BMR can be multiplied by illness factors of between 1.2 and 2.0, depending on the individual case.

A severely debilitated animal should not be overfed, as starvation decreases metabolic rate and the risk of inducing or worsening hepatic lipidosis is high. It is recommended to start with approximately 50% of daily requirement and increase gradually to 100% over 3–5 days.

If caecotrophy is absent or reduced, extra B vitamins can be given.

Nasogastric intubation

This is well tolerated and extremely useful for assisted feeding of anorexic animals.

1. Restrain the rabbit securely on a non-slip surface or by wrapping in a towel.
2. Place a few drops of local anaesthetic eyedrops into the nostril or place a small amount of lignocaine gel on the end of the tube.
3. Using a 5–8 French urinary catheter, measure the tube length from the nose to the caudal end of the sternum.
4. Elevate the rabbit's head and insert the tube into the ventral nasal meatus, aiming ventrally and medially.
5. As the tube approaches the back of the pharynx, flex the head so that the tube passes into the oesophagus.
6. *Always ensure correct placement by taking a radiograph*. Rabbits often do not cough if the tube passes into the trachea.
7. Suture or glue the tube to the top of the head.

Anaesthesia and analgesia

Rabbits have an unnecessary reputation for being difficult to anaesthetize. With the correct techniques, there is no reason why rabbits should not be anaesthetized safely and successfully. The main problems are their high susceptibility to stress and underlying respiratory disease.

Preoperative care

It is not necessary to fast rabbits before anaesthesia, as they are unable to vomit, but they can safely be fasted for 2–4 hours to reduce gut fill. Anaesthetic candidates are often dehydrated and hypoglycaemic (if anorexic for any reason) and this must be corrected first (see Figure 8.16). Rabbits with overt respiratory disease are a high risk, and ideally this should be treated before anaesthesia is attempted. Many pet rabbits have inapparent lung disease and damage due to *Pasteurella* infection.

Anaesthesia

Premedication is essential in rabbits as they are easily stressed. A high percentage have serum atropinesterase, so glycopyrrolate at 0.01 mg/kg s.c. can be used as an anticholinergic. Suitable premedicants are fentanyl/fluanisone, medetomidine, xylazine, acepromazine, diazepam or midazolam (Figure 8.17).

Drug	
Acepromazine	0.1– 0.5 mg/kg i.m.
Fentanyl/fluanisone	0.2–0.5 ml/kg (Hypnorm® licensed for rabbits in UK)
Medetomidine	0.25–0.5 mg/kg
Midazolam/diazepam	0.5–2.0 mg/kg (licensed for human use)
Buprenorphine	0.05–0.1 mg/kg tid
Butorphanol	0.1–0.5 mg/kg every 4 hours
Ketamine	25–50 mg/kg
Ketamine/medetomidine	15 mg/kg s.c. + 0.25 mg/kg s.c.
Ketamine/medetomidine/ butorphanol	15 mg/kg s.c. + 0.25 mg/kg s.c. + 0.4 mg/kg s.c.
Ketamine/xylazine	35 mg/kg i.m. + 5 mg/kg i.m.
Xylazine	5 mg/kg i.m.
Meloxicam	0.2 mg/kg orally sid
Ketoprofen	3 mg/kg i.m. sid–bid
Carprofen	4–5 mg/kg sid

Figure 8.17 Sedatives, analgesics and anaesthetics.

Induction using a face mask without prior use of premedication should be avoided. Rabbits hold their breath when exposed to all volatile agents, even at low concentrations, for periods up to 2 minutes. Stress releases catecholamines, and halothane sensitizes the myocardium to these, which is a lethal combination.

Fentanyl/fluanisone or another premedicant, followed by mask induction, results in a smooth onset of anaesthesia. Alternatively, an injectable combination can be used: fentanyl/fluanisone plus midazolam gives 30–40 minutes of surgical anaesthesia. Partial reversal with retention of analgesia can be achieved with buprenorphine or butorphanol.

Another good combination is medetomidine plus ketamine, to which butorphanol can also be added. The addition of butorphanol prolongs anaesthetic time from about 30 to about 80 minutes. This combination can be partially reversed with atipamezole at 1 mg/kg.

When using an injectable regimen it is prudent to administer oxygen concurrently by face mask. Rabbits are easily intubated by either direct visualization or a blind technique (see below). An Ayres T-piece circuit or Bain circuit should be used.

Intubation

Always allow the rabbit to breathe 100% oxygen for 3–4 minutes before intubation is attempted.

With all techniques, never force the tube into the larynx, as this will cause haemorrhage and oedema.

Direct visualization

1. Place the anaesthetized rabbit in dorsal recumbency. Extend the neck. Grasp the tongue gently, retract and hold to one side.

2. Visualize the larynx using a Wisconsin size 1 laryngoscope and insert a 2.5–3 mm endotracheal tube.

Alternatively:

1. Place the anaesthetized rabbit in sternal recumbency. Grasp the back of the head and extend the neck so that the nose is pointing vertically.
2. Visualize the larynx using an otoscope.
3. Place the introducer into the larynx through the otoscope.
4. Remove the otoscope and introduce the endotracheal tube gently over the introducer.
5. Remove the introducer.

Blind technique

1. Hold the anaesthetized rabbit in sternal recumbency with head and neck extended vertically.
2. Pass the endotracheal tube over the tongue and advance it until exhalation is heard loudly (place end of tube to the ear), or until presence of condensation at each breath is observed if using a clear tube.
3. Advance the tube gently as the rabbit inhales, and the tub will pass into the trachea.

Monitoring

Depth of anaesthesia should be monitored by use of the ear pinch. Standard monitoring equipment (ECG, pulse oximeter) should be used wherever possible. Eye position is not useful in the rabbit, and the palpebral reflex is not lost until the animal is dangerously deep.

Postoperative care

This is as for any other species.

- Rabbits should be kept warm but not over-hot
- Handling should be minimized during the recovery period
- Continued fluid therapy may be necessary, and the rabbit should be monitored closely until it is eating again. Force feeding may be required
- After intra-abdominal surgery, gut stasis can be a problem and the use of metoclopramide and/or cisapride is indicated.

Analgesia

Alleviation of postoperative pain is essential, and very important in encouraging the animal to eat and drink again. Buprenorphine and butorphanol (see Figure 8.17) are useful opioid agents and will reverse the respiratory and cardiovascular depressant effects of fentanyl while maintaining analgesia. The NSAID carprofen is also highly effective.

Common surgical procedures

Special considerations

Suture material often provokes a marked caseous and suppurative inflammatory response in rabbits. Modern monofilament absorbable suture materials are preferable to catgut for this reason. Subcuticular sutures for skin closure are recommended, as skin sutures are invariably chewed and Elizabethan collars poorly tolerated. Alternatively, tissue glue or skin staples can be used.

Rabbits are very prone to the formation of intra-abdominal adhesions and great care must be taken not to damage, desiccate or irritate abdominal organs. Verapamil (a calcium channel blocker) is reported to be of use in the prevention of adhesion formation (200 µg/kg orally or slowly i.v. at surgery and then every 8 hours for up to nine doses).

Dentistry

Grinding

Established tooth overgrowth may be helped by repeating mechanical tooth grinding at intervals of 4–6 weeks. Radiographic assessment of tooth roots is essential in all cases before undertaking treatment.

Trimming incisors: In the unlikely event that problems are restricted to the incisor teeth, these can easily be trimmed back to a normal length and shape or, if repeated treatment is needed, extracted. Incisor trimming can be performed without difficulty in conscious animals using either high- or low-speed dental equipment. A high-speed cutting burr rotating at 200,000–400,000 times a second will cut the teeth with minimal effort. Low-speed burrs or the more dangerous diamond disc can be used but they are less efficient.

Under no circumstances should teeth be clipped, as this leaves sharp edges and longitudinal cracks in the teeth and will often expose the pulp. Clipping also releases a considerable amount of energy into the tooth, concussing the pulp, and damages the pulp, periodontal and periapical tissues.

Grinding cheek teeth: It is possible to grind down elongated cheek tooth crowns but this requires general anaesthesia. As oral access is limited, even when using mouth gags and cheek dilators, a straight low-speed dental handpiece fitted with a soft-tissue protector and an extra long shanked burr is required. There is no point in simply removing sharp edges or 'points', as this does not address the main problem – tooth elongation. By taking the exposed crowns down to the correct height, the spikes will also be removed and the teeth will start erupting again, provided there are minimal apical changes.

Rasps are unsuitable for use on the teeth as they apply too much force, often tearing the periodontal ligament and on occasion ripping teeth out of the jaw.

Chewing efficiency is greatly reduced by coronal reduction of the cheek teeth as it temporarily removes the transverse occlusal ridging and also because it takes some time for the jaw muscles to recover their ability to contract fully. By the time the muscles have recovered, the teeth may have erupted back to their pre-treatment length and so repeated treatment is often necessary.

Caries: Early caries lesions may be eliminated by burring away the affected tissue but they will reform unless the diet is corrected. Also, the coronal reduction may result in abnormal wear of opposing teeth.

Periodontal treatment
Periodontal pockets deeper than 3 mm are difficult to clean in rabbits. Standard subgingival curettes may be used but small dental excavators are often more effective. Deeper pocketing is usually associated with abscessation, in which case the tooth will need extracting. This will also result in abnormal wear of opposing teeth.

Extraction
Extraction of healthy rabbit teeth is straightforward but diseased teeth are generally elongated with deformed roots (see Figures 8.12 and 8.13), complicating extraction. Provided the embedded tooth structure has remained relatively normal, the periodontal ligament can be sectioned and torn, using commercial or custom-made instruments with a standard luxation technique. Once loosened, the tooth should be intruded into its alveolus and manipulated to help to destroy any remaining germinal tissue prior to removal. The pulp should remain in the extracted tooth. If not, the germinal tissues are probably intact and should be actively curetted using a sterile instrument. If the germinal tissues are left intact the tooth will regrow, possibly as a normal tooth but more likely with gross deformity, in some cases forming a pseudo-odontoma within the jaw bone.

Castration
Castration will prevent aggression, urine spraying in the house and unwanted litters. The testicles descend into the scrotum at about 3–4 months of age. The procedure is simple: a scrotal skin incision is made and the skin is peeled back away from the tunic; then a closed technique with a transfixing suture is placed above the testicle. Alternatively an open technique can be used. The tunic should be stitched. A large fat pad in the inguinal canal usually prevents herniation of abdominal contents but this should not be relied on.

Ovariohysterectomy
Routine ovariohysterectomy of young female rabbits at about 6 months of age will prevent aggression and territorial behaviour; it will also prevent uterine hyperplasia and adenocarcinoma in later life. A ventral midline approach should be made. The mesometrium is the principal site of fat storage in the doe, which can make identification and ligation of blood vessels difficult. The uterus is often quite friable, especially if the doe is pseudopregnant, and uterine vessels should be ligated. There are often several ovarian vessels to ligate, but these are usually small. A single transfixing suture should be placed just caudal to the two cervices.

Abscesses
Complete surgical removal of abscesses is the treatment of choice wherever possible. The thick capsule must be removed in its entirety. If this is not possible, aggressive surgical debridement should be attempted. The use of antibiotic-impregnated methyl methacrylate has been reported to be of use in the treatment of bony abscesses and osteomyelitis but calcium hydroxide can be associated with severe tissue damage. Injection of gentamicin into the capsule wall has also been reported to be effective.

Drug formulary

Drug	Dose
Antibacterials	
Cephalexin	11–22 mg/kg (may cause enteritis)
Doxycycline	2.5 mg/kg bid
Enrofloxacin	5–10 mg/kg bid (Baytril licensed for rabbits in UK)
Fusidic acid ophthalmic drops	1 drop sid or bid for staphylococcal infections (Fucithalmic Vet licensed for rabbits in UK)
Gentamicin ophthalmic solution	1 or 2 drops tid (Tiacil licensed for rabbits in UK)
Metronidazole	20 mg/kg bid
Penicillin	40,000 IU/kg every 7 days for rabbit syphilis
Sulphadimethoxine	15 mg/kg orally bid for 10 days (coccidiosis)
Trimethoprim/sulphadiazine	30 mg/kg bid
Antiparasitics	
Albendazole	15 mg/kg sid
Fenbendazole	10–20 mg/kg orally every 2 weeks, 10–20 mg/kg orally daily for *Encephalitozoon cuniculi*
Ivermectin	0.2–0.4 mg/kg every 7–14 days
Miscellaneous	
Barium	10–14 ml/kg orally (GI studies)
Cholestyramine	2 g orally sid (human licence)
Cisapride	0.5 mg/kg bid (human licence)
Dexamethasone	2–4 mg/kg s.c., i.v. (shock); 0.2 mg/kg s.c., i.m. (anti-inflammatory)
Glycopyrrolate	0.01–0.02 mg/kg s.c. (human licence)
Metaclopramide	0.2–0.5 mg/kg bid
Oxytocin	0.1–3.0 IU/kg
Stilboestrol	0.5 mg 1 or 2 times a week

Figure 8.18 Drug formulary for the rabbit. All drugs are licensed for veterinary use unless otherwise stated.

References and further reading

Brown SA (1993) Incisor removal in the rabbit. *Proceedings of the North American Veterinary Conference 1993*, pp.791–792

Bryer LW (1957) An experimental evaluation of the physiology of tooth eruption. *International Dental Journal* **7**, 432–478

Burling K, Murphy CJ, da Silva Curiel J, Koblik P and Bellhorn RW (1991) Anatomy of the rabbit nasolacrimal duct and its clinical implications. *Progress in Veterinary and Comparative Ophthalmology* **1**, 33–40

Carpenter JW, Mashima TY and Rupiper DJ (1996) *Exotic Animal Formulary*. Greystone Publications, Manhattan, Kansas

Crossley DA (1995) Clinical aspects of lagomorph dental anatomy: the rabbit (*Oryctolagus cuniculus*). *Journal of Veterinary Dentistry* **4**, 131–135

Flecknell P (1996) *Laboratory Animal Anaesthesia, 2nd edn.* Academic Press, London

Flecknell P (2000) *Manual of Rabbit Medicine and Surgery*. BSAVA Publications, Gloucester

Harcourt-Brown FM (1995) A review of clinical conditions in pet rabbits associated with their teeth. *Veterinary Record*, **137**, 341–346

Harkness JE and Wagner JE. (1995) *The Biology and Medicine of Rabbits and Rodents, 4th edn.* Lea & Febiger, Philadelphia

Hillyer EV (1994) Pet rabbits. In: *Exotic Pet Medicine II. Veterinary Clinics of North America: Small Animal Practice* **24**(1) 25–66

Hillyer and Quesenberry (1997) *Ferrets, Rabbits and Rodents. Clinical Medicine and Surgery*. WB Saunders, Philadelphia

Kertesz, P (1993) Dental diseases and their treatments in captive wild animals. In: *A Colour Atlas of Veterinary Dentistry and Oral Surgery*. Wolfe Publishing, London

Laber-Laird K, Swindle MM and Flecknell P (1996) *Handbook of Rodent and Rabbit Medicine*. Pergamon, Oxford

Lobprise HB and Wiggs RB (1991) Dental and oral disease in lagomorphs. *Journal of Veterinary Dentistry*, **8(2)**, 11–17

Okerman L (1994) *Diseases of Domestic Rabbits, 2nd edn.* Blackwell Scientific, Oxford

Paul-Murphy J and Ramer JC (1998) Urgent care of the pet rabbit. In: *Critical Care. Veterinary Clinics of North America: Exotic Animal Practice* **1**(1), 127–152

Ramer JC, Paul-Murphy J and Benson KG (1999). Evaluating and stabilising critically ill rabbits. Parts I and II. *Compendium on Continuing Education for the Practicing Veterinarian* **21**, 30–40 and 116–125

Steenkamp G and Crossley DA (1999) Incisor tooth regrowth in a rabbit following complete extraction. *Veterinary Record* **145**, 585–586

Swartout MS and Gerken DF (1987) Lead-induced toxicosis in two domestic rabbits. *Journal of the American Veterinary Medical Association* **191**, 717–719

Suter C, Muller-Doblies UU, Hatt J-M, *et al.* (2001) Prevention and treatment of *Encephalitozoon cuniculi* infection in rabbits with fenbendazole. *Veterinary Record* **148**, 478–480

Wiggs RB and Lobprise HB (1995) Dentistry in pet lagomorphs and rodents. In: *Manual of Small Animal Dentistry, 2nd edn*, ed. DA Crossley and S Penman, pp. 68–92. BSAVA Publications, Cheltenham

Wiggs RB and Lobprise HB (1997) Diseases in rodents and lagomorphs. In: *Veterinary Dentistry, Principles and Practice*, ed. RB Wiggs and HB Lobprise, pp. 518–537. Lippincott-Raven, Philadelphia

9

Ferrets

Nico J. Schoemaker

Introduction

Ferrets are kept for many purposes, particularly hunting. Besides hunting rabbits in the field, ferrets can be used to control rat populations in areas where shooting is too risky, e.g. in buildings. The latter was the original reason why ferrets were taken to the USA, though there are now many states where 'working' is not allowed. Ferrets are increasingly being kept as pets.

Many people believe that the ferret *Mustela putorius furo* should not be kept in captivity. This animal, however, can be considered a domesticated creature of which no wild counterpart exists. Its closest relatives in the wild are the European polecat *Mustela putorius* and possibly the Steppe polecat *M. eversmanni*. Aristophanes (c. 450 BC) was probably the first to describe an animal which may have been a ferret in one of his comedies. In the literature from 2000 years ago both Strabo and Pliny describe the use of ferrets for hunting rabbits (Thomson, 1951).

Biology

The ferret is a carnivore with an average bodyweight of 1200 grams in hobs (males) and 600 grams in jills (females). Chapter 1 discusses ferret anatomy and physiology and there is a good overview in Fox (1998).

Although most of the ferret's biological features can be compared with the other pet carnivores, there are some differences. Compared with the cat, the ferret's reproductive season is even more influenced by the length of the day. In order to ovulate, jills need vaginal stimulation and they also need to be dragged around by the male. The lifespan is a little shorter than that of the dog and cat, but much longer than for most other small mammal pets. Figure 9.1 gives an overview of most of the biological data of the ferret.

Husbandry

Housing
The size of a ferret cage is not important as long as the owners regularly let their animals play, under supervision, outside the cage. Most importantly it should be well built, as ferrets are good at escaping. It should be high enough to allow the ferret to stand on its

Life expectancy	8–10 years (max. 15 years)
Average bodyweight hob	1200 g
Average bodyweight jill	600 g
Sexual maturity	First spring (March) after birth
Breeding season (Northern hemisphere)	March–September
Breeding season (Southern hemisphere)	August–January
Gestation period	41–42 days
Average litter size	8
Weight at birth	8–10 g
Eyes open at age	4–5 weeks
Eruption of deciduous teeth	3–4 weeks
Eruption of permanent teeth	7–10 weeks
Weaning age	6–8 (preferably 8) weeks
Heart rate	200–250 beats per minute
Respiratory rate	33–36 breaths per minute
Rectal temperature	38.8°C (range 37.8–40°C)

Figure 9.1 Biological data for ferrets.

hindlegs to investigate its surroundings, and it should be big enough to provide a sleeping area (nest box), a litter box, a feeding area and some room to play. Mesh or solid materials can be used for the bottom of the cage. In cages with solid bottoms litter boxes should be placed away from the food and water and sleeping area. Water can be provided in either a bowl or a bottle. Most owners prefer bottles because ferrets tend to play with bowls and make a mess. Bottles should be thoroughly cleaned and refilled daily. Food can be provided in a bowl attached to the cage or in a bowl heavy enough to prevent the ferret from tipping it up. The sleeping area should be some kind of box for them to hide in. Cloths, towels or old T-shirts can be used for bedding material. Hay, straw and wood shavings are not recommended as inhalation of dust may lead to chronic irritation of the upper respiratory tract (Jenkins and Brown, 1993). Ferrets can be housed either inside or outside. When housed outdoors ferrets should be provided with protection against the elements. The resting area should be dry and clean and give them enough insulation against freezing conditions.

Under supervision ferrets can be kept with dogs and cats but not with rabbits or rodents.

Diet

The ferret is a carnivore and can therefore be maintained on a good quality high protein diet. The fat content can vary from 9% to 28%, but both the carbohydrate and fibre fraction should be low. Specific ferret diets as well as good quality cat diets, commercially available in the past decade, are suitable for ferrets. Some ferrets fed specific diets seem to have firmer stools that smell less strongly. Although ferrets can be fed canned products, dry pellets are preferred. These stay fresh longer and seem to decrease the amount of dental calculi formed. Fresh water should be available, especially when pellets are fed. Because ferrets have a short gut and a fast gut transit time they should be fed *ad libitum*. Ferrets may also be fed the traditional and more natural diet of whole rodents or rabbits [Editor].

Handling and restraint

Most pet ferrets are used to being handled, so the risk of being bitten is no greater than with a cat or dog. Ferrets should be picked up by placing one hand around the thorax and supporting the hindlegs with the other hand (Figure 9.2). Ferrets struggle if their hindlegs are held too firmly. If struggling is excessive the neck should be gripped more firmly. Scruffing of the loose skin at the back of the neck may be necessary for restraining difficult ferrets. Ferrets can be distracted by applying a liquid diet to the abdomen; most owners can manage to clip the nails of their pets while they are licking the food.

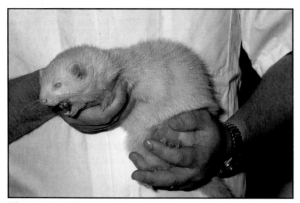

Figure 9.2 Gentle restraint around the neck, with support of the hindlegs, is usually sufficient to carry a ferret.

Diagnostic approach

Physical examination

Physical examination of the ferret is basically similar to that of the dog and cat. Some features, such as the peripheral pulse, however, are almost impossible to check.

As with any consultation a thorough case history is mandatory. Alertness and attitude should then be assessed. In the carrier the ferret may appear quite sleepy, but once out of the carrier it should be highly active. Ferrets normally arch their backs when they walk or run.

Handling of the ferret may alter its body temperature, heart rate and respiratory frequency. The author prefers to measure respiratory rate prior to handling. Heart rate measurement necessitates handing. The rectal temperature can then be measured, preferably with a digital thermometer. Reference values can be found in Figure 9.1.

Checking the hydration status of any small mammal is one of the most important features of a physical examination, and can be performed by assessing: the skin turgor of the upper eyelids; skin tenting in the neck; and the moistness of the oral mucosa. While checking the oral mucosa, attention should also be paid to the teeth, which should be free from tartar.

Since ferrets often have ear mites, special attention should be paid to the external ear canals. The neck, axillary, inguinal and popliteal lymph nodes should be checked. They may appear enlarged in overweight animals. If they are also firm, a fine needle aspirate should be taken to check for lymphoma. Both auscultation of the thorax as well as an abdominal palpation are finally included in the standard physical examination. An enlarged spleen is a common finding on palpation.

Sample collection

Blood

As a general rule blood comprising 1% of the bodyweight of a healthy ferret can be collected, although usually far less is necessary. Most laboratories can do haematology and full biochemical analysis with 2 ml of blood.

Techniques for bleeding, such as toenail clipping and cardiac or periorbital puncture, should be considered obsolete today. Much better locations are the lateral saphenous vein or cephalic vein for small amounts of blood (up to 1 ml) and the jugular vein or the cranial vena cava for larger amounts. The author prefers a 26 gauge needle and a 2 ml or 5 ml syringe for drawing blood. The jugular vein is approached as for cats and can be performed in docile ferrets without anaesthesia (Figure 9.3). The cranial vena cava approach is best performed under isoflurane anaesthesia, although this is not necessary in debilitated ferrets. Isoflurane anaesthesia can artificially lower the red blood cell count and PCV by up to 40%. Changes in plasma protein and the white blood cell count are not seen. Red cell changes return to normal after approximately 45 minutes of anaesthesia [Editor].

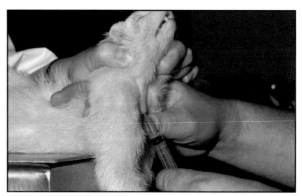

Figure 9.3 In docile ferrets blood may be collected from the jugular vein in a manner similar to that in cats and dogs.

No premedication is necessary. The ferret should be placed in dorsal recumbency and the needle inserted into the thoracic inlet just cranial to the connection between the manubrium and the first rib and then directed towards the contralateral hindleg at a 30 degree angle (Figure 9.4). As the heart is located relatively caudally within the thoracic cavity and the needle is only 1.2 cm long, there is no risk of cardiac puncture from this technique.

Figure 9.5 shows reference ranges for haematological and biochemical parameters.

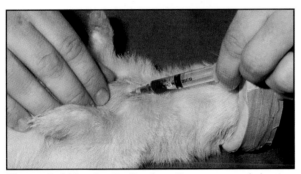

Figure 9.4 Blood collection from the vena cava is best performed in an anaesthetized ferret.

Parameter (SI units)	Range	Mean
WBC (x 10⁹/l)	2–10	5.7
PCV (%)	36–53	47.3
Heterophils (%)	13–48	28.2
Lymphocytes (%)	40–82	53.8
Monocytes (%)	7–9	6.9
Eosinophils (%)	2–8	5.02
Basophils (%)	0–3	1
Blood urea nitrogen (mmol/l)	0.2–16.1	10.4
Creatinine (μmol/l)	8.8–106	53
Alkaline phosphatase (IU/l)	14–144	41
Alanine aminotranferase (IU/l)	48–292	138
Aspartate aminotransferase (IU/l)	46–118	68.3
Lactate dehydrogenase (IU/l)	222–377	278
Bile acids (μmol/l)	1–28	9.1
Creatine kinase (IU/l)	98–564	245
Glucose (mmol/l)	6.66–7.99	6.69
Calcium (mmol/l)	1.9–2.4	2.04
Total protein (g/l)	43–60	52
Albumin (g/l)	34–48	39
Globulins (g/l)	2–24	13

Figure 9.5 Reference ranges for haematological and biochemical parameters in the ferret. Data from Fudge (2000).

Common conditions

Viral diseases

Canine distemper
On a worldwide basis canine distemper (caused by a paramyxovirus) is the most serious viral infection of ferrets and is almost always fatal. The disease is seldom seen in ferrets nowadays owing to vaccination.

The classic symptoms are dermatitis on the lips and chin and around the inguinal region, 7–9 days after infection. Other common signs are mucopurulent ocular and nasal discharge, pyrexia (over 40°C), sneezing, coughing and anorexia. Just as in dogs, ferrets can develop hyperkeratosis of the footpads (hardpad).

Diagnosis is based on fluorescent antibody tests on conjunctival smears and/or brain tissue. As vaccination is performed with a modified live virus, vaccinated ferrets give a positive result with this test and therefore only non-vaccinated ferrets should be tested.

The USA is the only country with a registered canine distemper vaccine (Fervac-D, United Vaccines, Madison, WI) available for use in ferrets. Some veterinary surgeons have reported adverse reactions to this vaccine. Standard modified live vaccines developed for use in dogs can be used provided they are derived from non-ferret cell lines, as ferrets subjected to these can develop distemper from the vaccine. Manufacturers will provide veterinarians with data on the use of their products in ferrets. Many of these products have been used safely in hundreds of ferrets.

Influenza
Ferrets are highly susceptible to several strains of human influenza virus and therefore influenza should be considered a zoonosis. Humans can infect ferrets and *vice versa*. Veterinarians or staff with minor symptoms of influenza either should not treat ferrets or should wear a mask to prevent the spread of the virus.

Many of the symptoms of influenza are similar to those of canine distemper but less severe. Nasal discharge is mucoserous instead of mucopurulent, there is more sneezing and coughing and the fever is usually over before the animal is presented to the veterinary surgeon. Just as in humans, the infection is self-limiting and usually not fatal.

Aleutian disease
Aleutian disease is caused by a parvovirus, unrelated to that causing bloody diarrhoea in dogs. Of the Mustelidae the mink is the most susceptible, but a ferret-specific strain has been found (Porter *et al.*, 1982). As no vaccine is available to prevent infection, mink farms routinely check their animals for antibodies. Aleutian disease is considered more of a problem in the UK than elsewhere. Although infection has been suspected several times in the Netherlands, the diagnosis was only confirmed once. Aleutian disease has been diagnosed in ferrets in the USA, and screening of 500 clinically normal ferrets housed in shelters in northern America resulted in the detection of antibodies against Aleutian disease in about 10% of the animals.

Aleutian disease is an immune complex-mediated condition, resulting in multiple organ failure. Clinical signs in mink include wasting, hepatomegaly, splenomegaly, melaena, recurrent fevers and eventually hindleg paralysis and other neurological signs. Most mink die within 5 months of infection. Ferrets seldom develop such severe symptoms. Although serum countercurrent immunoelectrophoresis is necessary to confirm the diagnosis, a hypergammaglobulinaemia together with chronic wasting signs suggests Aleutian disease (Figure 9.6).

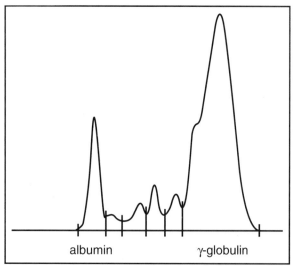

albumin   γ-globulin

Figure 9.6 Protein electrophoresis of a blood sample from a ferret with Aleutian disease. Note the extremely high concentration of gamma-globulin.

As with almost all viral infections there is no specific treatment, but antibiotics and steroids have been reported to give some relief.

Parasitic infestations

Ear mites

The ear mite *Otodectes cynotis* is the most common ectoparasite found on ferrets (Figure 9.7). Massive infestations can cause pruritus, but many ferrets have low-grade infestations without showing many signs. Mites may be seen during a routine otoscopic examination but can also be easily overlooked. The best diagnostic technique is to place a sample scraped from the ear canal on to a microscope slide with potassium hydroxide (KOH). The mites can be seen moving around.

Reports of treatment with subcutaneous injections of ivermectin have shown it to be ineffective and in some instances tissue necrosis has occurred. Application of ivermectin or fipronil drops within the ear canals seems to work well. Recent trials with the topical application of selamectin at the base of the skull have shown promising results. Although no side effects have been reported in ferrets with either fipronil or selamectin, these drugs are not registered for use in ferrets. An advantage of topical selamectin is that it does not need to be administered within the ear canal and there is therefore no risk of an ototoxic effect if the eardrum is not intact.

Fleas (*Ctenocephalides felis*)

Ferrets are just as sensitive to flea infestations as are dogs and cats and the clinical manifestations are similar, although the author has never seen or heard of flea allergy in ferrets. Just as in dogs and cats, treatment of the environment is just as, if not more, important than treatment of the ferret alone. Sprays used on dogs or cats are suitable. Owners who regularly wash their ferrets use a flea shampoo containing permethrin for this purpose. Fipronil or selamectin can also be used for flea control.

Worms

Usually ferrets are free of gastrointestinal parasites. Routine deworming is therefore not recommended. If worm eggs are found in the faeces, ivermectin (0.2 mg/kg i.m.) can be given. The new avermectin, selamectin, can also be used for endoparasitic infestations. Therefore this drug can be used in young animals for the combined control of ear mite and possible worm infestations.

Endocrine disease

Persistent oestrus

Female ferrets (jills) are seasonal breeders and come into oestrus under the influence of light. Day lengths exceeding 12 hours induce oestrus, which continues until the day lengths decrease again to less than 12 hours. Therefore under natural light conditions the oestrous season is approximately from March until September. A firm stimulant, in the form of dragging by the scruff of the neck and mating, is necessary for ovulation. If the jill is not mated, she will not ovulate, as ferrets are induced ovulators. This results in increased oestradiol levels. Oestradiol levels remain high until the end of the oestrous season. Continued high levels of oestradiol can lead to alopecia (Figure 9.8) and bone marrow suppression, resulting in a

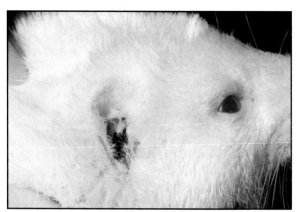

Figure 9.7 Ferrets with ear mite infestations have a crusty black secretion in the outer ear canal.

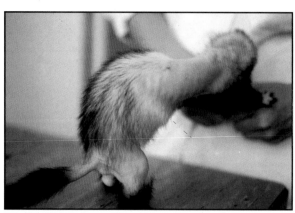

Figure 9.8 Ferrets with persistent oestrus show symmetrical alopecia and swelling of the vulva.

pancytopenia and eventual death. Some ferrets show this pancytopenia within the first oestrous season. The best preventive measure is neutering the ferret within its first year before the oestrous season has begun (usually January and February). Alternatively, proligestone (50 mg/kg i.m.) can be given.

Insulinoma

Insulinomas, small tumours of the pancreatic beta cells resulting in hypoglycaemia, are a common finding in ferrets. Insulinomas are equally distributed among the sexes, and animals are affected at a median age of 5 years (range 2–8 years). Symptoms vary from slight incoordination and weakness in the hindlimbs to complete collapse and coma. Episodes of salivation and a glazed look may be noticed by owners. These are most often seen when the ferret has not eaten for some time. They do not usually last long and clear up when the ferret is given food or a calorie-rich beverage. Insulinomas are commonly found incidentally during surgery for other conditions such as hyperadrenocorticism. Diagnosis is usually based on serum glucose levels lower than 3.4 mmol/l (60 mg/dl). When plasma insulin levels are measured they are usually increased, although this is not always the case.

Surgery is the best treatment option, as this removes the excess insulin. Tumours are, however, small (5–7 mm) and sometimes difficult to remove (Figure 9.9); they may be undetectable at surgery. Diabetes mellitus can occur if too much pancreas is removed. This should be avoided as the medical management of insulinomas is far easier than that of diabetes mellitus. Although adenocarcinomas of the pancreas have been reported, most insulinomas are benign. If an owner refuses surgery, diazoxide (5–30 mg/kg bid orally), an insulin inhibiting agent, or prednisolone (0.2–1 mg/kg sid orally) may be prescribed. The author prefers diazoxide because this agent has the most specific effect.

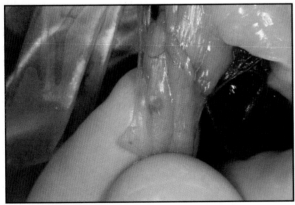

Figure 9.9 Insulinomas are usually no bigger than 3 mm in diameter.

Prognosis is considered better in ferrets than in dogs. Metastases are seldom found in ferrets in the Netherlands whereas insulinomas almost always metastasize in dogs. A literature survey (unpublished data) revealed that insulinomas have already metastasized in 46% of cases by the time of surgery. Although metastases are rare in ferrets, multiple tumours and recurrent signs are common. Recurrent signs are probably due to the development of new tumours rather than to metastasis of the earlier tumour. Animals remain disease-free for about 10 months after surgery, and the average survival time is 1.5 years.

Hyperadrenocorticism

Although hyperadrenocorticism is now considered one of the most common diseases in ferrets, it was first reported as recently as 1987 (Fox et al., 1987). Since that time a lot of research has been done, especially in the USA. Results have shown that hyperadrenocorticism in ferrets is different from that in dogs, cats and humans. In the latter groups increased plasma cortisol levels are characteristic of Cushing's disease, whereas in ferrets androstenedione, 17-hydroxyprogesterone and oestradiol plasma concentrations are increased but not cortisol.

Researchers in the USA have hypothesized that adrenal tumours may develop in ferrets due to early neutering. This theory is based on reports of adrenal tumours developing in certain strains of mice after early castration. Ferrets are commonly neutered in the USA at 6 weeks of age. Because hyperadrenocorticism is common in the Netherlands and ferrets there are neutered at a much older age (>6 months), the author does not believe that the neutering has to occur at an early age for the tumour to develop. It is, however, likely that neutering does play a part in the aetiology of hyperadrenocorticism. A temporal correlation has been found between the time of neutering and the time of hyperadrenocorticism being diagnosed (Schoemaker et al., 2000). Also reports from the USA show that the gonadotrophin-releasing hormone (GnRH)-analogue leuprolide acetate can control the signs of hyperadrenocorticism. Large-scale research on this subject is ongoing. It is hypothesized that the negative feedback of testosterone and oestradiol on hypothalamic GnRH is lost due to castration. This results in an uninhibited secretion of GnRH followed by the secretion of luteinizing hormone and follicle-stimulating hormone. These hormones, together or separately, continuously stimulate the adrenal glands, resulting in hyperplasia and tumour formation.

The most prominent signs of hyperadrenocorticism in ferrets are symmetrical alopecia (Figure 9.10), vulvar swelling in neutered jills, and pruritus of unknown origin. No sex predilection could be found in a study in the Netherlands. Diagnosis is based on clinical signs, ultrasonography and surgery of the adrenal gland followed by histological confirmation. In the USA a serum adrenal panel is performed at the University of Tennessee. This panel consists of androstenedione, oestradiol, 17-hydroxyprogesterone and dehydroepiandrosterone sulphate. An increase in one or more of these hormones is considered diagnostic for hyperadrenocorticism. In the author's

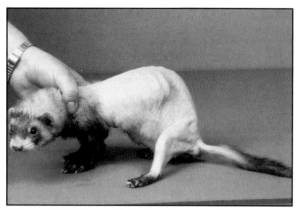

Figure 9.10 Symmetrical alopecia is a typical presentation in ferrets with hyperadrenocorticism.

opinion androstenedione is the most sensitive indicator of these hormones. The most likely differential diagnosis is a non-ovariectomized jill or remnant ovaries, which cannot be differentiated by using the hormone panel.

Surgery is the treatment of choice: the left adrenal gland can be fairly easily removed whereas the right adrenal gland is attached to the caudal vena cava, making resection difficult. Bilateral tumours may occur, resulting in a treatment dilemma. Usually in such cases all of the left adrenal gland and part of the right adrenal gland are removed. Some veterinary surgeons remove both adrenal glands and supplement the ferrets postoperatively in a manner similar to that for dogs.

Many pathologists classify the tumours into three categories: hyperplasia, adenoma or carcinoma. This classification, however, is subjective. Differentiation between hyperplasia and adenoma is a functional differentiation. Only hyperplasia can return to normal function whereas adenoma cannot. Carcinoma suggests the potential for metastasis, although this hardly ever occurs. Tumours that do metastasize have a totally different aspect (Figure 9.11).

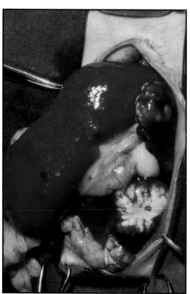

Figure 9.11 The large white masses in this ferret proved to be metastasized adrenal tumours. Note the large spleen, which is commonly found in ferrets.

Diabetes mellitus

Diabetes mellitus has been documented in ferrets but is considered rare. It is most often seen after debulking of the pancreas for the removal of insulinomas. Clinical signs are identical to those in dogs and cats, with polyuria and polydipsia the most prominent signs. Plasma glucose concentrations above 22 mmol/l are considered suspicious for diabetes mellitus. Regulation has been attempted, starting with 0.1 IU of insulin twice daily (Hillyer and Quesenberry, 1997).

Cardiovascular disease

Congestive cardiomyopathy is a common cardiac disease of ferrets. Clinical signs are often non-specific and include lethargy and dyspnoea. Physical examination may reveal tachycardia, a systolic murmur and muffled heart sounds. Both pleural effusion and ascites can be seen with cardiomyopathy. Ultrasonography is the best diagnostic technique, showing results similar to other species (increased ventricular dimensions, decreased fractional shortening and enlarged left atrium).

Treatment is similar to that for other species. When ascites or pleural effusion is present frusemide (2–4 mg/kg bid) is indicated. Although some veterinarians prefer to remove these fluids, severe hypotension may occur, and much protein is lost. Therefore only a small amount of fluid should be removed to improve respiration. To improve cardiac function either digoxin (0.01 mg/kg sid–tid) or enalapril (0.5 mg/kg sid) can be given.

Lymphoma

Lymphomas are the third most common tumours found in ferrets after insulinomas and tumours of the adrenal glands. Lymphomas occur in both juvenile and adult ferrets. The disease is much more aggressive in juveniles than it is in adults. Preliminary data suggest that the juvenile form may be caused by a virus (Erdman *et al.*, 1995).

Symptoms are often non-specific and may include loss of appetite, weight loss and enlargement of the peripheral lymph nodes. These symptoms may wax and wane for years. More severe symptoms, as seen in juvenile ferrets, may include dyspnoea and coughing caused by pleural effusion.

An absolute lymphocyte count of 3.5×10^9/l or more or a relative count greater than 60% of the total white blood cell count is suggestive of lymphoma. Lymphoblastic leukaemias have also been diagnosed in ferrets. Although radiography can detect pleural effusion and masses in the anterior mediastinum, ultrasonography is more precise for diagnosing individual masses and can also detect masses in the abdomen. Ultrasonography is also useful as a guiding tool for taking samples by fine-needle aspiration biopsy. These samples are essential for confirming the diagnosis, but false negative results (reactive lymph node) do occur. A full thickness biopsy or surgical removal of enlarged external lymph nodes is therefore recommended.

Lymphomas of juvenile and young adult ferrets are often immunoblastic with a high mitotic index, whereas those of adults are mixed cell lymphomas with a much lower mitotic index.

Because symptoms wax and wane the most effective treatment is difficult to determine. Initially ferrets often respond well to glucocorticosteroids. Different chemotherapy protocols have also been developed, with mixed results. A period of remission can be achieved, but a cure is not likely. Recently a ferret was successfully treated with radiotherapy (Orcutt, 2000).

Splenomegaly

Splenomegaly is a common finding in ferrets but is seldom of clinical importance. It can be found in healthy ferrets and in animals with seemingly unrelated diseases. During abdominal palpation the spleen can easily be detected and in severe cases extend all the way to the pelvic inlet. In contrast to hypersplenism, the total blood count and differentiation of ferrets with splenomegaly does not show any abnormalities. The most common histological diagnosis of these enlarged spleens is extramedullary haematopoiesis. Tumours of the spleen, however, do occur. Therefore, when a ferret is presented with non-specific symptoms and a large spleen is palpable, abdominal ultrasonography is recommended. In cases of lymphoma the spleen usually has an irregular aspect on ultrasonography. An ultrasound-guided biopsy is mandatory to confirm the diagnosis prior to surgery. The only indication for splenectomy is if the spleen contains a tumour (lymphoma) or there is discomfort.

Supportive care

Drug administration

Tablets and capsules are not easily accepted by ferrets. Capsules are usually too big for them to swallow and fall apart, and because ferrets have a low bodyweight no commercial capsule contains the right amount of drug. Tablets can be split into quarters for more accurate dosing, although most tablets are still too concentrated for use in ferrets. This author prefers potions and suspensions for oral treatment. They are easily accepted by ferrets and can be accurately dosed. Practices dealing with ferrets and other small exotics should keep a stock of methylcellulose for the preparation of suspensions.

Injection sites

Ferrets can receive intramuscular injections, but total muscle mass is a limiting factor. If injections have to be given, the subcutaneous route is preferred.

Although the intravenous and intraosseous routes are the most direct for fluid therapy, the subcutaneous and intraperitoneal routes are suitable for most ferrets.

Catheterization

The lateral saphenous vein and cephalic vein are suitable for the placement of indwelling catheters.

Anaesthesia and analgesia

Sedation and light anaesthesia

For non-painful simple procedures, such as taking blood from the vena cava or ultrasonography of the adrenal gland, ferrets can be simply sedated with isoflurane. Sedation or light anaesthesia by mask induction with 100% oxygen and 4% isoflurane and maintenance with 2% isoflurane enables procedures to be performed quickly and often with little stress. Ferrets awake quickly from anaesthesia so owners can take their pet home soon after the procedure.

Medetomidine can also be given: 80–100 μg/kg is usually sufficient for sedation of about 30 minutes. Atipamezole can be used to reverse the effects of medetomidine; a practical dosage is 2.5 times that of medetomidine in micrograms (i.e. half the volume dose).

Because ferrets have a relatively fast gastrointestinal transit time, a fasting period of only about 4 hours prior to sedation or anaesthesia is necessary.

Anaesthesia

The standard anaesthesia protocol used at Utrecht University for ferrets is to premedicate with 100 μg/kg medetomidine followed by the placement of a catheter in the cephalic vein through which the ferret is induced with 1 to 3 mg/kg propofol. Anaesthesia is maintained with isoflurane. Ferrets are always intubated (inner diameter 2–2.5 mm) during long surgical procedures.

Different combinations of injectable anaesthesia agents have been investigated (Ko *et al.*, 1997). A practical combination is medetomidine and ketamine 0.08 and 5 mg/kg, respectively.

Ferrets should be kept warm both during and after anaesthesia as hypothermia can occur easily.

Analgesia

The use of analgesics is an important part of good veterinary practice. During general anaesthesia both ketamine and medetomidine provide analgesia, but the addition of buprenorphine may reduce the dosages of ketamine and medetomidine necessary.

The new analgesics meloxicam (0.2 mg/kg orally) and carprofen (1–5 mg/kg orally) have proven to be useful in ferrets.

Common surgical procedures

Castration

Castration of male ferrets reduces their dominant character, but most importantly reduces the secretion of their sebaceous glands during the breeding season, resulting in less odour. Both open and closed techniques have been described for castration. The author prefers the open technique in which the spermatic cord and vessels are ligated with 4-0 monofilament. The scrotal sac does not need to be closed.

Ovariohysterectomy

As mentioned above, jills that are not bred should be neutered to prevent bone marrow suppression during a prolonged oestrous period. In the USA, ferrets in breeding farms are neutered at 4–6 weeks. In Europe most ferrets are neutered just prior to their first oestrus, when they are 6–9 months of age.

The technique is similar to that in cats. A complicating factor in ferrets is the large amount of fat in the mesovarium. This might be one of the reasons why a fair number of remnant ovaries are seen in the Netherlands. At Utrecht University we advise incisions of at least 3 or 4 cm so that there is good vision during surgery.

Removal of foreign bodies

Ingestion of foreign bodies should be considered in any lethargic ferret that has anorexia and diarrhoea. Although vomiting may occur, it may not be mentioned by the owner. In most cases the foreign bodies contain rubber because ferrets seem to like its taste.

Diagnosis by abdominal palpation is possible when a foreign body is stuck in the small intestine but may be difficult if the object is still in the stomach. Radiographs and ultrasonograms can help to confirm the diagnosis. The ferret must be stabilized prior to surgery.

A midline approach can be used to inspect the gastrointestinal tract, followed by a gastrotomy or enterotomy similar to that in other small species. The stomach can be closed in two layers with 3-0 or 4-0 monofilament, and the intestines can be closed in one layer with 4-0 to 5-0 monofilament. Water and liquid food can be given again after 12–24 hours.

Removal of anal glands

In the USA most ferrets are bred in large breeding farms where they are neutered and have their anal glands removed at 6 weeks of age. Anal glands are removed because of the false belief that they are responsible for the ferret's strong odour (in fact it is the sebaceous glands). Unless for medical reasons, it is illegal to remove the anal glands from ferrets in the UK and the Netherlands.

Euthanasia

The author prefers to sedate animals prior to euthanasia because most agents used for euthanasia are irritating to the tissues and ferrets may react to them. Most owners also appreciate seeing their animals sedated. If no postmortem examination of the peritoneal cavity is necessary an intraperitoneal injection with any of the available agents may be given. Cardiac puncture may be too distressing to perform in the presence of the owner (for humane reasons, this technique should only be performed in a sedated or anaesthetized animal). If postmortem examination is required, an intravenous injection is mandatory.

Drug formulary

Drug	Dose
Analgesics	
Butorphanol	0.1–0.5 mg/kg s.c. or i.m. every 4 hours
Buprenorphine	0.01–0.03 mg/kg s.c. or i.m. bid–tid
Carprofen	1–5 mg/kg orally or s.c.
Meloxicam	0.1–0.2 mg/kg orally
Antibacterial agents	
Amoxicillin (+ clavulanic acid)	10–20 mg/kg orally or s.c. sid–bid
Cephalexin	15–25 mg/kg orally bid–tid
Chloramphenicol	50 mg/kg orally, s.c. or i.m. bid
Enrofloxacin	5–15 mg/kg orally, s.c. or i.m. bid
Metronidazole	10–20 mg/kg orally bid
Oxytetracycline	20 mg/kg orally tid
Penicillin G procaine	20,000 IU/kg i.m. bid
Tetracycline	25 mg/kg orally bid–tid
Trimethoprim–sulphonamides	15–30 mg/kg orally or s.c. bid
Tylosin	10 mg/kg orally bid
Antifungal agents	
Griseofulvin	25 mg/kg orally sid
Antiparasitic agents	
Ivermectin 1% (1:10 diluted in propylene glycol)	0.2–0.4 mg/kg topically
Fipronil	2 drops in each ear
Pyrethrin products	applied topically
Selamectin	applied topically
Other agents	
Cimetidine	10 mg/kg orally, s.c., i.m. or i.v. tid
Cisapride	0.5 mg/kg orally tid
Diazoxide	5–30 mg/kg orally bid
Digoxin	0.005–0.01 mg/kg orally sid–tid
Enalapril	0.25–0.5 mg/kg orally every 24–48 hours
Frusemide	1–4 mg/kg orally, s.c., i.m. or i.v. bid–tid
GnRH (leuprolide acetate)	0.1 mg/kg i.m. once per month
HCG	100 IU i.m.; repeat in 2 wks
Metoclopramide	0.2–1 mg/kg orally or s.c. tid–qid
Prednisolone	0.2–1 mg/kg orally sid
Proligestone	50 mg/kg i.m. once
Propranolol	0.5–2 mg/kg orally or s.c. sid–bid

Figure 9.12 Drug formulary for the ferret. (Data from Hillyer and Quesenberry, 1997).

References and further reading

Erdman SE, Reimann KA, Moore FM *et al.* (1995) Transmission of a chronic lymphoproliferative syndrome in ferrets. *Laboratory Investigation* **72,** 539–546
Fox JG (1998) *Biology and Diseases of the Ferret, 2nd edn.* Williams and Wilkins, London

Fox JG, Pequet-Goad ME, Garibaldi BA and Wiest LM (1987) Hyperadrenocorticism in a ferret. *Journal of the American Veterinary Medical Association* **191,** 343–344

Fudge AM (2000) *Laboratory Medicine; Avian and Exotic Pets.* WB Saunders, Philadelphia

Jenkins JR and Brown SA (1993) *A Practitioner's Guide to Rabbits and Ferrets.* American Animal Hospital Association

Ko JC, Heaton-Jones TG and Nicklin CF (1997) Evaluation of the sedative and cardiorespiratory effects of medetomidine, medetomidine-butorphanol, medetomidine-ketamine, and medetomidine-butorphanol-ketamine in ferrets. *Journal of the American Animal Hospital Association* **33(5),** 438–448

Orcutt C (2000) Presented at ICE 2000, Fort Lauderdale, May 2000

Porter HG, Porter DD and Larsen AE (1982) Aleutian disease in ferrets. *Infections and Immunity* **36,** 379–386

Hillyer EV and Quesenberry KE (1997) *Ferrets, Rabbits and Rodents: Clinical Medicine and Surgery.* WB Saunders, Philadelphia

Schoemaker NJ, Schuurmans M, Moorman H and Lumeij JT (2000) Correlation between age at neutering and age at onset of hyperadrenocorticism in ferrets. *Journal of the American Veterinary Medical Association* **15,** 216(2):195–197

Thomson APD (1951) A history of the ferret. *Journal of the History of Medicine and Allied Sciences* **6,** 471

10

Other small mammals

Cathy A. Johnson-Delaney

Introduction

A number of exotic small mammals have become popular as pets in the United States over the past few years. Only one of the species is native to the United States: the prairie dog *Cynomys ludovicianus*, which until recently was always wild-caught for the pet trade. The sugar glider *Petaurus breviceps* is native to New Guinea and Australia, with founding stock being wild-caught and imported recently. The African pygmy hedgehog *Atelerix albiventris* was imported from New Zealand (where it had been introduced into the wild and is considered a pest species) and Africa. Importation of this hedgehog for the pet trade has ceased, as it is possibly a carrier of foot-and-mouth disease from countries of origin; all the animals currently available in the pet trade are domestically raised. Other recent additions to the pet trade include the South American 'Brazilian' short-tailed opossum *Monodelphis domestica*, the degu *Octodon degus* and the duprasi or fat-tailed gerbil *Pachyuromys duprasi*, all of which are fairly docile but non-domesticated animals that may challenge practitioners.

Pet stores that sell exotic small mammals are required to be registered by the US Department of Agriculture and regularly inspected. Veterinarians must know their local, state and national laws pertaining to owning, breeding, selling and transporting these different species, as owners frequently ask for services such as health certificates for shipment. While practitioners are not regulatory enforcers, they should not knowingly perpetrate illegalities in the pet trade. When presented with an animal that is not legal in the locale, the duty of the practitioner is to provide veterinary care for that animal and to educate the owner.

Sugar glider *Petaurus breviceps*

The sugar glider is a marsupial and is native to New Guinea and Australia, with at least seven recognized subspecies. The habitats are primarily open forest – either tropical or coastal, or dry inland sclerophyll tropical forest. The animals are nocturnal and arboreal; they nest in leaf-lined tree holes with up to six other adults and young.

Gliding distance can be up to 50 m. The gliding membrane (patagium) extends from the fifth digit of the forepaws to the ankles. The first and second digit of the forepaws to the ankles. The first and second digit of the hindfeet are partially fused (syndactylous). The tail is well furred and weakly prehensile.

The female has the typical marsupial bilobed uterus with lateral vaginas and central birth canal. The pouch contains two teats and two offspring are common. Males have a forked penis and mid-ventral scrotum. In captivity, sugar gliders will breed throughout the year and produce two litters per year on average. Biological data are summarized in Figure 10.1.

Lifespan	In wild: 4–5 years (up to 9 years recorded) In captivity: 12–14 years (optimum diet and husbandry)
Weight	Varies for different subspecies. Larger: male 115–160 g, female 95–135 g
Length	Head and body 120–132 mm; tail 150–480 mm
Body temperature	Average 32°C
Sexual maturity	Female 8–12 months; male 12–14 months
Gestation period	16 days; fetus then migrates to pouch
Litter size	1–2
Weaning age	Joeys leave pouch at about 70 days; independent at 17 weeks but may remain in parental nest

Figure 10.1 Biological data for the sugar glider.

Behaviour

Males develop a scent gland on the forehead and may rub this on the female's chest. Males also have scent glands on the chest, and anal glands. Both sexes scent-mark territory with secretions from scent glands; in addition the female uses urine to mark territory. The female's scent glands are within the pouch and she will secrete and increase marking to indicate breeding readiness to the male.

Sugar gliders are quite vocal, with a whole series of alarm yaps and screams. They are highly social animals and should not be kept as a solitary pet: they become clinically depressed when housed singly. Self-mutilation is not uncommon in solitary gliders. Those without proper socialization or exercise and territory space may become aggressive.

- Adult males need adequate territories and will fight if there is not enough distance between nest boxes
- All sugar gliders may fight and become irritable at the beginning of breeding

- Males without adequate stimulation frequently become aggressive towards humans. Neutering may help but they will continue to scent-mark and will not be 'human-socialized' like a domesticated animal.

Housing

Enclosures should be a minimum of 2 m wide × 2 m long and at least 1.8 m high. Bird cages are not suitable. Supplemental heating is usually necessary for a healthy glider, as home temperatures are at the low end of their metabolic tolerance and comfort zone. Sugar gliders become almost torpid during the day (their night) or if they are too cold, and can be extremely difficult to rouse.

The animals need large areas for activity and exercise – ideally the freedom of a whole room, fitted with vertical 'trees'. This may be impractical in a typical home and many owners are reluctant to allow such freedom because gliders scent-mark and are active at night.

Diet

The natural diet in the wet season (winter) is primarily the sugary sap or gum of eucalypts and acacias, and nectar from flowers of eucalypts, banksias, acacias and several types of native apple. For the rest of the year, sugar gliders are mainly insectivorous and the diet includes a range of insects and arachnids and also small vertebrates. They have specialized incisors for gouging the bark of trees.

Small insects trapped in wattle or acacia gum (a carbohydrate-rich sap) are consumed. Favourite trees include the Australian 'bloodwood', the red sap of which crystallizes, mixes with the decaying pulp of the tree, and attracts termite and ant activity. Other favourite tree species have a yellowish sap that produces 'manna', a deposit of white encrusting sugars, from wounds made by sap-sucking insects, birds, squirrel gliders or possums. The sugar glider has been observed to eat honeydew, secreted by sap-sucking insects.

Despite published advice, sugar gliders do not rely on nuts, grains or seeds. The diet for a captive sugar glider should contain a variety of foods appropriate for insectivores – at least 50% of total intake, particularly if they are active breeders. Most of the remaining 50% should be sources of fruit sugars, preferably in the form of a sap or nectar (there is no proof that commercial lorikeet nectars are adequate for gliders). A small amount of fruit can be given as a treat. The diet should be offered in fresh portions in the evening.

Australian rehabilitators set up outdoor lights to attract insects as a major portion of the diet, with an artificial nectar (either Leadbeater's Mix or one designed for honey-eating possums) as the other major portion, and occasional small pieces of fruit as treats.

In the absence of a very large variety of insects, a zoo-formula insectivore food can be used but this should be supplemented with pet-industry insects raised on a commercial cricket diet or enriched feed and dusted with complete vitamin/mineral powders. Insects, such as mealworms (large or small), crickets, waxworms and moths, and spiders can be offered. Suggested diets are given in Figure 10.2.

Diet 1 (Johnson-Delaney)

For one glider portion (fed in evening):

- Leadbeater's Mix (50% of diet)
  - 150 ml warm water
  - 150 ml honey
  - One shelled, boiled egg
  - 25 g high-protein baby cereal
  - 1 tsp vitamin/mineral supplement

Mix warm water and honey. In separate container, blend egg until homogenized. Gradually add water/honey, then vitamin powder, then baby cereal, blending after each addition until smooth. Keep refrigerated until served.

- Insectivore/carnivore diet (50% of total diet)
- Treat foods: various fruits, chopped; may add bee pollen, vitamin/mineral supplement.

Diet 2 (Booth)

Offer a total of 15–20% of bodyweight daily. Select one diet from each of the following groups each day. (Animals will benefit from a regular supply of vitamin/mineral-enriched insects.)

- Group 1
  - Insects: 75% moths, crickets, beetles; 25% fly pupae, mealworms
  - Meat mix: commercial small carnivore or insectivore mix
- Group 2
  - Nectar mix: 1.5 cups fructose, 1.5 cups sucrose (brown sugar), 0.5 cup glucose made up to 2 l with warm water; commercially available mixes have the advantage of some vitamin/mineral additives.
  - Dry lorikeet mix: 4 cups rolled oats, 1 cup wheat germ, 1 cup brown sugar, 0.5 cup glucose, 0.5 cup raisins or sultanas
- Group 3
  - Fruit and vegetables: select from diced apple, nectarine, melons, grapes, raisins, sultana, figs, tomato, sweet corn kernels, sweet potato, beans, shredded carrot, butternut pumpkin.
  - Greens: mixed sprouts, lettuce, broccoli, parsley, with a vitamin/mineral supplement at manufacturer's directions.

Figure 10.2 Suggested diets for sugar gliders.

The portion size for one glider is roughly a table-spoonful of insects (e.g. about a dozen small mealworms or four small or two large waxworms) and a tablespoon-ful of nectar, with fresh water always available. Portion size may be increased or decreased depending on activity level and reproductive or growth conditions.

If fruit is fed as a treat, a variety should be offered, chopped together in small pieces to reduce the glider's ability to pick out only its favourite parts. A small amount of multiple vitamin/mineral powder should be mixed through the fruit. Bee pollen may be dusted over any fruit given.

Techniques

Restraint of a sugar glider is demonstrated in Figure 10.3.

Blood sampling

Blood draw sites for smaller volumes are the cephalic, lateral saphenous, femoral, ventral coccygeal or lateral tail vein or medial tibial artery. Tail vessels are more easily utilized if the tail is warmed and the vessels dilated, as with rodents. The jugular and cranial vena

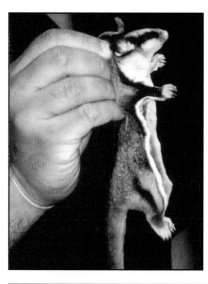

Figure 10.3
Restraint of a
sugar glider.
(Courtesy of
Robert Ness.)

cava can be used for larger volumes (up to 1 ml in adults) but general anaesthetic with isoflurane is required.

Injection sites

- Intramuscular injection sites include the quadriceps and biceps/triceps
- Subcutaneous injections are given in the scapular area as in other animals but fluids may end up pooling in the gliding membrane
- The saphenous vein has been used for intravenous injections.

Common conditions

In general, physiological parameters such as complete blood counts, serum chemistries and urinalysis follow those of other carnivorous species. Medications safe for ferrets or cats have been used with apparent efficacy. Differential diagnoses are summarized in Figure 10.4.

Clinical signs/disease	Aetiology	Diagnostics	Therapy
Weakness, ataxia, paresis/paralysis, weight loss, muscle wasting, lethargy, reluctance to move, soft jaws/teeth, neurological signs including tremor, osteomalacia, osteoporosis, encephalomalacia, encephalitis	Improper diet: deficiencies of calcium, protein, vitamins A, E, D, etc. Excesses of sugar, carbohydrates, fats. Ambient temperature too cool adding to stress of malnourishment. Infections: *Listeria, Baylisascaris,* bacterial encephalitis from systemic infection	CBC, chemistry panel; radiographs. Dietary, husbandry history. *Listeria:* possible serology, culture of CSF; necropsy/histopathology may be necessary for diagnosis of nervous system disease	Immediate therapy: NSAIDS and/or analgesics, parenteral calcium, fluids; gavage feed with high protein/calcium-rich food. Vitamin/mineral supplementation. Correct diet to include calcium-rich insects, protein; decrease sugars, fats. Increase ambient temperature, provide exercise. Physical therapy may be needed initially. For *Listeria:* penicillin, antibiotics as indicated from antibiogram; zoonotic potential! *Baylisascaris:* ivermectin, eliminate exposure to raccoons, skunks
Behavioural: self-injurious (SIB), overgrooming, aggressiveness, cannibalism of young	Stress, improper husbandry, lack of social interactions. SIB most often seen in solitary pets. Lack of space, areas for exercise, adult males confined together, incompatible pairs, etc.	Husbandry history, including habitat information, ambient temperatures, exercise, environmental enrichment; social structure. If wounds, culture/sensitivity. CBC/chemistry, radiology to ascertain general health	Treat wounds as in other animals: NSAIDS, analgesics, antimicrobials. Correct deficiencies of husbandry, social patterns. Anti-depressant medical therapy and/or benzodiazepines if SIB, overgrooming continue. Neuter overly aggressive males
Cataracts	Vitamin A deficiency, hyperglycaemia (dietary or diabetes), congenital/hereditary?	History including diet, husbandry. CBC/chemistry, urinalysis, ophthalmic examination. Check pedigree, breeding history	Cataract removal may be possible. Correct diet to lower blood sugar. If true diabetes, manage as in cats. If possibly genetic, do not breed
Urinary tract disease: penile prolapse, necrosis; male urinary tract blockage; bladder rupture; uroliths/cystitis with haematuria, stranguria, crystalluria; pyelonephritis/nephritis, renal disease/failure	Ascending bacterial infection from cloaca. Lack of territory/furnishings to mark so urine retention; subclinical dehydration (chronic); improper diet (mineral balance, water/electrolytes, ash content?); lack of exercise, poor overall body condition; age	CBC, chemistry panel, urinalysis (cystocentesis), culture and sensitivity of urine; radiographs, excretory urogram; diet, husbandry history	Blocked males: relieve blockage via catheterization, flushing, urethrostomy (as in cats), cystotomy for urolith removal; NSAIDS, analgesics, fluid therapy, antimicrobial therapy. Correct diet, husbandry. Treat renal disease/failure as in other animals: fluid administration, phosphorus binding agent, vitamin B complex, potassium, dietary modifications
Gastrointestinal: rectal prolapse (usually marked tenesmus), diarrhoea, enteritis/enteropathy	Bacterial (*E. coli, Clostridium* etc.); parasitic (nematode, cestode, protozoal including giardia), dietary; foreign body ingestion. Prolapses exacerbated by abdominal muscle weakness, overall health, pregnancy, age	Faecal flotation, direct smear, Gram stain, culture and sensitivity; CBC/chemistry panel, radiographs (contrast study), diet, husbandry history including breeding status	Appropriate antimicrobials depending on faecal exam, culture, aetiology. Surgical correction of prolapse; NSAIDS, analgesics, fluid therapy, nutritional support; enterotomy if foreign body/obstruction. Adjunctive therapy of intestinal protectants: bismuth subsalicylate
Poor hair coat, sebaceous gland/pouch dermatitis	General poor health, dietary/husbandry deficiency, lack of grooming. Pouch infections: bacterial, candida	Diet/husbandry history; dermatitis: skin scraping/biopsy; culture and sensitivity	Correct diet/husbandry, antimicrobials as indicated. Topical corticosteroids, antihistamines and/or NSAIDS
Ear margin canker	Mite with secondary bacterial infection	Scraping, culture and sensitivity	Ivermectin; appropriate topical antimicrobial, NSAIDS or anti-inflammatory if pruritic
Reproductive: weak, not thriving, dying joeys; infertility, pouch/reproductive tract infections; mastitis	Inadequate nutrition of dam, overbreeding (too many litters/year), poor husbandry, chronic bacterial/yeast infection of dam; retained/mummified fetus	Diet/husbandry history; CBC/chemistry, radiographs; cytology of milk, urogenital mucosa; culture and sensitivity of exudates/reproductive tract/pouch	Correct diet/husbandry, appropriate antimicrobials, calcium, fluids; hold out of breeding until healthy; check male for bacterial/yeast infection
Trauma: wounds, fractures	Attacks from mate/rival, other pets; falls/injuries due to confinement, poor body condition	Radiographs, CBC/chemistry panel to check general health; if wounds infected, culture and sensitivity	Appropriate antimicrobial, wound care as in other animals; NSAIDS, analgesics. Fracture repair similar to birds/small mammals. Correct diet/husbandry

Figure 10.4 Diseases of the sugar glider.

Nutritional disorders

By far the largest number of clinical problems in sugar gliders can be attributed to improper diet and husbandry. Signs include: weakness, ataxia, paresis/paralysis, weight loss, muscle wasting, lethargy, inability to support own weight, reluctance to move, often coupled with hypothermia, dehydration, soft jaws/teeth, neurological signs including tremor, osteomalacia, osteoporosis and encephalomalacia.

The diet of most pet gliders seems to be deficient in protein, vitamins and minerals. Animals presented with the above signs are often being fed table fruits, seeds, nuts, human foods and possibly some mealworms, on a basis of free choice. Commercial glider products and marketed 'home recipe' diets have not undergone feeding trials and many are not quality controlled for guaranteed analysis. These dietary deficiencies are unnecessary, as the nutritional needs of sugar gliders have been extensively studied and are known.

Therapy consists of supportive care, diet adjustment, supplementation with calcium and other deficient vitamins and minerals, and the use of analgesics in the case of osteomalacia or osteoporosis where the glider exhibits painful responses while trying to walk. Pathological fractures should be handled as in other small mammals. A review of the habitat and improvement of husbandry should accompany diet adjustment and parenteral support.

Cataracts

Cataracts may have a genetic cause as well as a nutritional or possibly infectious one. They are seen particularly when the mother has been pushed for breeding and when she is on an inadequate diet or one high in sugars. Many marsupials do not handle hyperglycaemia well. Vitamin A deficiency has been proposed as part of the aetiology. The role of pouch infections, particularly candidiasis, has not been investigated but many breeding females have yeast or fungal pouch infections. A thorough physical examination of the dam and any breeding or genetics records may help to prevent cataract development in infant gliders.

Gastrointestinal disease

Gliders have been presented with rectal prolapse, diarrhoea and bacterial or protozoal enteritis. Stool culture, flotation, direct smear and Gram staining are diagnostic tools to determine the underlying disease condition. *Giardia* spp. can cause diarrhoea, which may be intermittent.

Improper diet consistency seems to contribute to prolapse, and weakened muscle tone is a contributory factor. The prolapse should be reduced gently and the cloacal opening temporarily decreased with two vertical sutures rather than a purse-string suture. Magnification is needed, to ensure that the urogenital slit is not sutured closed. Antimicrobial therapy, bismuth subsalicylate, anti-inflammatory medication and an analgesic are administered.

Urinary tract disorders

These include penile prolapse, necrosis, male urinary tract blockage, bladder rupture with subsequent peritonitis, pyelonephritis/nephritis and renal disease/failure.

Most cases seem to be in gliders on a diet of fruit and catfood, rather than on a diet of Leadbeater's mix and insectivore food supplemented with live prey, plus adequate environmental heat.

If the penis has become necrotic, the glider may already be toxic or septicaemic and in renal compromise. Urethrostomy following penile amputation may be tried. A lacrimal cannula is of the appropriate size to open the urethra but the damage may have extended further proximally. Treatment is antimicrobial therapy along with an NSAID, an analgesic and fluid therapy but the prognosis is poor.

Skin problems

Gliders are frequently presented with poor hair coats and glands with sebaceous build-up. Dietary insufficiencies and husbandry deficiencies are usually the cause, and the signs regress with correction.

Ear margin canker has been reported and a mite seen upon skin scraping. The condition responds to ivermectin at 200 µg/kg bodyweight administered topically or subcutaneously. If not treated early, secondary bacterial infections may need to be treated with systemic antibiotics. Once the infestation or infection has cleared, there may be scarring of the pinna.

Reproductive problems

These include joeys that are weak, not thriving or dying, which may be due to inadequate nutrition of the dam, infection of the pouch or reproductive tract, mastitis, poor parental care or overbreeding. Some breeders pull joeys early to force a second birthing within a year period, or even more frequently, as gliders can be continuous breeders. In the wild, joeys usually stay with the parents an entire year.

A full health examination is recommended prior to breeding. This should include:

- Blood tests (check calcium)
- Pouch swab for yeast or bacteria
- Faecal parasite examination
- Urinalysis (may pick up subclinical urogenital tract infections)
- Radiographs to assess bone density.

A review of the husbandry and diet will help owners to rear healthy joeys.

Trauma

Gliders may be wounded by other pets in the household, particularly cats. Gliders have also been injured when given free exercise at home by crashing into furnishings and walls, or being burned by landing on the top of lamps and light bulbs. Fractures due to falling because of overall weakness are not uncommon. Wounds and injuries can be managed as in other small mammals.

Surgical procedures

In most cases surgical techniques follow the same guidelines as for other small mammals. General anaesthesia is best accomplished with isoflurane and can be maintained as in other small mammals. Sugar gliders are adept at suture removal unless adequate analgesic is provided and the sutures are buried.

Orchidectomy

Orchidectomy is slightly different, because of the different marsupial anatomy. The testicles in the scrotum are attached via a short stalk to the mid-ventral body wall.

1. Make an incision longitudinal and parallel to and running along the stalk.
2. Use blunt dissection to expose the blood supply and vas deferens.
3. Ligate the blood supply and vas deferens.
4. Remove the scrotal sac.
5. Close the skin with subcuticular buried sutures.

Analgesics

Postoperative analgesics include:

- Butorphanol (0.1–0.5 mg/kg, given every 6–8 hours as needed, i.m., s.c. or orally)
- Flunixin (1 mg/kg every 12–24 hours as needed, for up to 3 days.

Flunixin is an NSAID and helps with postoperative inflammation as well as providing some degree of analgesia. Butorphanol and flunixin can be administered concurrently.

Prairie dog *Cynomys ludovicianus*

The black-tailed prairie dog (Figure 10.5) is native to North America. It is diurnal; it does not truly hibernate but may have dormant periods in inclement weather. Vocalizations include a 'bark' when excited, and various chatters and growls. Prairie dogs are social animals and live in large communities or 'towns' in the wild. They require companionship; they do not do well as solitary animals and may develop behavioural abnormalities, including self-mutilation and aggressiveness towards humans. Digging is a primary activity. They are not agile climbers, but many will try to climb in a household environment.

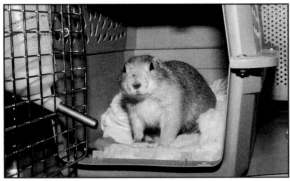

Figure 10.5 Prairie dog.

As wild resources dwindle, some captive-bred animals are becoming available, but many prairie dogs offered for sale have been taken from the wild as pups in the burrow, pulled out by means of large vacuum devices.

- Prairie dogs have open-rooted incisors
- The nails are long for digging and need frequent trimming
- They have trigonal anal sac ducts which appear as white papillae beside the anus
- The testicles descend relatively late and are more prominent during the breeding season. There is no distinct scrotal sac; the testicles only descend into an inguinal position
- They are hindgut fermenters and require adequate roughage in the diet
- They are monoestrous and seasonal breeders for 2–3 weeks (January to March in US latitudes)
- They have one litter per year.

Biological data are summarized in Figure 10.6.

Weight	0.5–2.2 kg (males larger than females)
Sexual maturity	2–3 years of age
Gestation period	30–35 days
Litter size	2–10 (average 5)
Weaning age	6 weeks

Figure 10.6 Biological data for the black-tailed prairie dog.

Housing

Prairie dogs should be housed in large wire cages suitable for rabbits or guinea pigs, with deep substrate bedding of wood shavings, shredded newspaper or similar product for digging. Provision of PVC pipes simulates the tunnels they would normally build. The preferred environmental temperature range is 18–24°C.

Diet

- Prairie dogs should be fed unlimited grass hay
- As juveniles, they may also be fed pelleted chows and alfalfa, *ad libitum*
- As adults, or if the juvenile becomes obese, access to pelleted chows should be limited to one or two rodent chow blocks per week, with no alfalfa hay
- Small amounts of various fresh greens can be offered as treats
- As prairie dogs will eat almost anything, owners should resist feeding them items such as peanuts, raisins, french fries, cereal, bread and dog biscuits.

Techniques

Blood collection is from the lateral or medial saphenous, cephalic or jugular vein or cranial vena cava, with the latter two under isoflurane aanesthesia delivered via nose cone.

Injection sites are as for the guinea pig.

Common conditions

Therapeutics that seem efficacious and non-toxic are those used for the guinea pig or chinchilla. Normal stools are similar to those of a guinea pig, which are dry and oval shaped. Urine is alkaline (pH 8–9) and clear yellow.

Because of the possibility of the prairie dog being wild-caught, the practitioner should screen the animal for parasites such as pulmonary mites (*Pneumocoptes penrosei*) as well as potentially zoonotic diseases that wild prairie dogs have been shown to carry, such as *Yersinia pestis*.

Differential diagnoses are summarized in Figure 10.7.

Obesity and dormancy

Common clinical conditions include obesity (in large part due to improper and excessive diet plus lack of exercise) and dormancy (because the home temperature has dropped below 16°C for several days, coupled with decreased light). The dormant prairie dog may have elevated blood urea nitrogen levels, be slightly dehydrated and slightly hypothermic, but will rouse with warming and administration of warmed subcutaneous fluids.

Dental disease

Dental disease is common and includes fractured teeth, root abscesses, and malocclusions associated with loss or overgrowth. Maxillary teeth may abscess into the nasal cavities and sinuses, resulting in upper respiratory tract disease.

Dental neoplasia (odontoma) has been associated with chronic dental disease or mouth trauma from chewing on inappropriate objects, such as cage bars. Radiographs as well as a thorough dental examination under isoflurane anaesthesia are necessary to determine the condition of the tooth roots and bone. Prairie dogs can be intubated with a 2.0 or 2.5 mm endotracheal tube using a blind technique or with the aid of a laryngoscope. Removal of diseased teeth along with the creation of permanent openings in the nasal bones caudal to a tumour mass have been tried as treatment but usually the condition is progressive. Antibiotic therapy along with NSAID treatment has helped symptomatically.

Respiratory disease

Prairie dogs suffering from upper respiratory tract disease may be presented with open-mouthed breathing (Figure 10.8). As well as maxillary teeth abscesses and neoplasia, causes of dyspnoea include *Pasteurella multocida* pneumonia, sinusitis and rhinitis. Pulmonary

Clinical signs/disease	Aetiology	Diagnostics	Therapy
Obesity (fatty liver, lethargy)	Overfeeding and/or improper foods; initiation of winter dormancy; lack of exercise	Diet history, ambient temperature/husbandry. CBC/chemistry panel. Radiographs, ultrasound of liver	Correct diet (hay-based). Decrease total quantity. Light/temperature correction. Exercise. If liver disease, supportive care as appropriate. To rouse from dormant condition, warmed subcutaneous fluids, increase light
Dental disease: fractured teeth, malocclusion, tooth root abscesses, oral swellings/neoplasia	Fractured teeth: falls, chewing on bars/toys, trauma; abscesses may be due to improper wear, punctures from food/foreign objects; neoplasia (odontomas) possible aetiology includes repeated mouth trauma	Oral examination under sedation; head radiographs, endoscopy of nasal cavity	Remove abscessed teeth; trim malocclusive teeth; surgical excision of some neoplasias possible; correct diet for tooth wear; appropriate antimicrobials including periodontal/intra-abscess PMMA bead pack; NSAIDS, analgesics as necessary
Open-mouthed breathing/dyspnoea; possible nasal/ocular discharge	Rule out oral, maxillary odontoma/neoplasia; nasolacrimal duct infection/blockage from tooth root abscess; sinus infection; severe respiratory tract infection	Radiographs, ophthalmic exam including nasolacrimal flush; culture and sensitivity of exudates; thorough oral examination	Flush nasolacrimal duct if possible; remove abscessed teeth, provide drainage. Treatment as above for oral abscesses. Surgical excision of odontoma/neoplasia may be possible. Appropriate antimicrobials, NSAIDS, analgesics
Dyspnoea, with/without sinusitis, rhinitis	*Pasteurella multocida*; pulmonary mites (*Pneumocoptes penrosei*)	Culture and sensitivity, cytology of tracheal/sinus wash; radiographs. CBC, chemistry	Appropriate antibiotic (fluoroquinolones first choice), ivermectin for mites; supportive care including nebulization, bronchodilators, NSAIDS, topical ophthalmic preparations for sinuses
Trauma: fractures, torn nails	Falls, injuries from other pets, nails caught in carpets	Radiographs for fractures	Trim nails, repair fractures with guidelines used for rabbits, guinea pigs
Self-injurious behaviour: wounding, self-amputation. Seen most frequently if solitary	Improper husbandry and lack of social stimulation, boredom, stereotypical behavior. Wounds may become secondarily infected, painful	Assess husbandry. Radiographs if severe, bone involved. Culture and sensitivity of infected wounds	Provide companionship, social stimulation, enriched environment (large, ability to dig). Wound treatment as in rabbits, guinea pigs. Benzodiazepines may be needed to control SIB
Pododermatitis	Poor husbandry: dirty, wet bedding; obese, inactive animal	Radiograph to assess bone involvement; culture and sensitivity of edges of lesions	Treat as in guinea pigs: remove exudate, appropriate antimicrobials, soft bandages, soft flooring; NSAIDS, supportive care. Correct sanitation/husbandry
Neurological signs: ataxia, torticollis, stumbling, seizures	*Baylisascaris* sp. infection; heavy metal toxicosis (lead, zinc)	*Baylisascaris*: history of wild-caught or housed in caging used by skunks/raccoons. CT or MRI for antemortem Dx, usually made at necropsy. Heavy metal: history of objects chewed on: blood lead, zinc levels, evidence metal particulates in GI tract radiographs	No treatment for *Baylisascaris* although ivermectin has been tried. Heavy metal: chelation therapy with Ca-EDTA or d-penicillamine as in other species. Remove dangerous toys, objects

Figure 10.7 Diseases of the prairie dog.

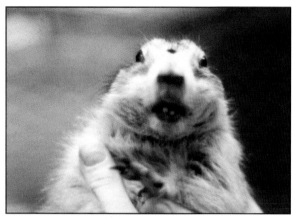

Figure 10.8 Prairie dog presenting with open-mouthed breathing, a sign of upper respiratory tract or dental disease.

mites (*Pneumocoptes penrosei*) found in wild-caught prairie dogs may also cause nasal occlusion. These can be diagnosed on cytology of a tracheal wash. Ivermectin at 200–500 µg/kg every 14 days for three treatments has been tried to treat this condition.

Neurological disease
Neurological signs including ataxia, torticollis, stumbling and seizures have been reported in pet prairie dogs. *Baylisascaris* spp. have been implicated, particularly if the pet was wild-caught or if it was housed in caging previously used for skunks or raccoons; the parasite is absent from the UK. There is no treatment. Diagnosis may be aided by computerized tomography or magnetic resonance imaging for inflammatory lesions in the brain, but definitive diagnosis is made at necropsy.

Skin problems
Pododermatitis has been seen similar to that in guinea pigs and is the result of poor husbandry – dirty, wet bedding along with obesity and inactivity.

Trauma
Trauma is frequently seen, including vertebral and long-bone fractures from falling in a home environment. Self-inflicted wounds, including amputation and subsequent osteomyelitis, have been seen in solitary prairie dogs.

Toxicosis
Heavy metal toxicosis is not uncommon and animals may present with vague neurological or gastrointestinal signs. Both zinc and lead toxicosis have been reported. Prairie dogs frequently chew on their caging, which may contain high levels of zinc. Metal densities may or may not be present in the gastrointestinal tract on radiography. Chelation is with calcium EDTA at 30 mg/kg s.c. every 12 hours for 3–5 days or D-penicillamine at 30–55 mg/kg orally every 12 hours for 1–2 weeks.

Surgical procedures
Many pet prairie dogs are presented for ovariohysterectomy (which is similar to that for a guinea pig or rabbit) or castration. It is preferable to perform these surgeries during the spring or summer, in the first year of life as there is less body fat. Intradermal or subcuticular sutures should be used to close incisions.

Testicles may be found lateral to the penis. A separate skin incision is made over each testicle. The spermatic cord and vessels are best clamped and ligated using a closed technique, because of the open inguinal ring.

If the testicles have not descended, a caudal coeliotomy is performed. The spermatic cords are located between the colon and bladder in a location analogous to the uterus in the female. The spermatic cord is retracted, which allows the testicle to be exteriorized. The vas deferens and vessels are ligated and transected. Closure is routine.

African pygmy hedgehog *Atelerix albiventris*

The African pygmy hedgehog (Figure 10.9) ranges across equatorial and central Africa. It is quite different from the larger, brown European hedgehog and it does not hibernate. Females weigh 250–400g and males 500–600g (non-obese adults).

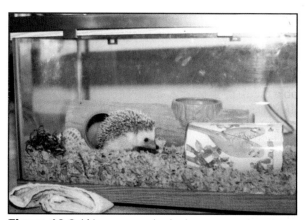

Figure 10.9 African pygmy hedgehog.

Behaviour
Pygmy hedgehogs are nocturnal and solitary. As pets, they will dig, hide, forage and use exercise wheels. Wheels should have flat slats, as hedgehogs may fall through wire rodent wheels; they should also be washable, as the animals tend to defecate while using a wheel.

They are a non-domesticated species and readily display defensive actions and vocalizations (hissing and fussing). They have a moderate tolerance of handling but are more comfortable if handled when very young; then they will allow stroking of the face and underside.

Anting or annointing behaviour is exhibited when an unknown object, odour or other stimulus is encountered. The hedgehog will salivate and place this foam on its quills. Pet hedgehogs can be rinsed off under warm water and allowed to dry in a warm box with towels. Some hedgehogs like to swim and take baths in warm, shallow water but keeping them warm after wetting is essential.

Housing
Cage walls should be smooth and high to prevent escape. The caging should not be made of wire, as this

would catch their feet and legs. Many owners let their hedgehogs roam the house in the evening and the animals can be allowed out of their cage for supervised exercise in the house as long as crevices, heating vents and spaces under appliances or furniture are blocked, as hedgehogs can wedge themselves into small spaces and frequently get their legs and feet caught. Other pets should be confined.

Bedding in the cage should be at least 10 cm deep and kept clean and dry. Most home temperatures are too cool for pygmy hedgehogs: ambient temperatures should be kept at 24–30°C, with the aid of heating pads, heating platforms, infrared emitters or radiant heating units as necessary.

Cage accessories should include a hide box, log, exercise wheel and litter pan (some will use a certain corner, as they tend to be latrine animals). Dishes should be heavy crocks or large flat dishes that cannot tip. Water can be provided in a sipper tube or crock dish, depending on what the hedgehog learned to drink from during weaning. A pan or shallow tub filled with warm water for swimming can be offered.

Most pygmy hedgehogs are kept in housing that is too small and does not provide space for digging and exercise; even a 25 gallon aquarium does not have adequate space or height for a wheel. Hedgehogs seem to enjoy sunshine and grass (provided there are no pesticides or fertilizers) and it is probably acceptable to take them outdoors in very warm weather but they should be supervised and there should be no dogs or cats in the vicinity. Perimeter enclosure fencing of the type used for guinea pigs is useful, as long as the hedgehog is unable to climb it or dig under it.

Diet

Hedgehogs are insectivores and omnivores in the wild. Diets should be relatively high in protein and low in fat. There are several formulations on the market specifically for pet hedgehogs but most are based on feline formulations and there are no published dietary studies on the nutritional requirements of the pygmy hedgehog. A suggested diet is given in Figure 10.10.

Per night:
• 2 tablespoons dry, reduced-calorie catfood or mixture of dry/canned food or good insectivore diet
• 1–2 tablespoons thawed mixed frozen vegetables sprinkled with a complete vitamin/mineral powder or calcium carbonate.
Several times a week:
• Three to five insects
• To a volume of 1–2 teaspoons: babyfood meats or stews (without onion), hard-boiled egg, waxworms, mealworms, pinky mice, horsemeat, various other worms/insects.
Insects and worms should be dusted with a calcium supplement.

Figure 10.10 An appropriate diet for a pygmy hedgehog.

Food should not be provided *ad libitum* but should be limited to what an adult animal will consume by dawn. Despite veterinary warnings about overfeeding, most pet hedgehogs presented are obese. To prevent obesity, it is also recommended that owners weigh their hedgehogs frequently.

Crickets and other 'clean' insects and worms sold in pet shops can be fed in limited numbers to add interest; they also encourage exercise, as the hedgehog must hunt and forage for them. The insects should be fed calcium-fortified cricket food for several days prior to being offered to the hedgehog.

Although hedgehogs love mealworms, these contain a fairly high level of fat and the number should be limited to one giant mealworm or half a teaspoon of small worms, three to five times a week. Worms and live foods can be hidden in the bedding to promote foraging behaviour.

The idea of unlimited bowls of catfood being appropriate for hedgehogs is incorrect: many cases of cystitis or urolithiasis have been reported in hedgehogs on catfood diets, which resolve when the animals are placed on a more appropriate insectivore diet. Feline urinary/cystitis diets have been used for short-term therapy during conversion to an insectivore diet. Some hedgehogs are resistant to dietary changes but the following method is successful:

- Pulverize everything, mix together, and slowly increase proportion of insectivore diet
- Only offer food at night and remove anything left in the morning, ensuring that the hedgehog will be hungry by the next evening and more receptive to any food offered.

Restraint and handling

- Subdued lights, quiet and a towelled surface may help
- Gloves are recommended
- A clear acrylic tube may help to visualize the patient
- Light sedation with isoflurane may ultimately be needed to do a proper examination. It is usually less stressful than forcing them to uncurl.

There are many techniques to uncurl a hedgehog:

- Mantle scruffing: gather up the mantle longitudinally and gently squeeze, causing the hedgehog to uncurl. This may be too stressful if the hedgehog is presented with respiratory difficulties or is ill
- Hanging up by the hindfeet: the hedgehog is slowly pushed to the edge of the table with someone crouched below with a towel in case the hedgehog jumps or rolls off; a second person gently prods it towards the edge. Usually the hedgehog will uncurl to prevent itself falling: quickly grab its hindlegs and hold it up by them, with the head down. Some animals soon learn this trick and will roll up while hung up. With others, it will work once or twice
- Put the animal in a bucket with about 2 cm of warm water and grab the legs (not recommended for an obviously ill hedgehog)
- Put the animal on its back when it is in a ball, then stand back and quietly wait: the hedgehog will unroll as it turns itself over and it may be possible to grab it as it does so.

When the animal unfurls, a hand positioned under its jaw will keep its head out for oral medications.

Techniques

Blood sampling
The saphenous or cephalic veins are accessible for amounts up to 0.5 ml. In thinner hedgehogs it is possible to access the jugular vein. The cranial vena cava can be accessed for larger amounts.

Injection sites
The mantle is largely muscle. On top of that is the subcutaneous organized fat and dermis.

- Subcutaneous injections can reliably be placed in the flank area at the junction of the furred skin and mantle.
- Intramuscular injections can be delivered into the orbicularis muscle of the mantle, or the thigh muscles
- True subcutaneous or even intramuscular injections can be done with a 9 cm spinal needle to enter deep past the spines. With muscles contracted and the hedgehog rolled into a ball, it is actually easier to inject deeper.

Radiography
On all views, the mantle is prominent.

- Spondylosis is commonly seen in geriatric hedgehogs
- Attention should be paid to the liver size and density
- Bones are fairly dense and 'stocky'
- The heart lies fairly cranially in the thoracic cavity
- The liver usually lies totally within the rib cage.

Regular examination
Husbandry, diet, behaviour and handling should be reviewed with the owner on first visit and annually. Physical examination may need to be completed under isoflurane anaesthesia. A fresh stool sample should be examined for parasite ova and protozoans. Optional tests include *Salmonella* culture, skin scrapings for fungal and bacterial culture, and blood sampling. Anaesthesia will be needed for full dental examination and cleaning, nail trimming (toenails need trimming, as they can get caught in carpet and cause lameness) and radiography.

Common conditions
Differential diagnoses are summarized in Figure 10.11.

Clinical signs/disease	Aetiology	Diagnostics	Therapy
Obesity	Overeating, incorrect diet, lack of exercise, ambient temperature too cold	CBC, chemistry panel, radiographs	Correct diet, amount. Provide exercise, proper ambient temperature
Liver disease: hepatitis, hepatosis, hepatic lipidosis, neoplasia	Chronic obesity, fatty diet, liver toxins, chronic bacterial infection, possible human herpes virus infection; genetic predisposition	CBC, chemistry panel, radiographs, liver biopsy, ultrasound	Dietary correction, antimicrobials, possible excision of nodular neoplasia; supportive care, fluids, vitamin B complex, vitamin K, milk thistle, lactulose, S-adenosylmethionine
Flaky skin, dermatitis, breaking quills, alopecia	Ectoparasites (psoroptic, sarcoptic, demodectic mites; fleas); bacterial infection; dermatophytes	Skin scraping, cytology, biopsy. Culture and sensitivity if secondary bacterial infection; fungal culture	Ivermectin, repeated treatments. Appropriate antimicrobial/antifungal therapy as indicated. Thorough cleaning of environment
Wounds, fractures	Trauma from other hedgehogs, other pets; falling, being stepped on	Radiographs if fractures, culture and sensitivity of wound if infected	Manage as in other small mammals: appropriate antimicrobials, lesion repair, fracture repair; NSAIDS, analgesics
Gastroenteritis, vomiting, diarrhoea	Bacterial, protozoal, nematode infestation, endotoxins, foreign body ingestion, neoplasia	CBC, chemistry panel, faecal flotation, smear, Gram stain, culture and sensitivity (*Salmonella* screen), radiographs, contrast series	Appropriate antimicrobials, antiparasitics; supportive care (fluids, nutritional support to avoid hepatic lipidosis); protectants (bismuth subsalicylate), metoclopramide for acute emesis; antidiarrhoeal medications such as loperamide. If *Salmonella*, public health significance, follow reporting rules
Weight loss, wasting, abdominal enlargement, lumps/nodules including oral lesions	Neoplasias – various organs	CBC, chemistry panel, radiographs, ultrasonography, laparotomy; biopsy, histopathology, necropsy	Surgical excision if possible; otherwise symptomatic supportive care, NSAIDS, analgesics, control secondary infections
Neurological disease: ataxia, paresis/paralysis, muscle wasting, knuckling, severe weakness	Too cold (ambient temperature below 18–20°C); trauma, neoplasia, spondylosis, arthritis, encephalitis, demyelination (possibly viral?), hepatic encephalopathy	Husbandry history, body temperature; CBC, chemistry panel, radiographs, ultrasonography (liver/tumour biopsy). Diagnosis may be at necropsy with histopathology	Warm up, improve husbandry. Antimicrobials if bacterial encephalitis. Supportive care, physical therapy. NSAIDS, analgesics, nutraceuticals for arthritis
Alopecia, pendulous abdomen, PU/PD, polyphagia	Cushing's disease	Cortisol level, CBC, chemistry, urinalysis, low-dose dexamethasone test	Therapy as in other mammals?
Dyspnoea, exercise intolerance, cyanosis, coughing, abdominal enlargement	Pneumonia: *Bordetella bronchiseptica*, *Pasteurella multocida*, *Mycoplasma* spp.; environmental chilling, malnutrition, secondary to other systemic disease; irritation/aerosols/toxins, dusts (wet cedar bedding, smoke, carpet cleaners, etc); lung parasites; neoplasia. Cardiomyopathy, congestive heart failure	Auscultation, radiology, tracheal wash/culture and sensitivity, cytology. CBC, chemistry panel. Husbandry history. ECG, abdominocentesis and analysis if ascites; pulse oximetry to assess oxygenation. Neoplasia: biopsy, ultrasonography, histopathology	Antimicrobials, NSAIDS, bronchodilators, remove environmental stresses, irritants. Nebulization. Ivermectin if lung mites. Cardiomyopathy, CHF medication pending diagnosis: enalapril, digoxin, frusemide, potassium supplementation, diet/exercise plan
Haemorrhage, petechiation, wasting, pale mucous membranes	Eosinophilic leukaemia, anaemias, thrombocytopenia, liver disease	CBC, chemistry, bone marrow aspiration, histopathology, liver biopsy	Vitamin K, B complexes, treat liver disease. Neoplasia – treat as in cats????

Figure 10.11 Diseases of the African pygmy hedgehog.

Dental disease

Hedgehogs have fairly small canine teeth and the incisors are angled forward. They are closed-rooted and do not grow continuously. Full oral examinations should be done frequently. Dental disease is fairly common and includes significant plaque, gingivitis and oral neoplasia. Tartar-control cat-treats are well accepted. The teeth can be brushed using pet-formulated products, as for other 'carnivores'.

Gastrointestinal disease

Gastroenteritis of suspected bacterial or parasitic aetiology or foreign body ingestion has been reported. Pygmy hedgehogs have been found to carry *Salmonella* serotype Tilene, which has been reported as a zoonotic agent causing illness in humans.

Internal parasites include *Crenosoma* and *Capillaria* species in animals imported from New Zealand. The literature documents a whole host of recorded parasites from hedgehogs collected in Africa.

In addition to obesity, hepatitis, hepatosis and lipidosis are fairly common. Human herpes simplex I can cause a chronic hepatitis. Liver disease must be considered prior to any surgery and clotting ability should be checked. So far, clinical chemistries seem moderately sensitive in indicating liver disease, though a fair amount of damage may have occurred before enzymes show any elevation. Conversely, if the liver is end-stage, enzymes may be extremely low.

Progression of liver disease may be slowed by putting an obese hedgehog on a weight-reduction diet. This should proceed slowly, following the same cautions as in weight loss plans for obese cats. Conceivably a hedgehog with hepatic lipidosis that becomes anorexic could experience the same difficulties as seen in cats. Oral alimentation supplementation is difficult, though hedgehogs can often be tempted with live foods. Liver biopsies can be done fairly easily, augmented with endoscopic approach.

Respiratory disease

Bacterial agents causing pneumonia include *Bordetella bronchiseptica*, *Pasteurella multocida* and *Mycoplasma* spp. These may be exacerbated by environmental stress from chilling, systemic disease, irritation from aerosols or toxins, lung parasites and neoplasia. Diagnosis is by auscultation, radiographs, endoscopy, tracheal wash, culture and cytology. Treatments follow guidelines for other animals: raise ambient temperature (27–30°C) and give oxygen, antimicrobials, bronchodilators and nebulization. Administration of medications must not be stressful.

Haematological disorders

These have been poorly characterized in African pygmy hedgehogs but the author has diagnosed cases of eosinophilic leukaemia, anaemias, thrombocytopenias, and prolonged bleeding times associated with liver disease. Malnutrition, liver disease and neoplasia are possible aetiologies.

Urogenital problems

Normal urine is yellow and clear (pH 5–6.5, 'carnivore' parameters).

Renal diseases include glomerulosclerosis, nephritis and end-stage kidneys in animals older than 2 years. The role of nephrotoxins is unknown. Cystitis and urolithiasis have been seen, particularly in hedgehogs on catfood-based diets. Preputial injuries with urethral irritation have been seen. Guidelines for treatments of the above conditions follow those for the same diseases in dogs and cats. Switching hedgehogs to a hedgehog insectivore diet instead of catfood makes a difference – recurrences of urolithiasis are rare on a proper insectivore diet.

Neurological disease

While many hedgehogs presented with severe ataxia or paresis or paralysis are showing the effects of being kept in environments that are too cold, several actual pathological processes have been noted. Trauma, neoplasia, spondylosis and arthritis need to be ruled out.

There seems to be a demyelinating paralysis that was first noted in the UK in wild European hedgehogs: a number of hedgehogs developed ataxia and paresis slowly, eventually becoming paraplegic, with urine retention. No other neurological deficit was noted. The clinical course lasted for 1–2 weeks. On histopathology, demyelination was the major sign. In mice, a similar condition is induced by a picornavirus (Theiler's virus-induced demyelinating disease of mice, a model for multiple sclerosis). It is unknown at this time whether hedgehogs are being affected by a virus. Theiler's virus can infect other rodents and a possible receptor has been found in dogs. Full histopathology of the nervous system of any affected hedgehogs is needed, along with virology to discover whether this is what is happening in the pet hedgehog.

Skin problems

Ectoparasites (psoroptic, sarcoptic and demodectic mites and fleas) are common, as are subsequent deep and superficial dermatophyte infections (Figure 10.12).

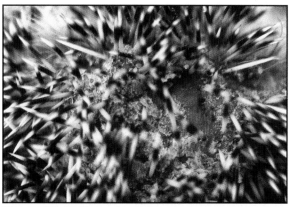

Figure 10.12 Mange in a pygmy hedgehog.

The psoroptid mite *Caparinia tripilis*, which is not zoonotic, is commonly found on pygmy hedgehogs in Europe and in New Zealand, where it is extremely common, with severe infestations. The mite burrows deeply into the skin. The condition can be debilitating, with the hedgehog so denuded that it does not survive the winter. Coinfestation with the sarcoptid mite *Notoedres muris* is common. Dermatophyte infections are usually secondary and deep, so biopsy may be the better diagnostic test. There is a higher incidence of severe infestations in dense populations, which may limit wild and feral populations.

N. muris generally causes crusting and surface lesions, as it burrows fairly superficially into the skin. It is common in New Zealand, where severe infestations are found. Diagnosis is by microscopic examination of skin scrapings or skin biopsies.

Ivermectin has been used as treatment for both species at 200–500 μg/kg topically or subcutaneously. Repeated administrations are usually needed to eliminate *C. tripilis*.

When treating the mites, the ear canals should always be checked. They may be totally impacted with mites and debris, which must be mechanically removed. Ivermectin in propylene glycol can be administered topically at 400 μg/kg partial dose in each ear, and the remainder either by subcutaneous injection or applied topically.

Pyoderma caused by *Staphylococcus aureus* has been reported as being fatal to a litter of neonatal hedgehogs.

Other

Cushing's disease as a result of an adrenal tumour has been diagnosed, with clinical signs of pendulous abdomen, alopecia, neutrophilia, polyuria, polydipsia and polyphagia. The diagnosis was confirmed with a low-dose dexamethasone suppression test using canine guidelines. The animal died before any therapy began.

Neoplasias are common. Meibomian cysts have been seen. Trauma is seen, particularly if more than one hedgehog vies for territory.

Analgesics, anaesthetics and therapeutics

- Butorphanol: 0.05–0.1 mg/kg every 8–12 hours i.m. or s.c.
- Buprenorphine: 0.01–0.5 mg/kg every 8–12 hours i.m. or s.c.
- Flunixin: 0.03 mg/kg as needed every 8 hours i.m.; or 0.3 mg/kg every 24 hours s.c.

Other therapeutics are based on dosages used in ferrets. Fluid therapy is administered based on 50–100 ml/kg per 24 hours. Injections should not be given into the mantle fat layer as absorption rates are unknown.

Surgery

Orchidectomy

The testicles are abdominal and have large fat bodies associated with the epididymis. The incision site for orchidectomy should be just off midline. In an obese hedgehog, two incisions may be necessary.

South American (Brazilian) short-tailed opossum
Monodelphis domestica

The short-tailed opossum (Figure 10.13) is from eastern and central Brazil, Bolivia and Paraguay. It has been used extensively as a laboratory animal. Biological data are summarized in Figure 10.14.

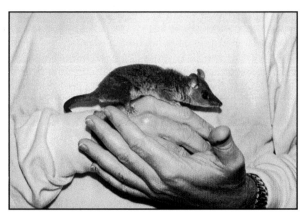

Figure 10.13 Short-tailed opossum.

Weight	Male 90–150 g; female, 80–100 g
Length	Head and body 110–200 mm; tail 45–80 mm
Sexual maturity	4–5 months
Gestation period	14–15 days
Litter size	5–12
Weaning age	About 50 days

Figure 10.14 Biological data for the short-tailed opossum.

The tail is about half as long as the head and body, but always shorter than the body alone, and sparsely haired. It is prehensile and is used by the opossum to carry bedding and other items to be dragged back into the nest. The pouch is not developed. The mammae are arranged in a circle on the abdomen and number 8–14.

Breeding occurs throughout the year in tropical ranges. Neonates cling to the nipples of the mother; later they ride on her back and flanks. These opossums may have up to four litters annually. Breeding has occurred at up to 39 months of age in males, 28 months in females. Oestrus lasts 3–12 days but may vary up to 1 month.

Behaviour

Short-tailed opossums usually dwell on the ground but can climb. Nests are usually built in hollow logs. The animals are basically nocturnal but, as pets, they do spend time interacting with owners during the day. They will use rat wheels for exercise. In South America they live in human dwellings, where they are welcome as they destroy rodents, insects and arachnids such as scorpions. Individuals are highly intolerant of each other, though conflicts rarely result in serious injury.

Diet

In laboratory facilities, short-tailed opossums are fed a pelleted fox diet, insects and pinky mice. They are fed in the evening. Live foods are let loose in the cage and fruit can be placed on branches to encourage foraging and exercise. Suggested daily diets are given in Figure 10.15.

Diet 1 (adapted from the National Zoo)
1 teaspoon of a blended meat mixture comprising: • 1 cup chopped, cooked lean meat (horse or beef) • One hard-boiled egg yolk • 1 tablespoon wheatgerm flakes • 2 teaspoons powdered milk • $^1/_2$ teaspoon multivitamin supplement. This mixture is supplemented daily with: • 1 cm cube of fresh fruit (kiwi, orange, apple, grape, banana) • 1 cm cube of commercial marmoset diet • One or two calcium gut-loaded crickets, one large mealworm and six small mealworms OR two large mealworms OR ten small mealworms.

Diet 2
• 1 teaspoon commercial insectivore diet (hedgehog) • $^1/_2$ teaspoon cooked meat (turkey, chicken, beef, deboned fish) sprinkled with multivitamin/mineral supplement • 1 cm cube of fresh fruit (kiwi, orange, apple, grape, banana) sprinkled with multivitamin/mineral supplement • One or two calcium gut-loaded crickets • One large mealworm and six small mealworms OR two large mealworms OR ten small mealworms. In addition, three to five times per week: • $^1/_4$ teaspoon hard-boiled egg (chop white and yolk together, sprinkle with vitamin/mineral supplement) • $^1/_4$ teaspoon cottage cheese.

Figure 10.15 Daily diets for short-tailed opossum.

Techniques

Blood samples may be drawn from the ventral tail artery or lateral tail vein. In the laboratory, cardiocentesis is usually done, but this is not recommended in pets as it occasionally leads to acute haemorrhage and death.

Common conditions

In general, short-tailed opossums are fairly hardy. In pets, malnutrition, obesity, chilling, injury from falling or handling, and mange mite have been seen. Differential diagnoses for this species are summarized in Figure 10.16.

The principal spontaneous disease problems occur in the digestive system and most diagnoses are lesions of the liver. The most common cause of death from digestive system disease is rectal prolapse. Neoplasia is found most frequently in the digestive system – mainly in the liver, followed by the pancreas. Another frequent disease is enteritis of the small intestine with gaseous distension. They are prone to atherosclerosis following hyperlipidaemia and hypercholesterolaemia.

The second most common system in which lesions are diagnosed is the urogenital system, with the kidney most frequently affected (with nephritis).

The most common neoplasm is pituitary adenoma (prolactinoma), followed by uterine leiomyoma, skin lipomas, adrenal gland phaeochromocytomas and liver carcinomas. Most of these are found in opossums older than 22 months.

Cardiovascular disease is fairly common, with congestive heart failure developing in males more frequently than in females. Heart disease is generally found in animals averaging 37 months of age.

Clinical signs/disease	Aetiology	Diagnostics	Therapy
Rectal prolapse	Enteritis/enteropathy, lack of dietary roughage; phenomenon of ageing, particularly aged females	Faecal flotation/smear, Gram stain; culture. Review of diet; cloacal examination, cytology	Surgical reduction of prolapse, cloacal suture similar to birds – avoid urogenital slits. Antimicrobials, NSAIDS, analgesics, treat underlying enteropathy. Increase roughage in diet
Gastrointestinal distension, ileus; diarrhoea	Bacterial, dietary, rarely protozoal	Faecal cytology, Gram stain, culture and sensitivity; diet review, radiographs	Appropriate antimicrobial, bismuth subsalicylate, NSAIDS, analgesics, fluid therapy, nutritional support
Neoplasia: weight loss or gain, abdominal enlargement, dyspnoea, exercise intolerance	Ageing plays role; liver, pancreas most common	Radiographs, laparotomy, biopsy	Supportive care if excision not possible
Nephritis, pyelonephritis, nephrosis: signs include PU/PD, haematuria, pyuria	Bacterial, ascending from cloaca, reproductive tract	Urinalysis with cytology, culture and sensitivity, CBC, chemistry panel, radiographs; renal biopsy, histopathology	Appropriate antimicrobials, fluid therapy, potassium/electrolyte correction, phosphorus inhibitor, diet modification
Alopecia, particularly on rump, back	Endocrine neoplasia (pituitary adenoma, prolactinoma)	Serum prolactin, oestradiol levels; rule out other causes alopecia; skin biopsy	Leuprolide acetate depot(?); anti-prolactin drugs
Alopecia, with/without pruritis	Ectoparasites: mites, fleas	Skin scraping, observation, biopsy	Ivermectin for mites; flea control of other pets in household
Cardiomyopathy; congestive heart failure: exercise intolerance, cold extremities, cyanosis, dyspnoea, ascites	Ageing? Diet?	Auscultation, radiographs, abdominocentesis and analysis, CBC/chemistry panel	Enalapril, frusemide, potassium supplementation, digitalis may be indicated; supportive care, as in other marsupials
Wounds, lacerations, fractures	Falls, fighting with mates/other opossums	Radiographs to assess fractures; if wounds infected, culture and sensitivity, Gram stain	As in other small mammals: appropriate antimicrobials, NSAIDS, analgesics. Separate incompatible animals

Figure 10.16 Diseases of the short-tailed opossum.

Degu *Octodon degus*

The degu (Figure 10.17), a hystricomorph rodent, is native to northern and central Chile on the West Andean slopes up to 1200 m. Its coat is grey/brown with creamy yellow underparts. The tip of its tail has a black brush and it may slip the fur, exposing the vertebrae (which the animal will bite off, with little bleeding); the section will not be replaced. Thus, as with the chinchilla, restraint should not be by the tail. The claw of the fifth digit is reduced and there are comblike bristles over the claws of the hindfeet. Biological data are summarized in Figure 10.18.

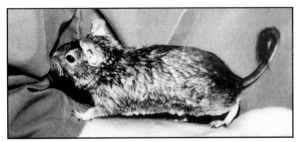

Figure 10.17 Degu.

Lifespan	7 years is the record in captivity
Weight	170–300 g
Length	Head and body 125–195 mm; tail 105–165 mm
Sexual maturity	Average 6 months
Gestation period	Average 90 days
Litter size	1–10 (average 6.8 in captivity)
Weaning	4 weeks of age

Figure 10.18 Biological data for the degu.

The degu is diurnal and active throughout year. Vocalizations include soft chortles and whistles. There is strong social organization based on group territoriality and the animals live in colonies and construct burrows; the females rear their young in a communal burrow. In captivity, degus should be kept socially in pairs or groups.

Degus will breed at any time of year and have multiple litters. There is no regular oestrous cycle but it appears that the female requires the presence of a male to induce ovulation. Neonates weigh 14 g and their eyes may not open for 2–3 days.

Housing

Caging is as for the chinchilla, with tunnelling and a burrow or nest box, sufficient bedding for digging and stockpiling food (they store food for the winter) and space for an exercise wheel. They will utilize a sipper-tube water bottle and might use chinchilla dustbaths. Normal home temperatures seem to be adequate but overheating (> 30°C) should be avoided.

Diet

Degus are herbivorous and are hindgut fermenters. The natural diet includes grass, leaves, bark, herbs, seeds, fruits, fresh cattle/horse droppings during dry season and crops. In captivity, the diet should include rodent chow (one to five cubes per week) and grass hay, with occasional small amounts of a variety of fresh greens. Nutritional requirements for maintenance and reproduction have been published in the laboratory animal literature (the animals are used as models for circadian rhythm, sleep biology and jet-lag studies).

Techniques and therapy

Blood sampling, injection sites, techniques for clinical manipulation and therapy can be based on those used for guinea pigs and chinchillas.

Duprasi (fat-tailed gerbil) *Pachyuromys duprasi*

The duprasi or fat-tailed gerbil is native to the hamada (patches of vegetation) of the northern Sahara Desert from western Morocco to Egypt. Its coat is yellow-grey to buffy brown, with white feet and underparts, a white spot behind each ear and a bicoloured club-shaped tail. It has well developed claws on the front feet and its open-rooted upper incisors are slightly grooved. Biological data are summarized in Figure 10.19.

Lifespan	Average 3 years (4 years 5 months recorded)
Weight	60–90 g
Length	Head and body 105–135 mm; tail 45–60 mm
Sexual maturity	$2\frac{1}{2}$–$3\frac{1}{2}$ months
Gestation period	19–22 days
Litter size	3–6

Figure 10.19 Biological data for the duprasi.

It is insectivorous and the diet can be similar to that of the African pygmy hedgehog except that it can be fed *ad libitum* unless the animal becomes obese (Figure 10.20) – which it will do on the seed/grain-based diets commonly sold for gerbils and hamsters.

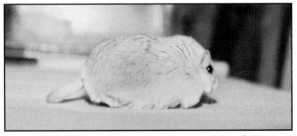

Figure 10.20 Fat-tailed gerbil showing signs of obesity.

Blood-sampling and injection sites are as for domestic gerbils and hamsters. Medications and dosages for hamsters seem to be effective and safe for duprasi but no pharmacological trials have been documented. Isoflurane delivered via nose cone is the preferred anaesthetic.

The major disease problems seen so far include obesity, malnutrition, trauma, diarrhoea and enteropathy (probably associated with bacterial pathogens) and dental malocclusion of the incisors. Differential diagnoses of diseases in the duprasi are summarized in Figure 10.21.

Clinical signs/disease	Aetiology	Diagnostics	Therapy
Obesity, malnutrition	Improper diet, too much carbohydrate, fat; lack of exercise	CBC/chemistry panel; radiographs	Correct diet/husbandry. Provide exercise, live insects
Trauma: wounds, fractures	Attacks from other pets; being dropped/mishandled	Radiographs, culture and sensitivity if wounds infected	Appropriate antimicrobial, wound care as in other animals; NSAIDS, analgesics. Fracture repair similar to birds/small mammals. Correct diet/husbandry
Diarrhoea, enteropathy	Bacterial infections, ingestion of foreign bodies	Faecal examination, culture and sensitivity; radiographs, CBC/chemistry panel	Appropriate antimicrobial therapy, NSAIDS/GI protectants, fluid therapy, supportive care. If foreign body impaction, enterotomy
Malocclusion	Dental trauma, tooth root infection	Radiographs, history, oral examination	Trim teeth, treat underlying cause: infection: antimicrobials; NSAIDS to stop osteomyelitis

Figure 10.21 Diseases of the duprasi.

References and further reading

Mench JA and Kreger MD (1996) Ethical and welfare issues associated with keeping wild mammals in captivity. In: *Wild Mammals in Captivity*, eds Kleiman DG *et al.*, pp. 5–15. University of Chicago Press, Chicago, Illinois

Sugar gliders
Bernard JB, Allen ME and Ullrey DE (1997) Feeding captive insectivorous animals: nutritional aspects of insects as food. *AZA Nutrition Advisory Group Handbook, Fact Sheet 003*. Association of Zoos and Aquariums, Wheeling, West Virginia
Booth RJ (2000) General husbandry and medical care of sugar gliders. In: *Kirk's Current Veterinary Therapy XIII Small Animal Practice*, ed. JD Bonagura, pp. 1157–1163. WB Saunders, Philadelphia
Johnson SD (1997) Orchiectomy of the mature sugar glider. *Exotic Pet Practice* **2**, 71
Johnson-Delaney CA (1997) Pocket pets: essentials for the small animal practitioner. In: *Exotic Pet Conference Proceedings*, pp. 21–37. Texas A & M University, College Station, Texas
Johnson-Delaney CA (1998) The marsupial pet: sugar gliders, exotic possums, and wallabies. In: *Proceedings of the Annual Conference of the Association of Avian Veterinarians*, pp. 329–339. St Paul, Minnesota
Johnson-Delaney CA (2000) Therapeutics of companion exotic marsupials. *Veterinary Clinics of North America: Exotic Animal Practice* **3**, 173–181
Johnson-Delaney CA (2000) Medical update for sugar gliders. *Exotic DVM* **2.3**, 91–93
Ness RD (1999) Clinical pathology and sample collection of exotic small mammals. *Veterinary Clinics of North America: Exotic Animal Practice* **2**, 591–620
Ness RD (2000) Sugar glider (*Petaurus breviceps*): general husbandry and medicine. In: *Proceedings Knowledge 'Rains' in Portland, Clinical Cytology, Exotic Small Mammal Medicine and Management*, pp. 99–107. Association of Avian Veterinarians, Portland, Oregon
Smith A and Hume I (1996) *Possums and Gliders*. Surrey Beatty and Sons Pty Limited/Australian Mammal Society, Chipping Norton, New South Wales
Strahan R (ed.) (1995) *The Mammals of Australia*. Australian Museum/Reed Books, Chatsworth, New South Wales

Prairie dogs
Bennett RA (2000) Husbandry and medicine of prairie dogs. In: *Proceedings Knowledge 'Rains' in Portland, Clinical Cytology, Exotic Small Mammal Medicine and Management*, pp. 79–83. Association of Avian Veterinarians, Portland, Oregon
Johnson-Delaney CA (1996) Special rodents: prairie dogs. In: *Exotic Companion Medicine Handbook for Veterinarians*, pp. 18–25. Wingers Publishing/ZEN Publications, Lake Worth, Florida
Lightfoot TL (2000) Therapeutics of African pygmy hedgehogs and prairie dogs. *Veterinary Clinics of North America: Exotic Animal Practice* **3**, 155–172
Ness RD (1999) Clinical pathology and sample collection of exotic small mammals. *Veterinary Clinics of North America: Exotic Animal Practice* **2**, 591–620

Hedgehogs
Bennett RA (2000) Husbandry and medicine of hedgehogs. In: *Proceedings Knowledge 'Rains' in Portland, Clinical Cytology, Exotic Small Mammal Medicine and Management*, pp. 109–114. Association of Avian Veterinarians, Portland, Oregon
Hoefer HL (1994) Hedgehogs. *Veterinary Clinics of North America: Small Animal Practice* **24**, 113–120
Isenbugel E and Baumgartner RA (1993) Diseases of the hedgehog. In: *Zoo and Wild Animal Medicine Current Therapy 3*, ed. ME Fowler, pp. 294–303. WB Saunders, Philadelphia, Pennsylvania
Johnson-Delaney CA (1996, 1997) Hedgehogs. In: *Exotic Companion Medicine Handbook*, pp. 1–14. Wingers Publishing Inc./ZEN Publishing, Lake Worth, Florida
Lightfoot TL (2000) Therapeutics of African pygmy hedgehogs and prairie dogs. *Veterinary Clinics of North America: Exotic Animal Practice* **3**, 155–172
Ness RD (1999) Clinical pathology and sample collection of exotic small mammals. *Veterinary Clinics of North America: Exotic Animal Practice* **2**, 591–620
Reeve N (1994) *Hedgehogs*. T & AD Poyser, London

Short-tailed opossums
Cothran EG, Haines CK and VandeBerg JL (1990) Age effects on hematologic and serum chemical values in gray short-tailed opossums (*Monodelphis domestica*). *Laboratory Animal Science* **40**, 192–197
Fadem BH, Trupin GL, Maliniak E *et al.* (1982) Care and breeding of the gray, short-tailed opossum (*Monodelphis domestica*). *Laboratory Animal Science* **32**, 405–409
Field KJ and Griffith JW (1990) Corneal lesion in a grey short-tailed opossum. *Lab Animal* **19**, 19–20
Hubbard GB, Mahaney MC, Gleiser CA *et al.* (1997) Spontaneous pathology of the gray short-tailed opossum (*Monodelphis domestica*). *Laboratory Animal Science* **47**, 19–26
Keller LSF, Drozdowicz CK, Rice L *et al.* (1988) An evaluation of three anaesthetic regimes in the gray short-tailed opossum (*Monodelphis domestica*). *Laboratory Animals* **22**, 269–275
Kraus DB and Fadem BH (1987) Reproduction, development and physiology of the gray short-tailed opossum (*Monodelphis domestica*). *Laboratory Animal Science* **37**, 478–482

Degus
Johnson-Delaney CA (1997) Special rodents: degus. In: *Exotic Companion Medicine Handbook for Veterinarians*, pp. 27–32. Wingers Publishing/ZEN Publications, Lake Worth, Florida
Rush HG, Lee TM and Young AT (2000) Growth and reproductive performance of degus (*Octodon degus*) on commercial rodent diets. *Contemporary Topics* **39**, 104
Smith PC, Chrisp CE and Rush HG (2000) Parathyroid adenocarcinoma with metastasis and pulmonary adenocarcinoma in a degu (*Octodon degus*). *Contemporary Topics* **39**, 89

Duprasis
Johnson-Delaney CA (1997) Special rodents: duprasi. In: *Exotic Companion Medicine Handbook for Veterinarians*, pp. 34–37. Wingers Publishing/ZEN Publications, Lake Worth, Florida

11

Fancy pigs

David J. Taylor

Introduction

Fancy pigs may belong to conventional rare breeds such as the Tamworth or to one of a small number of exotic breeds such as the Vietnamese Potbellied or the Kune Kune from New Zealand (Figure 11.1). Some may be crosses between one of these and another domestic breed, or even with wild boar. All are domestic pigs; as such, they require care similar to that given to farmed pigs and are subject to the Diseases of Animals legislation.

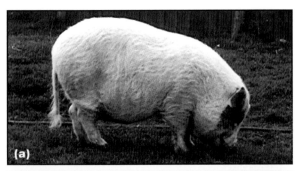

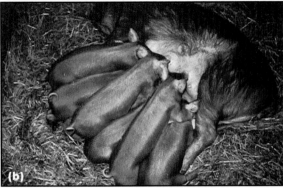

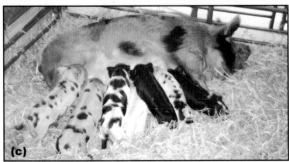

Figure 11.1 Some pigs kept as pets: (a) Vietnamese Potbellied; (b) Tamworth; (c) Kune Kune. (Courtesy of J. Carr)

Many pet pigs are kept in small numbers or singly and they may live in close proximity to their owners, even within the home. This proximity, and the bond between owner and pet, makes the management of disease a matter for individual assessment. The small numbers of pigs kept and their size (initially small but considerable when mature) lead to problems that are rarely experienced when diagnosing disease in farmed pigs.

Fancy pigs should be considered companion animals. The simplest procedures may be difficult to carry out in a newborn piglet or in a mature boar or sow, and owners may lack facilities for control or expertise in restraint. Diagnosis cannot always rely on texts that describe disease in farmed pigs, as they use features such as herd behaviour and skin colour changes (breeds such as the Vietnamese Potbellied often have dark skins), and rely on herd pathology (unlikely to be an option in pet pigs). Also, farmed pigs are generally younger than the presented pet pig. Some of the techniques used in many companion animals to supplement clinical examination, such as radiography and electrocardiography, may be difficult to carry out in the pig.

Thus, examination and diagnosis may be less simple than in the farmed animal and a wider range of medical and surgical procedures may be requested by the owner than are commonly provided for farmed pigs. Treatment of some conditions in pet pigs cannot be achieved using the pharmaceutical products intended for use in food animals, and veterinary surgeons may wish to use products not licensed for pigs (see Formulary at the end of this chapter). Before these products are used, the legal and technical position should be considered. Finally, the question of euthanasia and carcass disposal may pose problems in larger specimens, for both the owner and the veterinary surgeon.

Biology

The average lifespan for a pet pig is 10–15 years. Weaning age is 6–8 weeks, although in some cases piglets may need supplementary feeding even while suckling. The age of sexual maturity for male potbellied pigs is around 2 months of age, and that for females 3 months of age. This early maturation is a good reason for castration or spaying in the pet pig.

Biological data for pigs are summarized in Figure 11.2.

Body temperature	30°C
Lower critical point	38.4°C
Upper critical point	40°C
Respiratory rate (resting, 18°C)	20–30 breaths per minute; more in young (up to 50); less in old sows (13–15)
Heart rate (resting)	70–80 beats per minute; higher in young (200–280 newborn)
Average lifespan	10–15 years
Sexual maturity	2–4 months
Gestation	114 days
Weaning age	6–8 weeks

Figure 11.2 Biological data for pigs.

Husbandry

The pet pig has the same minimum requirements for space, environmental temperature, food, water, lighting, observation and other forms of care as the farmed breeds. The government's Welfare Codes provide guidance about these.

Housing

Housing can be relatively simple (Figure 11.3). Ideally, pet pigs should not be housed indoors. If they do live in the house, training should be given to ensure that they observe a lavatory area. Dunging and urination in a particular spot can be encouraged by making this area cooler than the remainder of the accommodation, by placing the water bowl or trough nearby, or by installing a low barrier over which the pig must step to leave the clean area.

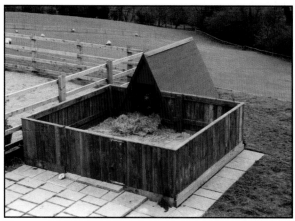

Figure 11.3 Simple outdoor enclosure for a pet pig. (Courtesy of J. Carr)

Figure 11.4 provides a guide to environmental temperatures for pet pigs. These temperatures should not fluctuate. In hot weather the pig will appreciate a water spray or wallow. Accommodation should be draught-free, and provision for heating (heat pads, heat lamps) should be made to prevent hypothermia in winter or where young animals are present. The provision of fresh, deep barley or oat straw will provide draught proofing and supplement the feed. As pet pigs

eat their straw, it should be replenished each evening to provide maximum insulation through the night. Outdoor enclosures can be fenced with commercial electric fencing or with pig wire netting supported by stout posts and stretched wire. Shade, shelter and water should always be available outdoors.

Minimum temperature requirements	
Adults	
In houses and yards	15–20°C
At farrowing	15–18°C
Piglets with the sow to 5 kg	25–30°C
Piglets 3–6 weeks, housed alone	27–32°C
Weaned pigs (6–12 weeks)	21–24°C
Growing animals (12–16 weeks)	15–21°C
Pigs (16–26 weeks)	13–18°C
Maximum temperature requirements	
Adults: In houses and yards	28°C (beyond this, cooling should be provided)

Figure 11.4 A guide to the temperatures required by fancy pigs.

Diet

Pet pigs are often bought or acquired as recently weaned or orphaned piglets but will grow considerably to reach adult size; their nutritional needs change as they grow. As piglets or weaners, a commercial creep or weaner ration is advisable, as it is formulated carefully for young animals. As the animal becomes more robust (by 10–12 weeks of age) these diets can be replaced by a commercial grower ration. Finisher rations should be avoided as they lead to too fast a growth rate. Finally, by 6 months of age, the pig can be given commercial sow meal or sow rolls (large pellets designed for outdoor pigs). Home-made diets must follow the same principles and contain easily digestible materials with relatively high protein content for young piglets (rolled oats, milk powder, barley meal), gradually lowering the amount of protein and carbohydrate with age until adults have a relatively fibrous diet. Dietary supplementation with household scraps is not advised, as the presence of meat or contact with meat may lead to infection with diseases such as swine fever and foot and mouth disease and lead to compulsory slaughter. Adult pigs can be fed fruit and potatoes.

Baby pigs fed on inadequate diets, mature pot-bellied pigs kept outdoors (where quantities fed may be inadequate for winter maintenance) and animals receiving incomplete diets consisting of bread or grain meal without adequate balancing nutrients may all be predisposed to problems. Adults are often overweight and should be fed to maintain good, but not fat, body condition. Restriction of the diet physically will lead to rooting and to behavioural disturbances. The quantity of food given can be maintained to provide satisfaction by using horse pellets, which have a higher fibre content, or by offering fibrous feeds including good straw. This low-energy diet should not be given to animals at risk of hypothermia.

Breeding

Potbellied pigs mature early (see above) and mixed-sex pairs of weaners can soon mature and mate. The young piglets may be a surprise to the owners, who may not have prepared nesting or farrowing areas or be ready to support young litters. This, coupled with the youth of the sow, often produces disappointing results and high mortality.

The period of gestation in pet pigs is the same as in the commercial breeds (114 days), but where breeding pairs are kept together the service date is not always known. As a result, it may be necessary to watch for nesting behaviour, enlargement of the udder or slackening of the vulva, and to ensure that the sow is in a warm sheltered place separate from the boar.

Handling and restraint

Physical restraint may be by use of a snare of stout cord (Figure 11.5). The snare (a running loop) should be placed over the upper jaw, pulled well back into the lateral commissures of the lips and then tightened with the knot over the centre of the upper jaw. Care should be taken to ensure that the noose does not tighten around the sensitive fleshy end of the snout and that it is supported by the bones of the maxilla and premaxilla. This method may not be possible for pigs with short snouts.

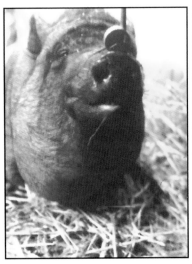

Figure 11.5
Physical restraint may be by use of a snare of stout cord. The pig also has a large *Actinobacillus suis* abscess on the right lower jaw which was surgically removed. (Courtesy of J. Carr)

The owner must be made aware that this procedure is to take place. Snared animals remain still and pull back by reflex against the cord and so can easily be examined single-handed. Vocalization soon dies away. When examination is complete, the snare is released by loosening it at the knot on the snout and the pig merely grunts and walks away.

Small pigs may be restrained manually, but piglets should be picked up only when the sow is in a farrowing crate or shut outside the pen, as she may be very protective.

Chemical restraint of pigs by sedation is possible, using azaperone, but priapism may occur in large boars at levels above 1 mg/kg.

Diagnostic approach

Most pet pigs are examined during home visits but some examinations take place in the surgery. In the UK, movement of pigs should always be carried out under licence (Movement and Sale of Pigs Order, 1975), obtainable from the Police or relevant Ministry.

History

The history is extremely important, as the presenting signs may be difficult to interpret or may be no longer present at examination. The factors to be considered include:

- Breed (or cross)
- Age
- Numbers of animals present on the premises
- Type of housing (outdoor and indoor pigs may suffer from different conditions)
- Access to toxic materials, such as rat poison or lead
- Physical trauma related to the environment or to companion pigs
- Type of food
- Past inappetence
- Lameness
- Nervous signs
- Discharges
- Diarrhoea
- Reproductive abnormalities.

Inspection and examination

Protective clothing may be required – boots, washable or disposable overalls, and a head covering if the animal is housed indoors. Disinfectant that conforms to the criteria of the Disinfectants Orders should be made up ready to disinfect footwear after the visit. The examination of breeding stock may be dangerous and a pig board (a square or rectangular board with a handle grip at the top) should be carried in order to approach the animal safely.

Inspection of the pig in its own environment and from outside the pen is of considerable value and should include:

- Bodily condition
- Presence of inappetence
- Lameness
- Nervous signs
- Increased respiratory rates
- Discharges
- Diarrhoea
- Skin conditions
- Injuries.

It is important to observe the behaviour of the pig towards its environment:

- If the temperature is too low or if fever is present, the animal will shiver or attempt to bury itself in any bedding present
- Where the environmental temperature is too high, the animal will attempt to wallow and, where no water or mud is available, will roll in faeces and urine in an attempt to cool off.

Physical examination (Figure 11.6) may be possible without restraint, simply by examining the animal in its environment. The examination should be carried out with as little disturbance to the pig as possible. Pigs are extremely vocal and the owner may be distressed by the noise resulting from rough or injudicious handling. When physical restraint is necessary for general or specific examinations, the reason should be given and the procedure carefully explained before restraint begins.

Examination of the restrained pig should include the areas outlined in Figure 11.7. Further examination may be carried out by using a speculum to examine the vagina, or, when farrowing difficulties are encountered, manual examination may be carried out by those with small hands (gloved). Ultrasound has been used to locate the site of fractures, to detect pericarditis and cystic ovaries, and to detect pregnancy and visualize the contents of the pregnant uterus. A number of commercial pregnancy testing devices are available.

Rectal temperatures	Can be taken by inserting thermometer and following pig, holding thermometer in rectum against tail. Animal often defecates following this procedure and faeces can be examined
Urine	May be obtained or inspected by alert practitioner, as pigs frequently urinate immediately when they stand up
Skin	Appearance and any lesions present may be recorded Pallor in dark-skinned animals best observed by examining mucous membranes, (e.g. mouth, vulva)
Nervous signs	Tremor, convulsions, etc. identified and site of nervous lesions assessed in paralysed animals
Feet and legs	More difficult to assess – pigs resent feet and legs being held
Mouth and eyes	Conjunctival discharge and straightness of snout noted
Auscultation of chest	Possible but available lung field small and vocalization often obscures lung sounds Heart more easily examined; apex beat easily seen in young or thin pigs but must be examined in sows

Figure 11.6 Physical examination.

Eyes	Conjunctivitis
Nose	Nasal discharge
Mouth and snout	Ulcers
Ears	Crusting and evidence of mange Record necrosis of pinna, bite marks, ulceration, thickening of pinna, presence of waxy deposits within external auditory meatus
Face	Oedema of skin of forehead or eyes Bite marks on face or cheeks of piglets
Mouth, teeth, tonsils	Examine mouth of conscious pig with gag and torch (mouth is too long and dangerous to attempt examination without gag). Pig gags are metal, shaped like tuning forks with a cross-piece; they vary in size to suit piglets or adults
Skin	Wounds and lesions (e.g. erysipelas); not easily seen in brown pigs – run hand across skin of back and hams to check for presence of raised rhomboid lesions Colour of the skin can indicate systemic conditions in white pigs In potbellied pigs, pallor, congestion and jaundice may only be visible in mouth, sclera of eye or the lips of vulva Various degrees of scaliness of skin may indicate presence of sarcoptic mange (intensely irritant), vitamin deficiency or infection (e.g. exudative epidermitis in piglets); axilla and belly should be checked for these as well as back Tail should be checked for biting
Anus	Prolapse, diarrhoea or constipation Diarrhoea may be white in sucking piglets or brown and watery, contain fresh or altered blood (black faeces), mucus and necrotic material in older pigs – all of diagnostic importance
Vulva	Hypertrophy, masculinization, evidence of biting, discharge Where pig dehydrated, crystalline deposits on lips Oestrus results in swelling of vulva; can be confirmed by gentle back pressure when sow will stand
Udder	Teats should be regular with no everted nipples Sows in milk: feel both sides of mammary ridge and confirm presence of mastitis by feeling hardening of glands; litter will be thin and hungry if no supplementary feeding Udder may be overstocked if small litter but involution of unwanted glands soon occurs
Testicles	Size and evenness
Prepuce lining	By eversion
Penis	By exteriorization to confirm integrity
Hernias	Confirm as such by reduction; record size and location – they may affect castration (inguinal) or transport (umbilical and inguinal)
Lameness	Important: animal should be seen to walk and any physical abnormalities of limbs felt Swollen joints checked for heat (suggests active infection) and for fluctuation of joint capsule Broken legs or epiphyseolysis (fracture of mid portion of femoral head) very difficult to detect Extreme muscular nature of pig limbs means that fractures may be self-supporting; existence of fracture and location may be hard to find

Figure 11.7 Examination of the restrained pig.

Diagnostic tests and techniques

The following samples may be taken for laboratory examination.

- *Nasal swabs*: taken from a restrained pig by holding its mouth shut and inserting a fine-wire swab (urethral or nasal) into the nares. The snout should be steadied and the swab slipped into the ventral portion of the nasal cavity when the nasal sphincter is opened for breathing. It should be withdrawn slowly so as not to cause damage
- *Tonsillar swabs*: require use of a gag
- *Ear scrapings and ear wax*: for diagnosis of mange mites; taken from inside of pinna
- *Skin scrapings*
- *Faecal samples*: taken from the rectum. If this is empty, stimulation with gloved finger will usually induce production of sample
- *Urine*: taken from gilts by catheterization
- *Vaginal samples*: by use of speculum
- *Blood samples*: taken by 'vacutainer' into suitable tube, using jugular vein (large pigs) or anterior vena cava (piglets). Sampling from these sites may require training.

Normal haematological and biochemical values are set out in Figure 11.8 and normal urine composition in Figure 11.9.

Parameter	Mean	Range	Units
Packed cell volume (PCV)	0.42	0.37–0.46	l/l
Red blood cells	7.0	6.5–8.0	10^{12}/l
White blood cells	18.0	10.0–23.0	10^9/l
Platelets	400.0	250.0–700.0	10^9/l
Haemoglobin	140	110–142	g/l
Calcium	2.70	2.4–3.0	mmol/l
Phosphorus	2.68	2.1–3.3	mmol/l
Sodium	152	133–171	mmol/l
Potassium	5.49	4.5–6.5	mmol/l
Chloride	nd	95–110	mmol/l
Bilirubin	2.1	0.1–4.1	mmol/l
Total protein	70.4	55.84–85.4	g/l
Urea	5.5	2.9–8.1	mmol/l
Glucose	5.18	4.0–6.36	mmol/l
Lactate	5.2	0–11.0	mmol/l
Alkaline phosphatase	215	140–190	IU/l
AST	17	9–25	IU/l
Creatine kinase	nd	0–800	IU/l
Cholesterol	nd	2.0–3.3	mmol/l
Gamma GT	nd	10–40	IU/l
GLDH	nd	0–5.5	IU/l

Figure 11.8 Normal haematological and biochemical values for the pig. These vary from breed to breed, and with age in some cases.
nd = no data available

Specific gravity	1.020
pH	5.5–7.5
Protein	None
Colour	Yellow to amber
Bacteria	< 10^4/ml

Figure 11.9 Urine composition in normal adults (based on sows).

Common conditions

Notifiable diseases

The possible presence of notifiable disease should always be considered (Figure 11.10), as some owners may be tempted to feed table scraps. Suspicion of any of these diseases should be notified to the relevant Ministry.

Disease	Signs
Foot and mouth disease and swine vesicular disease	Vesicles on snout or on coronary bands Lesions on feet extremely painful; pig very lame and may scream if moved As lesions on feet heal, may be thimbling of horn or symmetrical horizontal lesions around claws on all four feet Piglets may die suddenly
Aujeszky's disease	Difficult to identify but may give rise to abortion in sows or nervous signs with high pig mortality in freshly introduced infections
Swine fevers	May present as dullness, inappetence, high fever, congestion and petechiation of skin, unsteadiness of gait, rapidly progressing to death Conjuctival discharge, raised respiratory rate, diarrhoea may occur Congestion of skin may not be evident in dark-skinned pigs Death common
Anthrax	Unusual in any pig May be seen as fever, localized swelling of neck, bloody diarrhoea, or sudden death

Figure 11.10 Notifiable diseases in the UK.

Non-notifiable diseases

Many of the pigs presented for consultation will be adult or independent and solitary or in non-breeding pairs or groups. Because of single housing, small numbers and extensive conditions, pet pigs are not affected by many of the infections that cause clinical disease in commercially farmed pigs. For example, enzootic pneumonia and the porcine reproductive and respiratory syndrome (PRRS) rarely cause clinical disease. Lack of appetite and dullness may be present in adult pigs. Figure 11.11 suggests possible differential diagnoses for a range of clinical signs.

The reproducing family group, farrowing problems and problems in the suckling piglet may be encountered less frequently and are considered separately below.

Skin disease

Erysipelas

Characteristic raised diamond skin lesions may not be visible on dark-skinned pigs but may be readily felt. The pig becomes lame, with hot swollen joints. Treatment is with parenteral penicillin. All pigs should be vaccinated.

Ringworm

Ringworm may be difficult to identify. Both *Trichophyton mentagrophytes* and *Microsporum canis* may occur in pet pigs but the brown greasy lesions may not

Sign	Possible causes
Fever	Consider erysipelas
Fever, pneumonia, raised respiratory rate	Consider pasteurellosis, pleuropneumonia or influenza Pasteurellosis, pleuropneumonia: treat with parenteral oxytetracycline or specialist antibiotic (ceftiofur). Prevention of pleuropneumonia: vaccination Influenza: dramatic course of disease, associated with depression, conjunctival discharge, coughing and sneezing, congestion of extremities; followed by spontaneous recovery
Fever and diarrhoea	Consider salmonellosis Faeces may contain necrotic material and occasionally be tinged with fresh blood but rarely contain mucus Treatment: injection with enrofloxacin, trimethoprim sulphonamide, apramycin, spectinomycin
Diarrhoea without fever	Swine dysentery in adult pigs: can be distinguished in early cases by presence of fresh blood and mucus, later containing necrotic material Spirochaetal diarrhoea: may be difficult to identify (resembles mild swine dysentery) Treatment for both diseases: parenteral lincomycin or tiamulin followed by course of drug in water Worm infestations (*Trichuris suis, Oesophagostomum* spp.) and cocciodiosis may be causes of featureless diarrhoea in adults. Treatment: conventional wormers (parenteral ivermectin or doramectin may be preferable to ensure compliance)
Profuse rapidly spreading	Sudden acute diarrhoea may be viral in origin; may be transmissible gastroenteritis, porcine epidemic diarrhoea or rotavirus Usually spontaneous recovery in adults
Black faeces and pallor	Consider proliferative enteropathy or gastric ulceration Treatment: gastric ulceration symptomatically but proliferative enteropathy parenterally or oral tetracycline
Nervous signs and fever	Glasser's disease, streptococcal meningitis or swine fevers Streptococcal meningitis: parenteral penicillins (but animal may remain paralysed or with some degree of residual nervous dysfunction); nurse and reassess at 3-day intervals; rehydration with physiological saline from flutter valve into rectum; euthanase if paralysis persists but not necessary if partially dysfunctional unless physical damage occurring
Depression and subnormal temperature	Hypothermia in outdoor-housed adults or young pigs in cold weather Housing within normal temperature range and provision of food may restore (some potbellied pigs do not recover) Congestive cardiac failure: congestion of ears and extremities in white or partially white pigs but not visible in potbellied – may require auscultation and examination of mucous membranes Ultrasound to identify cardiac changes and distinguish between fibrous pericarditis, vegetative endocarditis and uncomplicated heart failure. Euthanasia recommended for first two

Figure 11.11 Differential diagnoses.

be apparent on brown pigs and suspicion may develop only after human infection. *M. canis* infections can be identified using a Wood's lamp but this will not identify other species. Treatment is with enilconazole or natamycin or by thorough washing with hexetidine. The housing should also be washed down to prevent re-infection.

Mange

Mange is easily identified by the characteristic flaky skin lesions (Figure 11.12) and the scratching and rubbing behaviour (mange-free animals rarely scratch and rub and do not rub the hairs off their flanks or break the skin by rubbing). As the diagnosis of mange may not be acceptable to the owner, examination of the inside of the ear canal for wax crusts and the demonstration of mange mites from these or from an ear scraping may be required. Treatment should be carried out on all pigs on the premises with ivermectin or doramectin by injection, unless numbers and facilities allow the use of in-feed or cutaneous products. Two injections 18 days apart should eradicate the mite.

Lice

Lice may be seen as adults moving on white pigs and as egg cases on the neck hairs of brown or black pigs. Ivermectin and doramectin injection should control.

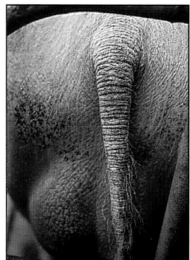

Figure 11.12 Chronic rubbing associated with mange in this boar has resulted in very scaly skin on the back and along the tail head. The mites may be difficult to find in this area, but are readily found in an ear wax sample. (Courtesy of J. Carr)

Scurf

Scurfy skins may result from essential fatty acid deficiencies and can be corrected by adding a little cod liver oil or margarine to the diet.

Wounds

Wounds and biting will be obvious. In outdoor systems, these may result from attack by birds such as magpies and crows; pigs may need to be protected by netting.

Musculoskeletal disease

Lameness may occur in pet pigs and is particularly noticeable in animals that regularly walk with their owners. The major problems are foot abscess, arthritis and some cases of osteoarthrosis. In all cases, care should be taken not to allow a lame pig to suffer. Many of the problems of intensively housed pigs, such as osteochondrosis, bursitis and sole erosion, are absent but the last two occasionally occur in animals kept on hard surfaces.

Foot abscess and arthritis are easily recognizable:

- Foot abscess: inspection after cleaning the foot
- Arthritis: localization of lameness to affected region of leg, followed by inspection and palpation.

Treatment of both conditions depends on the stage of the disease. In early disease, when swollen joints are hot and fluid-filled (in streptococcal infection, Glasser's disease and erysipelas), antimicrobial treatment is possible. Parenteral penicillin can be used and successful treatment rapidly leads to the disappearance of clinical signs. As infection is not immediately eliminated, the treatment should be repeated until a full course has been given (3–7 days).

Treatment may eliminate heat without eliminating swelling and loss of function. Function may then be restored by using a non-steroidal anti-inflammatory such as meloxicam. This approach may be used in cases of chronic arthritis.

Where foot abscess is at an early stage and the tracks of pus from the coronary band are small, prolonged treatment coupled with bathing and local poulticing may relieve the condition. If treatment is unsuccessful, the infected digit should be removed under general anaesthetic, the wound bandaged and the animal kept on a clean floor to protect the healing foot.

Problems of breeding animals and young litters

As pet piglets are relatively small, obstetrical problems are uncommon but manual interference may be required on occasion.

- After birth, it is essential that the piglets take colostrum and are warm enough. It may be difficult to arrange a creep area and hypothermia is a major cause of loss at this stage
- Crushing by the sow is also common.

Hypoglycaemia

Shivering, depression followed by convulsions and air hunger suggest the presence of hypoglycaemia. Piglets may be restored by 50 ml intraperitoneal 5% glucose saline solution and heat.

Mastitis and agalactia

These can be detected by feeling both sides of the mammary ridge for hardness. They can be managed by giving oxytocin intravenously or intramuscularly to encourage milk let-down. A milk substitute should be provided for the young piglets if the mother has insufficient milk. Where the sow is also depressed or fevered and where there is vulval discharge, a course of antimicrobial such as penicillin and streptomycin, ampicillin or tetracycline should be given parenterally.

Small litters and infertility

Sometimes pet pigs produce small litters or do not breed regularly. When this occurs, infertility can be investigated.

- *Condition*: animals should be in normal bodily condition and not overfat
- *Return to service after normal oestrus and service*: there may have been inadequate penetration. Supervised services may be required and the fertility of the boar should be checked
- *Oestrus not observed*: the season should be considered – pigs may not show oestrus in very hot or cold weather or in winter. If this is not the case and the female external genitalia are normal, cystic ovaries may be present and injection with gonadotrophins may be required. Has the gilt or sow been spayed?
- *Boar fails to mount*: may be a penile lesion, arthritis of the legs or spine or testicular damage
- *Mummified piglets or small litters*: parvovirus could be the cause. Breeding gilts and sows should be vaccinated against parvovirus.

Problems of suckling pigs and young weaners

Congenital abnormalities

Common congenital abnormalities in newborn pigs include umbilical and inguinal hernias, atresia ani (where there is failure of the anus to open) and hermaphroditism.

- If congenital tremor is seen in the UK, the Ministry should be informed in case classical swine fever is present
- Piglets born with splayleg must be managed carefully, ensuring that they can feed and do not get caught in bedding. The splayed limbs may be taped together for 2–3 days to enable them to move and suck.

Escherichia coli septicaemia

Piglets may die from *E. coli* septicaemia within the first day or so of birth. Treatment is by parenteral antimicrobial injection with ampicillin, enrofloxacin or trimethoprim sulphonamide.

Diarrhoea

Neonatal diarrhoea occurs in cold damp conditions. Oral treatment and oral rehydration should be given. Oral treatment in suckling pigs is by means of piglet pumps or oral dosers containing antimicrobials such as neomycin or trimethoprim–sulphonamide and delivering a daily measured dose. Vaccination of the sow and colostral ingestion may prevent the diarrhoea.

Diarrhoea may occur later in the suckling period and be caused by rotavirus and coccidians. These diarrhoeas are rarely fatal and can be managed by providing electrolyte solution for the piglets to drink and maintaining a warm, draught-free environment.

Progressive atrophic rhinitis

Sneezing may be evidence of progressive atrophic rhinitis, which later causes shortening and diversion of the snout. The disease can be treated and the bony changes prevented by injection with trimethoprim sulphonamide at 3, 10 and 21 days of age. Vaccination of the sow will prevent.

Streptococcal joint ill

Lameness and meningitis can occur at two distinct periods in the suckling period:

- At 7–10 days, the soft hot swollen joints may be due to *Streptococcus suis* Type 1. Prompt treatment with penicillin will cure the disease and subsequent litters born to the same sow can be treated just before the disease is due to develop, thus eliminating the developing infection
- From 3 weeks onward, Glasser's disease may be responsible and may be treated using tetracyclines parenterally or in water. A combined enzootic pneumonia and *Haemophilus parasuis* vaccine is available.

Umbilical abscesses

Umbilical abscesses may result from infection of the cord at birth but only become apparent from 7 to 10 days of age. Affected pigs grow slowly and may develop arthritis and more generalized infection. Well established abscesses do not always respond to treatment and may represent a cause of continued ill-health. They may be prevented to some extent if the navels of newborn piglets are dipped in an iodophor disinfectant.

Skin conditions

- Scabby cheeks may be due to fighting: the udder should be examined to eliminate mastitis as a contributory cause
- Generalized exudative change on the skin from 7–10 days of age onward: probably exudative epidermitis. Early erythema and brown flakes on skin may be difficult to identify in dark-coloured piglets. Treatment: bathing in hexetidine and parenteral treatment with semi-synthetic penicillins or lincomycin
- Localized 2 cm raised lesions on back: may be pig pox
- Expanding scabby circles on belly from 6 weeks onward: usually pityriasis rosea, a congenital condition that eventually disappears.

Piglet anaemia

Pet pigs are rarely weaned before 6–8 weeks of age. Those that are reared indoors may develop iron-deficiency anaemia and should be given iron supplementation. Affected piglets are usually at least 3 weeks of age and pale (the mucous membranes should be checked) and have a prominent apex beat. Parenteral iron injections should be given within 3–4 days of birth but oral supplementation with iron or access to soil should be ensured. If peat is used as a source of iron, it should be pasteurized to prevent tuberculosis.

Post-weaning *E. coli* diarrhoea

Weaning may be accompanied by post-weaning *E. coli* diarrhoea as the piglet adapts to a solid diet or when the animal is rehomed. Oral fluid replacement therapy should be given in all cases and an oral antimicrobial such as neomycin, amoxycillin clavulanate or trimethoprim sulphonamide should be given to severely affected piglets by oral doser or in water. Warm dry draught-free accommodation should be provided and an easily digestible diet made available to recently weaned animals.

Sudden death

Sudden death may occur in pigs of any age. A post-mortem examination may be carried out but consideration should be given to the subsequent disposal of the carcass. In many cases the cause will be obvious: a twisted bowel, mulberry heart disease, vegetative endocarditis, cystitis or pneumonia. The risk to other animals can then be assessed and preventive measures taken to safeguard them.

Supportive care

Treatment can be administered by the following routes:

- Oral: in feed, water or as oral dosers for piglets
- Parenteral: by intramuscular injection in the neck behind the ear
- Intravenously: in the lateral ear vein.

Supportive treatments are summarized in Figure 11.13.

Colostrum substitute	Can be given to piglets by stomach tube (see product leaflets)
Sow milk replacer for orphan and weak piglets	From agricultural chemists and feed merchants
Oral fluid replacement	Make up and provide in tube drinker therapy
Creep feeds	To ensure proper nutrition of sucking or orphaned piglets
Colitis diets	Commercially available; reduce diarrhoea in weaned pigs
Sow rolls	Satisfactory way of feeding outdoor animals
Iron dextran preparations for piglets	1 ml by deep i.m. injection into hindlimb at 3 days of age

Figure 11.13 Supportive treatments.

Anaesthesia

- Pigs can be sedated using azaperone (1–2 mg/kg)
- For full anaesthesia, azaperone at 1–8 mg/kg (usually 4 mg/kg) is given and 20 minutes later intravenous anaesthesia is given via the lateral ear vein

- Intravenous anaesthesia can be induced with pentobarbitone, ketamine (2–5 mg/kg) and alphaxalone/alphadolone (Saffan®) (2 mg/kg) and can be maintained for short procedures such as castration in adults or inguinal hernia repair
- Anaesthesia can be maintained for longer procedures using halothane or isoflurane. There is a slight risk of susceptibility to halothane in some breeds and a blood sample may be tested for the presence of the gene governing susceptibility
- Intubation may be difficult in pigs. If doubtful about tracheal intubation, a T-shaped nasal tube can be used instead.

Figure 11.14 shows an anaesthetized pig stabilized using intranasal intubation attached to a circle anaesthetic machine.

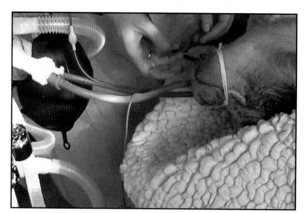

Figure 11.14 Anaesthetized pig stabilized using intranasal intubation attached to a circle anaesthetic machine. The cuffs are inflated inside the nostril and the pig's mouth held closed by a tape to reduce mouth breathing. (Courtesy of J. Carr)

Pigs that have been anaesthetized should be allowed to recover on their own in sternal recumbency and should not be returned until completely recovered. If they form part of a group, reintroduction should be watched or azaperone given to the whole group to prevent fighting.

Common surgical procedures

The pet pig can be offered a greater range of surgical procedures than the commercial animal because the degree of attention and nursing it can be given is far greater. Some routine procedures are required because pet pigs live to maturity close to their owners. Examples include castration, spaying and detusking boars. All surgical procedures should be performed under general anaesthetic for humane reasons and to avoid the distress and vocalization resulting from restraint.

Castration

Castration is essential in pet pigs not intended for breeding. As inguinal hernias are common, their presence requires general anaesthetic and simultaneous hernia repair (see below). If there is no hernia, anaesthesia is not required by law in the UK in piglets under 14 days old (castration can be carried out by two people, one holding the hindlegs of the piglet while the other carries out the procedure); however, anaesthesia is recommended.

1. Clean and disinfect the scrotum.
2. With a scalpel, cut the skin over the line of the testicle and cut the tunica vaginalis.
3. Remove the testicle and cut free from the tunica.
4. Pull the spermatic cord away.
5. The second testicle can be removed through the same incision or through a separate incision.
6. The wound may be powdered with antimicrobial wound powder and is best left open but may be stitched.

Piglets may be given antimicrobial agents parenterally. The wounds heal rapidly but any puffiness or evidence of infection should be investigated and treated immediately.

Castration in adult boars must be carried out under anaesthetic:

- Boars may be anaesthetized as described above or by direct injection of the testicle with pentobarbitone (45 mg/kg)
- The skin of the scrotum is clipped and prepared rapidly and the testicles removed, as with smaller animals
- Pulling the spermatic cord free is not possible without considerable force and damage, so it should be cut above the rete testis and transfixed
- If both testes are removed through a midline incision, the muscular layers may be closed using catgut and the skin using vicryl
- Infection control should be ensured as in piglets.

Ovariohysterectomy

This is carried out from the midline. The middle uterine artery must be ligated separately and the uterine body transfixed (Figure 11.15). Females should not be spayed while in oestrus.

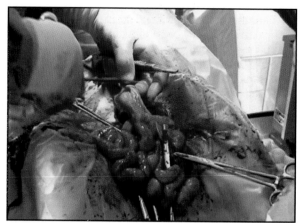

Figure 11.15 Spay. The uterine body is being clamped following exteriorization of the ovaries and uterine horns. Note that pigs have very long uterine horns. (Courtesy of J. Carr)

Inguinal hernia repair

Hernias are usually repaired at castration. General anaesthesia is required and the skin should be prepared.

1. A single incision is made between the inguinal ring and the testicles in the midline and the entire processus vaginalis containing the testicle is dissected bluntly.
2. Herniated intestine is pushed back into the abdomen and the processus vaginalis is twisted to keep it there.
3. The processus vaginalis is then transfixed by a retaining suture at the inguinal ring and the entire processus vaginalis and testicle are removed.
4. The same procedure is repeated on the other side to avoid herniation.

Rectal prolapse

Rectal prolapse is not uncommon. Where pigs are kept alone, damage may be minimal and only result from the animal backing into obstacles. Where others are kept with it, the prolapse may be bitten. The animal should be anaesthetized, the prolapse cleaned and replaced or amputated and stitched and then secured with a purse-string suture. Alternatively the corrugated plastic hose treatment of Douglas (1985) can be used:

1. Insert an 18–20 cm helical corrugated plastic tube (diameter 1.5 cm for weaners and fatteners, 2–3 cm for sows) into the prolapse.
2. Place heavy-duty rubber bands over the prolapse near the anal ring.
3. Tube and prolapse drop off after 5–7 days.

Uterine prolapse

Uterine prolapse may occur after farrowing. Animals may be distressed and in shock. Fluid replacement can aid recovery but may be possible only while the animal is under anaesthesia. The litter should be supported

1. Where possible, anaesthetize the animal. Place an intravenous catheter (5 mm) or a 16 or 18 gauge needle in the ear vein and stitch into place.
2. Give physiological saline 20–40 ml/kg/hour to stabilize the sow, followed by 4–10 ml saline which may contain glucose.
3. Clean the prolapse with cold water and repair it. The pig may need to be held up by its rear legs in sternal recumbency to slip the uterus in more easily, beginning at the horn tips. If oedema is too great for the uterus to be replaced, hypertonic solutions may reduce the volume, or an abdominal incision may be carried out to pull the uterus inside.
4. Remove any remaining piglets.
5. Amputate the uterus if too badly damaged.
6. After all remaining uterine tissue has been replaced, it is held in place by a vulval purse-string suture.

Caesarian section

- Anaesthesia and rehydration are essential
- The incision should be high on the flank to avoid interfering with the udder

- Piglets can be removed easily. They should be freed from membranes and persuaded to breathe (they may require vigorous resuscitation) and then have their navels clamped or tied
- Repair of the uterus and the flank incision is straightforward
- Piglets should receive colostrum before any milk supplement is given and then receive support such as warmth and supplementary food if required.

Tusk removal

The tusks of mature boars are dangerous. The boar can be anaesthetized and the tusks removed entirely by opening the alveolus and removing tusk and entire alveolar sac, closing it with a suture; or the tusks can simply be sawn off as a short-term solution.

Amputation of a digit

Removal of a digit from an animal with a foot abscess is commonly performed. General anaesthesia is preferred to any form of local anaesthesia.

1. Clean the affected foot and assess the extent of the damage. If infection has extended beyond the fetlock, the foot may not be operable. The same applies if the other claw is unable to support the pig.
2. Place a tourniquet above the operation site to reduce bleeding.
3. Cut the skin of the affected claw at the level of the mid second phalanx. Then cut the bone, using an obstetrical wire or bone saw.
4. Remove the second phalanx completely and close the wound.
5. A drain may be inserted and the wound packed and bandaged.
6. Healing occurs in 7–10 days.

Euthanasia

Euthanasia is usually by means of barbiturate overdose and is best administered intravenously by way of the lateral ear vein. It may be given into the anterior vena cava in small pigs but this requires a reliable assistant. Those using barbiturate for euthanasia should be aware that it inhibits respiration in the pig: the surgeon should be absolutely certain that the heart has stopped before leaving the animal.

Carcass disposal is normally by collection by the local pet cemetery company. Burial of all but the smallest pigs is usually impractical, and cremation is the preferred method of disposal of the bodies of pet pigs.

Drug formulary

The products listed are those used specifically for disease in pigs. They may need to be ordered, or are not readily available, in small animal practices.

Drug	Dose
Antibacterials	
Injectable:	
Ceftiofur	3 mg/kg daily for pleuropneumonia and pasteurellosis
Enrofloxacin	5 mg/kg daily for 5 days
Apramycin	20 mg/kg by injection, followed by course of the drug in water
Lincomycin	11 mg/kg by injection, followed by course of the drug in water
Tiamulin	10 mg/kg by injection, followed by course of the drug in water
Oral dosers for the sucking pig and young weaner:	
Amoxycillin	Clamoxyl Oral Multidoser: 1 dose twice daily to 7 kg; 2 doses twice daily 7–15 kg
Apramycin	10–20 mg/kg daily
Enrofloxacin	1 ml/3 kg, 3 ml/10 kg daily
Neomycin	Neobiotic Pump (Pharmacia & Upjohn): 1 dose per 5.5 kg daily for 5–7 days Orojet N (Fort Dodge): 1 ml/5 kg twice daily for 3–4 days
Spectinomycin	Spectam Scourhalt (CEVA): 1 pump twice daily
Trimethoprim sulphonamide	1.1 ml/2 kg daily for up to 5 days
Anthelmintics and antiparasitic agents	
Ivermectin	300 µg/kg
Doramectin	0.3 mg/kg
Antifungals	
Natamycin	Topical, licensed for horses and cattle but not pigs
Enilconazole	Topical, licensed for horses and cattle but not pigs
Drugs for manipulation of breeding	
Oxytocin	2–10 IU (0.2–1.0 ml) by deep intramuscular injection for fast action Where action need not be fast: s.c. will suffice For i.v.: give 25% of the dose diluted 1:10 with water
Gonadotrophins	5 ml i.m. at base of ear with needle horizontal Oestrus should occur within 5 days of injection Anoestrous gilts may respond to single injection at 5 months of age Same dose may be used for anoestrous sows and may cure cystic ovaries
Sedatives	
Azaperone	40 mg/ml To prevent aggression at mixing, savaging of litter: i.m. injection at 1 ml/20 kg (2 mg/kg) For boars in transport: 1 mg/kg Premedication for general anaesthesia: 0.5–1 ml/20 kg (1–2 mg/kg)
Vaccines (Vaccine pack sizes often too large for small number of individuals involved)	
Erysipelas: Erysorb Parvo, Erysorb Plus, Porcilis Ery, Porcilis Ery+Parvo, Intervet; Suvaxyn Erysipelas, Fort Dodge	
Parvovirus: Erysorb Parvo, Porcilis Ery+Parvo, Intervet; Suvaxyn Parvo, Suvaxyn Parvo 2, Fort Dodge	
Progressive atrophic rhinitis: Porcilis AR-T, Intervet	
Neonatal *E. coli*: Colisorb, Porcilis Porcol 5, Intervet; Gletvax 6, Schering Plough; Suvaxyn E. coli P4, Fort Dodge	
Glasser's disease: Suvaxyn M.HYO – Parasuis, Fort Dodge	
Pleuropneumonia: Suvaxyn App, Fort Dodge	

Figure 11.16 Drug formulary for pet pigs.

References and further reading

Carr J (2001) Reproductive surgery in the pet pig. *In Practice* **23**, 98–101
Douglas RGA (1985) A simple method for correcting rectal prolapse in pigs. *Veterinary Record* **117**, 129
Codes of Recommendations for the Welfare of Livestock. Pigs. MAFF, Department of Agriculture and Fisheries for Scotland and Welsh Office (1986, reprinted 2000)
Muirhead MR and Alexander TJL (1997) *Managing Pig Health and Treatment of Disease.* 5M Enterprises, Sheffield
Reeves D (1993) *Care and Management of Miniature Pet Pigs.* Veterinary Practice Publishing Company, Santa Barbara
Straw BE, D'Allaire S, Mengeling WL and Taylor DJ (eds) (1999) *Diseases of Swine, 8th edn.* Iowa State University Press, Ames, Iowa
Taylor DJ (1999) *Pig Diseases, 7th edn.* Available from DJ Taylor, 31 North Birbiston Rd, Lennoxtown, Glasgow G66 7LZ

Acknowledgement

We are grateful to Professor John Carr of Iowa State University for providing illustrations.

Website

Potbellied Pig Club UK
http://www.welcome.to/potbelliedpigs.pa

12

Primates

Susan M. Thornton

Introduction

Primates as pets are relatively uncommon in the UK. The common marmoset *Callithrix jacchus* is the species most likely to be seen in general practice, as this is the only simian that does not require a licence under the Dangerous Wild Animals Act 1976 (as amended by the Dangerous Wild Animals Act 1976 (Modification) Order 1984). Squirrel monkeys (*Saimiri* spp.), capuchins (*Cebus* spp.) and other marmosets and tamarins are rarely seen as pets but will be covered in this chapter as they are commonly seen in private collections and small zoos.

Biology

Biological data for these species are summarized in Figure 12.2 and normal haematological and biochemical data are summarized in Figure 12.3. Old World monkeys and the greater and lesser apes are beyond the remit of this chapter but occasional references will be made to them.

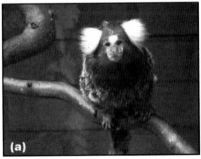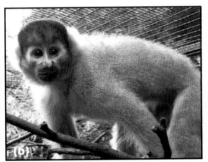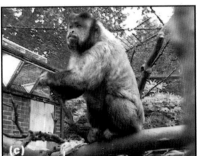

Figure 12.1 Some captive primates: (a) common marmoset; (b) squirrel monkey; (c) capuchin.

	Common marmoset	Squirrel monkey	Capuchin monkey	Tamarin
Lifespan	15–20 years	30 years	50 years	15–20 years
Weight Male Female	350–400 g 350–400 g	600–1100 g 500–700 g	3.5–3.9 kg 2.5–3 kg	600–800 g 600–800 g
Respiratory rate	50–70 breaths/minute	30–50 breaths/minute	30–50 breaths/minute	50–70 breaths/minute
Heart rate	200–350 beats/minute	200–350 beats/minute	165–225 beats/minute	200–350 beats/minute
Rectal temperature	39–40°C	37–38.5°C	37–38.5°C	39–40°C
Sexual maturity Male Female	15–24 months 14–24 months	5 years 3 years	8 years 4 years	24 months 18 months
Monogamous/polygamous	Usually monogamous	Polygamous	Polygamous	Permanent pair bond
Interbirth interval	6 months	1 year	2 years	6 months
Length of gestation	130–150 days	152–168 days	180 days	128 days
Litter size	1–4 (av. 2)	1	1 (twins very rare)	1–2 (very rarely 3)
Birthweight	35–40 g	100 g	200–250 g	50 g
Weaning age	2–3 months	6 months	9 months	2–3 months
Wild groupings	Family groups of 4–15 with dominant pair. Usually only the dominant female breeds	30–40	3–30 with a dominant male	Family groups of 2–11 with dominant pair. Usually only the dominant female mates

Figure 12.2 Biological data for primates.

	Common marmoset	Squirrel monkey	Capuchin monkey	Tamarin
Haematology				
PCV l/l	0.45–0.48	0.43–0.56	0.45–0.53	0.45
RBC (10¹²/l)	6.9	7.1–10.9	6	6.6
Hb (g/dl)	15.1–15.5	12.9–17.0	14–17	15.5
WBC (10⁹/l)	7–12	5.1–10.9	5–24	12.6–14.4
Neutrophils (%)	28–55	36–66	55	43–64
Lymphocytes (%)	43–67	27–55	41	34–49
Monocytes (%)	0.4–2.1	0–6.0	1.8	2.0–5.0
Eosinophils (%)	0.5–0.6	0–11.0	1.6	1.0–1.2
Basophils (%)	0.3–1.3	<1	<1	0.1
Platelets (10⁹/l)	390–490	112	108–187	331–650
Biochemistry				
ALT IU/l	9.5–10.2	59–99		7–14
AST IU/l	160–182	56–118		49–59
Bilirubin (μmol/l)	8.5–10.3	1.7–9.0		2.4–4.4
BUN (mmol/l)	9.64	8.21–13.92	8.57–15.71	2.14–4.28
Calcium (mmol/l)	2.4–2.6	2.1–2.4	2.5	2.5
Cholesterol (mmol/l)	1.4–6.4	3.3–5.4	4.4–6.6	1.8
Glucose (mmol/l)	7.0–8.3	2.9–6.0	2.4–5.2	6.9–10.5
LDH (IU/l)	799	271–490		
Phosphorus (mmol/l)	0.5–3.3	1.1–2.5	2.3	1.0–1.9
Protein (g/l)	70	69–81	75–87	62–86

Figure 12.3 Normal haematological and biochemical values for primates.

Husbandry

Housing

Primates do best in large aviary-type outdoor enclosures with heated indoor accommodation. If the ambient temperature drops below 15°C at night, it is recommended that supplementary heat be used in the nest box. If it drops to below 15°C during the day, a 'hot spot' up to 29°C should be provided for basking.

The design of the housing should take into consideration the group size, behaviour and social organization of the species. For example, the minimum cage size for a pair of marmosets is 1.5 m × 1.5 m × 2 m. The wire mesh should be welded stainless steel (not chicken wire) with a mesh size suitable for the size of primate: it should not be big enough for a primate to put its arm through, as the animal may seriously injure itself and would also be able to grab at people and possibly inflict injury on them.

Housing and food store areas should be designed to prevent access by rodents, wild birds and cats. Mice are a possible source of lymphocytic choriomeningitis virus, the cause of fatal callitrichid hepatitis. Rodents and wild birds are carriers of *Yersinia pseudotuberculosis*, which is passed in the faeces, and contamination of food with this organism has caused multiple and sporadic deaths in primates from the New and Old World. Cats are potential carriers of *Toxoplasma gondii*, which has caused multiple deaths in colonies of primates, especially squirrel monkeys.

- Primates require a complex and stimulating environment and should not be housed alone for long periods

- It is important that natural social structures be taken into account when housing more than a pair of animals
- For group-housed primates, areas must be designed to allow animals to avoid visual contact with others so that hierarchical stress can be minimized
- Primates are very destructive
- Cage furniture should be easily cleaned or replaced
- Any live plants used must not be toxic
- Locks must be escape-proof
- Humidity should be maintained at approximately 50–60%, as low humidity can cause skin problems and can be detrimental to infants. A substrate of moist peat helps to maintain a high humidity.

Multi-species housing is generally a compromise. For example, it can be difficult to manage balanced diets, especially when species of differing sizes are housed together. There are also disease problems; in particular, mixing or even keeping squirrel monkeys and other cebids in close proximity to callitrichids should be avoided, since a number of fatal herpes viruses are carried by cebids.

Hygiene

The close relatedness of primates to humans means that high standards of hygiene are probably more important in the care and keeping of primates than any other pet. Frequent hand washing is probably the single most important measure to reduce or prevent the spread of infection. Disposable latex gloves should be worn when cleaning primate cages as well as when handling primates and their food dishes. Owners rarely wear gloves but they should be encouraged to do so.

It is of utmost importance that veterinary and nursing staff should wear gloves and consider contamination of the environment when a primate has visited the surgery.

Disinfectants, both viricidal and bactericidal, should be used and these should be well rinsed away with water after use, to avoid contact with the animals.

Veterinary surgeons who have clients with primates should consider ensuring that all staff are vaccinated against possible primate diseases (they should also encourage the owners to consider this). Vaccinations could include tetanus, polio, measles, hepatitis B, influenza and tuberculosis. Conversely, primates are very susceptible to human diseases and owners should be made aware that relatively minor diseases in a human can be devastating in non-human primates.

Nutrition

Primates are omnivorous. In the wild they would eat fruits, gums and saps, invertebrates (e.g. insects and snails) and small vertebrates (e.g. birds, snakes, lizards, frogs and rodents). In captivity, poor nutrition (including selective feeding of fruits), along with physiological stress factors, can lead to nutritional bone disease, scurvy, diarrhoea, colitis and wasting disease.

Commercial diets of primate pellets and gum substitutes are available and a variety of fruits should be given. By way of example, Figure 12.4 gives details of a diet that is perfectly balanced for squirrel monkeys: it was initially designed for a group of animals suffering from nutritional bone disease and also proved to be highly successful in maintaining their continuing health.

- Morning feed:
  - 100 g Trio Munch primate pellets (Mazuri)
  - 10 ml Ribena Toothkind, diluted with water, for soaking the Trio Munch
- Afternoon feed:
  - 20 g mealworms
  - 20 g peanuts
  - 20 g whole hardboiled egg
  - 20 g grapes
  - 20 g apple, with skin
  - 20 g banana
  - 25 g minced beef

Figure 12.4 Balanced diet for squirrel monkeys (amounts are for three adults).

All primates require dietary vitamin C, which should be adequately available from fresh fruits and vegetables. New World primates require vitamin D_3 and it appears that callitrichids in particular may have higher requirements for vitamin D_3 than humans and other primates. For this reason, indoor exhibits should be furnished with ultraviolet light (UV-B) or the animals should be supplemented with vitamin D_3. A sufficient level of supplementation for an adult common marmoset would be 250 IU/day.

Sufficient dietary protein is also required, as calcium transported in the body is protein-bound. Dietary protein should be as much as 27% dry matter in juveniles and breeding females. This level is often not achieved because of an excess of fruit consumption.

- Mice should never be fed to callitrichids as a protein source, as they can carry lymphocytic choriomeningitis virus, the agent causing callitrichid hepatitis, which has a high mortality rate
- When pellets are fed, their low palatability leads them to be ignored by the primates if there is sufficient other food to provide the required energy
- Invertebrates are often fed as enrichment for primates and it is important that they are gut-loaded with a calcium supplement.

Contraception

Primates can be prolific breeders in captivity and owners often request control of breeding. If contraception is required, the method that causes least disruption of the social hierarchy and is also the least invasive is vasectomy of the male. Castration, using the open method followed by subcuticular sutures, has been used in group situations before sexual maturity of the young males. This has led to the males continuing to live in the group as low-ranking animals with no signs of hierarchical problems associated with maturity.

Contraception for female primates has been implemented with various drugs, such as melangoestrol acetate, medroxyprogesterone acetate and laevonorgoestrol, but all have side effects. There have been records of successful breeding after removal of implants but the consensus in the zoo world is that permanent sterilization is preferable if breeding is not required and that hormonal manipulation should only be used if there is a very good reason for it.

Hand rearing

Hand rearing is labour intensive and the young animal's future must be considered before it is attempted. Primates are social animals and imprinted primates can have great difficulty in adapting to life with other primates. Rearing more than one primate at a time helps (e.g. handrearing twins) but the sooner the infants are introduced to other group members, the better. This can be done by attaching a hand-rearing cage to the main enclosure that houses the group, so that the rearer does not need to enter the main cage when dealing with the infant. This is preferable to placing the rearing cage within the main enclosure as, until the infant is feeding well, its distress call could lead to attacks on the rearer by the rest of the group.

Figure 12.5 gives guidelines for hand rearing. A number of different methods have been used and Hearn and Burden (1979) reported that when triplets are born it is possible to rear them 'collaboratively' so that the weakest is not dropped in the first week. One young was removed in turn at 0900 hours daily and placed in an incubator (25–30°C, relative humidity 80%) with a furry toy as a surrogate mother. The isolated neonate was hand-fed for 24 hours before being exchanged for another. This allowed the parents to cope with only two young at a time and also enabled the three youngsters to grow up as primates.

Guidelines
• Only one person to be responsible for one animal during the critical initial 7 days
• Animals to be kept warm at all times. It is generally impossible to maintain a constant ambient temperature but a heat pad or baby's electric blanket can be used, with a hot water bottle for transport
• Supply tissue for animal to cling to. A surrogate mother (small soft toy) is ideal if the animal is strong enough to cling to it
• Siblings best kept together, again with surrogate mother
• Feed using 1 ml syringe with lacrymal cannula attached (cut down to size), doll's bottle or kitten feeder. Babies suck at their own rate if the milk is dropped on their lips at the front of the mouth.

Feeding solutions
• Glucose: 1 teaspoon glucose in 28 ml sterile water
• SMA (baby milk solution): 1 dessertspoon SMA in 28 ml sterile water
• SMA + Casilan: 1 dessertspoon Casilan (mixed to a paste in cold water and made up to 28 ml with boiling water) + 1 dessertspoon SMA; generally $\frac{1}{2}$ teaspoon glucose powder is added to each 28 ml solution
• SMA + $\frac{1}{2}$ Casilan: as above but with only 1 teaspoon Casilan
• Farex Solution, SMA + Casilan Sol: As above plus 1 dessertspoon of Farex
• $\frac{1}{2}$ Farex Solution + Casilan Sol: As above plus 1 teaspoon of Farex
• Vitamin Solution: 2 ml water + 0.1 ml Cytacon + 0.1 ml ABIDEC
(ABIDEC™: multivitamin solution, Pfizer; Casilan™: protein multivitamin concentrate, Heinz; Cytacon B12™: vitamin B_{12} solution, Goldshield Pharmaceuticals; Farex™: baby cereal, Heinz; SMA™: powdered baby milk, SMA Nutrition.)

Protocol

• Day 1 (at 2-hour intervals):
  – Feed 1 glucose (0.3–0.5 ml) (tamarins 0.6–0.1 ml)
  – Feed 2 $\frac{1}{2}$ glucose + $\frac{1}{2}$ SMA Solution
  – Feed 3 $\frac{1}{2}$ glucose + $\frac{1}{2}$ SMA Solution
  – Continue SMA feed at 2-hourly intervals.

• Day 2 (0800, 1000, 1200): SMA + $\frac{1}{2}$ Casilan (this feed continued at 2-hour intervals until 2400, but with one feed of Vitamin Solution at 2000 to prevent dehydration)
• Days 3–7: 2-hourly feeds of SMA + Casilan with one feed per day of Vitamin Solution
• Weeks 2–3 (0800, 1000, 1200, 1500, 1800, 2100, 2400): all feeds SMA + Casilan with one feed per day of Vitamin Solution. Vitamin D_3 given twice a week (suspended in arachis oil) before feeding. About 800 IU per week. Add Farex from days 19–20. Three feeds per day consist of $\frac{1}{2}$ Farex Solution

• Week 4
  – 0900: Farex Solution
  – 1200: SMA + Casilan
  – 1500: Farex Solution
  – 1800: Vitamin Solution + $\frac{1}{4}$ SMA + $\frac{1}{4}$ Casilan
  – 2100: Farex Solution
  – 2400: SMA + Casilan.

Notes
• Tamarins may become constipated with Casilan. If this occurs, remove it from the mixture
• After each feed, the animal's back should be rubbed and its genitals gently wiped with warm moist cotton wool to encourage urination and defecation. They begin urinating and defecating spontaneously at about 14 days. They usually pass urine and faeces at each feed. Passing nothing at one feed is not a cause for concern but passing no urine or faeces at two consecutive feeds might indicate a problem
• Tempt with soft fruits (e.g. banana and grapes) until the animal is feeding for itself by about 5 weeks. Then offer ground soaked primate pellet. Animal should be feeding independently by 6 weeks of age
• Bodyweight should show a steady increase by the end of the first week.

Figure 12.5 Hand rearing guidelines for common marmosets and tamarins used at Battersea Park Children's Zoo by Denise Todd (pers. comm.). They follow those produced for the Zoological Society of London and the Primate Society of Great Britain.

Microchips

If more than a pair of primates are kept, the use of microchips is probably the best method for identification of individuals. The site for microchipping is usually between the shoulder blades and the use of tissue glue reduces the likelihood of early loss of the microchip. Tattoos on the inner thigh can be difficult to read and require handling of the animal, whereas a microchip can be read from a short distance, which is less stressful for an animal not used to being handled.

Handling and restraint

Care must be taken when handling primates because they may harbour zoonoses (disposable latex gloves should always be worn) and can inflict serious bites. Leather gloves or gauntlets are often required but even with this protection the longer canines relative to the length of the incisors means that the teeth can penetrate the leather. After restraint, the animal should be prevented from biting the leather as this can lead to tooth damage.

Figure 12.6 illustrates examples of handling methods. Other types of restraint include crush cages, nets and soft brooms (Sainsbury *et al.*, 1989).

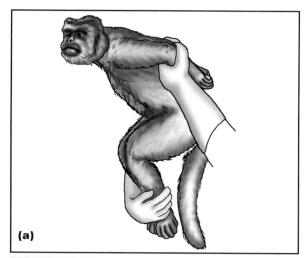
(a)

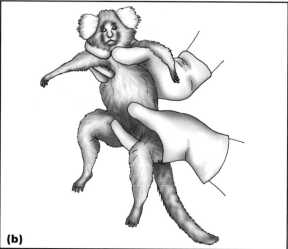
(b)

Figure 12.6 (a) Method of restraint for a capuchin-sized monkey. (b) Handling a marmoset in the correct manner.

Diagnostic approach

Sample collection

Blood
Blood is most easily collected from the femoral vein using a 1 ml or 2 ml syringe with a 25 or 27 gauge needle. The femoral artery should be palpated. The vein is medial to the artery. Haematoma formation is possible following femoral blood sampling; digital pressure applied on removal of the needle is necessary.

Radiography
Radiography must be carried out under general anaesthesia. In New World primates it is most often required to assess the quality of the skeleton. A normal bone and graduated metal wedge are used to aid the assessment of the density of the skeleton. If the thorax is to be evaluated, the position of choice is to lay the animal in ventral recumbency and tie the elbows together when pulled cranially as far as possible. This will straighten the scapulae and remove them from the area required.

Common conditions

Dental disease
Periodontal disease is common in captive primates. There are a number of possible reasons for this. Nutrition is likely to be a prime factor but teeth may also be damaged during manual restraint, when primates will often bite hard on the gauntlet worn by the handler.

The most common presenting sign is a swelling of the face seen just below the eye in the case of an upper canine tooth root abscess. Initially this should be treated with antibiotics but then the underlying cause must be addressed. This may mean root canal treatment, if the expertise and facilities are available, or simply removing the tooth. Primates cope extremely well even if virtually all the teeth are lost due to periodontal disease, though care should be taken to feed softened food or food that is presented in small pieces. Abnormal tooth eruption and 'floating teeth' in the jaw are usually secondary to nutritional bone disease.

Nutritional diseases

Nutritional bone disease
Incorrect nutrition is probably linked to the commonest cause of disease in pet New World Primates: nutritional bone disease (NBD), or fibrous osteodystrophy (Figure 12.7).

Clinical signs of NBD include lethargy, anorexia, pain, inability to jump (often called cage paralysis), pathological fractures, vertebral damage and spinal cord compression, faecal impaction and facial deformity (rubber jaw). The causes include:

- Dietary calcium to phosphorus ratio < 1
- Lack of dietary vitamin D$_3$ or lack of access to ultraviolet light
- Low dietary protein.

Treatment of NBD should be attempted only after an assessment of the clinical signs and the radiographs. Once vertebrae have collapsed, causing compression

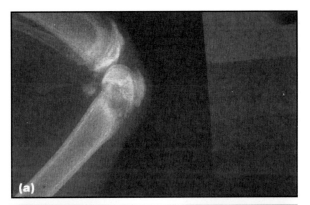
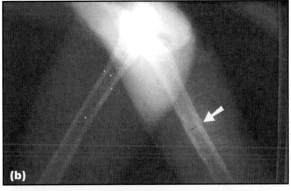
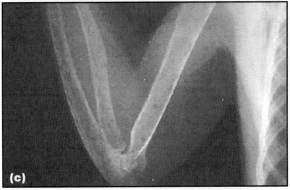
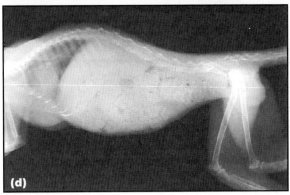

Figure 12.7 Nutritional bone disease (NBD). (a) Stifle joint of a red-faced spider monkey. Note the extreme widening of the growth plates. Although the cortices appear thick at first glance, they are poorly mineralized. The skeleton of this animal increased in density after increasing the calcium and protein in its diet. (b) Pathological folding fracture (arrowed) in the mid-shaft of the femur in a juvenile white-faced saki monkey. Again, the cortices are wide but poorly mineralized. (c) Arm of a common marmoset, showing severe NBD. The cortices are extremely ragged and poorly mineralized. (d) Faecal impaction associated with moderate NBD in a common marmoset.

of the spinal cord, the prognosis is very poor. Generally, pathological fractures of the long bones heal well if the animal is confined to a small cage and given extra calcium, vitamin D$_3$ and protein. (For the animal's mental wellbeing, its cage may be placed adjacent to its cagemates, or even within their cage.) The skeleton should be re-evaluated after 6 weeks and then again after 6 months. The use of splints and other forms of fixation is not recommended, as this places stresses at new points and usually leads to further fractures.

Scurvy

Clinical signs of dietary vitamin C deficiency include haemorrhage from gums and pain on movement; lesions include haemorrhages in the subcutis and skeletal muscle around joints and on all serosal surfaces. Supplementary vitamin C (250 mg) in a child's chewable tablet can be offered but adequate fresh fruits and vegetables usually suffice.

Viral diseases

Herpes viruses

Squirrel monkeys are the reservoir host for *Herpesvirus tamarinus*, an alpha herpes virus (Herpes T or *H. platyrrhinae*). Another alpha herpes virus, *Herpes simplex*, is the cause of cold sores in humans and has been implicated in fatalities in callitrichids associated with owners or keepers with open herpetic lip or mouth ulcers. These viruses can cause acute disseminated disease characterized by oral and cutaneous ulceration, lethargy and death in several days.

Latent gamma herpes viruses include *Herpesvirus saimiri* in squirrel monkeys and *Herpesvirus ateles* in spider monkeys (*Ateles* spp.). The human herpes Epstein–Barr virus (EBV, or human herpes virus-4) can experimentally induce lymphoproliferative conditions in callitrichids and potentially cause lymphomatous conditions in these species (Montali and Bush, 1999).

Lymphocytic choriomeningitis virus (LCMV)

LCMV causes callitrichid hepatitis. It presents acutely, with lethargy, anorexia, elevated liver enzymes with or without jaundice, and seizures. Mortality rates are high. It is commonly associated with the primates eating mice, either as part of their diet or through catching wild rodents in their cages.

Measles

Measles, a morbillivirus, can be asymptomatic in primates but can also be a fatal disease, particularly in New World primates. Clinical signs include oedema of the upper eyelids and progressive lethargy, culminating in death within 8–18 hours. Some animals show a mucous nasal discharge, facial erythema and oedema, with maculopapules on the lips. Interstitial and bronchopneumonia is also a common finding.

Antibiotics for the secondary bacterial infection and other supportive treatment may be worthwhile, as some animals will seroconvert and survive. Human gammaglobulin and human measles vaccine have been used prophylactically (see Vaccination).

Poliomyelitis

Clinical poliomyelitis has been reported in chimpanzee, gorilla and orang-utan. Although other species are known to be susceptible experimentally, this is beyond the remit of this chapter but see Vaccination section.

Bacterial diseases

Yersinia

Yersinia pseudotuberculosis, spread by rodents and birds in their faeces, causes sporadic or high mortalities in callitrichids and other primates. Fatalities can occur at any time of year but a feature of this Gram-negative bacterium is that it grows well in cold temperatures and so it is common for outbreaks to occur in the early autumn, when the temperature drops and levels of *Y. pseudotuberculosis* build up in the environment. The route of infection is oral.

Usually the first sign of the disease is death. The usual finding on postmortem is severe multiple abscessation throughout the liver and perhaps the intestines. The lesions contain massive colonies of the organism. Prophylactic treatment of the remaining animals is often carried out using amoxycillin with clavulanic acid.

Bacterial diarrhoea

Diarrhoea caused by *Salmonella*, *Campylobacter* and *Shigella* spp. can occur in primates and should be ruled out in cases of enteric disease. All three are zoonotic but good standards of hygiene should be sufficient to prevent transmission of disease. Treatment should be based on sensitivity tests. Paediatric oral electrolyte solutions are usually well tolerated.

Pneumonia

Bordetella bronchiseptica, *Klebsiella pneumoniae* and *Pasteurella* spp. are relatively common causes of pneumonia in primates.

Tetanus

Clinical tetanus has been reported in wild and captive macaques, squirrel monkeys, guenons, callitrichids and other species and is generally fatal (see Vaccination).

Parasitic diseases

See Figure 12.10 for a summary of antiparasitic drugs.

Protozoa

Toxoplasma gondii: Disease caused by *T. gondii* occurs sporadically in primates but can have high mortality rates. Often sudden death is the first clinical sign but respiratory distress may be seen from pulmonary oedema. Primates may become infected by one of two sources: cat faeces or wild rodents. Prevention through cat and rodent control is the key to dealing with this infection.

Contamination of feed or housing with cat faeces will lead to the ingestion of sporulated oocysts. The sporozoites rapidly penetrate the intestinal wall and spread to other organs haematogenously. The invasive and proliferative stage is the tachyzoite: on entering the target cell it multiplies asexually by budding (endodyogyny); when 8–16 tachyzoites have accumulated, the cell ruptures and new cells are infected. This acute phase of toxoplasmosis causes the fatalities.

A primate catching and eating a wild rodent also eats bradyzoites and tachyzoites in the flesh. The cycle of infection is similar to that following oocyst ingestion.

Enteric flagellates: These frequently occur in large numbers in primate diarrhoea and are often non-pathogenic. A monkey strain of *Entamoeba histolytica* (the cause of amoebic dysentery in humans) can cause diarrhoea in primates and can also infect humans. Motile organisms and cysts of *E. histolytica* may be detected in smears from faeces and may be the cause if diarrhoea is present, but differentiation from less pathogenic species is a specialist task. Primates are usually treated with metronidazole but even the human paediatric preparations taste foul and it can be difficult to dose primates with this drug.

Helminths

Acanthocephala: The thorny-headed worm *Prosthenorchis elegans* has caused fatal peritonitis from gastric penetration in collections of callitrichids. The intermediate host is the cockroach, and pest control is an essential part of controlling this parasite. Treatment with mebendazole (up to 100 mg/kg bodyweight for alternate weeks) with surgical removal of adult and juvenile worms embedded in the intestine has been reported (Wolf *et al.*, 1990).

Tapeworms: Hydatidosis has been found in captive primates both incidentally and causing death. Control of the carnivore hosts and preventing faecal contamination of food and the environment are required.

Nematodes: Several nematodes have been associated with morbidity and mortality in primates. *Pterygodermatites nycticebi*, a spirurid nematode, causes profound weakness, anaemia and hypoproteinaemia in heavily infested animals. The cockroach is an intermediate host. Regular faecal screening of callitrichids for spirurid eggs and biannual prophylaxis with mebendazole at 40 mg/kg, combined with a rigorous cockroach extermination programme, have achieved effective control of *P. nycticebi*. Two other pathogenic spirurid nematodes that are rare in the UK but could be found in a newly imported primate are *Trichospirura leptostoma* (found in the pancreatic duct of callitrichids and usually considered incidental but it has been implicated in wasting marmoset syndrome) and *Gongylonema pulchrum*, which affects the oral cavity and has been reported as clinically important in Goeldi's monkeys and pygmy marmosets. Diagnosis is by faecal flotation or oral cavity scrape for the eggs of *G. pulchrum*. Treatment with fenbendazole (40–60 mg/kg orally for 5 consecutive days) or ivermectin (200 µg/kg s.c.) is reported to be effective for the intestinal and pancreatic spirurids. *G. pulchrum* is more resistant to treatment and may need mebendazole (70 mg/kg daily for

3 consecutive days monthly, quarterly or biannually depending on the degree of infection) in association with rigorous pest control.

Miscellaneous conditions

Wounds
Bite wounds are a common finding in primates. Fighting may occur when new groupings are set up or during normal hierarchical disputes. Generally it is best to leave wounds to heal by second intention, as a primate bite is a dirty bite and usually leads to infection. Even deep gaping wounds are best cleaned, debrided of necrotic tissue and left to heal.

Often the first sign that there has been a fight is the swelling caused by an abscess. This can be lanced under anaesthetic and antibiotics given orally (e.g. amoxycillin and clavulanic acid).

On occasions it may be necessary to amputate fingers and tails after fights. These can be difficult to manage, as the primate often interferes with the wound. Wherever possible, the use of subcuticular sutures is likely to give the best results. Some primates will tolerate a light dressing but others often remove dressings. Carprofen as a single dose is useful when a wound appears painful.

Acute gastric dilation
An outbreak of this condition has been reported following antimicrobial therapy and it has also been seen after a sudden change of diet in long-term captive animals. It has been associated with an overgrowth of *Clostridium perfringens*. The condition is rapidly fatal but may be relieved in the early stages by passing a stomach tube and lavaging the stomach contents.

Intussusception and rectal prolapse
This condition is likely to be seen in cases of severe diarrhoea. An intussusception may be palpated manually and requires urgent surgical intervention. Rectal prolapse can be treated with a purse-string suture but both conditions require the underlying cause to be identified and removed.

Wasting marmoset syndrome
This probably has a multifactorial aetiology. Possible causes include poor nutrition, selective feeding of fruits by the primate or physiological stress factors. Improving nutrition and environment is of importance. The skeletal calcium levels should be evaluated: if they are shown to be poor, an increase in dietary calcium as well as an increase in protein intake may be successful in treating the problem. Infection with the parasite *Trichospirura leptostoma* in the pancreatic duct of callitrichids is usually considered incidental but it has been implicated in wasting marmoset syndrome.

Vaccination

Tetanus
The most common vaccination in primates is for tetanus protection: 40 IU of human tetanus toxoid given three times at intervals of 2–3 months is likely to be sufficient for years of protection. Intramuscular

boosters are usually given after 5 years and at 10-year intervals thereafter. The triple vaccine known as DPT or DTP (diphtheria, tetanus and pertussis) should not be used; a large number of adverse reactions have been recorded in non-human primates and they are not particularly susceptible to diphtheria or pertussis.

Measles

For vaccination against measles a human live hyper-attenuated monovalent vaccine should be used intramuscularly at 6 months of age and boosted at 12 months. (Apes should be given a single dose at 15 months of age or over.)

Hepatitis B virus

Hepatitis B virus is most commonly seen in Old World primates, particularly gibbons, but if a carrier is detected the in-contact animals can be vaccinated with hepatitis B vaccine (e.g. Engerix B, SmithKline Beecham, Welwyn Garden City, Hertfordshire). This course of action is probably only possible for a few zoos capable of coping with the extra zoonotic risks. It is unlikely that this would be wise for a pet primate carrying hepatitis B virus. If vaccination is carried out, the antibody titre should be tested to ensure a good response to the vaccine.

Mumps and rubella

Mumps and rubella (German measles) are primarily subclinical diseases in non-human primates and therefore vaccination is not required.

Poliomyelitis

For apes, three doses of live oral trivalent polio vaccine (containing attenuated strains of poliomyelitis virus, types 1, 2 and 3) are given at 1-month intervals. This may be started at 2 months of age (or earlier if a particularly high risk exists). Oral boosters are given after 5 years and at 10-year intervals thereafter. It is important to give the oral polio vaccine to all animals in a group at the same time, particularly with the first dose of any course.

An alternative strategy is to use the enhanced potency inactivated polio vaccine (eIPV) containing polio viruses of all three types inactivated by formaldehyde. Three doses of 0.5 ml are given by subcutaneous injection at monthly intervals, starting at 2 months of age or above. Booster doses of eIPV are given after 5 years and at 10-year intervals thereafter (J. Lewis, pers. comm.)

Anaesthesia

Small marmosets and tamarins can be placed in a chamber for induction of anaesthesia with isoflurane, or manually restrained and masked down with isoflurane. Details of anaesthetic agents (including dose rates, routes and comments) are given in Figure 12.8.

During anaesthesia and on recovery it is important to keep the primate warm, especially small monkeys. Recovery in a small cage on a covered heat pad until the animal is fully awake will remove the risks of climbing and falling. Larger animals can be given a straw bed for warmth and protection. It is important for their psychological wellbeing to return them to their group as soon as possible.

Common surgical procedures

Caesarean section

This is probably one of the most common surgical procedures carried out in pet primates, particularly common marmosets. It is generally believed that poor nutrition (either obesity or calcium deficiency) contributes to this problem.

Primates usually give birth during the night and so if a primate is obviously still straining to pass a fetus in the morning it should be considered an emergency. This is one of the few occasions when the use of isoflurane by mask for induction is indicated.

The female should be given subcutaneous fluids at the start of the procedure (Figure 12.9). Intravenous fluids can more easily be used in the larger primates. The choice of site must take account of how long setting up the intravenous line will take compared with the whole procedure.

Analgesia is also given. Some favour the use of carprofen as a single dose given at the start of the procedure; others favour buprenorphine.

1. The animal should be intubated and placed in dorsal recumbency
2. The site for laparotomy is ventral midline just cranial to the pubis; care must be taken not to incise beyond the abdominal musculature, which is extremely thin
3. The uterus can be exteriorized and the fetus removed after incision through the uterine wall, taking care to keep away from the neck of the bladder (which could become compromised in the suturing of the uterus)
4. The uterus is closed in a standard two-layer continuous inverting pattern; the linea alba is closed using absorbable suture material in a simple interrupted pattern; and the skin is closed with a subcuticular layer followed by interrupted mattress sutures.

The wound is less likely to be interfered with if this pattern of suturing is used. Problems often occur when simple interrupted skin sutures are used, especially if a subcuticular layer is omitted.

If the baby is delivered alive, attempts are often made to return it to the mother as this should result in a psychologically normal primate. Whether the attempt is likely to succeed or not becomes very obvious once the mother awakes and reacts to the youngster.

In general, if space permits, the female is allowed to recover for 5–10 days before being returned to the group. This enables close monitoring of the wound. Sometimes the female may have to be returned on the same day but care must be taken to observe the wound.

Vasectomy

Prior to elective surgery the animal should be starved. When the procedure is to be carried out in the morning, food and water are removed from marmosets and tamarins first thing in the morning and surgery takes place 2–3 hours later. Larger primates are starved overnight but allowed access to water, which is then removed first thing in the morning.

Agent	Dose rate	Route	Usage	Comments
Acepromazine maleate	0.5–1.0 mg/kg	Orally, s.c., i.m.	Rare	Can be used as a pre-anaesthetic or a tranquillizer
Alphaxalone/alphadolone	8 mg/kg 12–18 mg/kg 18–25 mg/kg	i.m.	Uncommon due to volume required	Light sedation Deep sedation to light surgical anaesthesia Surgical anaesthesia. Can be topped up
Diazepam	0.5–1.0 mg/kg 0.25–0.5 mg/kg	Orally i.m. / i.v.	Uncommon	Sedation; give in small amount of food or drink 30–60 min prior to anaesthesia. Degree of sedation variable, recovery prolonged
Isoflurane	Can be masked down with 4% isoflurane but best if sedated first to reduce stress	Mask/ET tube	Very common	Lignocaine (lidocaine) on tube or sprayed on to glottis required to prevent laryngeal spasm. Primates have a short neck and care must be taken not to reach the tracheal bifurcation
Ketamine hydrochloride	5–15 mg/kg	i.m.	Common	Produces restraint sufficient for handling, blood sampling and clinical examination. Generally animals are not relaxed sufficiently for radiography. Causes seizures in lemurs
Ketamine/diazepam	15 mg/kg (K) 1 mg/kg (D)	i.m.	Common	Anaesthesia
Ketamine/medetomidine	10–15 mg/kg (K) 0.1 mg/kg (M) Lower doses are required in large primates (e.g. Great Apes)	i.m.	Common	Light anaesthesia. Can be topped up or further supplemented with isoflurane anaesthetic. Topping up with a half dose of ketamine is also common. Reversal of the medetomidine with atipamezole 0.5 mg/kg leads to fast smooth recovery. Rarely causes vomition on induction
Ketamine/xylazine	10 mg/kg (K) 0.5 mg/kg (X)	i.m.	Rare, has been superseded by ketamine/medetomidine combination	Often causes vomition on induction. The xylazine component can be reversed with atipamezole
Propofol	5–10 mg/kg	i.v.	Rare because of the need to administer i.v.	Can be given as a continuous infusion. May cause a period of apnoea and therefore the primate should be intubated
Tiletamine/zolazepam	2–10 mg/kg	i.m.	Not licensed in UK Can use with a special treatment authorization from the VMD	Commonly used in the USA

Figure 12.8 Anaesthetics for use in primates.

Common marmoset	15–20 ml
Squirrel monkey	30–60 ml male 25–35 ml female
Capuchin monkey	175–190 ml male 125–150 ml female
Tamarin	30–40 ml

Figure 12.9 Quantities for subcutaneous fluid therapy (approximately 5% bodyweight).

1. The animal is anaesthetized and placed in dorsal recumbency
2. Hair is plucked from the incision site in the ventral midline cranial to the scrotum (the use of clippers can lead to skin damage, which impairs healing)
3. The surgical site is prepared as normal and a 1 cm skin incision is made in the ventral midline over the pubic symphysis, approximately 1 cm cranial to the cranial border of the scrotum
4. Blunt dissection to the right or left of the midline exposes the spermatic sacs (the spermatic cord, vaginal tunic and overlying fascia)
5. The body of the sac is dissected free and exteriorized
6. Blunt dissection allows the freeing of the off-white ductus deferens, which must be carefully separated from its closely associated artery
7. The ductus deferens is ligated twice with non-absorbable suture material and a section is removed from between the ligatures (it is wise to send the dissected piece of ductus for histological examination – at least until the veterinary surgeon is familiar with the procedure, when it is wise to keep the pieces in formalin in case of any future problems)
8. The wound is sutured with a subcuticular suture (e.g. 3/0 Vicryl) and the skin is closed with either surgical adhesive or a single mattress suture.

A single dose of carprofen at the start of the procedure is recommended.

Drug formulary

Drug	Dose	Comments
Antimicrobial and antifungal agents		
Amoxicillin	11 mg/kg orally bid 11 mg/kg s.c., i.m. sid	
Amoxicillin and clavulanic acid	15 mg/kg orally bid	
Amphotericin B	0.25–1.0 mg/kg i.v. sid	
Ceftazidime	50 mg/kg i.m., i.v. tid	
Cephalexin	20 mg/kg orally bid	
Chloramphenicol	50 mg/kg orally bid 50–100 mg/kg orally, s.c., i.v. tid 20 mg/kg i.m. bid	
Clindamycin	10 mg/kg orally bid	
Ciprofloxacin	16–20 mg/kg orally bid	Paediatric suspension available. Not clear if side effects are as bad as with enrofloxacin but should be considered likely
Doxycycline	3–4 mg/kg orally bid	
Enrofloxacin	5 mg/kg orally, i.m., s.c. sid	In humans this causes night sweats, bitter taste and hallucinations. It is not clear whether primates have similar side effects but it should be used only if sensitivity testing indicates that there is no other choice
Erythromycin	10 mg/kg orally tid 10 mg/kg i.m. bid	
Gentamicin	1–2 mg/kg i.m., i.v. tid 2–3 mg/kg i.m., i.v. bid	
Griseofulvin	20 mg/kg orally sid 200 mg/kg orally every 10 days	
Lincomycin	5–10 mg/kg i.m. bid	
Methicillin sodium	50 mg/kg i.m. bid	
Neomycin	10 mg/kg i.m., orally sid	
Nitrofurantoin	2–4 mg/kg orally tid	
Nystatin	200,000 units per animal orally every 6 hours	Gastrointestinal candidiasis; continue 48 hours after clinical recovery
Oxytetracycline	10 mg/kg s.c., i.m. sid	
Penicillin G, benzathine	40,000 IU/kg i.m. every 72 hours	
Pencillin G, procaine	20,000 IU/kg i.m. bid	
Piperacillin sodium	80–100 mg/kg i.m., i.v. tid 100–150 mg/kg i.m., i.v. bid	
Sulphasalazine	30 mg/kg orally bid	
Tetracycline	20–25 mg/kg orally every 8–12 hours 25 mg/kg i.m., i.v. bid	
Trimethoprim/sulphadiazine	15 mg/kg orally bid 30 mg/kg s.c. sid	
Antiparasitic agents		
Albendazole	25 mg/kg orally bid × 5 days	*Filaroides*
Clindamycin	12.5–25 mg/kg orally bid	*Toxoplasma*
Doxycycline	5 mg/kg orally bid × 1 day then 2.5 mg/kg sid	*Balantidium*
Fenbendazole	40–60 mg/kg orally sid × 3 days 50 mg/kg orally sid × 14 days	Gastrointestinal nematodes *Filaroides*
Ivermectin	0.2 mg/kg orally, s.c., i.m.	
Levamisole	5 mg/kg orally, repeat in 3 weeks 10 mg/kg orally	*Strongyloides, Filaroides, Trichuris*
Mebendazole	40 mg/kg orally sid × 3 days (up to 70 mg/kg for *Gongylonema*) Repeat frequency depending on species and level of infestation	*Strongyloides, Trichuris, Pterygodermatitis, Gongylonema*
Metronidazole	17.5–25 mg/kg orally bid × 10 days 30–50 mg/kg orally bid × 5–10 days	Enteric flagellates and amoebae *Balantidium coli*
Moxidectin	0.2 mg/kg orally, s.c.	Useful to treat *Trichuris* sp.
Piperazine	65 mg/kg orally sid × 10 days	
Praziquantel	40 mg/kg orally, i.m. 15–20 mg/kg orally, i.m.	Trematodes Some cestodes
Pyrantel pamoate	11 mg/kg orally once	*Necator*, pinworms
Sulphadiazine	100 mg/kg orally sid	*Toxoplasma* in New World primates
Thiabendazole	50 mg/kg orally sid × 2 days 75–100 mg/kg orally repeat in 3 weeks	*Strongyloides, Necator*

Figure 12.10 Drug formulary for primates. (continues)

Drug	Dose	Comments
Analgesics		
Aspirin (acetylsalicylic acid)	5–10 mg/kg orally every 4–6 hours	Analgesic, anti-inflammatory, anti-pyretic
Buprenorphine	0.01 mg/kg i.m., i.v. bid	Analgesic
Butorphanol	0.1–0.2 mg/kg i.m. every 12–48 hours	Analgesic
Carprofen	2–4 mg/kg	Analgesic, anti-inflammatory, anti-pyretic Can be used preoperatively. Half-life differs greatly with species Calculate dose frequency to clinical effect
Flunixin meglumine	0.3–1.0 mg/kg s.c., i.v. every 12–24 hours	Analgesic, anti-inflammatory, anti-pyretic
Paracetamol (acetominophen)	5–10 mg/kg orally every 6 hours	Analgesic, anti-inflammatory, anti-pyretic
Pethidine	2–4 mg/kg i.m. every 3–4 hours	Analgesic

Figure 12.10 continued Drug formulary for primates.

References and further reading

Ankel-Simons F (2000) *Primate Anatomy*, 2nd edn. Academic Press, London

Brack M (1987) *Agents Transmissible from Simians to Man*. Springer-Verlag, Berlin

Carpenter JW, Mashima TY and Rupiper DJ (1996) *Exotic Animal Formulary*, pp. 263–283

Hearn JP and Burden FJ (1979) Collaborative rearing of marmoset triplets. *Laboratory Animals* **13**, 131–133

Ialeggio M and Baker AJ (1995) Results of a preliminary study into wasting marmoset syndrome in callitrichid collections. In: *Proceedings of the First Annual Conference of the Nutrition Advisory Group of the American Zoo and Aquarium Association*, Ontario, Canada, pp. 148–158

Juan-Salles C, Ramos-Vara JA, Prats N, Sole-Nicolas J, Segales J and Marco AJ (1997) Spontaneous herpes simplex virus infection in common marmosets, *Callithrix jacchus*. *Journal of Veterinary Diagnostic Investigation* **9**, 341–345

Juan-Salles C, Prats N, Marco AJ, Ramos-Vara JA, Borras D and Fernandez J (1998) Fatal acute toxoplasmoses in three golden lion tamarins *Leontopithecus rosalia*. *Journal of Zoo and Wildlife Medicine* **29**(1), 55–60

Kirkwood JK and Stathatos K (1992) *Biology, Rearing, and Care of Young Primates*. Oxford University Press, Oxford

Montali RJ and Bush M (1999) Diseases of the Callitrichidae. In: *Zoo and Wild Animal Medicine: Current Therapy 4*, eds ME Fowler and RE Miller, pp. 369–376. WB Saunders, Philadelphia

Montali RJ, Scanga CA, Pernikoff D, Wessner DR, Ward R and Holmes KV (1993) A common-source outbreak of callitrichid hepatitis in captive tamarins and marmosets. *Journal of Infectious Disease* **167**, 946–950

Morris TH and David CL (1993) Illustrated guide to surgical technique for vasectomy of the common marmoset. *Laboratory Animals* **27**, 381–384

Nowak RM (1999) Primates. In: *Walker's Mammals of the World*, pp. 490–631. John Hopkins University Press, Baltimore, Maryland

Potkay S (1992) Diseases of the Callitrichidae: a review. *Journal of Medical Primatology* **21**, 189–236

Power ML, Oftedal OT, Savage A *et al.* (1997) Assessing vitamin D status of callitrichids:base-line data from wild cottontop tamarins *Sanguinus oedipus*, in Columbia. *Zoo Biology* **16**, 39–46

Primate Society of Great Britain (1987) *The Welfare of Pet Marmosets*. Universities Federation for Animal Welfare, Wheathampstead

Ramsey E and Montali RJ (1993) Viral hepatitis in New World primates. In: *Zoo and Wild Animal Medicine: Current Therapy 4*, eds ME Fowler and RE Miller, pp. 63–78. WB Saunders, Philadelphia

Sainsbury AW, Eaton BD and Cooper JE (1989) Restraint and anaesthesia of primates. *Veterinary Record* **125**, 640

Scanga CA, Holmes KV and Montali RJ (1993) Serological evidence of infection with lymphocytic choriomeningitis virus, the agent of callitrichid hepatitis, in primates in zoos, primate research centers and a natural reserve. *Journal of Zoo and Wildlife Medicine* **24**(4), 469–474

Shinki T, Shiina Y, Takahashi N, Tanioka Y, Koizumi H and Suda T (1983) Extremely high circulating levels of 1α,25-dihydroxy vitamin D3 in the marmoset, a New World monkey. *Biochemistry and Biophysics Research Communications* **114**, 452–457

Stein FJ, Lewis DH, Stott GG and Sis RF (1981) Acute gastric dilatation in common marmosets (*Callithrix jacchus*). *Laboratory Animal Science* **5**, 522–523

Ullrey DE and Bernard JB (1999) Vitamin D: metabolism, sources, unique problems in zoo animals, meeting needs. In: *Zoo and Wild Animal Medicine: Current Therapy 4*, eds ME Fowler and RE Miller, pp. 63–78. WB Saunders, Philadelphia

Wisman MA (1999) Nutrition and husbandry of callitrichids (marmosets and tamarins). *Veterinary Clinics of North America: Exotics* **2**, 209–240

Wolf P, Pond J and Meehan T (1990) Surgical removal of *Prosthenorchis elegans* from six species of Callitrichidae. *Annual Proceedings of the American Association of Zoo Veterinarians*, South Padre Island, Texas, pp. 95–97

Yamaguchi A, Kohno Y, Yamazaki T, *et al.* (1986) Bone in the marmoset: a resemblance to vitamin D dependent rickets, type II calcification. *Calcified Tissue International* **39**(1), 22–27

Zenker W (1996) Problems in management of captive callitrichids. In: *Proceedings of the First Scientific Meeting of the European Association of Zoo and Wildlife Veterinarians*, pp. 141–147

Acknowledgement

I should like to thank JCM Lewis and PA Cusdin for their critical review of the manuscript, S Elmhurst for producing the restraint figures and AW Sainsbury and the *Veterinary Record* for permission to adapt them.

Avian anatomy and physiology

Nigel Harcourt-Brown

Introduction

The current consensus puts the total number of avian species at slightly over 9220. Relatively few species, from only several families, are seen by the veterinary surgeon in general practice. Anatomy and physiology, as well as biochemistry, pathology and diseases, differ from family to family, as they do in mammals. This chapter is written to highlight the differences in birds when compared to mammals.

Integument

The outer surface of a bird is covered with feathers that form a continuous layer that insulates, protects, and enables the bird to fly. The skin is thinner and more fragile than mammalian skin.

The dermis is thinner than that of mammals. It contains the feather follicles; smooth muscles and elastic tendons, which move the feathers; it also contains blood vessels and nerves.

The subcutaneous layer contains fat, often as discrete fat bodies. This fat is useful for insulation and is an energy source in migrating birds. This layer also contains striated subcutaneous muscles. This complicated layer is responsible for feather movement.

Sebum and glands

The surface of the bird is completely covered with a layer of oil (sebum) that has antimicrobial properties, as well as keeping the skin supple and preventing dehydration.

At the base of the tail is the uropygial gland, which produces a water-repellent secretion. Ducks rely on this gland for waterproofing but in other birds, such as the pigeon *Columba livia*, only 7% of the sebum in the plumage is from the uropygial gland. Some birds, such as Amazon and *Pionus* parrots, do not have a preen gland at all. Preen gland secretions may be odorous or coloured.

Birds have no sweat glands, and no true cutaneous glands. Heat loss is accomplished through the feet, especially whilst flying, and the respiratory tract.

Specialized skin

The skin is modified in several areas of the body. The distal portion of the leg is usually covered with scaly skin. The scales (*scutes*) are of many different sizes. The skin on the underside of the foot overlies, and is closely attached to, the digital pads. Spurs are found on the caudal aspect of the leg on many game birds.

Feathers

Feathers are found on all birds in a huge variety of shapes and colours. The feather is a very complicated epidermal structure; it is a derivative of the epidermis and is formed in a follicle. The feathers are arranged in distinct areas known as feather tracts (*pterylae*); between these the featherless spaces (*apteriae*) may be bare or covered with semiplumes and down feathers; these are covered by overlying contour feathers. Figure 13.1 shows the position of primary and secondary feathers on a parrot's wing.

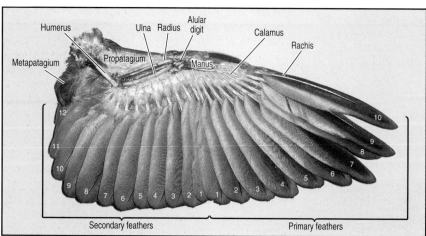

Figure 13.1 Ventral view of the left wing of a scaly-headed parrot *Pionus maximillianus*. The skin and muscles have been removed from the ventral aspect to reveal the bones and feathers and their calamus. A triangular portion of elastic skin, the propatagium, extends from the cranial aspect of the shoulder to the carpus and caudally to the elbow. This forms the leading edge of the wing.

Feather types

Contour feathers: These form the majority of the external plumage. Each feather has a long central stalk or *rachis*, on either side of which are the barbs. The barbs are further divided into the proximal and distal barbules, which hold on to their adjacent barbules with *hamuli* or hooklets. Contour feathers (Figure 13.2) cover most of the body; they are also the flight and tail feathers.

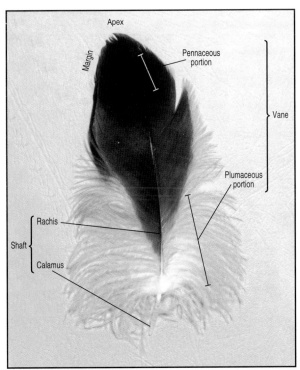

Figure 13.2 A ventral body contour feather from a lappet-faced vulture *Aegypius tracheliotus,* showing the outer surface.

Down feathers: These have a short rachis and long soft barbs. Down feathers are found under the contour feathers, where they form an insulating undercoat.

Semiplumes: These are a combination of the above two types, downy at the base and a contour feather at the tip. They are found along the margins of the contour feather tracts.

Powder down feathers: These are found in pigeons and parrots, and in some other families. These white feathers grow continuously and the barbs at the tip break off constantly. A fine white dust coats the whole bird and its surroundings; this is very obvious in white cockatoos.

Filoplumes: These are present in nearly all birds, though often not visible until the bird is plucked. The filoplume is a long spike with a tassel of barbs at its tip and is usually associated with a contour feather. Filoplumes are assumed to be sensory detectors and probably assess the strains and movement of the contour feathers, which is vital for flight. Each flight feather has a number (up to 10) of closely associated filoplumes.

Bristle feathers: These are the short spiky feathers around the eye in most species and the oral region in some. They are protective.

Feather colour

Coloration of the plumage is achieved in several ways:

- Brown, yellow, and black melanins are produced by melanocytes, e.g. Harris' hawk *Parabuteo unicinctus*
- Reds and yellows are produced from carotenoids such as carotenes and xanthophils, e.g. flamingos; these dietary pigments are dissolved in fat globules in the feather cells. Some reds are from porphyrins, e.g. turacos
- Greens are a product of physical interference by reflection of light through the feathers. Rarely, greens are produced by pigments, e.g. turacoverdin in Turacos
- White is due to reflection and refraction of light through airspaces in the feathers with no pigmentation
- Blue pigment is rare. The bright blue in budgerigars is due to the Tyndall effect: a scattering of light on particles <0.6 µm across, similar to the effect that produces the blue of the sky. Most parrots have green feathers that are a mixture of yellow carotenoids and the blue Tyndall effect; remove one of these colours and a blue or yellow feather results.

Moulting and regrowth

Some birds moult twice yearly and have breeding plumage different from their off-season plumage. Birds usually moult in a predictable sequence of feather loss. Wing and tail feathers are lost as mirror-image pairs. Large birds such as vultures take up to 4 years for a complete moult. Ducks lose all their wing feathers at once and cannot fly in this eclipse phase. Moulting frequently makes birds less active and they also require sufficient protein and especially sulphur-containing amino acids to regrow their feathers.

Feathers grow from a blood-filled shaft; when fully formed they are isolated from their blood supply and the feather is dead.

Beak

The horny beak or bill is a hard, tough epidermal structure. It consists of layers of keratin-filled cells that are mineralized with hydroxyapatite crystals, the whole being held to a layer of keratin, which is firmly bound to the periosteum over the bone of the beak. The most rostral portion of the beak can have a well developed superficial innervation, as in the ducks, or be completely inert. The beak grows continually through life both from a germinal layer corresponding to the coronary band and from a germinal layer over the supporting bone.

Claws

Claws are also heavily keratinized and mineralized. They are made of a dorsal thicker, harder, and more rapidly growing portion and a flat softer, ventral portion.

As the growth is greatest in the dorsal portion, the claw is curved and therefore is ideally suited for grasping. A vestigial claw may be found on the alula in some species, e.g. falcons.

Musculoskeletal system

The musculoskeletal system is so diverse and variable that many of its anatomical features have been used as a basis for taxonomic classification.

The skeleton (Figure 13.3) of the majority of birds is very light but is 'engineered' to be very strong. The bones of a frigate bird weigh less that its feathers. All the large bones are hollow and filled with either air or marrow. Cross struts are used to give strength.

Skull

The skull is a lightweight box and has two huge orbits.

The upper jaw is formed by the premaxilla and nasal bones and can be moved relative to the rest of the skull usually due to flexible elastic zones, except in parrots

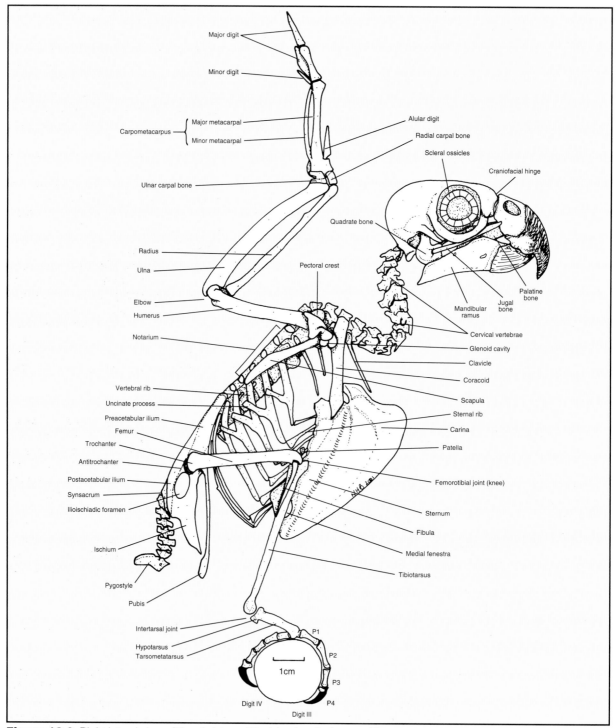

Figure 13.3 Right lateral view of the skeleton of the blue-headed parrot *Pionus menstruus*. The wing is elevated. The bird is in a normal perching position. © Nigel Harcourt-Brown

where there is a true joint. The lower jaw consists of two fused mandibles. The mandibles do not articulate directly with the skull but form a complex articulation with several small bones, which makes the upper and lower jaws move in concert. The complex movements of the upper and lower jaws, relative to each other, allow the beak to be used in many subtle ways other than a basic scissors movement.

The tongue is supported by the hyobranchial apparatus. Only parrots have intrinsic muscles in the tongue.

Vertebral column

The total number of vertebrae varies from 39 to 64. The fewest vertebrae occur in passerine birds, the most in swans and ratites. The vertebrae of the trunk are mainly fused. The *notarium* is formed from some of the thoracic vertebrae, and occasionally cervical vertebrae, fusing together into a single unit in the area over the lungs. One or two movable vertebrae are found caudal to the notarium and the remaining thoracic, lumbar and sacral vertebrae are fused to form the *synsacrum*.

The trunk of the bird is very inflexible. To compensate for this the jointed cervical region is relatively long. In swans there are 25 vertebrae; in most birds there are 14 or 15. All birds can rotate their head through 180 degrees. The caudal vertebrae are also freely movable. The vertebral column terminates with the pygostyle bone.

Ribs

The ribs articulate with the vertebrae and/or notarium. They support the sternum. The sternum in birds is very well developed to accommodate the pectoral muscles and support the thoracic girdle.

Thoracic girdle and wings

The thoracic girdle consists of the scapula, clavicle and coracoid bones. The coracoid acts as a strut, holding the wing at a constant distance from the sternum. The scapula is adjacent to the ribs, and the left and right clavicles are fused into a structure known as the *furcula*. The furcula acts as a spring and stores energy during the downbeat as it is compressed. These three bones are joined at their proximal ends to articulate with the head of the humerus; in their jointed articular surface they form the triosseal foramen. The tendon of the supracoracoideus muscle passes through this foramen to the humerus.

The wing bones are the humerus, radius and ulna, and a complex of bones – the *manus*. The manus has been reduced; there are only two free carpal bones; the remainder and the metacarpals are fused to form the carpometacarpus. There are only three digits: the alula digit, the major digit and the minor digit. The bones are constructed and held by ligaments so that when flexed the wing is very mobile but when extended the wing only moves at the shoulder joint.

Wing muscles and flight

The wing has its main muscle mass on the sternum. The pectoral muscle contracts to cause the down stroke of the wing. During normal flapping flight the supracoracoideus muscle rotates the humerus to make the wing elevate its leading edge. This allows the bird to maintain its position in the air between down strokes.

During slow flight and take off, the shoulder muscles elevate the wing. The elbow joint has a wide range of movements when flexed, and the radius and ulna pronate and supinate. When the wing is extended the elbow joint 'locks' and cannot be moved except for flexion; the same can be said for the carpus.

Pelvis and legs

The pelvis is formed by fusion of the ilium, ischium, and pubis. The pelvis is also fused to the synsacrum. The acetabulum is not a bony cup but has a bony rim. Caudodorsal to the acetabulum is the antitrochanter, which articulates with the trochanter of the femur and prevents abduction of the limb when in a normal standing position.

The main muscle mass of the pelvic limb is close to the body, as it is in the thoracic wing. The muscles that move the distal joints have long tendons of insertion. The pelvic limb has a locking mechanism in the digits where the flexor tendons have a ratchet that prevents them from moving when the muscle is tensed and the toes are flexed and gripping.

The pelvic limb is formed by: the femur; the tibiotarsus, which is the tibia fused to the proximal row of tarsal bones, and fibula; the tarsometatarsus, which is the distal row of tarsal bones combined with the fused second, third and fourth metatarsal bones; a free first metatarsal bone; and a variable number of digits – from 2 to 4.

Bone structure and growth

Growth and ossification take place from a cartilaginous area at each end of the bone. There is no radiographically obvious growth plate, as there is in a mammal, because the epiphysis is not ossified as the bones grows. Medullary bone is labile bone that occurs only in female birds in the reproductive phase. Phases of formation and destruction alternate during the laying cycle. The formation of medullary bone is controlled by oestrogens and androgens.

Muscle types

Muscle fibres in birds are of two types: red and white. Red fibres contain relatively large amounts of myoglobin and, in comparison with the white fibres, they have more mitochondria and lipid globules and greater vascularity. Red fibres use fat for their energy source and they are therefore more efficient than the white, glycogen-using fibres. Red fibres are less prone to muscle fatigue and are considered to be predominantly adapted for sustained effort. However, all muscle masses in birds are a mixture of red and white fibres in different proportions. In some muscles the distribution seems related to function but not in others.

Digestive system

Oesophagus and crop

The oesophagus usually lies on the right side of the neck. The oesophagus lies in voluminous folds in many species, to accommodate food, but is often modified at the thoracic inlet to form the crop (Figure 13.4). The crop is absent in some groups, such as owls and penguins. Peristaltic waves move the food down the oesophagus and also around the crop.

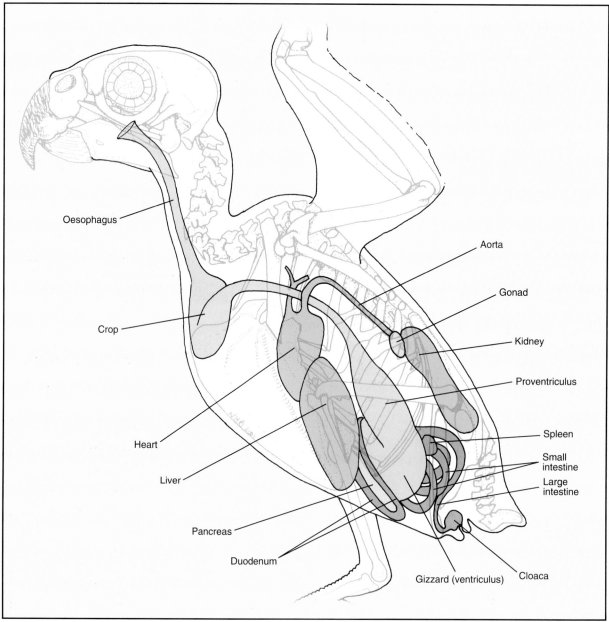

Figure 13.4 Left lateral view of the viscera of the blue-headed parrot. © Nigel Harcourt-Brown

The crop does not play any significant role in chemical digestion but produces 'crop milk' in pigeons. The milk contains 7–12% fat and 13–18% protein but lacks calcium and carbohydrates. The production of crop milk is controlled by prolactin.

Stomach

The stomach is divided into a proventriculus and ventriculus (gizzard) (see Figure 13.4). Cranially the proventriculus is glandular; caudally it is muscular. The intermediate zone opens into the gizzard.

In carnivores and fish-eaters the gizzard is uniformly muscular and resembles a mammalian stomach. In birds that eat soft food the gizzard is a storage organ and gastric juice causes proteolysis. In seed-eaters the gizzard is extremely muscular

and has internal and external adaptations for grinding food with grit. The internal surface is covered with the cuticle (koilin layer).

The pyloric part of the stomach is sandwiched between the muscular part of the gizzard and the duodenum. It contains endocrine cells.

In turkeys and parrots radiographic studies have shown that the food is propelled in alternate directions between the proventriculus and the gizzard in a series of cycles. In raptors the indigestible parts of the diet are rolled into a pellet that is regurgitated.

Intestine

The duodenum is a U-shaped loop of bowel (see Figure 13.4). The jejunum and the ileum are arranged in a series of coils. The intestinal arrangements are specific and have been used taxonomically. At the junction between the ileum and the jejunum is the vitelline diverticulum: the remnant of the yolk sac and the yolk duct. Chemical digestion and absorption of food takes place in the small intestine.

The large bowel consists of a short rectum and paired caeca. In some species the caeca are well developed and in others they are vestigial. The caeca arise at the junction between the jejunum and the rectum. The caecal contents are voided separately from the normal intestinal contents as a dark brown, glutinous mass.

Pancreas

The pancreas lies in the loop of the duodenum (see Figure 13.4) and secretes the same exocrine digestive enzymes as in mammals: amylase, lipase and proteases including trypsin. It also produces insulin and glucagon, although insulin has little effect on glucose metabolism, which is mainly controlled by steroid hormones.

Liver

The liver has right and left lobes; in most species the right lobe is larger. The gall bladder is absent in some species, including many parrots.

Urinary system

The kidneys are large and lie symmetrically in the renal fossae of the synsacrum (see Figure 13.4). Each kidney is divided into cranial, middle and caudal divisions. Each division has many lobules that may be seen as small lumps on the renal surface; the lobule is the fundamental unit of the kidney. The blood supply to the kidney is very complex (Figure 13.5).

Excretion

Birds, like reptiles, are uricotelic, i.e. uric acid rather than urea is the end point of nitrogen metabolism. The uric acid is formed in the liver and, although some is excreted through glomerular filtration, 90% is actively secreted by renal tubular secretion.

There are two types of nephron. One is found in the medulla of the lobule and has a well developed glomerulus plus a loop of Henle. This is known as a mammalian-type nephron. The other is found in the cortex of the lobule and has a less developed glomerulus and no loop of Henle; it is known as a reptilian-type nephron.

The renal portal veins and efferent venous flow from the glomerulus form the peritubular capillary plexus.

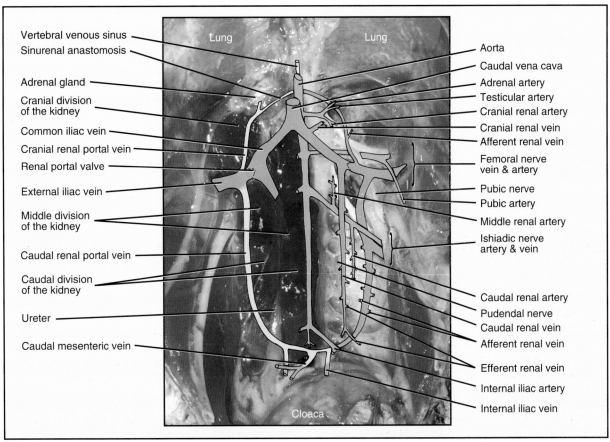

Figure 13.5 The blood supply to the kidney. A ventral view of the pelvic region of a grey parrot *Psittacus erithacus*. The right kidney remains *in situ*; the left kidney was removed to reveal the lumbosacral plexus. The nerves leave the synsacrum and run between the kidney and the pelvis. Arteries are shown in red and veins in blue; in life they are mostly surrounded by kidney tissue and thus are represented as a drawing. Each kidney has an arterial supply and matching venous drainage but the kidney is also supplied from a complete venous ring: the venous portal system. Two thirds of the blood entering the kidney is from the venous system. The direction and quantity of blood flowing through this ring, and therefore entering the kidney for waste product removal, can be altered by the renal portal valves that are controlled by the autonomic nervous system. © Nigel Harcourt-Brown

This plexus surrounds the proximal tubules, and urates are removed from the venous blood and secreted into the proximal tubule.

The urine is a mixture of colloids in mucus and water. It flows down the ureter and enters the urodeum – the terminal portion of the cloaca. The urine may then be transferred by retroperistalsis to the coprodeum and up into the rectum as far as the caeca. It is stored in the bowel until defecation. During this time water and some of the solutes are reabsorbed as required by the coprodeum and the bowel.

Marine birds (and some others) have a supraorbital gland capable of secreting sufficient salt to allow birds to drink seawater. They lose up to 75% of the sodium via these salt glands.

Reproductive system

Male

The male reproductive organs are a pair of equally active testes. In many birds the right testis is considerably smaller than the left. The testes vary greatly in size and vascularity during the reproductive cycle. They produce sperm, which is collected in the epididymis and emptied into the convoluted ductus deferens. The ductus deferens enlarges distally into a sperm receptacle in many species. There are no accessory genital glands.

Female

Usually only the left side of the female reproductive tract is fully and functionally developed. Some species, such as falcons, have a partly developed right ovary.

The blood supply to the ovary is large and the vessels are quite short. The ovary is closely attached to the body wall, next to the adrenal gland and cranial division of the kidney. The ovary has many obvious follicles; these are small in immature birds and enlarged by yolk in breeding adults.

Egg production

The follicle contains a large primary oocyte surrounded by a multi-layered wall that is potentially divided by the stigma. At ovulation the stigma splits and the (secondary) oocyte is 'grabbed' by the infundibulum. The oviduct, which is supported by dorsal and ventral ligaments, has five parts:

- The *infundibulum* picks up the oocyte and surrounds it with a first layer of albumen (egg white). There is a period of about 15 minutes between the oocyte being released from the ovary and being covered with albumen, when the oocyte can be fertilized by sperm
- The egg passes through the *magnum* where the rest of the albumen is added
- In the *isthmus* the shell membranes are produced
- The egg then enters the *shell gland* where it spends 80% of its time in the oviduct. First, the egg absorbs water and enlarges. Then the calcium carbonate and protein shell is produced,

covered by a cuticle that givies the egg its shiny appearance. The shell contains thousands of tiny pores, allowing the embryo to respire
- The final part of the oviduct is the muscular *vagina;* in many species this has spermatic fossulae capable of sperm storage. In many species, such as budgerigars, viable sperm can be stored and released for several weeks. After mating, some of the sperm is stored; some is able to reach the infundibulum within a few minutes.

Cloaca

The cloaca is the terminal portion of the urinary, reproductive and alimentary tracts (see Figure 13.5) . It has three compartments.

In many birds the rectum becomes the coprodeum with no special junction, except in ostriches and ducks. Villi line the coprodeum in some species and not in others. The urodeum is the middle and smallest compartment. It is separated from the other compartments by two circular mucosal folds. If the coprodeum is full of faeces it can empty by eversion of the urocoprodeal fold through the urodeum to the outside. Faeces do not have to travel through the urodeum and proctodeum. The coprourodeal fold will also close during egg-laying.

The ureter and reproductive ducts open into the urodeum, the ureters open relatively dorsally.

The vas deferens opens through a small papilla. A similar papilla is seen in immature female fowl, ducks, and penguins. It is retained into maturity in penguins and, as it is smaller than the male papilla, it can be used to determine the sex of the birds.

The left oviduct develops with a membrane over the opening that usually disappears when the bird is mature. The right oviduct is permanently sealed.

The proctodeum is short and can contain a variety of potentially tumescent structures.

Ratites, such as the ostrich, and ducks have an erectile phallus; the erection is effected by lymphatic fluid. Many other species have lymphatic folds and phallic bodies. The cloacal bursa (bursa of Fabricius) opens into the proctodeum in young birds (see Lymphatic system).

Cardiovascular system

Heart

The heart of birds is relatively much larger and beats faster than that of mammals. For example, a hummingbird's heart is 2.5% of its total bodyweight (compared with 0.5% in a mouse) and can beat 1000 times a minute. Birds have a high cardiac output, seven times greater in a budgerigar than in a man or dog at maximum exercise. This high cardiac output is combined with a high arterial pressure: 180/140 is usual in a chicken; 180/135 in a pigeon; 180/130 in a starling.

The four-chambered heart lies ventral to the lungs, surrounded by pericardium and the liver. The right atrioventricular valve is a muscular flap; other valves are similar to those of mammals.

Blood vessels

There is a similar system of arteries and veins as in mammals, though there are many species differences. The jugular anastomosis allows the blood in the left jugular vein to be shunted to the right; the right jugular vein is usually much larger and the left jugular vein is occasionally absent.

Lymphatic system

Birds have a well developed lymphatic system. Lymphatic vessels return extravascular fluids to the circulating blood. There are fewer valves than in mammals and lymphatic hearts can be found in the abdomen of some families. The lymphatic ducts drain into the venae cavae.

Lymphoid tissue is found in several areas that are different from mammals. The thymus is multilobed and runs along the neck. The thymus produces mainly T lymphocytes and some B lymphocytes. The cloacal bursa is unique to birds; it is a dorsomedial diverticulum in the proctodeum. It may be a substantial organ or a thin-walled sac as in parrots. The bursa is the source of the majority of the B lymphocytes. The bursa involutes slowly and is usually just a remnant of tissue by the time the bird is mature. True lymph nodes are rare in birds; when they do occur they are in a pair near the thyroid and a pair near the kidneys. There are mural lymphoid nodules in the walls of the lymphatics, and also there are some solitary aggregates of lymphoid tissue e.g. the caecal tonsils. The spleen phagocytoses erythrocytes, produces lymphocytes and antibodies but is not erythropoietic.

Respiratory system

The body of the bird contains the viscera within their peritoneal cavities (see Figure 13.4) and a number of air-filled sacs (Figure 13.6). There is no diaphragm.

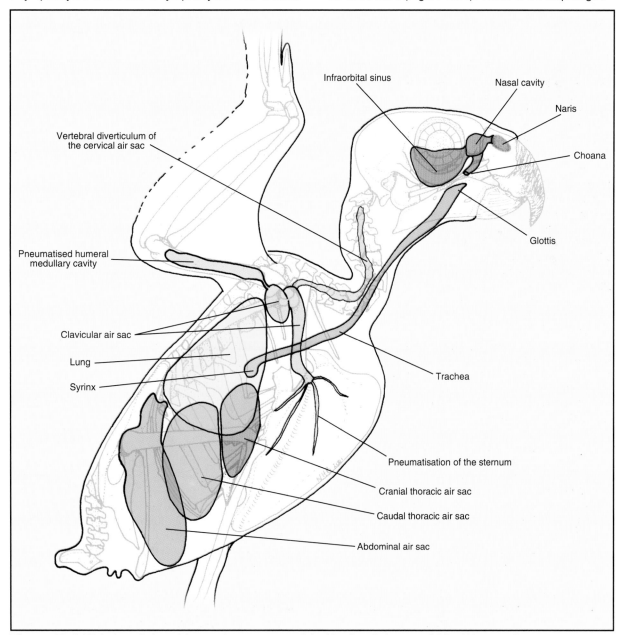

Figure 13.6 Right lateral view of the respiratory organs of the blue-headed parrot. © Nigel Harcourt-Brown

Lungs and air sacs

The two lungs are a mass of interconnected airways that commence at the primary bronchus and finish via holes (*ostia*) that enter the air sacs (Figure 13.7). There are eight air sacs: 1 cervical; 1 clavicular; 2 cranial thoracic; 2 caudal thoracic; and 2 abdominal. The cervical and clavicular sacs enter the vertebrae, humerus and other soft tissue structures mainly outside the main body cavity. Caudoventral to the lungs are the thoracic and abdominal sacs. The abdominal air sacs also extend into the femur and around the kidneys. The exact structure of the sacs and the pneumatization of the body differ between species, e.g. the femur is pneumatized in birds of prey but not in parrots. The air sacs have two principal functions: reduction of the bird's weight; and ventilation by acting as bellows to pull air through the lungs. Respiratory movements elevate and depress the sternum and also expand and contract the rib cage. This expands and contracts the air-filled sacs but does not change the volume of the lungs.

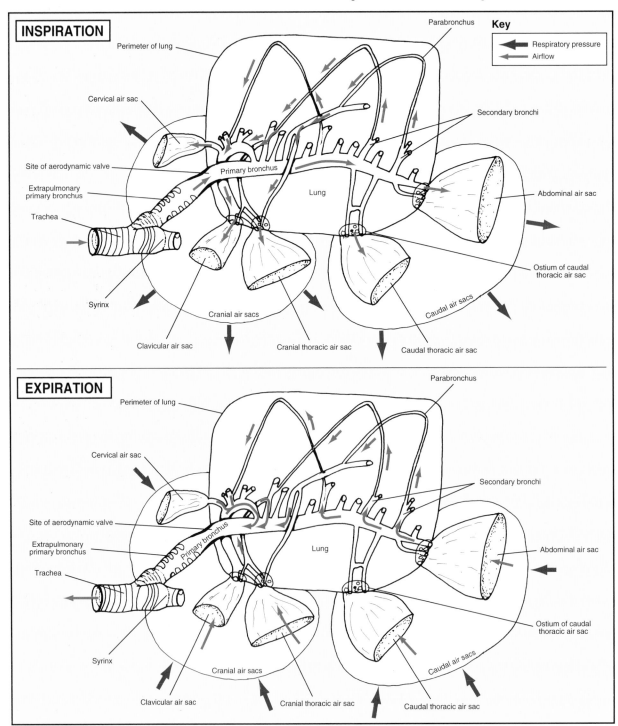

Figure 13.7 Movement of air through the lung of a bird. Inspiratory movements increase air sac volumes and expiratory movements decrease them. The volume and shape of the lung remains the same. Because of the arrangement of the parabronchi and the possible presence of an aerodynamic valve, the air is moved unidirectionally through the parabronchi and therefore the area of gaseous exchange. © Nigel Harcourt-Brown

Upper respiratory tract

The upper respiratory tract provides a filter system of nostril and concha to warm, moisten, and filter the air. The nasal passages connect to an extensive air-filled infraorbital sinus. The air passes through a slit in the roof of the mouth (*choana*) to the larynx.

The larynx can open and shut but has no ability to make noises. The trachea consists of complete tracheal rings and can be complicated either by bullae, or a long sinuous path, to aid vocalization. The trachea divides at the syrinx. Vocalization is produced principally in the syrinx, which has a structure and musculature so complicated and variable that it is widely used for taxonomy.

The syrinx gives rise to two primary bronchi, one supplying each lung. The primary bronchi divide into smaller and smaller airways, all of which are variously interconnected but finally pass through the lung to empty into the air sacs. This complex system of airways, plus an aerodynamic valve, allows a unidirectional path through the majority of the lung tissue for the majority of the air (see Figure 13.7). The final unit of gaseous exchange is the smallest section of the airway: the air capillary. The air capillaries form an anastomosing three-dimensional network of airways through which the air flows. The air capillaries are intimately entwined with the blood capillary network.

Central nervous system

The CNS of birds is similar to that of mammals. The brain is not as large comparatively as the mammalian brain, but is larger than the reptilian brain. There is a very poorly developed cerebral cortex. The rostral colliculus (optic lobe) is huge and the total cross-sectional area of the optic nerve is greater than that of the cervical spinal cord. The olfactory region is poorly developed except in kiwis and some other birds, e.g. turkey vulture *Cathartes aura*.

The spinal chord is morphologically similar to that of all other vertebrates. It is surrounded by the meninges. The epidural space is filled with a gelatinous rather than liquid substance. A large venous sinus runs along the dorsal aspect of the vertebral canal and is voluminous in the area of the medulla oblongata. The spinal cord runs the full length of the neural canal and gives off its nerves laterally. There is no cauda equina.

The wing is supplied from a brachial plexus and the pelvic limb from a lumbosacral plexus. The brachial plexus gives rise to both a ventral and dorsal fascicle, so that all the wing is surrounded with nerves, whereas most of the leg has a caudolateral supply.

Sense organs

Eyes

The eye is huge in most species of bird. Prey species, e.g. pigeons, tend to have narrow heads with the eyes set laterally (visual field 300 degrees); predatory species, e.g. owls, tend to have their eyes facing rostrally in a broad head (visual field 150 degrees). The eye has a small anterior chamber covered with cornea. The posterior chamber is much larger and can vary in shape. Tubular eyes are usual for night vision; diurnal birds with wide heads have a globular eye and narrow-headed birds have a flat eye. These shapes allow the retina to have all-round visual acuity, unlike in mammals, which have a single region of acute vision. The eyeball is supported by bony scleral ossicles adjacent to the cornea. The ciliary body suspends the lens and contains two striated muscles, the anterior and posterior sclerocorneal muscles.

Accommodation is effected in one of three ways. In many birds the posterior sclerocorneal muscle forces the ciliary body against the lens and increases the curvature of the lens. In owls and hawks the anterior sclerocorneal muscle is well developed and distorts the cornea by pulling the sclerocorneal junction. In many diving birds the iris is forced against the lens, causing the lens to bulge through the pupil. As the muscles of the eye are striated muscle, including that controlling the iris, birds have conscious control over their iris and accommodation. Many parrots use their iris as a behavioural signal, especially Amazon parrots.

The retina consists of a large number of cones and some rods, giving excellent visual acuity and good night vision. For example, the American kestrel *Falco sparverius* can see a 2 mm insect from a perch 18 metres away.

Most non-predatory birds look closely at an object by turning their head and using a single eye. Whilst flying, many birds are able to view the ground and the horizon at the same time, with both in focus even though they are different distances away from the bird. Not only does this use different parts of the retina, but the visual impulses also go to different parts of the brain.

The pecten is a thin black structure found in the posterior chamber. It tends to be small and simple in nocturnal birds and large and complex in diurnal birds. It is a highly vascular structure that has been considered to be part of the image analysing system but has also been shown that it has a nutritive function within the posterior chamber. This is important as the retina is relatively avascular.

There is a transparent nictitating membrane that protects the eye. It is moved voluntarily by two muscles under the control of the sixth cranial nerve. There is a gland associated with the membrane and as the membrane sweeps across the eye it distributes secretions from this gland.

Ears

The ear is not as well developed as the eye, except in some species such as owls. The facial disc of an owl is an acoustic organ and in many species the ears are asymmetrical to help with directional finding. Diving birds have the ear canal reduced and protected with strong feathers.

References and further reading

Baumel JJ (1993) *Handbook of Avian Anatomy: Nomina Anatomica Avium, 2nd edn.* Nuttall Ornithological Club, Harvard University, Massachusetts *[Extremely useful: the fundamental anatomical text as it standardizes and defines the names of anatomical structures.]*

Brown RE, Kovacs CE, Butler JP *et al.* (1995) The avian lung: is there an aerodynamic expiratory valve. *The Journal of Experimental Biology* **198**, 2349–2357

King AS and McLelland J. (1984) *Birds: their Structure and Function.* Baillière Tindall, London *[An affordable and very good, anatomical overview]*

McLelland J (1990) *A Colour Atlas of Avian Anatomy.* Wolfe Publishing, Aylesbury *[A very useful book using high quality photographs to give an excellent guide to general avian anatomy.]*

Poore SO, Ashcroft A, Sanchez-Haiman A and Goslow GE (1997) The contractile properties of the m. supracoracoideus in the pigeon and starling: a case for long axis rotation of the humerus. *The Journal of Experimental Biology* **200,** 2987–3002

Whittow GC (2000) *Sturkie's Avian Physiology, 5ᵗʰ edn.* Academic Press, Harcourt Science and Technology Company, San Diego, California

Avian imaging

Claudia Hochleithner, Manfred Hochleithner and Andreas Artmann

In small animal practice the number of avian clients is increasing, and owners expect the same efforts of investigation for their birds that are used for dogs and cats. Radiography, ultrasonography (despite limiting factors) and new techniques such as computed tomography (CT) are performed.

Patient preparation

To limit the stress on the bird during these procedures and to standardize the positioning while performing radiography, ultrasonography or CT, the birds are anaesthetized. The authors use isoflurane. Depending on the size of the bird, 0.5–1 litre of oxygen flow is used; anaesthesia is induced with 5% isoflurane and maintained with 1–2% isoflurane during the procedure.

Radiography

It is possible to use the same X-ray machine and developing system for avian clients as for dogs and cats. Preferably, single-emulsion film and single-screen rare earth systems, as used for mammography, should be used. These allow greater detail, although they require increased exposure times.

Views and positioning
Two views should generally be taken: ventrodorsal and lateral. In severely ill birds with suspected heavy metal intoxication it may be advantageous to put the conscious bird on the screen and take one exposure just to detect the radiodense particles.

Ventrodorsal view
The bird is restrained in dorsal recumbency. The wings are spread at 90 degrees from the body and held in place, fixed by sandbags or lead gloves. The legs are pulled caudally and parallel to the body and fixed with tapes. In this position, the spine and the sternum are superimposed and the scapulae, acetabula and femurs are parallel (Figure 13.8a).

Lateral view
A left-to-right lateral view is preferred. The wings are extended dorsally and fixed in position. Both legs are extended caudally and fixed. Figure 13.8b shows a lateral radiograph of a normal pigeon.

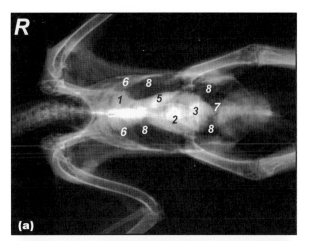

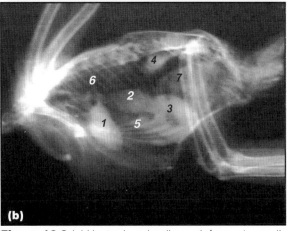

Figure 13.8 (a) Ventrodorsal radiograph from a 'normal' bird. (b) Lateral radiograph from a 'normal' bird. 1 = heart; 2 = proventriculus; 3 = ventriculus; 4 = kidneys; 5 = liver; 6 = lung; 7 = intestine; 8 = airsac.

Clinical findings
The quality of the radiograph should first be assessed for exact positioning of the patient and level of the exposure. In order not to miss any important changes, the entire radiograph should be studied and not just the suspected lesion.

Musculoskeletal system

Skeleton: The skeleton is checked for changes in normal anatomy, dislocations and fractures. Changes in bone density and deformation due to poor husbandry or malnutrition can be seen, especially in young birds (hypovitaminosis D, calcium and phosphorus imbalance). In females bone density is increased prior to ovulation (polyostotic hyperostosis). Prolonged or abnormally elevated oestrogen levels also cause a diffusely increased medullary bone density. Figure 13.9 shows diffuse increased bone density in the head of a mynah bird due to osteosarcoma.

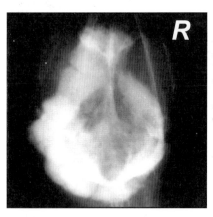

Figure 13.9 Diffuse increased bone density in the head of a mynah bird. Histology showed osteosarcoma.

The architecture of the bone should be evaluated and lesions and their distribution investigated. Fractures should be assessed for: location; whether simple or comminuted; articular involvement; the density of the bone; whether there is a periosteal reaction; soft tissue involvement; and whether the fracture is open or closed.

Soft tissue: Soft tissue masses may be seen on radiographs in connection with abscesses, haematomas, tumours, or swelling in connection with fractures.

Respiratory system
High-quality radiographs are necessary to detect the sometimes very subtle lesions in connection with diseases of the respiratory system. The normal syrinx is difficult to visualize. The lung parenchyma has a honeycombed structure and the bronchioles can be visualized as transverse, linear structures.

Bacterial or fungal infections (Figure 13.10) are the most common cause of pathological changes in the respiratory tract. Hypovitaminosis A also plays a leading role in the pathogenesis of respiratory diseases.

Changes in the diameter of the trachea, intraluminal soft tissue masses and obstructions, especially in the region of the syrinx, can be diagnosed radiographically. Shadows in the lungfield are visualized in the ventrodorsal view, mainly in the caudal part of the lung.

The air sacs give a negative contrast for the coelomic cavity. Their size varies between inspiration and expiration. Radiographic changes in connection with inflamed air sacs show as fine lines across the air sacs, with increased opacity. They are best detected with lateral radiography.

Cardiovascular system
The size and shape of the heart varies with the species of bird and the phase of respiration and cardiac cycle. In psittacine birds the lateral margin of the heart and liver create an hourglass shape.

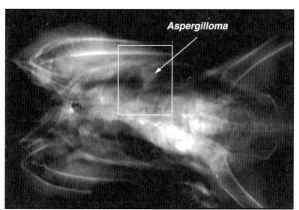

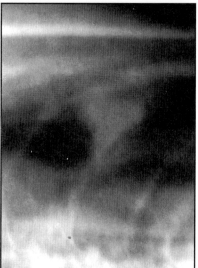

Figure 13.10 Ventrodorsal view of a buzzard and detail. Aspergillomas are usually best seen in the lateral view. The caudal thoracic and abdominal airsacs are usually most affected. This bird had no clinical signs and the disease was detected during endoscopy for sexing.

The most common radiographic change seen is cardiomegaly caused by cardiomyopathy, valvular degeneration or endocarditis, but microcardia can also be found in connection with hypovolaemia or endotoxic shock. Arteriosclerosis with mineralization of the great vessels can be diagnosed, especially in older birds (Figure 13.11).

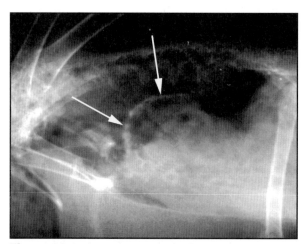

Figure 13.11 Lateral radiograph of a 35-year-old blue-fronted Amazon parrot, showing arteriosclerosis and mineralization of the great vessels.

Coelomic cavity and gastrointestinal system

Liver: The shadow of the liver should not extend laterally past a line drawn from the coracoid to the acetabulum. The size should be investigated in the ventrodorsal view on inspiration. Hepatomegaly (Figure 13.12) is a common finding on radiographs in connection with loss of the hourglass waist, rounding of liver lobe margins, and extension of the liver lobes laterally and caudally. The aetiology of enlargement of the liver may be infectious (viral, e.g. Pacheco's disease; bacterial; chlamydiosis; mycobacteriosis), metabolic (fatty liver degeneration, lipidosis, haemochromatosis in mynah birds) or neoplastic.

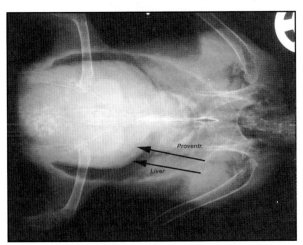

Figure 13.12 Ventrodorsal view of a 28-year-old female blue-fronted Amazon parrot. She weighed 654 g and she was on a 100% sunflower seed diet.

Spleen: The spleen can be visualized in the ventrodorsal view as a rounded structure between the proventriculus and ventriculus. If visible in the lateral view, it overlaps the caudal end of the proventriculus. Causes of splenomegaly may be infectious (chlamydiosis, viral, bacterial or mycobacterial), metabolic or neoplastic (lymphoma).

Alimentary tract: The alimentary tract can be investigated with plain radiographs or with barium contrast studies. The presence of gas in the intestine of birds is not considered normal. Any changes in the diameter, abnormal fluid or gas-filled bowel loops or compressions from the surrounding organs can be seen on radiographs and differentiated with positive contrast studies. Dilation of the crop (Figure 13.13), proventriculus and ventriculus can be seen in connection with parasitic, bacterial and fungal infections, but also in connection with neuropathic gastric dilation. Radiodense foreign bodies (e.g. zippers, heavy metals) can be easily localized (Figures 13.14 and 13.15).

Enlargement or dilation of the cloaca can be seen with plain radiography but it is helpful to perform retrograde contrast studies (positive, Figure 13.16; or negative) to find the cause (e.g. soft-shelled eggs, papillomas, neoplasms).

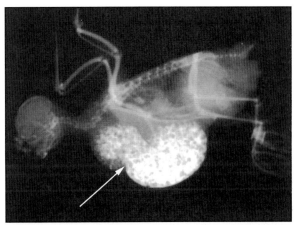

Figure 13.13 Contrast study of the gastrointestinal tract in a female budgerigar with a history of emesis. The radiograph was taken 30 minutes after administration of 2 mm of barium sulphate via a feeding tube. The arrow shows the normal extent of the crop in a budgerigar. The diagnosis was crop dilation. There is also diffuse increased medullary bone density (osteopetrosis).

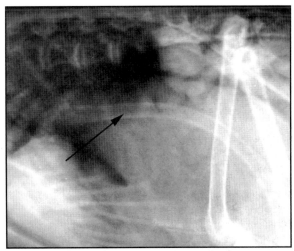

Figure 13.14 Foreign body in a 7-week-old hyacinth macaw. The plastic feeding tube was removed using an endoscope.

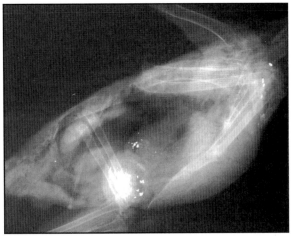

Figure 13.15 Heavy metal objects are easily detected by radiography. Correct positioning is not vital for this if the bird's health precludes it.

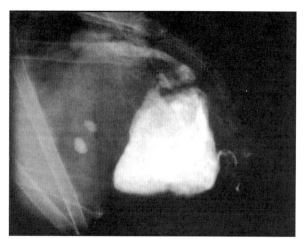

Figure 13.16 Positive contrast study of the cloaca of a female African grey parrot. The bird had a cloacal dilation associated with neuropathy but the proventriculus and ventriculus showed very few pathological changes.

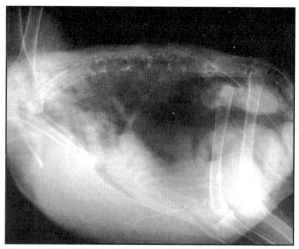

Figure 13.17 There is increased kidney density in connection with nephromegaly. This may occur in various kidney diseases and also as a result of dehydration.

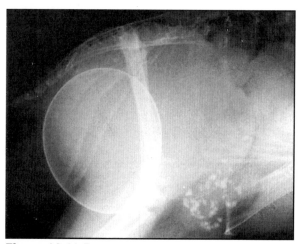

Figure 13.18 Eggs are easily visualized on radiography because of the minerals in the shells.

Changes in the location of the gastrointestinal tract can be caused by intra-abdominal masses of different origins. Tract displacement can give a clue as to which organ is enlarged. Enlargement of the spleen, testicles or ovaries and kidneys dislocate the gastrointestinal tract ventrally and either cranially or caudally. A displacement of the proventriculus and ventriculus to the dorsal and caudodorsal position can be caused by hepatomegaly. Fluid in the abdomen results in a homogeneous appearance in the intestinal peritoneal cavity. In these cases ultrasonography is indicated where the fluid acts as contrast medium and aids diagnosis.

Kidneys: On lateral view the kidneys are surrounded by air, which gives a negative contrast. Dorsally the kidneys are attached to the synsacrum and have smoothly rounded cranial and caudal divisions. In the lateral view the kidneys are superimposed. Therefore, the density and size of the kidneys should be investigated in the ventrodorsal view, although normal kidneys are hard to see. Bilateral symmetrical enlargement of the kidneys can be found in connection with infections, metabolic diseases, postrenal obstructions and neoplasia (lymphoreticular). Increased density in connection with nephromegaly (Figure 13.17) can also be seen in cases of dehydration. Unilateral or localized enlargement can be seen in cases of neoplasia, cysts or abscesses.

Reproductive system: Tumours of the spleen, testicles, ovaries or oviduct can be misinterpreted as kidney tumours. The only way to diagnose the origin is to perform a laparoscopy. Inflammation or enlargement of the testicles is hardly seen on radiographs; therefore the diagnostic tool of choice is also laparoscopy. In females, retained eggs, cystic ovaries or oviduct, and egg yolk peritonitis can be diagnosed from specific changes on radiography. Eggs can be easily visualized due to the mineralized shell (Figure 13.18) and the number of eggs retained can be evaluated. However, ultrasonography is the diagnostic tool of choice in those cases with suspected soft-shelled eggs or multilayered eggs, and for differentiating the origin of any peritonitis or abdominal effusion.

Contrast studies

Patient preparation
A severely ill bird should be stabilized before performing contrast studies, as there will be a higher frequency of sedation and radiography procedures. Contrast suspensions are hypertonic and might cause dehydration. It should be borne in mind that most of the drugs used for anaesthesia may slow the passage of contrast medium, which could be misinterpreted as pathological. Survey radiographs should always be performed prior to any contrast study.

Techniques
The most important contrast studies performed in avian patients are gastrointestinal positive contrast studies. Barium follow-through studies should be performed in cases of vomiting and diarrhoea (acute or chronic, not responsive to treatment), suspected obstructions, displacement of abdominal organs, suspected perforation, ingested foreign bodies, haemorrhagic diarrhoea and weight loss of unknown origin.

It is best to perform these studies with an empty gastrointestinal tract. Normally 4 hours of fasting should be enough and will not harm even very small birds. Depending on the size and age of the bird, as well as the specific diet (e.g. seeds, pellets, fruits), changes in gut motility and gastrointestinal transit time can be evaluated. Some drugs influence gut motility and thus transit time.

Commercially available barium sulphate solutions can be used in birds, either in the concentration provided or diluted with water. Depending on the size of the bird, 20–30 ml of contrast medium should be administered. In juvenile birds barium should be warmed before being administered into the crop, similar to tube feeding.

The frequency and number of radiographs depends on the species and the indication. The first radiograph should be taken immediately after administration, to visualize the crop. Further radiographs should be taken at 30-minute, 1-, 2-, 4-, 8- and 24-hour intervals, depending on the lesion suspected.

It is also possible to obtain double-contrast studies of the crop (ingluviography) with half air and half barium, to visualize changes where only the crop is involved. It is important to administer the air first to prevent air bubbles mixing with the barium solution.

Clinical findings

The radiographic changes in contrast studies in birds are quite similar to those found in dogs and cats. Mechanical and functional ileus can be differentiated by the region where the contrast medium is stopped and how the lumen is dilated. In neuropathic gastric dilation, functional ileus is the most frequent radiographic change, with uniform distension, especially of the proventriculus and ventriculus, and also sometimes the intestine. Intoxications (e.g. lead), inflammation and some drugs can also cause functional ileus.

Mechanical obstructions can be diagnosed due to foreign bodies, parasites, intraluminal masses (e.g. neoplasms, intussusception, papillomas) and extraluminal masses compressing the lumen of the gastrointestinal tract.

Enlargement of intra-abdominal organs leads to displacement of the gastrointestinal tract. Enlargement of the liver dislocates the proventriculus to the dorsal region and the ventriculus to the caudodorsal part of the radiograph in the laterolateral view. Spleen, gonads and kidney enlargements push the intestine to the ventral portion. With hernias the intestine is dislocated to the ventral part of the abdomen (with dilation of the abdominal wall).

Intravenous excretory urography and other special contrast techniques such as rhinosinography, angiography, irrigoscopy and myelography are also possible, but are not of the same importance as in small mammals.

Ultrasonography

The authors use the same ultrasound machine that is used for small mammals. The probes used for birds are 5 or 7.5 MHz switchable sector transducers. Stand-off pads are used, or latex gloves filled with lubricating jelly will also do a perfect job. As with all special investigations, it is important to know the anatomy of the animal.

One of the limiting factors in ultrasonography is air. This causes total reflection of the ultrasound with distal extinction of the beam, which means that the organs cannot be visualized. Due to the air sacs in birds, the window for visualizing the internal organs is very small.

The following access points are possible in birds:

- Cranioventral behind the xiphoid
- Caudoventral in the pelvis
- Lateral parasternally (almost impossible in psittacines)
- Transintestinal (with special high-frequency longitudinal transducers).

Indications

Ultrasonography is used for diagnosing:

- The origin of abdominal enlargements found on clinical examination or in radiographs, e.g. ascites, tumours or enlargement of organs
- Changes of the echotexture of the different organs, e.g. tumours, cysts, fatty degeneration
- In female birds to investigate the function of the ovary and in egg binding to visualize the quality of the shell and detect multilayered eggs
- Cloacal papillomatosis, using contrast studies
- Many kinds of tumour of the skin, soft tissue or bone.

Patient preparation

The authors recommend isoflurane anaesthesia to limit stress and to standardize positioning. The bird is normally held in dorsal recumbency. If the bird has suspected ascites or cardiac or respiratory distress, it is held in an upright position. Although ascitic fluid gives a wonderful contrast medium for ultrasonography, great care must be taken with these birds because the possibility of respiratory distress is very high due to the small space for ventilation.

The feathers are separated and lubricating jelly is placed on the window. As the lubricating jelly could cool the bird, it is important to do the procedure as quickly as possible and preferably to warm up the jelly or put the bird on a heating pad.

Clinical findings

Liver

It is useful to investigate the liver in longitudinal and transverse sections. The normal pattern of the liver is homogeneous and slightly granulated. The vessels can be visualized within the liver tissue. The liver is checked for size and shape, and for any changes in texture. As there are species and individual differences, it is not easy to give exact measurements of the normal organ. If the caudal margin reaches far caudal of the xiphoid process, one can say that it is enlarged. Radiography can be used to confirm this as it is not possible to visualize the whole liver using ultrasound since it is overlapped by the gastroduodenal tract.

Changes in the pattern of the liver can either be focal parenchymal abnormalities or diffuse changes, quite similar to those found in small mammals.

Focal parenchymal changes: Cysts have thin hyperechoic walls and anechoic internal echoes, with strong distal acoustic enhancement. Haematomas and abscesses with their different appearance as found in small mammals can also be distinguished, as can necrosis and neoplasia.

Diffuse liver changes: Those of fatty liver degeneration are seen as increased liver echogenicity (Figures 13.19 and 13.20). This is the most frequent finding in patients at the authors' clinic. Diffuse neoplastic involvement appears as uneven echogenicity throughout either a part of the liver or the whole organ.

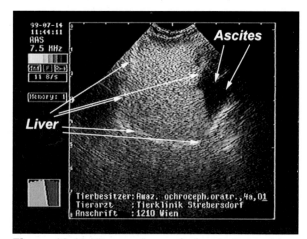

Figure 13.19 Ultrasound scan of a female 4-year-old double yellow-headed Amazon parrot with hepatomegaly, fatty liver disease (higher echogenicity of the liver) and ascites (anechoic region) due to malfunction of the liver.

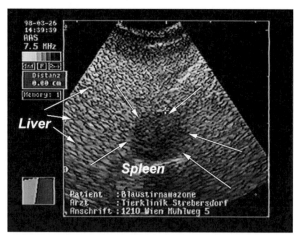

Figure 13.20 Ultrasound scan of an 8-year-old blue-fronted Amazon parrot with fatty liver degeneration and splenomegaly due to chlamydiosis.

Ascites: This can also be diagnosed in connection with liver diseases (see Figure 13.19), especially in mynah birds with haemosiderosis or haemochromatosis. The organs can be visualized very easily, as opposed to the findings on radiography.

Spleen

The echopattern of the spleen appears slightly more echoic than the liver. The size and shape depends on the species of bird. Normally the spleen is not easy to visualize, as it lies between the triangle of the proventriculus and ventriculus and is therefore overlapped by them. If the spleen is enlarged in cases of infection (e.g. chlamydiosis, bacterial or viral infections), it can be visualized behind the liver with the beam directed to the right laterodorsal side. These changes can be seen as homogeneous enlargements (see Figure 13.20). Tumours can be investigated as focal parenchymal changes with a nonhomogeneous pattern.

Alimentary tract

It is easier to investigate the alimentary tract if it is filled with fluid or is empty, as food particles and gas will compromise the image. Barium given for prior radiographic contrast studies will diminish the possibility of ultrasonography. Therefore, it should be kept in mind that if both ultrasound and contrast studies are to be performed, ultrasonography should be performed *before* barium is administered.

Sand and stones can be visualized in the ventriculus as hyperechoic particles with acoustic shadowing. The proventriculus can be seen cranial to the ventriculus as a round or oval shape, depending on the direction of the scan (longitudinal or transverse). The content is highly echoic with distal shadowing. Enlargements of the proventriculus, as seen in infectious diseases such as in neuropathic gastric dilation, can be visualized. Changes in motility and diameter can also be seen.

The intestine can be distinguished due to its peristaltic movement and the highly echoic content, either round or longitudinally scanned. It is not possible to distinguish the typical five layers found in small mammals. The duodenal loop can be distinguished because of the U-shape, but it is not very easy to see the pancreas in between the loop.

Access for cloacal investigation is caudoventral in the pelvis. Changes in the cloaca, as seen in papillomatosis, can be investigated using fluids or lubricating jelly as contrast medium to fill the cloaca.

Kidneys

It is not normally possible to visualize avian kidneys through transabdominal ultrasonography, as they are overlapped by airsacs and intestine. Only if the kidneys are enlarged can changes such as cysts (Figure 13.21) or tumours with a non-homogeneous pattern be diagnosed.

Reproductive system

With transintestinal scanners inactive gonads can be visualized.

Yolk in the first stage has an anechoic pattern; as it develops its echogenicity increases. In the magnum portion of the uterus, the yolk becomes surrounded by anechoic albumin. Depending on the stage of calcification, a highly echogenic shell can be visualized; total absorption of the ultrasound beam will make it impossible to differentiate any inner

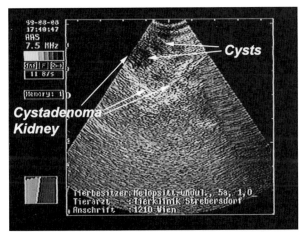

Figure 13.21 Ultrasound scan of a male 5-year-old budgerigar with enlarged kidneys due to a cystadenoma. The kidney tissue itself has a homgeneous pattern. Within the kidneys a few anechoic round structures (cysts) of different sizes can be differentiated. On histology, the cystadenoma was benign.

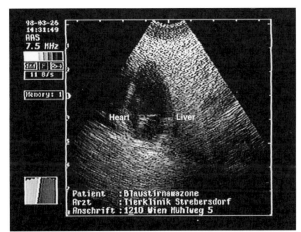

Figure 13.23 Ultrasound scan of an 8-year-old blue-fronted Amazon parrot. The left ventricle (peak) of the heart can be distinguished close to the transducer and a small portion of the right ventricle and part of the left atrium can be seen. The parrot had fatty liver degeneration.

structures. Multilayered eggs, soft-shelled eggs and eggs with abnormal shell structure can be differentiated by their typical appearance.

Cystic ovaries appear as round, anechoic structures with distal enhancement (increased brightness underneath the anechoic structure of the cysts). Ascites with higher echogenic particles in the liquid can be seen in connection with egg yolk peritonitis (Figure 13.22).

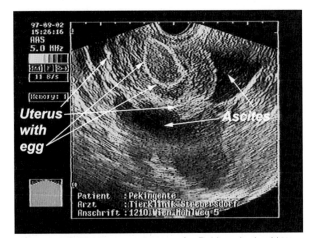

Figure 13.22 Ultrasound scan of a Peking duck with egg binding and egg yolk peritonitis. Two ruptured eggs can be seen: one in the uterus and one in the abdominal cavity. Within the uterus wall, inflammatory material is visualized as a highly echoic, slightly inhomogeneous area; a small portion of a non-calcified egg can be differentiated. Within the anechoic ascitic fluid are small particles of highly echogenic inflammatory material.

Small tumours of the testes and ovaries are difficult to diagnose with ultrasonography. Laparoscopy will give better results.

Heart
Figure 13.23 shows the ultrasonic appearance of the heart in an Amazon parrot.

Enlargement and effusions of the pericardium may be visualized using the ultrasound window behind the xiphoid in psittacine birds. In pigeons and chickens the right lateral approach is also possible. The naturally high heart rate of the patient has to be kept in mind when evaluating echocardiography; some machines are not fast enough to image the heart.

Soft tissue
Tumours of the skin and surrounding tissue can be evaluated for echogenicity (homogeneous, heterogeneous), shape and growth, and measurements can be made (multiple investigations for prognosis). It is helpful to use stand-off pads for this procedure. Results of the investigation can help in diagnosis and prognosis for possible surgery, and also in evaluation further treatment for recurring tumours.

Computed tomography (CT)

This allows superior imaging of three-dimensional structures compared with conventional radiography. The high level of differentiation of soft tissue and the absence of superimpositions of overlying structures are major advantages of this technique. Furthermore, the stored data make later reworking possible.

The region of interest can be shown in various planes and with various degrees of contrast. It is also possible to measure the density, in Hounsfield units (HU), of special areas, thus providing additional information for differentiation of various tissues and pathological alterations. Special programs allow a three-dimensional reconstruction.

As birds require isoflurane anaesthesia during CT, the procedure should not be prolonged. The use of 'helical scanning' is recommended. With this technology, a CT examination takes about 1 minute, depending on the dimension of the region of interest and the thickness of the cross-sections.

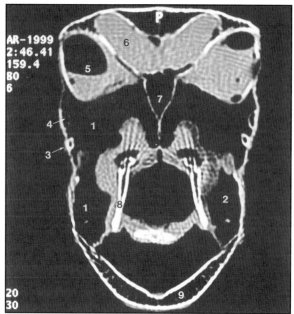

Figure 13.24 Transverse cross-sectional CT image of the pars infraorbitalis of the sinus paranasalis of a greenwing macaw (*Ara chloroptera*). 1 = pars infraorbitalis; 2 = mandibular recess; 3 = arcus jugale; 4 = arcus infraorbitalis osseus; 5 = eye (globe); 6 = brain (encephalon); 7 = interorbital septum; 8 = os platinum; 9 = mandible.

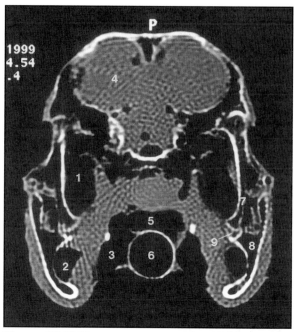

Figure 13.25 Transverse cross-sectional CT image of the pars quadrata of the sinus paranasalis of a greenwing macaw (*Ara chloroptera*). 1 = pars quadrata; 2 = mandibular recess; 3 = paratracheal recess; 4 = brain (encephalon); 5 = oesophagus; 6 = trachea; 7 = os quadratum; 8 = mandible; 9 = quadratomandibular joint.

Ventral recumbency is the preferred position. Transverse cross-sections provide detailed information and bilateral comparison, but more 'slices' are needed than for longitudinal scans. Conventional (incremental) CT means a higher cost and a longer examination time. Depending on the anatomical location, longitudinal sections may provide a better overview.

CT is useful for examining the avian respiratory tract. It allows an early and more exact diagnosis of pulmonary and air sac diseases. It is also possible to get reliable diagnosis of pathological processes occurring within the complex paranasal sinuses (of parrots) and to determine their exact location (Figures 13.24 and 13.25).

CT is also of great help in diagnosing diseases of the eye and brain. As CT becomes increasingly available, we can soon expect further indications.

References and further reading

Artmann A (2000) *Schnittbildanatomie der Kopf- und Harlsrgion der Gattung Ara unter besonderer Berücksichtigung des paranasalen Sinussystems.* Inaugural Dissertation Veterinärmedizinische Universität Wien

Enders F *et al.* (1993) Sonographic evaluation of liver diseases in birds. *Proceedings of the 1993 European Conference on Avian Medicine and Surgery*, pp. 155–163

Forbes NA (1996) Respiratory problems. In: *Manual of Psittacine Birds*, ed. PH Beynon *et al.* pp. 147–157. BSAVA Publications, Cheltenham

Fritsch R and Gerwing M (1993) *Sonografie bei Hund and Katze.* Enke, Stuttgart

Hathcock JT and Stickle RL (1993) Principles and concepts of computed tomography, *Veterinary Clinics of North America, Small Animal Practice* **23**, 399–415

Henninger W (1997) Computer- und Resonanztomographie, klinische Indikationen bei Haustieren. In: *Handlexikon der Tierärztlichen Praxis*, ed. E Wiesner, pp. 161j–161zj. Enke, Stuttgart

Hildebrand TB *et al.* (1997) Transintestinal sonography (TSI) in common quail. *Proceedings of the 4th Conference of the EAAV*, pp 26–27

Krautwald-Junghanns ME (1997) *Computertomographie des aviären Respirationstraktes. 1.Aufl.* Blackwell, Berlin

Krautwald-Junghanns ME *et al.* (1991) Diagnostic use of ultrasonography in birds, *Proceedings of the Association of Avian Veterinarians*, pp. 269–275

Krautwald-Junghanns ME and Enders F (1997) Ultrasonography. In: *Avian Medicine and Surgery*, ed. RB Altmann *et al.*, pp. 200–209. WB Saunders, Philadelphia

McMillan MC (1994) Imaging techniques. In: *Avian Medicine: Principles and Applications*, ed. BW Ritchie *et al.*, pp. 247–326. Wingers Publishing, Lake Worth, Florida

Nyland TG and Mattson JS (1995) *Veterinary Diagnostic Ultrasound.* WB Saunders, Philadelphia

Pohlmeyer K and Kummerfeld N (1989) Morphologie der Nasenhöhle und der Nasennebenhöhlen sowie ihre klinische Bedeutung bei Grosspapageien. *Kleintierpraxis* **34**, pp. 127–133

Thielebein J *et al.* (1996) Ultrasonographische Verlaufskontrolle der saisonalen Hodenveränderungen bei Gantern während einer Reproduktionsperiode. *Abstracts zum Dreiländertreffen Ultraschall 1996*, p. 88

14

Cage and aviary birds

Michael Stanford

Introduction

Over the past decade cage and aviary birds have dramatically increased in popularity as pets. Most noticeably, parrots are being bred and hand-reared in large numbers, producing both tame and interesting pets. Owners now have an increased expectation from their veterinary surgeons, as the birds seen may vary from a £15 budgerigar to a £2000 macaw. A range of pet birds is illustrated in Figure 14.1.

Biology

Figure 14.2 gives basic information about the most commonly kept species. Weight ranges and crop capacities are included to aid calculations of dosage and fluid therapy.

Husbandry

Housing

The Wildlife and Countryside Act 1981 covers bird cages. They must be of adequate size to allow the bird to extend and stretch its wings fully. Cheaper cages are often made from galvanized metal, which can lead to zinc poisoning. Perches must be provided, as most birds have a psychological need to perch. The perches supplied with most cages are, however, often made from plastic or wooden dowels, which are too smooth and

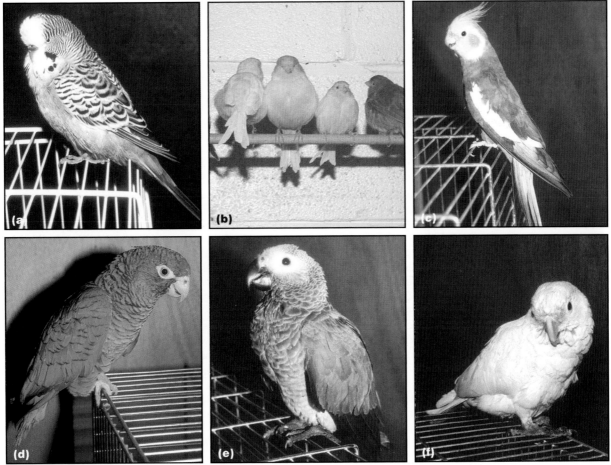

Figure 14.1 A variety of cage and aviary birds: (a) budgerigar; (b) canaries; (c) cockatiel; (d) Amazon parrot; (e) African grey parrot; (f) cockatoo.

Species	Mean weight (g) (ranges in parentheses)	Crop capacity (ml)	Comments
Zebra finch *Peophilia guttata*	15 (10–18)	0.5	Small short-lived seed-eater. Usually treat flock, not individuals.
Canary *Serinus canaria*	20 (15–40)	0.5–1.0	Kept for singing or bird shows.
Budgerigar *Melopsittacus undulatus*	50 (30–90)	1.0–2.0	Still most popular caged bird. Good talker. Commonly obese.
Cockatiel *Nymphicus hollandicus*	90 (70–110)	2.0–4.0	Common parakeet. Can be hand-reared, producing a tame bird.
Senegal parrot *Piocephalus senegalus*	130 (125–155)	5.0	Dwarf African parrot. Shy, nervous bird; good pet if hand-reared.
Sun conure *Aratinga solstitialis*	110 (90–130)	5.0	South American dwarf parrot. Colourful but noisy pet.
Red lory *Eos bornea*	100 (90–125)	NA	Brilliantly coloured nectar eater. Not ideal pet bird; difficult to keep.
African grey parrot *Psittacus erithacus*	450 (350–600)	10–15	Most popular pet parrot. Bred in UK in large numbers. Can be aggressive.
Blue-fronted Amazon parrot *Amazona aestiva*	450 (400–550)	10–15	Popular South American parrot. Gentler than African grey. Poor talker.
Lesser sulphur-crested cockatoo *Cacatua sulphurea*	250 (200–320)	10.0	Full of character but noisy. Often develop behavioural problems.
Umbrella cockatoo *Cacatua alba*	750 (600–950)	15–20	Not recommended as pet due to excessive noise and behavioural problems.
Blue and gold macaw *Ara ararauna*	1000 (1000–1500)	20	Large colourful bird. Intelligent pet. Bred in UK in large numbers.
Indian hill mynah *Gracula religiosa*	150 (90–200)	NA	Eats insectivorous mixtures. Excellent mimic. Messy.

Figure 14.2 Common cagebirds: mean weight and crop capacity. NA = not available.

usually too small in diameter for the bird to use properly. This can lead to problems with overgrown nails and skin lesions to the feet due to epithelial degeneration. Perches should be rough natural branches from non-poisonous trees – fruit trees are ideal.

Birds must have constant access to clean water and fresh food. Daily bathing by spraying the birds or providing a bath encourages preening, reduces feather dust and keeps the plumage in good condition. It is essential to allow tame birds out to exercise regularly. (Aviary birds are generally more fit and less fat than caged birds.) Toys (zinc-free) should be provided for all caged birds, especially the larger psittacine birds, to prevent boredom. Wing clipping is not recommended, especially in young birds, as this may to lead to severe psychological problems and feather disorders. Harnesses and corrective training should be used as an alternative to wing clipping.

Air quality is an important factor. Dusty conditions (which can considerably increase the chance of respiratory disease, particularly aspergillosis), excessive tobacco smoke and fumes from cooking utensils made from Teflon® should be avoided.

Diet

Most diseased birds are malnourished to some degree, and many ailments occur as a direct result of poor diet. Even with minor ailments it is always important to take a full dietary history and to try to correct the diet if possible.

Dietary requirements and recommendations for cage and aviary birds are listed in Figure 14.3. Fruit, vegetables and seed should always be fresh and fit for human consumption, as many cases of aspergillosis and bacterial infections can be traced back to a contaminated food source. Properly prepared pellet diets are becoming more popular with the owners of larger psittacines, although their availability is limited in some countries. The birds should always be provided with the correct avian vitamin supplement for the species.

The author recommends a home-made diet of pulses (Figure 14.4) for the larger psittacine birds, based on the following recipe:

1. Soak a mixture of pulses (soya beans, mung beans, black-eye beans, chickpeas) for 24–48 hours until they are just sprouting, then rinse thoroughly.
2. Add an equal weight of carrots, apples and fresh green vegetables.
3. Add a specific avian vitamin supplement, as recommended by the manufacturer.

This pulse and vegetable mixture should ideally form 70% of the diet, with the remaining 30% being made up of good quality seed mixtures or complete diets.

It is often vital to try to alter an owner's conception of what makes a 'good' parrot diet. If not, parrots often become fixated on poor quality seed mixtures, which can result in malnutrition.

Microchipping

Microchipping may be carried out to identify birds for a variety of reasons. The system used in the UK is the same as that marketed for dogs and cats. It is mainly

Type of bird	Common dietary problems	Recommended diet
Small psittacines, e.g. budgerigars, cockatiels, lovebirds	Usually fed seed mixtures with poor nutrient content, potentially contaminated with fungi or bacteria. Obesity is common due to high-fat diet and lack of exercise. Can become fixated on individual seed varieties, leading to malnutrition. Lack of fresh vegetable matter leads to lack of essential proteins, vitamins and minerals.	Good branded boxed diet with a large variety of seeds – cleaner than cheaper varieties and with a better nutrient content. Offer sprouted seed mixtures at least twice a week. Offer grated carrot, apple and fresh chickweed. Supplement with an avian vitamin supplement.
Passerines, e.g. finches, canaries	Fed dusty, poor quality seed mixtures with no vitamin supplementation or fresh food. Diet deficient in major vitamins, minerals and protein.	Clean, preferably branded, boxes of seed. Offer sprouted seed twice a week. Augment with an avian vitamin supplement.
Large psittacines, e.g. Amazons, African greys, cockatoos, conures, macaws	Most parrots are fed on pet shop seed mixtures and fruit combinations, which lead to severe malnutrition from a diet high in fat but low in protein, vitamins and minerals. Birds become fixated on individual seeds, usually sunflower. Commercial seed mixtures are generally of poor quality and may harbour pathogens (e.g. *Aspergillus*). Temperate fruits commonly used in the UK are poor nutrient sources for psittacines; due to lack of ultraviolet light, birds lack vitamin D_3, which is not present in this traditional diet.	Vital to convert parrot to a diet based on 20–25% human-quality seed, 40% sprouted seed and pulses, and 40% vegetable matter, with an avian vitamin supplement. Modern pellet diets are ideal, although palatability is a problem. Pigmented vegetables are a better food source than fruit. African grey parrots must be supplemented with a calcium source.
Insectivores, e.g. mynah birds, touracos	Usually fed branded dried diets. Bacterial contamination of the diet is common. Hypovitaminosis K and iron storage disease are common and considered to be related to diet.	Fresh food wherever possible, e.g. mealworms and crickets. Use a diet low in iron. Augment with correct vitamin supplement to provide vitamin K.
Nectar-eating birds, e.g. lories, lorikeets, toucans	Home-made nectar diets are often fed (due to lack of commercial alternatives) using honey and evaporated milk plus vitamin supplementation. These diets tend to be poorly balanced. Bacterial and yeast contamination soon occurs.	Commercial nectar diets plus fresh ripe fruit.

Figure 14.3 Dietary problems and recommendations for cage and aviary birds.

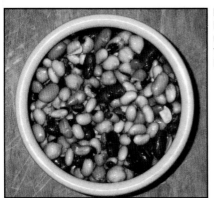

Figure 14.4 Pulse mixture recommended for psittacine birds.

used for valuable birds and may be a legal requirement. The operator must ensure that the bird is firmly cast on its back in a towel, with the legs, wings and beak completely under control. The microchip should be placed in the left pectoral muscle (see Figure 14.16) rather than subcutaneously. Tissue glue or a stitch may be used to repair the wound. To avoid the problem of haemorrhaging from the pectoral muscle, firm pressure must be applied after injecting the chip. Some veterinary surgeons may prefer to anaesthetize the bird prior to microchipping, but this is not the author's preference.

Sexing

Most common psittacine birds are sexually monomorphic. Exceptions are budgerigars (males have a blue cere and females a brown one) and cockatoos (females have a red iris, although this is not 100% conclusive). Aviculturists sex stock in several ways.

Endoscopy

Endoscopic (surgical) sexing may be carried out under anaesthesia by an experienced avian veterinary surgeon. The technique allows visualization of the testes or ovary. It has the advantage of predicting the sexual maturity of the bird (most parrots do not reach maturity until 5–6 years of age) but the disadvantage of being an invasive procedure.

DNA

Laboratory testing of DNA from feather, pulp or blood is a non-invasive procedure, and owners can often take the samples themselves. Several breast feathers should be plucked from the bird and, preferably, an EDTA sample of blood taken. This test only distinguishes sex and gives no indication of maturity.

Handling and restraint

Dim lighting calms birds and makes catching them easier. All obstructions, such as toys, should be removed from the cage. Gloves should not be used as they reduce dexterity. For larger parrots a towel is the best protection (Figure 14.5) and for smaller birds a clean handkerchief. The catching technique is the same for all birds: the bird should be gripped firmly around the neck, with the thumb and forefinger beneath the lower mandible to prevent biting. With larger birds the other hand can be used to immobilize the wings. Always ensure that the bird is held safely before removing it from its cage.

Many parrots are now bred in captivity and hand-reared, which makes handling easier. Even tame birds, however, should be held properly as they will bite if

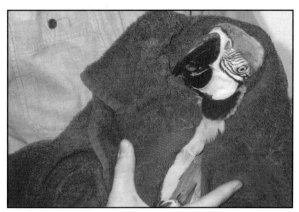

Figure 14.5 Holding a macaw for examination.

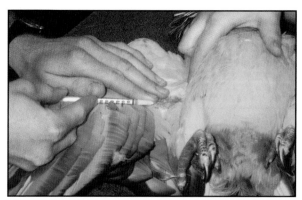

Figure 14.6 Taking a blood sample from the brachial vein of a macaw.

afraid. When dealing with a tame parrot, it is advisable to handle it out of sight of the owner; if the bird associates a 'bad' experience with the owner this can lead to behavioural problems.

Diagnostic approach

Clinical examination

Clinical examination should follow the same protocol as for other animals: a careful history is taken, followed by full clinical examination and relevant laboratory tests. The author uses the following regimen:

1. Examine the nares for discharges.
2. Examine the eyes for swellings, conjunctivitis or discharges.
3. Examine the mouth for lesions such as tongue abscesses or fungal plaques.
4. Examine the choanal slit: an auroscope is vital when looking for signs of discharges and inflammation.
5. Palpate the crop for signs of swelling, impaction, foreign bodies or problems with emptying.
6. Auscultate the dorsum for lung sounds, the ventral abdomen for air sacs and the pectorals for the heart.
7. Palpate the abdomen for masses.
8. Examine the long bones of the wings for deformity.
9. Examine the feet.

Sample collection

See Chapter 16 on Birds of prey for the methods used for flushing sinuses and tracheal washes for obtaining samples.

Blood

Blood samples should be taken from the jugular or brachial vein with a 25–27 gauge needle (Figure 14.6). Blood can be taken from the metatarsal vein in larger birds. Blood samples taken from clipping the toenails should be avoided due to poor quality and contamination. For routine profiles the blood should be preserved in heparin. Sample volume should be between 0.5 and 1.0 ml. Blood volume is 10% of bodyweight so it is safe to take 2 ml from a parrot weighing 300 g. Haematoma formation can be a problem but can be avoided by applying pressure to the venepuncture site for 2 minutes after taking the sample.

Clinical pathology

Laboratory tests are increasingly required to aid or confirm diagnosis. Laboratories familiar with birds should always be used, as samples are often small and specialist knowledge is required. The laboratory will usually advise on sample collection and interpretation of results, as there are large variations in biochemical and haematological data between avian species (Figure 14.7).

Common conditions

Beak problems

Common disorders of the beak include congenital abnormalities, overgrowth, fractures and infections (Figure 14.8).

Gastrointestinal disease

The clinical signs, causes and treatment of common diseases of the gastrointestinal system are listed in Figure 14.9.

Respiratory disease

The clinical signs, causes and treatment of common diseases of the upper and lower respiratory tracts are listed in Figure 14.10.

Viral diseases

In the past decade the domestic parrot market has suffered from several viral diseases that have caused substantial losses in young birds. Adult birds carry many of these diseases asymptomatically. It is not the scope of this book to discuss these in detail but the reader should be aware of those diseases listed in Figure 14.11.

Psittacosis

Psittacosis (chlamydiosis), caused by *Chlamydia psittaci*, is still an ongoing problem in the pet trade and should always be considered when dealing with a sick caged bird. It is a potentially zoonotic condition and care must be taken when postmortem examinations are performed. The common signs are depression, sinusitis, conjunctivitis, respiratory problems, green diarrhoea and death. Definitive diagnosis on a live bird is difficult; the best test is currently considered

Parameter (units)	Blue-fronted Amazon[a]	African grey parrot[a]	Blue and gold macaw[a]	Umbrella cockatoo[a]	Lesser sulphur-crested cockatoo[b]	Budgerigar[a]	Cockatiel[a]	Sun conure[a]	Mynah bird[a]	Red lorry[b]	Senegal parrot[a]
WBC (x10^9/l)	5.0–17.0	6.0–13.0	5.1–17.5	3.9–13.5	9.0–16.0	3.0–8.0	4.29–8.16	7.3–16.4	3.57–17.67	8.0–13.0	5.6–14.0
RBC (x10^{12}/l)	1.96–2.50	3.0–3.6	2.0–3.4	2.3–3.4	2.0–3.4	3.77–4.6	3.47–4.11	3.58–4.25	2.77–4.59	3.25–3.95	2.07–3.96
PCV (%)	0.41–0.53	0.45–0.53	0.33–0.47	0.45–0.53	0.45–0.56	0.43–0.56	0.45–0.56	0.46–0.53	0.40–0.48	0.41–0.55	0.41–0.51
Haemoglobin (g/dl)	12.7–16.5	14.2–17.1	8.0–13.9	14.0–20.4	13.0–21.0	12.0–16.0	8.3–15.9	12.0–17.0	11.3–16.9	10.8–14.7	10.5–16.1
Heterophils: %	31–71	45–73	45–75	40–55	44–79	45–70	40–60			39–60	
(x10^9/l)		4.27–6.93	2.2–10.7	2.8–11.0			1.56–5.13	1.46–8.84	1.1–5.6		2.8–9.6
Lymphocytes: %	20–67	19–50	20–50	20–50	21–56	20–45	20–72			22–69	
(x10^9/l)		1.8–4.8	1.0–6.9	0.9–3.0			0.8–3.93	1.06–10.17	0.25–11.8		1.2–5.0
Monocytes: %	0–2	0–2	0–2	0–2	0–2	0–5	1.0–6.0			0–2	
(x10^9/l)		<1.9	<1.4	<0.6			0.2–0.6	<1.27	<1.06		<1.3
Eosinophils: %	0–1	0–1	0–1	0–2	0–2	0–1	0–1			0–3	
(x10^9/l)		<–0.85	<0.40	<0.6			<0.1	<0.72	<1.27		<0.28
Basophils: %	0–2	0–1	0–1	0–1	0–1	0–5	0–1			0–3	
(x10^9/l)		<0.85	<0.40	<0.3			<0.1	<0.31	<1.6		<1.3
Total protein (g/l)	33.0–53.0	27.0–44.0	33.0–53.0	28.0–43.0	28.0–46.0	25.0–45.0	15.0–29.0	26.0–40.0	33.0–49.0	49.0–78.0	23.0–31.0
Albumin (g/l)	12.0–22.0	9.0–18.0	13.0–19.0	9.0–15.0	14.0–24.0	9.0–12.0	7.0–13.0	12.0–16.0	14.0–26.0	13.0–21.0	10.0–14.0
Globulins (g/l)		12.0–36.0	15.0–27.0	12.0–34.0	8.0–30.0	7.0–15.0	4.0–16.0	17.0–21.0		18.0–38.0	11.0–23.0
Uric acid (µmol/l)	77.7–333	100–500	109–231	190–327	123–638	390–890	141–519	131–688	218–690	119–703	183–489
Calcium (mmol/l)	1.87–2.42	1.65–2.68	2.2–2.8	1.9–2.2	2.02–2.57	1.6–2.2	1.7–2.36	1.8–3.2	1.83–3.15	2.0–2.87	1.7–2.35
Aspartate aminotransferase (IU/l)	35–200	<125	58–206	32–180	134–276	251–531	140–273	181–311	204–386	141–369	143–255
CK (IU/l)	64–322	140–411	61–531	27–253	157–408	357–817	187–935	120–358	289–951	178–396	<699
Bile acids (µmol/l)	<80	<80	<80	<80	24–95	32–117	34–112	<90	30–96	20–97	<80
Zinc (mmol/l)	31.4	31.4	31.4	31.4	31.4	31.4	31.4	31.4	31.4	31.4	31.4

Figure 14.7 Normal ranges for haematological and biochemical parameters for a variety of cage and aviary birds. [a] Values from MEDLAB, Tarporley, Cheshire; [b] data from Fudge (2000).

Overgrowth
Common in smaller psittacines. Frequently require repeated trimming with cuticle clipper or, preferably, burring with a dental drill. Attempt to remodel beak if there is any sign of malocclusion. Always check for evidence of parasites (e.g. *Cnemidocoptes*) affecting development of beak and treat accordingly.
Fractures
Common due to trauma or fighting between larger psittacines. Control pain initially and stabilize bird with fluids. Repair small fractures with cyanoacrylate glue after cleaning site. Larger fractures require cross pinning; referral is recommended.
Sometimes beaks are completely removed and referral for prosthesis fixation is required.
Congenital abnormality
Common in larger psittacines. Abnormalities can be corrected by tension band techniques (malocclusion) or prostheses are available; must be performed in most cases before 10 weeks of age to be successful.
Infection
Candida spp.

Figure 14.8 Common conditions of the beak.

Condition	Aetiology	Diagnostic investigations	Treatment
Regurgitation	Crop infection, especially candidiasis or trichomoniasis. Crop impaction. Foreign bodies. Heavy metal poisoning. Proventricular dilatation disease. Systemic disease.	Physical examination including crop palpation, endoscopy or auroscopy, crop washes, barium meal.	Fluid therapy vital. Specific treatment for infections. Surgery to remove impactions; probiotics on recovery.
Blood in droppings	Cloacal prolapse or egg bound. Papilloma. Cloacal calculi. Endoparasites. Severe bacterial infection.	Cloacal palpation, microbiology, endoscopy, auroscopy, contrast radiography.	Identify prolapses and replace with purse string suture. Treat infections. Provide fluid therapy. Correct egg laying problems.
Watery droppings	Dietary changes or stress. Endoparasites, coccidians, bacteria, viruses. Systemic disease.	Microbiology, parasitology, blood tests.	Give probiotics. Treat specific infections. Provide fluids. Correct diet.
Undigested food	Proventricular dilation disease. Intestinal, pancreatic and liver disease.	Viral testing, haematology, biochemistry.	Provide nutritional support. Treat specific disease. Cull viraemic birds.
Discoloured faeces	Green indicates possible hepatic problems. Brown indicates possible bacterial enteritis. Red or pink can indicate heavy metal problems	Microbiology, biochemistry.	Treat specific disease. Provide fluids and nutritional support.
Discoloured urates	Bright green suggests liver disease (e.g. due to *Chlamydia*). Brown or hameorrhagic suggests bacterial infections. Pink indicates heavy metals. Variable colour changes with viral disease.	Viral testing, biochemistry.	Provide nutritional support. Treat specific disease. Give probiotics.

Figure 14.9 Gastrointestinal problems of cage and aviary birds.

Clinical signs	Possible aetiology	Diagnostic investigations	Treatment
Upper respiratory tract			
Nasal exudate. Mouth breathing. Periorbital swelling. Head shaking. Dyspnoea. Sneezing.	Hypovitaminosis A. Infection (bacterial, viral, fungal, mycoplasma). Foreign bodies.	Choanal swabs, sinus flushing, radiography, rhinoscopy, viral isolation.	Flush sinuses (see Chapter 16). Provide antibiotics, vitamin A. Debride solid abscesses. Give mucolytics.
Lower respiratory tract			
Dyspnoea. Tail bobbing. Inspiratory effort. Inappetence. Abdominal breathing.	Bacteria, viruses, fungi (aspergillosis), *Chlamydia*, parasites, yeasts.	Haematology, radiography, endoscopy, tracheal swabs, tracheal washes.	Treat for specific infections. Nebulize. Intratracheal wash.

Figure 14.10 Respiratory tract problems of cage and aviary birds.

Disease	Common clinical signs	Diagnostic investigations	Treatment
Psittacine beak and feather disease	Feather and beak problems. Depressed chicks. Secondary infections due to immunosuppression. Death in young birds.	Testing of blood or feather pulp for viral DNA.	Supply good plane of nutrition and probiotics. Separate and retest birds in 6 weeks; cull any birds still viraemic.
Proventricular dilation disease (macaw wasting disease)	Regurgitation, loss of weight, passing undigested food. Chronic disease. Death.	Contrast radiography. Proventricular or crop biopsy is most useful.	None known at present time. Provide nutrition via crop tube. Cull affected birds once diagnosis is confirmed.
Polyomavirus (budgie fledgling disease)	Diarrhoea. Paralysis. Feather problems, with badly deformed feather growth. Depression. Death. Infects all psittacines; usually affects chicks but can kill adults.	PCR for viral DNA.	No treatment.

Figure 14.11 Common avian viral diseases.

to be a PCR test of faeces that have been pooled for 3 days. Several rapid antibody–antigen tests are available too, but they seem less reliable. *Owners should always be warned about the zoonotic risk, and culling rather than treating pets must be considered.* All treatments should continue for at least 6 weeks and then a second test should be performed. Doxycycline is the drug of choice, preferably by injection. Enrofloxacin is also effective by injection or gavage. *Never guarantee that a bird is 'chlamydia-free' only that it gave a negative result at the time of testing, stating the test.*

Eggs and egg laying problems

Female birds may experience problems with overproduction of eggs, with egg laying, or with egg quality (Figure 14.12).

Feather plucking

Feather plucking is an extremely complex and multifactorial problem, which should always be investigated thoroughly and in a logical fashion. It is vital to decide whether the bird is plucking because of a physical illness or a neurosis. Most cases are related to diet or husbandry.

Investigation should proceed as follows:

- Clinical history: diet, environment, health status
- Clinical examination: distribution of plucking, feather examination. Is the bird ill?
- Blood testing: assess general health. Is there a physical illness, e.g. thyroid disease, hypocalcaemia, zinc poisoning?

- Behavioural history: when does plucking occur, where does plucking occur, is owner present, is the bird bored, is it properly trained?
- Feather examination, including culture: look for mites, signs of nutritional problems, 'stress marks' (culture should look for yeasts and fungi as well as bacteria)
- Faecal analysis: *Chlamydia*, parasites, giardiasis in cockatiels
- Virology: psittacine beak and feather disease, polyomavirus
- Skin biopsy and allergy testing: limited use at present time
- Radiography and endoscopy: useful if blood samples indicate physical disease, e.g. evidence of heavy metals, aspergillosis.

Figure 14.13 lists the treatment options for feather plucking.

Behavioural problems

With the more intelligent psittacine birds, it is important to ensure correct dominance training is being given to avoid undesirable behavioural problems (Welle, 1999).

The basic rules of behavioural training are to:

- Ensure humans are the flock leaders by dominating birds satisfactorily
- Always train on neutral territory, i.e. away from the cage
- Teach 'step up' and 'step down' commands for both training perches and hands
- Teach simple 'yes' and 'no' commands
- Punishments should not reward, e.g. shouting.

Condition	Clinical signs	Aetiology	Diagnostic investigations	Treatment
Egg binding	Depression. Straining, blood-stained faeces.	Low calcium intake. Overproduction of eggs.	Palpation, radiography, blood tests for hypocalcaemia.	Provide oxytocin, calcium. Manually express eggs or remove them surgically. Ovariohysterectomy.
Egg overproduction (common in cockatiels)		Hormone imbalance.	Blood test for hypocalcaemia.	Hysterectomy. Proligesterone injections.
Prolapsed oviduct	Depression. Obvious prolapse.	Straining. Egg binding.	Palpation, radiography.	Replace, with purse string suture.
Poor quality eggs	Soft shells, odd-shaped eggs	Low calcium intake, poor husbandry.	Egg examination, radiography.	Improve plane of nutrition, especially to balance calcium and vitamin D3 status.

Figure 14.12 Problems of eggs and egg laying.

Treatment	Comments
Treat any specific disease found by investigative tests	Infections (viral, bacterial, mycoses) Imp wing-clipped birds or pluck damaged feathers. Heavy metal poisoning. Hypocalcaemia. Internal or external parasites. Hypothyroidism. Trauma from other birds. Hepatomegaly or internal masses.
Improve plane of nutrition	Useful in most feather pluckers, vital in some (see Figure 14.3).
Improve environment	Provide ultraviolet light equivalent to birds' natural photoperiod. Spray or bathe daily. Provide toys. Provide nesting box for privacy. Spend more time with bird.
Use neck brace	Useful for assessing feather regrowth; leave on until feathers regrow. Do not use as an alternative to diagnosis.
Behavioural modification	Make sure bird is correctly trained; do not punish feather pluckers as they see it as a reward (see Behavioural problems).
Drug therapy	Only use as a last resort after all other avenues have been explored, or to break plucking cycle in the short term, e.g. haloperidol or diazepam.

Figure 14.13 Treatments for feather plucking.

Condition	Clinical signs	Aetiology	Diagnostic investigations	Treatment
Polydipsia	Excessive drinking	Dietary changes. Renal disease. Hepatic disease. Diabetes mellitus.	Urine analysis, haematology, biochemistry.	Correct diet. Treat specific disease.
Convulsions	Seizures, collapse, wings stretched out	Metabolic imbalances. Poisoning. Infection. Trauma. Nutritional.	Haematology, biochemistry, radiography, clinical history.	Correct metabolic imbalances. Correct diet. Treat specific disease.
Difficulty in perching	Resting feet. Resting on floor of cage	Renal problems. Overgrown nails. Infected feet. Neurological. Vitamin A deficiency.	Clinical examination, radiography.	Correct perches. Treat renal disease. Clip nails. Correct diet.
Heavy metal poisoning	Non-specific, dysphagia. Depression. Discoloured droppings. Regurgitation.	Zinc or lead from toys or cages	Radiography, haematology, biochemistry.	Chelation therapy. Remove metal objects; powder coat cages with a zinc-free powder coating.

Figure 14.14 Miscellaneous conditions.

Common behavioural problems are:

- Biting
- Excessive vocalization
- Neurosis and phobias about new objects
- 'One person' birds
- Feather plucking
- Separation anxiety
- Territorial behaviour.

Miscellaneous

Figure 14.14 lists some miscellaneous conditions found in birds.

Supportive care

Warming

Supplementary heat via a heat lamp or heat pad is essential as most sick birds are hypothermic. An ambient temperature of 40°C (normal body temperature is 38–42.5°C) is optimal. A standard garden propagator is a cheap method of providing controlled heat and humidity.

Fluid therapy

Most avian patients are dehydrated. Fluids via a crop tube or intravenous or intraosseous injection are advisable. Electrolyte solutions such as lactate or lactated Ringer's solution (10 ml/kg/min i.v. or i.o.) can be used. Specialized oral avian fluids are available and may supply essential amino acids and sugars.

Crop tubing is a vital procedure that should be learned by any veterinary surgeon who treats birds. The bird should be supported in a towel in the usual way and the tube passed over the tongue, avoiding the glottis, and into the oesophagus (Figure 14.15). To ensure the tube is in the crop, its presence can be felt in the neck area. Special crop tubes are available but in an emergency, drip set tubing or proprietary nasogastric tubes are a useful alternative.

Nutritional support

If the bird is eating, it is best to provide the diet it is used to rather than to make rapid changes. Most ill birds are anorexic and it is vital to supply nutrition by crop tube.

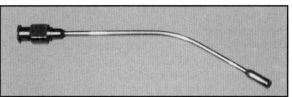

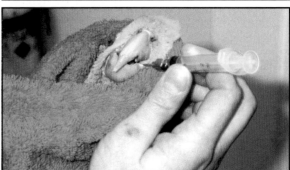

Figure 14.15 A crop tube plus its use in a parrot.

Baby food (e.g. vegetable or fruit puree) is a good rapid energy source. The baby food should be made up with a critical care solution and given by crop tube. Avian hand-rearing mixtures are also useful nutritional sources for sick adult birds.

Drug administration

Ideally a diagnosis should be made before starting treatment, as non-specific medical treatment, such as antibiotics, may be ineffective at best and harmful at worst by encouraging mycoses. Probiotics are useful during investigation. They are also useful for birds with mild illness or after courses of treatment with antibiotics. The formulary at the end of this chapter (Figure 14.19) suggests dose rates for the drugs most commonly used in avian medicine and found in most veterinary surgeries. The route of administration will vary with the type of drug used, severity of disease and owner compliance. It is usually preferable to give drugs to all but the smallest birds by injection.

Injection

Injections should be administered into the pectoral muscles (Figure 14.16). If the bird is being injected daily, injections should be alternated between the left

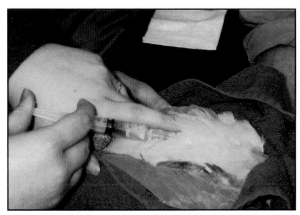

Figure 14.16 Pectoral muscles as injection site for drugs or microchip.

and right pectorals. Soft bills are often prone to clotting disorders due to iron storage disease, and haemorrhage at the site of an injection can be a problem.

Oral

Tablets can be crushed and mixed with a critical care solution or baby food and given by crop tube. Oral solutions should be given by crop tube. The success of drugs added to water is variable and is best avoided in most cases.

Nebulization

Nebulization of drugs is a useful technique for administering some drugs (e.g. tylosin) as it reduces the stress of handling. Nebulization increases the effectiveness of drugs in the respiratory system. Nebulizers for use by humans can now be bought cheaply and adapted to give the drug to birds in a covered cage or plastic tank (Figure 14.17).

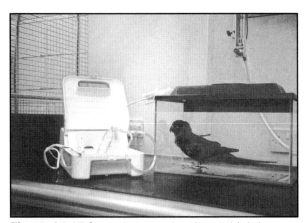

Figure 14.17 Some drugs can be given to birds by nebulization.

Anaesthesia

Gaseous anaesthesia

Gaseous anaesthesia is preferred to parenteral techniques. The technique of choice involves induction with 4–5% isoflurane by facemask at an oxygen flow rate of 1 litre per minute. Intubation with a paediatric endotracheal tube is important to allow

ventilation should apnoea occur. (Apnoea is a common problem in avian anaesthesia. The anaesthetist should be aware of this and, if it occurs, gently ventilate the bird, flushing the respiratory system with oxygen.) The tongue should be pulled forward with tissue forceps to allow visualization of the glottis and placement of the tube. Birds have complete tracheal rings, so care must be taken not to overinflate cuffed endotracheal tubes; uncuffed paediatric tubes are preferred.

Maintenance is usually with 2–3% isoflurane given via a T-piece circuit. Observation of the rate and depth of respiration and speed of third eyelid reflex aids in monitoring the depth of anaesthesia. The use of pulse oximeters via a cloacal probe is useful. The author does not recommend the routine use of nitrous oxide as it decreases the inspired oxygen concentrations in birds that already frequently have compromised respiratory function.

Heat should be supplied throughout the procedure and during recovery by heat pad or lamp.

Fluid therapy can be supplied throughout the procedure via an intravenous catheter (jugular or brachial vein) or an intraosseous needle (see Chapter 16). The use of oral or subcutaneous fluids postoperatively is advised. Birds should be cradled gently in a towel during recovery to prevent heat loss and trauma.

Although halothane may be used for avian anaesthesia, cardiac failure is relatively common so cannot be recommended except for emergency situations. Propofol is metabolized too rapidly by birds and there is evidence of too poor a safety margin for it to be a useful anaesthetic.

Local anaesthetics should be avoided due to toxicity problems.

Parenteral anaesthesia

If an injectable drug is used the bird must be weighed accurately to allow the correct dose to be calculated. Several drug combinations are in routine use (Figure 14.18).

Drug combination	Dose rate and route	Comments
Ketamine and medetomidine	1.5–2 mg/kg ketamine + 60–85 µg/kg medetomidine Reversed with atipamezole 250–380 µg/kg i.m.	Useful combination providing good sedation, analgesia, muscle relaxation and reversibility
Ketamine and xylazine	4.4 mg/kg ketamine i.v. + 2.2 mg/kg xylazine i.v. Reversed with atipamezole 250–380 µg/kg i.m.	Good surgical anaesthesia for short procedures. Must reverse or prolonged recovery becomes a problem
Ketamine and diazepam	25 mg/kg ketamine i.m. + 1–2 mg/kg diazepam i.m.	Useful sedative combination for minor procedures such as radiography; separate syringes must be used

Figure 14.18 Common parenteral drug combinations for anaesthesia of cage and aviary birds.

Endotracheal intubation should be used with parenteral anaesthesia so that supplementary oxygen can be supplied if required.

Basic surgical principles

Surgery in the avian patient follows the same principles as in other animals although it should be noted that specialized equipment and techniques are required for all but the most simple of procedures, so referral should be considered in most cases.

Basic principles are:

- The site should be prepared for surgery by plucking the minimum area possible and avoiding excessive wetting of the feathers to prevent excessive heat loss. For the same reason an antiseptic skin scrub without alcohol is preferred
- Control of haemorrhage during surgery is vital in the avian patient; radiosurgical units are useful
- The patient should be kept warm and surgery time kept to the absolute minimum

- Fine (4–0) absorbable suture materials seem to be non-irritant to the skin of avian patients
- Most fracture repairs require external or internal fixation using Kirshner wires, although many closed wing fractures heal satisfactorily with supportive bandaging
- Routine antibiosis and analgesia are used as required but care should be taken with excessive courses of antibiotic as they can lead to mycoses.

Drug formulary

Allometric scaling of doses is advised in all birds when calculating drug dosages, using the following formula:

$$E = (W/1000)^{0.75} \times D$$

where E = dose of drug in milligrams, W = bodyweight of bird in grams and D = dose recommended for cat or dog in mg/kg.

The drugs in bold type in Figure 14.19 indicate those most useful drugs in routine avian medicine as preferred by the author.

Drug	Dosage and route	Comments
Antimicrobials		
Amoxycillin	100 mg/kg orally bid	
Amoxycillin/clavulanic acid	**100 mg/kg i.m. sid, 100 mg/kg orally bid**	Useful for young birds
Clindamycin	100 mg/kg by mouth sid	For osteomyelitis give 150 mg/kg
Doxycycline	60–100 mg/kg i.m. every 5–7 days, 10 mg/kg i.m. sid, 20–50 mg/kg orally bid	For psittacosis give 75 mg/kg i.m. every 7 days for 6 weeks
Enrofloxacin	**5–15 mg/kg i.m. bid, 10 mg/kg orally bid, 100–200 mg/l drinking water (add blackcurrant juice to mask taste)**	**Well tolerated in psittacines. Often abused in aviculture and found on black market. Injection or gavage preferred. Can be irritant by injection**
Lincomycin	100 mg/kg i.m. bid, 75 mg/kg orally bid, 200 mg/l drinking water	Good for infected foot lesions
Metronidazole	50 mg/kg orally bid	Useful antiprotozoal
Oxytetracycline	50–100 mg/kg i.m. sid	
Trimethoprim/sulphonamide	10 mg/kg i.m. bid, 20–50 mg/kg orally bid, 1 g/l drinking water	Useful anticoccidial
Tylosin	30 mg/kg i.m. bid, 2 teaspoons per 4.5 litres drinking water	Mycoplasma
Antifungal agents		
Amphotericin B	**1 mg/kg orally bid for 5 days**	**Useful topical treatment for oral candida lesions. Can be nephrotoxic so ensure adequate hydration**
Enilconazole	1:50 dilution topically	Good topical treatment for mycotic infections
Itraconazole	**10 mg/kg orally bid for 3–12 weeks**	**African grey parrots do not seem to tolerate drug well. Best current drug for aspergillosis. Use long courses (6 weeks). Available commercially in liquid form for accurate oral dosing**
Ketoconazole	20 mg/kg orally bid	Potentially hepatotoxic but useful for aspergillosis in African grey parrots
Nystatin	300 000 IU/kg orally for 7–10 days	Only gut activity
Anti-inflammatories and analgesics		
Butorphanol	2–4 mg/kg i.v., i.m. or orally	
Carprofen	**5–10 mg/kg i.m. sid**	**Useful preoperative painkiller**
Dexamethasone	2–4 mg/kg i.m. sid	Use sparingly in avian medicine as predisposes to fungal infections
Ketoprofen	2 mg/kg i.m.	
Meloxicam	**0.1 mg/kg orally sid, 0.1–0.2 mg/kg i.m.**	**Easy to administer. Long courses seem to be well tolerated**
Prednisolone	2 mg/kg orally bid	Predisposes to mycoses so only use if absolutely necessary

Figure 14.19 Drug formulary for cage and aviary birds. (continues)   ▶

Drug	Dosage and route	Comments
Ectoparasiticides and endoparasiticides		
Fenbendazole	50–100 mg/kg orally sid, 10–20 mg daily for 5 days	High therapeutic index. Anthelmintic of choice by crop tube for larger species
Fipronil	One drop to skin on neck and under wings	Author's preferred ectoparasitic for psittacines. Well tolerated
Ivermectin	0.2 mg/kg orally or percutaneously	Useful, but toxicity problems especially by intramuscular routes
Levamisole	20 mg/kg orally for 3 days equivalent to 10 ml of 7.5% solution in 4.5 litres of water	Low therapeutic index
Hormones		
Medroxyprogesterone	20 mg/kg i.m. every 4 weeks	Useful for persistent egg laying in cockatiels
Megestrol acetate	2.5 mg/kg sid for 7 days then twice weekly	Useful for some feather plucking if a hormonal influence proven. Side effects can be severe unless care taken (diabetes-like conditions)
Oxytocin	2 IU/kg (0.2 ml)	For egg binding give with calcium borogluconate
Thyroxine	20–100 µg/kg orally bid	Monitor levels to avoid thyrotoxicosis
Miscellaneous drugs		
Allopurinol	10 mg/kg orally bid, 10 mg tablet/30 ml drinking water	For high uric acid concentration (gout)
Toltrazuril	7 mg/kg orally every 24 hours for 2–3 days or 75 mg/l drinking water 2 days weekly for 4–6 weeks	For coccidiosis refractory to other drugs
Calcium borogluconate 20%	1 ml/kg i.v. or i.m.	Used during egg laying problems, often in combination with oxytocin
Diazepam	0.5 mg/kg i.m. bid, 2–4 mg/kg orally bid	Anticonvulsant. Useful drug for feather pluckers, especially smaller psittacines (cockatiels)
Frusemide	0.1–0.2 mg/kg i.m. bid	
Haloperidol	0.2–0.4 mg/kg orally sid, 1–2 mg/kg i.m. every 14–21 days	Used in feather pluckers after full diagnostic investigation has indicated behavioural cause
Iodine	One drop in 250 ml water sid	Thyroid hyperplasia in budgerigars
Sodium calcium EDTA	30 mg/kg i.v. for 5 days	For zinc and lead poisoning
Vitamin A	20 000 IU i.m. weekly	For chronic respiratory disease

Figure 14.19 continued Drug formulary for cage and aviary birds.

References and further reading

Arnall L and Keymer IF (1975) *Bird Diseases*. Baillière Tindall, London

Beynon PH (1996) *Manual of Raptors, Pigeons and Waterfowl*. BSAVA Publications, Cheltenham

Beynon PH and Cooper JE (1994) *Manual of Exotic Pets*. BSAVA Publications, Cheltenham

Beynon PH, Forbes NA and Lawton MPC (1996) *Manual of Psittacine Birds*. BSAVA Publications, Cheltenham

Coles BH (1997) *Avian Medicine and Surgery*. Blackwell Science, Oxford

Forshaw JM and Cooper WT (1978) *Parrots of the World*. David and Charles, Newton Abbot

Fudge A (2000) Avian and exotic pets. *Laboratory Medicine: Avian and Exotic Pets*. WB Saunders, Philadelphia

Harrison GJ (1984) *The Veterinary Clinics of North America: Cage Bird Medicine*. Volume **14**

Harrison GJ and Harrison LR (1986) *Clinical Avian Medicine and Surgery*. WB Saunders, Philadelphia

King AS and McLelland J (1984) *Birds: their Structure and Function*. Baillière Tindall, London

Olsen GH and Orosz SE (2000) *Manual of Avian Medicine*. Mosby Inc., St Louis

Ritchie BW, Harrison GJ and Harrison LR (1994) *Avian Medicine, Principles and Application*. Wingers Publishing, Lake Worth, Florida

Welle KR (1998) Psittacine behaviour. *Proceedings of the Association of Avian Veterinarians, 1998*: 371–377

Welle KR (1999) A clinical approach to feather picking. *Proceedings of the Association of Avian Veterinarians, 1999*:119–124

Welle KR (1999) *Psittacine Behaviour Handbook*: Association of Avian Veterinarians Publication Office, Boca Raton, Florida

Useful additional resources

Association of Avian Veterinarians. AAV Central Office, PO Box 811720, Boca Raton, FL 33481, USA

British Veterinary Zoological Society (BVZS) c/o 7 Mansfield Street, London W1M 0AT

15

Pigeons

Sharon Redrobe

Introduction

The 313 species within the family Columbiformes vary from the sparrow-sized dwarf fruit dove *Ptilinopus naina* to the chicken-sized crowned pigeons *Goura* spp. of New Guinea (Figure 15.1). In general, 'pigeon' is the name given to larger species and 'dove' to smaller species. The most commonly kept member of the Columbiformes in captivity is the domestic pigeon, which is believed to derive from the rock dove *Columba livia*. Feral pigeons in the UK are, or are descended from, lost racing pigeons. Domestic pigeons are kept in a variety of forms, and over 200 fancy breeds now exist, including strains that have been developed for appearance, endurance flying, racing and meat production.

Many pigeon fanciers use various home remedies, sometimes including licensed drugs (anthelmintics, antibiotics, vaccines), before taking their sick birds to veterinary surgeons. Therefore the history taking must include treatment given by the owner. The rising value of racing show birds has increased the numbers presenting to veterinary surgeons in mainland Europe and will no doubt do so in the UK.

Biology

Figure 15.2 summarizes the biological data for pigeons.

Pigeons have special anatomical features: a vestigial caecum; no gall bladder; a vascular plexus extending from the cranium to the crop and base of the neck; absence of true powder down (the down is formed by the cells around growing feathers not by sheath or feather); a poorly developed or absent uropygeal (preen) gland; and fat quills in some breeds, e.g. Nuremburg swallows.

Rock doves nest and roost on cliffs, an instinct in feral pigeons that manifests as nesting and roosting on sheltered ledges on manmade structures. In their natural habitat pigeons usually live in pairs, feeding and roosting together, but they remain territorial and defend roosting spaces and nesting areas. Pairs are generally monogamous. Domestic pigeons are primarily seed-eaters but will take a wide range of grains, fruits, berries and vegetation and small snails and other molluscs.

Pigeons are well developed for navigation and orientation. This homing ability is thought to be a based on a combination of senses including the use of infra-acoustic waves, ultraviolet light, polarized light,

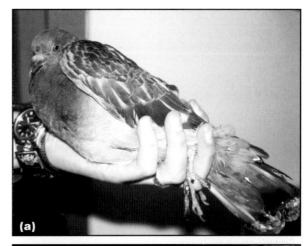
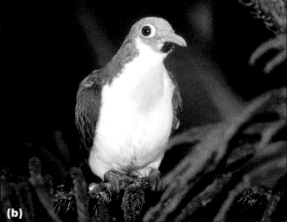
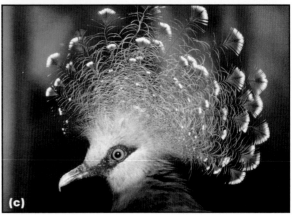

Figure 15.1 Types of pigeon. (a) Racing pigeon (courtesy of Emma Keeble); (b) Jambu fruit dove; (c) Victoria crowned pigeon.

Temperature	Average 40–41°C; the cloacal temperature ranges from 39.8 to 43.3°C and varies according to species and level of excitement (wood pigeon 41.8°C, African collared dove 41.0°C, mourning dove 42.6°C
Heart rate	180–250 beats per minute
Adult weight	350–550 g (racing pigeon, domestic pigeon)
Respiratory rate	25–30 breaths per minute
Water consumption	30–60 ml/day
Flight speed	100 km/h, height 5700 m, distance 500 or 1000 km
Blood volume	0.1–0.01 ml/g bodyweight
Moulting	August and September
Life expectancy	15–20 years
Food consumption	Average 10% of bodyweight per day
Prothrombin time	Average 15 seconds for undiluted pigeon plasma
Defecation rate	Fasted pigeons about 3 hours after consuming food
Gut transit times in common pigeon	Crop 3–17 hours, ventriculus 5–19 hours, intestine 9–14 hours
No. of clutches laid each year	2
Incubation period	17–18 days (both parents share incubation)
Crop milk secretion	By both parents at 14 days' incubation, stops at 10–13 days; 75–77% water, 11–13% protein, 5–7% fat, 1.2–1.8% mineral matter no carbohydrate, low in calcium, phosphorus, vitamins A and C
Young	Referred to as a nestling at 21 days old, squab up to 1 month and squeaker feathers at 1 or 2 months. Feathers appear at 6–7 days of age. Plumage growth is complete at 28–30 days. The first plumage is moulted at 6 weeks old
Sexual maturity	Average 5 months; breeding generally begins at 7–8

Figure 15.2 Biological data for pigeons.

changes in air pressure and perception of magnetic fields (iron oxide particles in the musculature of the cranium and neck allow the perception of small deviations in magnetic fields). Their ability to learn to perform tasks in the laboratory has led to their extensive use in behavioural and psychological studies.

Sexing
Endoscopy allows direct visualization of the gonads and hence sex determination. Sexing is also assisted by certain characteristics. For example, male red chequers, mealies and silvers have black flecking and the males strut up and down, turn 360 degrees, fan their tails and drag them along the floor when chasing or driving hens. Males produce a double coo and females a single one.

Husbandry

Housing
Pigeons can be housed in numbers up to 12. Cages should comprise a minimum area of 150,000 cm² plus 10,000 cm² for each additional bird. The minimum length of perch available should be 30 cm per bird and the food trough should allow 5 cm per bird.

Pigeons should be housed in large outdoor flights with free access to well ventilated draught-proof shelters with supplementary heating if necessary. Pigeons should not be housed in cages in which they cannot extend their wings; this prevents exercise and environmental stimulation and, in the UK, contravenes the Wildlife and Countryside Act 1981. Flights and aviaries should have a separate perching area for each bird. Pigeons produce considerable amounts of faeces, feather dust (keratinized scales) and debris, but daily cleaning of their housing and the use of minimal substrate can reduce the levels of dust and contamination. Good ventilation is also important in reducing dust levels. Allergic alveolitis (pigeon breeder's lung) is caused by frequent contact with feather dust in susceptible people.

Diet
Domestic or feral pigeons are omnivorous and so a mixed vegetable and animal protein diet is appropriate (Figure 15.3). Fruit doves require a fruit-based diet. Birds that are fed *ad libitum* and/or only allowed limited exercise tend to become fat, which can cause fertility problems. Oyster shell and mineral grit must be available at all times, and fresh water should be offered daily. Both the grit and water should be provided in covered containers to prevent fouling. Diet is often manipulated to improve racing performance. For example, an increased intake of fats helps in endurance races of 500 miles, whereas more carbohydrate allows better sprinting in races of 150 miles. Formulated complete diets are available. An unsupplemented diet of mixed grains results in poor fertility and increased morbidity and mortality of the squabs.

Captive breeding
Pedigree stocks are often maintained in pairs but racing stock are usually housed in groups, with a nesting area for each pair. Pigeons can be territorial and aggressive, sometimes causing fatal injuries in both males and females. Cock birds should be placed in the flight first, then the hens introduced once the cocks have established perching and nesting areas.

Female feral pigeons construct nests of twigs, grass and hay collected by the males. Earthenware nest pans or disposable *papier maché* nest pans should be provided, dusted with insecticidal powder before use. Small twigs and/or straw must be provided as nesting material to prevent pinwheel in squabs (see below). Two eggs are usually laid about 48 hours apart and 10–12 days after pairing. Incubation lasts for 17 or 18 days, and the squabs should be close ringed at 5–6 days old.

Component	Requirement per kg of feed
Crude protein (g)	30–150
Crude fat (g)	20–35
Crude fibre (g)	50
Metabolizable energy (ME)	12
Methionine (g)	3.5
Lysine (g)	8
Calcium (g)	10
Phosphorus (g)	6
Sodium (g)	1.5
Zinc (mg)	50
Iodine (mg)	1
Copper (mg)	2
Manganese (mg)	50
Vitamin A (IU)	7500
Vitamin D3 (IU)	750
Vitamin E (mg)	15
Vitamin K (mg)	3
Vitamin B1 (mg)	3.5
Vitamin B2 (mg)	3.5
Vitamin B6 (mg)	3.5
Vitamin B12 (μg)	15
Biotin (mg)	300
Choline (mg)	1000
Folic acid (mg)	1
Niacin (mg)	15
Pantothenic acid (mg)	15

Figure 15.3 Recommended diet for pigeons during racing, breeding and moulting. Data from Vogel *et al.* (1994).

At the end of the breeding season a clinical examination should be performed on the adults and offspring (Figure 15.4).

Pigeons should be rested and not allowed to breed all the year round.

Time of year	Disease	Treatment or control
Before racing season, before moulting, before breeding and 1 month before mating	Endoparasites Coccidiosis and toxoplasmosis Trichomoniasis	Febantel Ronidazole Sulphadimethoxine
During hatching	Trichomoniasis	Sulphadimethoxine
During weaning	Trichomoniasis Coccidiosis and toxoplasmosis	Sulphadimethoxine Ronidazole

Figure 15.4 Routine treatments for racing and breeding flocks. Drugs should be used consecutively, not at the same time.

Handling and restraint

Methods of handling vary according to the size of the bird and the handler's preference. Care must be taken to avoid constricting the breast muscles as that will impair breathing. The bite or peck from pigeons is usually not of concern to the handler as it rarely hurts, therefore the head may not require separate restraint. The body of the bird should be supported at all times and the wings held into the body to prevent flapping which can lead to overexertion and potential trauma to the wings.

One method is to grasp the pigeon from above and then wrap the hands around the body dorsally, keeping the wings restrained against the body (Figure 15.5). A light cloth may be used to restrain the wings; however, care must be taken to ensure that breast movement and hence ventilation is not impeded.

The 'racing pigeon hold' involves laying the feet through the first and second fingers of one hand, which is also supporting the breast and holding the wings (Figure 15.6). This technique is impractical in birds larger or smaller than the racing pigeon, or other particularly strong or non-tame pigeons of similar size.

Smaller birds, such as barbary doves, may simply be held cupped in the hands, with restraint focusing on holding the head around the neck lightly and using the cupped hands to restrain the wings.

Larger pigeons, e.g. the Victoria Crowned pigeon, require two hands to pick up the bird. One method of restraint of this size of pigeon is to tuck the bird under one arm so that the handler's arm and body are used to restrain the wings. The body is supported by one hand and the other used to restrain the head to prevent pecks to the face of the handler. Alternatively, the bird is restrained with the head facing to the rear, thereby avoiding the face of the handler. The legs are left free or held by the non-supporting hand.

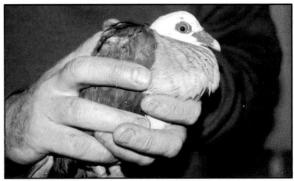

Figure 15.5 Restraint of a pink pigeon.

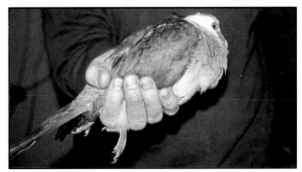

Figure 15.6 A pink pigeon in the 'racing pigeon hold'.

Diagnostic approach

The approach to a clinical case should begin with a thorough history and an assessment:

- Age and sex
- When and where the bird was obtained
- Previous medical problems
- Diet offered, including 'treats' and supplementation
- Other pets
- Photoperiod
- Electric or gas heating
- Access to fresh air and natural sunlight
- Provision of a bath or water spray.

Details of presenting problem should include:

- Duration and chronicity of problem
- Illness in other pets or family members
- Changes in appetite, thirst and droppings
- Coughing, sneezing, diarrhoea, vomiting
- Change in behaviour or voice
- Change in body posture
- Drowsiness
- Reproductive status.

Physical examination

Owners should be advised to bring their bird to the surgery in a cage not carry box to allow assessment of housing conditions and the bird at rest. Owners should be told to leave the cage uncleaned for 24 hours to allow examination of the volume and quality of the droppings. Birds should be examined in the cage or on a perch, not on the owner's shoulder or, initially, in the veterinary surgeon's hand.

The following should be borne in mind when examining birds at rest:

- Can the bird perch?
- Is it ruffled?
- Is it bright, alert and responsive?
- Respiratory rate
- Evidence of feather loss and change in colour (fret marks)
- Quality of the feathers, beak and nails
- Body posture: is the bird standing equally on both legs, are the wings at equal height?

Examination of the head, body, feathers, feet and wings may reveal abnormalities that suggest certain disease conditions (Figure 15.7).

Auscultation

Auscultation is generally only of value in large birds. A paediatric or infant head stethoscope is required. Lung fields can be heard over the back, where they adhere to the body wall. Normal respiratory sounds consist of a short loud inspiratory noise followed by a longer, lower pitch respiratory sound. Abnormal sounds include pleuritic rubs, rales, dull sounds and lack of sounds. Localization of lesions is difficult by auscultation; it is better by radiography.

Diagnostic tests and techniques

Blood sampling

Up to 1% of a bird's bodyweight can be collected for a blood sample, usually from the jugular, basilic or medial metatarsal vein. EDTA is the anticoagulant of choice, as heparin can cause clumping of the cells and

Examination	Abnormality	Clinical condition or cause
Head	Periocular swelling	Ocular or sinus disorder
Eyes	Epiphora, conjunctivitis, scabs, scars, pustules	Ocular or sinus disorder, *Mycoplasma*, poxvirus
Nares	Discharge (rhinitis), rhinoliths, enlarged orifice	Sinusitis, air sacculitis, hypovitaminosis A, severe rhinitis (bacterial, fungal)
Oral cavity	Excessive moisture, blunting choanal papillae, white plaques (removable), white or yellow fixed plaques	Inflammation, hypovitaminosis A, poxvirus, bacterial ulceration, trichomoniasis, candidiasis
Feathers	Dystrophic, broken, matted, chewed, plucked, missing	Self-trauma (discomfort, psychological), cage too small, seizures, cagemate (bullying, mating), endocrinopathy
Beak	Overgrowth, malocclusion	Cnemidocoptic mange, hypovitaminosis A
Pectoral muscles	Keel should only be felt with light pressure. Score prominence 0–4	Emaciation or obesity, superficial tumours
Abdomen	Enlargement	Liver enlargement, egg retention, excess fluid or solid mass
Wings	Abnormal position	Neoplasia, fracture (require radiography to differentiate), trauma
Legs	Distortion	Incorrect diet, fracture, neoplasia, arthritis, articular gout
Cloaca	External vent soiled, digital palpation	Gastrointestinal tract disease; differentiate between prolapse, impaction and tumour, papillomatosis, cloacoliths
Uropygeal gland	Increased size	Squamous cell carcinoma, adenoma, abscess (gland absent in some birds)
Feet	Nails overgrown or deformed, necrosis of digits, abnormal shape	Hypovitaminosis A, constriction by wire etc., frostbite, cnemidocoptic mange, bumblefoot

Figure 15.7 Clinical examination and common clinical conditions in pigeons.

alter staining characteristics. For small samples a full haematology and biochemistry profile is possible by taking 1 ml of heparin and making a fresh blood smear. No more than 10% of blood volume can be taken safely under most circumstances.

- Use the right jugular, cutaneous ulnar or metatarsal vein (Figure 15.8).
- Use a fresh drop of blood – intracellular parasites are surprisingly common, toxic heterophils indicate septicaemia and/or bacteraemia.

Figure 15.9 provides an interpretation of an avian haemogram.

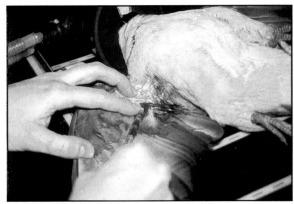

Figure 15.8 Taking a blood sample from the cutaneous ulnar vein (also known as the brachial vein).

Abnormal finding	Differential diagnosis
Regenerative (blood loss) anaemia	Trauma, parasites, coagulopathy, organic disease
Haemolytic anaemia	Red blood cell parasites, bacterial septicaemia, toxicity, immune-mediated
Non-regenerative anaemia	Chronic disease, hypothyroidism, toxicity, nutritional deficiencies, leukaemia
Leucocytosis	Infection, trauma, toxicity, haemorrhage, neoplasia, leukaemia
Heterophilia	Inflammation, stress response
Leucocytosis and heterophilia	Chlamydiosis, avian tuberculosis, aspergillosis
Immature heterophils	Severe inflammatory response
Toxic heterophils	Septicaemia, toxaemia
Leukopenia and heteropenia	Viral disease, overwhelming bacterial disease
Lymphocytosis	Infections
Monocytosis	Chlamydiosis, granulomas (bacterial, fungal), massive tissue necrosis
Thrombocytopenia	Severe septicaemia, rebound from blood loss

Figure 15.9 Interpretation of the avian haemogram.

Crop flush

Crop flushing is performed to examine the contents of the crop. The crop is flushed out with saline and the fluid sample centrifuged. The deposit can be examined in several ways, unstained for parasites or stained using Diff-Quick® or Gram stains. Crop crystals are

generally normal findings but can indicate hypovitaminosis A. *Alysiella* is common. A uniform bacterial population usually indicates an abnormality.

Cloacal swab or droppings

To obtain a cloacal sample, a moistened plastic- or wire-handled swab should be rubbed against the mucous membrane of the cloaca. This should be rolled on to a glass slide, air-dried and stained (Diff-Quick®, Gram, modified Ziehl–Nielsen). A normal test result in seed-eating birds yields a ratio of 80:20 Gram-positive to Gram-negative organisms. Gram staining detects bacteria, fungi and yeasts. If a few bacteria only are observed, then a smear should be obtained from fresh droppings. This should be checked for parasite eggs and oocysts by faecal flotation. The normal pH of the cloaca is 6.5–7.0. A basic pH (>7.5) encourages the growth of yeasts and Enterobacteriaceae.

Screening

Before new birds are introduced to the rest of the colony they should be placed in quarantine until the results of screening tests are known. Routine veterinary screening should also be performed on weaned squabs and annually on adult birds.

Screening comprises:

- A thorough clinical examination
- Full body radiography
- Full blood haematology (minimum recommendation red cell count, packed cell volume or haematocrit, haemoglobin, white cell count and differential)
- Blood biochemistry (minimum total protein, albumin, globulin, bile acids and uric acid)
- Crop washes and wet preparation for *Trichomonas* and *Candida*
- Choanal culture, including selective culture for *Salmonella* and *Campylobacter*
- Tests for *Chlamydia psittaci*; faecal antigen enzyme-linked immunosorbent assay (ELISA), polymerase chain reaction (PCR), serology for antibody
- Faecal parasitology
- External parasitology
- Serology for poxvirus, paramyxovirus-1.

Common conditions

Figure 15.10 lists the most common diseases of pigeons.

Respiratory disease

Signs of diseases of the respiratory system include acute or chronic dyspnoea, tail bobbing, increased abdominal effort, open mouth breathing, respiratory noise (unaided and with stethoscope), voice change, anorexia, decreased activity, decreased perching and a fluffed up appearance. A diagnostic investigation should include:

Disease	Aetiology	Clinical signs	Differential diagnosis	Diagnostic investigations	Treatment	Control and comments
Adenovirus	Adenovirus	Primary illness in young pigeons, hepatic necrosis symptoms		Liver biopsy (necrosis), serology	Supportive care	Young birds most susceptible
Ascaridiasis	Ascaris (?) columbae	Impaction, rupture of intestines, peritonitis, diarrhoea. Weight loss. Death		Faecal examination for parasites: thick-walled oval ova	Fenbendazole, levamisole, ivermectin	Young birds more susceptible in warm moist conditions
Aspergillosis	Aspergillus fumigatus	Weight loss, increased respiratory effort, lethargy, death		Culture from air sac or trachea serology	Itraconazole, clotrimazole, ketoconazole, amphotericin B	Cull infected birds, avoid mouldy food, improve hygiene and ventilation
Candidiasis	Candida albicans	Regurgitation, thickened crop (see trichomoniasis), distended crop, delayed emptying				Avoid poor hygiene, overcrowding, moist conditions
Capillariasis	Capillaria columbae, C. longicollis	Severe illness with diarrhoea, vomition, death (young birds), weight loss (adults)		Faecal examination for parasites: thick-walled bipolar ova	Fenbendazole, levamisole, ivermectin	
Coccidiosis	Eimeria labbeana, E. columbarum	Green diarrhoea. Catarrhal enteritis. Emaciated, stunted. Inappetence. Polydipsia		Coccidial oocysts seen on faecal examination or scrapings from intestine at postmortem examination	Sulphadimidine sodium, amprolium hydrochloride, clazuril, vitamin B supplementation	Role as primary pathogen in question. Check for stress or concurrent disease. Hygiene: especially affects birds aged 3–4 months (old birds may be carriers)
Colibacillosis	Escherichia coli	Anorexia, diarrhoea, lethargy, green droppings, reproductive failure	Salmonellosis	Isolation of organism from intestinal contents or crop	Antibiosis based on culture and sensitivity	Quarantine new stock, attention to strict hygiene
Hexamitiasis	Hexamita	Weight loss, diarrhoea		Detection of organism in fresh faeces	Dimetronidazole, metronidazole	Prevent faeco-oral contact, strict hygiene
Lice	Columbicola columbae and others	Feather damage	Mites, other ectoparasites	Microscopic examination of louse, feather, feather dust	Fipronil, ivermectin, bromocyclen	Infection usually an indication of other disease
Lipomas		Common in overweight birds – reduce fatty foods (e.g. sunflower seeds)		Biopsy	Surgical removal at veterinary surgeon's discretion	
Mites	Falculifer rostratis (small feather mite)	Feather damage, irritation of legs and face	Lice, other ectoparasites	Microscopic examination of mite, feather, feather dust	Fipronil, ivermectin, bromocyclen	Hygiene, especially for mites that survive off the bird
Neoplasia of uropygeal gland	Adenomas, adenocarcinomas		Impaction, abscess		Surgical removal advised	
Ornithosis complex	Chlamydia, Mycoplasma, Herpesvirus, other Gram-negative bacteria	Eye cold, 'one-eyed roup', conjunctivitis, often affects one eye		Isolation of organism from swab of affected area	Antibiosis based on culture and sensitivity (topical application most effective), supportive care	
Paramyxovirus	PMV-1	Polyuria (not diarrhoea), CNS signs, torticollis, incoordination, most appear well apart from CNS disturbance, may recover		Clinical signs, postmortem examination, serology	Supportive care, emergency vaccination of flock, routine vaccination programme	Prevention by vaccination and/or closed flock policy
Pigeon herpesvirus	PHV	Mild to necrotizing pharyngitis, oesophagitis, diphtheritic membranes, green droppings, anorexia, vomiting only in young birds		Liver biopsy (inclusion body hepatitis), clinical signs, serology	Supportive care	Lifelong carriers with intermittent shedding possible, young birds most susceptible
Pigeon malaria	Hemoproteus, rarely Plasmodium spp.	Lethargy, anaemia		Detection on fresh blood smear	Primaquine, quinacrine	Disease becomes clinical in stressed birds or those with concurrent disease. Control insect vectors (pigeon fly), minimize stress
Pinwheel		Affects squabs – feet cannot grip the substrate effectively so the legs become splayed and cannot support the bird		Clinical signs and husbandry factors (lack of or insufficient nesting substrate)	Any squabs that hatch with or develop splayed legs will never be able to walk and should be humanely euthanized	Pinwheel must be prevented by the provision of adequate nesting material
Poxvirus		Scabs and proliferations of beak, wattle, oral cavity, commissures of beak, feet and legs, conjunctivitis		Clinical signs, histology and electron microscopy of lesions	Supportive care, vaccination of stock, isolation of affected birds	Prevention by vaccination and control of insect vectors
Salmonellosis	Salmonella typhimurium var Copenhagen	Swollen wing and leg joints, anorexia, diarrhoea, lethargy, green droppings, reproductive failure	Colibacillosis	Swollen joints almost pathognomonic, isolation of organism from intestinal contents or crop	Antibiosis based on culture and sensitivity	Quarantine new stock, attention to strict hygiene
Tapeworm	Hymenolepis, Cotugnia	Weight loss. Lethargy		Faecal examination for parasites, tapeworm proglottids or ova	Dichlorphen, niclosamide	Control by elimination of intermediate hosts; molluscs; earthworms, various arthropods
Trichomoniasis	Trichomonas gallinae	'Canker', yellow caseous plaques on oral mucosa. Rarely omphalitis. Infection of liver and lung. Regurgitation, thickened crop (see trichomoniasis), distended crop, delayed emptying	Poxvirus, vitamin A deficiency	Scrape lesion and examine microscopically in saline	Dimetronidazole, metronidazole, febantel, ronidazole	Often with ornithosis complex and other diseases

Figure 15.10 Common diseases of pigeons.

- A blood sample: a complete blood count and biochemistry, *Aspergillus*, ELISA
- A faecal examination using Gram's method, wet preparation, PCR or serology for *Chlamydia*
- Transillumination of the neck
- A tracheal or lung wash using Gram's method, culture and sensitivity
- Radiography (Figure 15.11)
- Endoscopy of the upper respiratory tract, laparoscopy of the air sacs and abdominal organs (biopsy of the liver for *Chlamydia*).

Radiographic changes	Differential diagnosis
Blotchy pulmonary pattern	Parabronchial infiltrates
Non-distinct parabronchi	Exudate, haemorrhage, oedema
Abnormal or irregular pulmonary pattern	Fungal granuloma, abscess, tumour
Air sacculitis	Bacteria, fungae, hypovitaminosis A
Pulmonary masses	Fungal granuloma, abscess
Subcutaneous emphysema	Trauma to pneumatic bones, infraorbital sinus infection
Barrel-shaped cranial coelom at full inspiration	Air sac disease

Figure 15.11 Radiographic changes associated with respiratory disease.

Ornithosis (psittacosis)

Ornithosis or psittacosis is caused by infection with *Chlamydia psittaci*. Symptoms include:

- A listless and dull bird
- Respiratory signs (respiratory distress, respiratory clicks, auscultation, air sac infection)
- An enlarged liver and spleen on radiography
- Increased white blood cell count ($>25 \times 10^9$/l), especially if concurrent heterophilic left shift.

C. psittaci can be diagnosed from:

- Cloacal swabs by ELISA, PCR, or serology
- Findings at postmortem examination in in-contact birds: serous membranes thickened (air sacculitis, pericarditis)
- Signs of septicaemia in carcasses
- The presence of an enlarged spleen or liver (radiography, endoscopy, postmortem examination)
- Impression smear tests of parenchyma (liver, spleen, lung, kidney) and serosal (liver and spleen) surfaces with modified Ziehl-Nielsen for elementary bodies.

Owners should be warned that *C. psittaci* is potentially zoonotic so that they can make informed decisions about treatment or euthanasia. Symptoms in humans include headache, fever, confusion, myalgia, non-productive cough and lymphadenopathy. Immuno-compromised owners, e.g. those with HIV infection or on immunosuppressive drug treatment are particularly at risk. Strict hygiene standards should be adopted, e.g. washing hands with antiseptic after contact with affected birds and wearing a facemask.

Treatment should be started if ornthosis is suspected. Birds should be treated under quarantine conditions, with staff wearing plastic aprons, hats, masks and gloves. Parenteral treatment comprises doxycycline 2% 100 mg/kg i.m. (half dose either side of keel) and vitamin A injections. Birds should be treated for 45 days, with injections on days 1, 8, 15, 22, 28, 34, 40 and 45. ELISAs or PCR tests should be repeated (after stress or prednisolone) a few weeks after treatment. Doxycycline tablets can be crushed in lactulose for oral dosing.

Reproductive system

Egg retention

Egg retention is an avian emergency

Treatment involves warming the bird and increasing the humidity of the environment. Calcium treatment should be started within 60 minutes, then oxytocin. If the egg is not expelled, surgical access is usually made possible by this treatment.

Supportive care

Injection sites

Subcutaneous route: Small volumes may be injected into the dorsal caudal third of the neck. Large volumes may affect the jugular vein, the vagus nerve and the clavicular air sac. Larger volumes may be safely injected into subcutaneous tissue of the lateral thoracic wall.

It should be noted that members of the Columbiformes have a plexus of anastomosing vessels that extend from the cranium to the crop and base of the neck (the plexus arteriosus et venosus intracutaneous seu subcutaneous collaris). This plexus is important for sexual and territorial display and regulates body temperature in both sexes. Injections into or damage to this plexus, especially in hot weather or during display seasons, may result in fatal haemorrhage.

Intramuscular route: Small volumes may be injected into the iliotibialis muscle of the thigh and larger volumes into the pectoralis muscle. The injection site is in the cranial third of the muscle mass. Volumes are generally restricted to 0.5 ml in small birds.

Intravenous route: The ulnar, basilic or wing vein, positioned on the medial aspect of the elbow, may be used for intravenous injections. This vein is fragile and prone to haemorrhage after venepuncture. The medial metatarsal vein running along the medial aspect of the distal leg is often easily visualized. The jugular vein may be accessed in the neck, which runs in a line down to the base of the neck. It is hidden by feathers in many species, and plucking of the area is required to visualize the vein.

Intraosseous route: The intraosseous route is ideal for fluid administration in collapsed birds. Catheters may be placed in the distal radius or proximal tibia using the following procedure:

1. Prepare the site aseptically.
2. Inject local anaesthestic into the site (unless the animal is under general anaesthesia).

3. Introduce appropriately sized spinal needles or plain needles into the bone (size sufficient to enter medullary cavity based on knowledge or guided by size of cavity on radiography).
4. Flush with heparinized saline to ensure patency.
5. Secure in place with surgical cyanoacrylate adhesive or suture.
6. Attach short extension tube.
7. Bandage area to maintain cleanliness and to reduce mobility of the limb.

An aseptic technique should be used when giving drugs or fluids. The catheter should be filled with heparin or heparinized saline between use to prevent clot formation and should be flushed three times daily with heparinized saline when not in use.

Nursing

As part of the basic nursing care of sick birds, attention should be paid to:

- Nutrition – birds have a high energy requirement. If hepatic function is compromised, a fat-free energy source should be used (the alga *Spirulina* is an easily assimilable protein; the tablet should be crushed with water)
- Hydration – dehydrated birds should be gavaged with an electrolyte and probiotic solution
- Warming foods before administering via a crop tube (foods should not be overheated in a microwave or 'crop burn' may result)
- Probiotics – these are useful as stressed or ill birds often lose commensal bacteria from their short gastrointestinal tract
- Warmth – this should be provided without draughts (incubators are useful)
- Darkness and quiet – this tends to sedate birds and reduces stress.

Fluid therapy

If the packed cell volume is below 25 g/l a whole blood transfusion or colloid is required. Iron dextran and vitamin B injections may be given with the blood transfusion at 10% bodyweight as a bolus. If the packed cell volume is above 55–60 g/l the bird is dehydrated and should be given lactated Ringer's or Hartmann's solution at 10% of bodyweight as a bolus intravenously or subcutaneously. If glucose is below 180 g/l then 5% glucose saline should be given intravenously at 10% of bodyweight as a bolus.

Fluids should be warmed to 38–39°C. Lactated Ringer's solution and 5% dextrose are recommended solutions for fluid replacement. Fluids may be given via the intravenous or intraosseous route. Fluid requirements may be calculated as:

Estimated dehydration (%) × bodyweight (g) = fluid deficit (ml)

The requirement for maintenance fluids is 50 ml/kg per day. Half the fluid deficit should be replaced over the first 12–24 hours plus the ongoing maintenance requirements. The remainder of the deficit should be corrected over the next 48 hours. Bolus fluids for anaesthesia at a rate of 10 ml/kg may be given slowly over 5–7 minutes for relatively stress-free restraint for catheter placement. An intraosseous catheter may be placed aseptically into the ulna or tibiotarsus. The preferred sites for intravenous catheter placement in members of the Columbiformes are the right jugular or basilic (ulnar) veins.

Crop tubing

When force feeding or dosing birds food is introduced into the crop, not the stomach. Pigeons have small tongues and the beak can be held open with a finger.

1. Wrap the bird loosely in a towel and hold the bird around the neck with the left hand, so that it is facing you.
2. Insert a lubricated crop tube gently into the left corner of the mouth, slowly over the tongue to the back of the mouth and down into the crop. The tube is easily palpated in the crop through the skin when in place.
3. Fill the crop slowly.
4. Remove the tube gently.

Blood transfusion

Donor blood should be collected into acid citrate solution to give a concentration of 0.15 ml/ml of whole blood. Approximately 10–20% of the recipient blood volume may be given per transfusion via the intravenous or intraosseous route. Homologous blood transfusions are preferable to heterologous transfusions as the latter result in short erythrocyte survival times.

Anaesthesia and analgesia

Anaesthesia

A thorough clinical examination and accurate assessment of a bird's weight is essential before anaesthesia. The packed cell volume and concentrations of blood glucose and aspartate transaminase should be checked. Food should be withheld for 3–6 hours, or 1 hour in birds weighing under 100 g. Atropine 0.05–0.1 mg/kg (higher dose for small birds) may be used as a premedicant. Heat loss should be avoided by placing the bird on a pad with a surface temperature of 30°C and wrapping it in bubblewrap. Temperature should be monitored with an electronic rectal thermometer. As few feathers as possible should be gently plucked to avoid unnecessary heat loss and the site prepared with iodine solution not alcohol. An electrocardiograph with adhesive pads and respiratory monitors are useful for monitoring the effects of surgery and anaesthesia. An intravenous line should be established in the brachial vein. All anaesthetized birds should be intubated, size permitting, and flushed with oxygen every 5 minutes as they easily become hypercapnoeic. Birds should be positioned in sternal or lateral recumbency (Figure 15.12) as dorsal recumbency, although stable, compromises respiration by 10–60%. Quick position changes should be avoided as blood pressure can drop rapidly.

Isoflurane is the agent of choice for the induction and maintenance of general anaesthesia (Figure 15.13). ECG pads should be applied to the wings and feet. A pulse oximeter probe may be attached across the wing artery on the medial side of the wing, the metatarsal artery or across the tibiotarsus in small birds, or a rectal probe inserted a short distance in the cloaca.

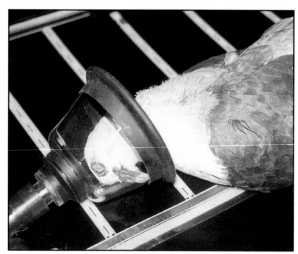

Figure 15.12 A pink pigeon undergoing gaseous anaesthesia.

Anaesthetic	Dosage	Comments
Isoflurane	Induction 4%, maintenance 2%, oxygen flow 1–2 l/min	Swift induction. Rapid recovery. 50% nitrous oxide reduces isoflurane dose required
Halothane	Induction 1%, increase to 3%, maintain at 1.5–3%	Cardiac failure if too rapid induction
Ketamine and diazepam or midazolam	25 mg/kg ketamine plus 2.5 mg/kg diazepam i.m.	20–30 minutes' deep sedation
Ketamine and medetomidine	3–7 mg/kg ketamine plus 75–150 mg/kg medetomidine i.m.	
Atipamezole	5 × medetomidine dose for reversal	
Propofol	3–5 mg/kg i.v.	Rapid recovery, care with transfer to gaseous anaesthetic

Figure 15.13 Anaesthetic dosages for pigeons.

Injectable combinations of agents used for anaesthesia include ketamine and xylazine and ketamine and medetomidine. Figure 15.14 lists the responses of anaesthetized birds according to depth of anaesthesia.

There is a wide variability in dosage required and safety between species and individuals birds. Members of the Columbiformes are sensitive to many local anaesthetic agents and may show adverse drug reactions or die.

Depth of anaesthesia	Responses of bird
Light plane	Absence of righting reflex, intact corneal palpebral and pedal reflexes
Surgical plane	Eyelids closed, pupils dilated
Too deep	Loss of corneal reflex, slow shallow respiration, respiratory arrest

Figure 15.14 Monitoring depth of anaesthesia in birds.

Analgesia

Several analgesics have been evaluated in psittacine birds (Figure 15.15). Many birds do not show obvious signs of pain such as depression or anorexia when subjected to suspected 'painful' stimuli, e.g. fractures, sinus curettage. However, although postoperative recovery is often speedier with perioperative analgesics there is a greater postoperative mortality.

Drug	Route	Dose
Flunixin meglumine	i.m. or i.v.	1–10 mg/kg sid
Butorphanol	i.m.	0.2–0.4 mg/kg (up to 10 × this dose)
Buprenorphine	i.m.	0.01–0.05 mg/kg

Figure 15.15 Analgesics commonly used in birds.

Common surgical procedures

Preparation of the skin

Feathers should be plucked to a distance of 2 or 3 cm around the surgical site. Water-soluble gel helps to keep down and contour feathers out of the surgical site. Clear plastic drapes allow more precise patient monitoring as respiratory movements can be seen easily. Avian skin is thinner than mammalian skin. The strongest areas are between rows of feathers (apteriae), and these should be used for anchoring sutures. Many capillaries are present so diathermy should be used for cutting or a precrush area incised with artery forceps. Radiosurgery is especially useful in birds. A suture of 3/0 and 5/0 polyglactin (Vicryl) in a mattress or continuous interlocking pattern is recommended. Large defects should be avoided as avian skin is inelastic. Tension-releasing incisions ('meshwork') are useful to aid closure in some cases.

Cannulation of infraorbital sinus

Cannulation of the infraorbital sinus is used for the treatment of sinusitis or rhinorrhoea. A swab should first be taken for antibiotic sensitivity. Light anaesthesia is required. A 20 gauge needle should be inserted into the angle dorsal to the angle of the mouth in a notch palpated through the skin (junction of premaxilla and maxillary bones) and advanced at a 45 degree angle (care being taken not to penetrate the orbit). Antibiotic should be injected and flushed, with the bird angled downwards as the fluid flows out of the choana and nares.

Cloacal prolapse

A cloacal prolapse should be examined urgently as it may result in occlusion of the ureters and colon.

A simple prolapse may be easily replaced: the prolapse should be cleaned, hydroscopic solution applied to reduce swelling, and lubricated and replaced gently. A thermometer is a useful retainer while placing a purse-string suture. Chromic catgut should be used on a round-bodied needle.

More complex prolapses require further surgery. The indications for cloacopexy include chronic cloacal prolapse, decreased sphincter tone and prolapse associated with reproductive disorders.

Percutaneous cloacopexy

For simple prolapses mattress sutures should be placed percutaneously on each side of the body wall through the body wall and urodeum. A probe placed per cloaca enables identification of the cloacal wall. Complications include entrapment of ureters or perforation of the rectum, duodenum or pancreas. Sutures may be removed after 2–4 weeks.

Rib cloacopexy

Rib cloacopexy is useful for a severe prolapse with distention of the cloaca. It may be performed by using a ventral midline or transverse abdominal coeliotomy. A Y-shaped coeliotomy provides the best exposure. A probe may be inserted into the cloaca to locate the wall. Fat from the ventral aspect of the cloaca must be removed to enable adhesions to form between the cloaca and body wall. The ribs should be manipulated caudally with the thumb, and the body wall reflected with the index finger to expose the ribs for suture placement. Two sutures should be preplaced around the last rib on each side and full thickness through the ventral aspect of the craniolateral wall of the urodeum on each side. When tied, there should be enough tension on the sutures to cause slight inversion of the vent. It is possible to suture to the caudal border of the sternum instead of the ribs. After the rib sutures have been placed, the body wall should be closed by incorporating cloacal wall sandwiched between the sides of the body wall.

Feather cysts

Feather cysts need to be differentiated from abscesses and neoplasia, so careful examination and biopsy is required. Cysts often occur as a result of trauma to the follicles caused by excessive preening, e.g. with mite infestation. Cysts can be treated by incision and evacuation or surgical excision. Cautery may be used to destroy the follicles to prevent recurrence. Fibrosed skin remains. If large areas of the skin have cysts, care is needed as avian skin is relatively inelastic. Closure of large defects requires tension-relieving techniques, such as the creation of skin meshes.

Dystocia

The diagnosis of dystocia is based on a history of passed eggs, clinical examination and radiography. Surgical correction is indicated if the bird is refractory to medical treatment or if the radiographs indicate oversized, malformed or fractured eggs.

A ventral midline incision should be made over the egg, avoiding the pubic artery over the pubic bone. The incision should run from the pubis to sternum. A flap or H-shaped incision aids access. The distended oviduct will be on the left. The dissection should proceed through the fat pad and down to the egg. Two sutures should be preplaced in the uterus, the uterus incised and the egg carefully removed. Sutures should be preplaced in the oviduct. If the egg breaks, the abdomen should be lavaged with warm fluid prior to closure. Egg peritonitis from broken eggs is a common sequel and carries a poor prognosis.

Salpingohysterectomy (hysterectomy or spay)

Salpingohysterectomy may be required to treat persistent egg laying, egg binding, diseased tissues or egg peritonitis.

The approach is via either a left lateral coeliotomy, as generally only the left ovary is functional, or a ventral midline approach. The ventriculus should be retracted ventrally and the oviduct positioned dorsally near the vena cava and iliac veins, being careful to avoid these. The ventral ligament of the oviduct should be bluntly dissected to allow the oviduct and uterus to be straightened into a linear configuration. The branch of the ovarian artery emerging from under the ovary should be coagulated and packed with Gelfoam/ Lysostypt if haemorrhage occurs. The infundibulum should be dissected free and the oviduct retracted ventrally and caudally to expose the dorsal ligament of the oviduct and the associated vascular arcade. To allow the oviduct and uterus to be dissected free the vessels within the dorsal ligament should be coagulated and clipped. The ureters may be identified as tubular white structures from the kidneys to the cloaca. The junction between the uterus and vagina (a short distance from the cloaca) should be clipped. If the clips are not secure they may leak cloacal contents into the coelom, causing peritonitis. The ovary should not be removed; it does not cycle if the entire shell gland has been removed.

Fractures

Midshaft fractures of the tibiotarsus are common in pigeons. Most heal within 3 weeks due to healing of the endosteum and periosteum. An Altman splint – two pieces of zinc oxide tape placed either side of joint and stuck together – prevents rotation. External fixator pins may be constructed from 21–23 gauge needles. Fractures of the humerus heal well if the wing is strapped in a folded position over the splint.

Air sac intubation

The abdominal air sacs can be intubated so that the bird breathes through this tube rather than through the trachea. This technique is useful for an emergency procedure, bypassing the trachea if it is blocked. The tube can also be used in preference to an endotracheal tube for introducing gaseous anaesthetics so that the head is free for surgery. Intubation of the air sacs should be performed as follows:

1. Pluck and aseptically prepare the site over the last rib on the right flank.
2. Enter the air sac by using blunt dissection where the sterile tube is to be introduced (an endotracheal tube or piece of intravenous drip tubing may be used).
3. Use surgical glue or a fingertrap suture to keep the tube in place.

If the bird relies on the tube to breathe postoperatively, then it must be checked frequently throughout the day to ensure its patency. When checking the tube, ensure that:

- The bird is breathing with little effort
- The tubing is fogging with each breath
- There is air movement, by holding a feather or hair against the tube
- There is no blood in the tube; blood may indicate damage to an internal organ from the tube so consider removing the tube and checking the bird before replacing it
- There is no air under the skin or any sign of infection around the tube.

Euthanasia

The preferred methods of euthanasia are by overdose with gaseous anaesthetic agents or intrahepatic injection of barbiturates.

Drug formulary

References and further reading

Hawes RO (1984) Pigeons. In: *Evolution of Domesticated Animals,* ed. IL Mason. London, Longman

Huber L (1994) Amelioration of laboratory conditions for pigeons (*Columba livia*). *Animal Welfare* **3**, 321–324

Hutchison RE (1999) Doves and pigeons. In: *The UFAW Handbook on the Care and Management of Laboratory Animals,* 7th edn, Vol 1: *Terrestrial Vertebrates,* pp.714–721. Blackwell Science, Oxford

Keymer IF (1991) Pigeons. In: *Manual of Exotic Pets,* ed. PH Beynon and JE Cooper, pp. 180–202. British Small Animal Veterinary Association, Cheltenham

Nepote K (1999a) Pigeon housing: practical considerations and welfare implications. *Laboratory Animal* **28**, 34–37

Nepote K (1999b) Pigeons as laboratory animals. *Poultry and Avian Biology Reviews* **10**, 109–115

Quesenberry K and Hillyer EV (1994) Supportive care and emergency therapy. In: *Avian Medicine, Principles and Applications,* ed. RW Ritchie, GJ Harrison and L Harrison, pp. 382–416. Wingers Publishing, Florida

Schmorrow DD and Ulrich RE (1991) Improving the housing and care of laboratory pigeons and rats. *Humane Innovations and Alternatives* **5**, 299–304

Vogel L, Gerlach H and Loffler M (1994). Columbiformes. In: *Avian Medicine: Principles and Application,* ed. Ritchie *et al.,* pp. 1200–1217. Wingers Publishing Inc., Lake Worth, Florida

Drug	Dose and route	Comments
Amino acids (methionine, choline) and B12	As directed	Moulting, convalescence, after antibiotics, supportive for liver disease
Amprolium 3.4%	28 ml per 4.5 l drinking water for 7 days	
Bromhexine	3–6 i.m. or 2 g 1% powder/l	Mucolytic and helps antibiotics penetrate respiratory mucosa
Calcium borogluconate 10%	1–5 ml/kg i.m. or s.c.	For egg retention and for hypocalcaemic tetany
Clazuril	5 mg/kg	
Delmadinone (Tardak)	0.02 ml/30 g i.m.	Coccidiosis
Dexamethasone 2 mg/ml	0.3–3 or 0.15–1.5 i.m. or i.v. bid	Shock or anti-inflammatory
Dimetronidazole	40 w/w at v 500 mg/l in drinking water for 7 days or 50 mg/kg orally	3 courses with 7-day intervals may be given, toxicity reported with overdoses or increased drinking in hot weather
Doxapram hydrochloride	5–10 i.m. or by drops to tongue	One drop for apnoea during GA and to speed recovery from ketamine anaesthesia
Doxycycline	15 mg/kg as 300 mg per 2 l drinking water for 5 days (make up fresh solution daily)	Bacterial respiratory disease, *Chlamydia,* sensitive ocular infections
Electrolytes and amino acids	As directed	Before or after racing, illness, breeding period
Febantel	30 mg/kg orally	Roundworm (*Ascaridia columbae*), hairworm (*Capillaria*), tapeworm, no problems with feather growth, no vomition
Fenbendazole	2.5% solution as 4 ml/kg feed for three days or 7.5 mg/kg single dose orally	Reversible feather abnormalities may occur with oral dose
Ivermectin	200 µg/kg single dose i.m. or s.c.	Toxicity reported, especially with overdosage
Levamisole	10–20 mg/kg single dose orally, repeated at 14-day intervals as required	Has a bitter taste, vomiting may occur 1–2 hours after treatment
Medroxyprogesterone acetate (5%)	5–10 i.m. or s.c. to suppress persistent ovulation, 30 to stop regurgitation	
Metronidazole	40 mg/kg orally for 5 days	
Oxytocin 10 IU/ml	3-5 IU i.m.	Once only for egg retention with calcium borogluconate
Ronidazole	10 mg/kg as tablet or 200 mg/2 l drinking water	Trichomoniasis Hexamitosis
Sulphadimethoxine	1000 mg per 2 l drinking water for 5–7 days	Coccidiosis and atoxoplasmosis (can be given throughout breeding season in infected flocks)
Sulphadimidine	15 ml of 33% solution in 4.5 l drinking water for 4 days	
Trimethoprim	400 mg into 2 l drinking water 5 days	May be repeated after 5 days in severe infections, salmonellosis, colibacillosis, sensitive infections of respiratory and gastrointestinal tract

Figure 15.16 Drug formulary for pigeons.

16

Birds of prey

John Chitty

Introduction

Falconry has been practised for many centuries, and diseases of birds of prey have been studied and documented for a long time; several Arabic treatises on the subject survive from the ninth century. Many birds of prey are now kept for private falconry, falconry displays, bird control (e.g. at airports and rubbish dumps) and breeding, as well as in zoological collections. Therefore veterinary clinics will see raptors from time to time and these are often presented in need of emergency stabilization following trauma or acute illness. Wild casualty birds are also frequently presented to clinics. Although this chapter will not specifically cover wildlife rehabilitation, many of the points raised will be applicable to both captive and wild raptors.

In the UK, it is illegal to take any raptor from the wild (alive or dead) and keep it, or any part of it, without a licence. If an injured wild raptor is taken, a licence should be obtained immediately from the Department of the Environment, Food and Rural Affairs (DEFRA), unless the bird is passed to a veterinary surgeon or to a person licensed to treat and release birds. An application to hold a bird unable to be released should be supported by a statement from a veterinary surgeon that the bird would not be able to survive in the wild if released.

Although there is no need to hold a formal licence to own or fly a bird of prey, there are specific legal requirements to register certain species:

- Under Section 7 of the Wildlife and Countryside Act 1981, any bird listed in Schedule 4 of the Act and kept in captivity must be registered with DETR (now DEFRA) and fitted with an official ring. Of the species listed, those most commonly encountered are the northern goshawk *Accipiter gentilis* and the merlin *Falco columbarius*
- From 1 April 1998 all species listed in Annex A of EC Regulation 338/97 require Article 10 Certificates if they are to be used commercially (e.g. public display, sale, or commercial breeding). The bird must be identified by a closed ring or microchip, and the application should be supported by information to prove that it was legally acquired. Zoological collections can apply for an Article 30

Certificate to cover all their birds for public display, but those used for commercial breeding still require an individual Article 10 Certificate. Species covered by this include most of those commonly used in falconry, with the exception of the Harris' hawk *Parabuteo unicinctus*
- If the bird is to be flown at birds not listed on Schedule 2 of the Wildlife and Countryside Act 1981, a quarry licence is required.

Biology

Birds of prey may be classed as raptors and form two groups:

- Diurnal – mainly the Falconiformes (e.g. hawks, falcons, eagles, vultures)
- Nocturnal – principally the Strigiformes (owls).

A wide range of species is kept in zoological collections, from the African pygmy falcons *Polihierax semitorquatus* to the Andean condor *Vultur gryphus*, but the range of those commonly used in falconry is much more limited (Figures 16.1 and 16.2). Typical bodyweights and other biological data for common species are given in Figures 16.3 and 16.4.

Eagles are used only occasionally. Owls are rarely flown at quarry but are frequently kept as breeding birds or as part of a growing 'pet' population.

Class	Examples
Hawks, or 'short-wings'	Harris' hawk *Parabuteo unicinctus*, the most commonly used falconry bird (Figure 16.2a); northern goshawk *Accipiter gentilis*; red-tailed hawk *Buteo jamaicensis*
Falcons, or 'long-wings'	Peregrine falcon *Falco peregrinus*; lanner *F.biarmicus* (Figure 16.2b); Saker *F. cherrug* (Figure 16.2c); merlin *F.columbarius* (Figure 16.2d)
Eagles	Golden eagle *Aquila chrysaetos*; Steppe eagle *A.nipalensis*; martial eagle *Polemactus bellicosus*
Owls	Eurasian eagle owl *Bubo bubo* (Figure 16.2e); Bengalese eagle owl (*B. bengalensis*); barn owl *Tyto alba*

Figure 16.1 Classification of falconry birds.

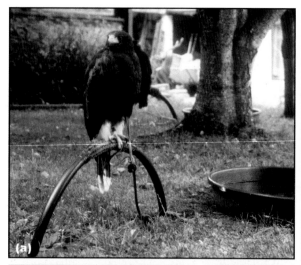
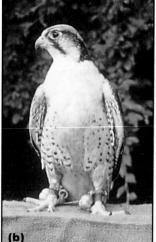
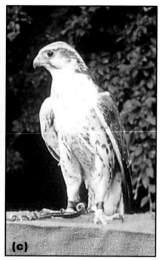
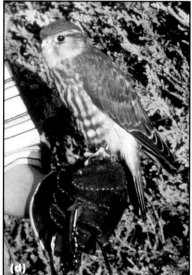
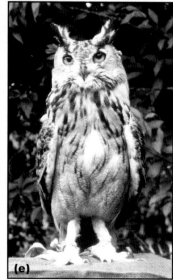

Figure 16.2 Some falconry species.
(a) Harris' hawk tethered on bow perch (note provision of water for bathing and drinking).
(b) Lanner. (c) Saker. (d) Merlin. (e) Eurasian eagle owl.

	Merlin	Peregrine falcon	Harris' hawk	Goshawk	Golden eagle	European eagle owl
Longevity	10–14 years	15–20 years	20–30 years	15–20 years	50–60 years	50–60 years
Age at sexual maturity	2 years	3+ years	3+ years	3+ years	5+ years	2+ years
Clutch size	2–7	2–6	2–4	2–5	1–3	2–4
Incubation period	28–32 days	29–32 days	28 days	35–38 days	43–45 days	32–35 days
Normal quarry	Skylark	Grouse, partridge, rook	Rabbit, pheasant	Rabbit, hare, gamebird	Rabbit, hare	Rarely used; rabbit?

Figure 16.3 Biological data for some common birds of prey.

Species	Male	Female
Merlin	160–170 g	220–250 g
Lanner	450–600 g	700–950 g
Peregrine	550–850 g	1110–1600 g
Saker	650–1000 g	950–1350 g
Harris' hawk	550–800 g	850–1300 g
Northern goshawk	650–850 g	950–1200 g
Golden eagle	2850–4500 g	3650–6700 g
Andean condor	11000–15000 g	8000–11000 g
Barn owl	200–400 g	350–500 g
Eurasian eagle owl	1500–2500 g	2250–3800 g

Figure 16.4 Typical bodyweights of common birds of prey.

Sexing

Sexual dimorphism is comparatively unusual in birds of prey, though there is often a size difference. Typically the female is larger than the male (though this may be reversed in the large vultures). The difference may be very marked; for example, in the peregrine, the falcon (female) is a third larger than the tiercel (male) (Figure 16.5). However, in some species, particularly the buzzards (*Buteo* spp.), there may be some overlap.

If there is doubt, sexing may be performed by laparoscopy or by DNA analysis (blood or feather).

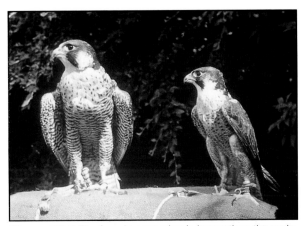

Figure 16.5 The female peregrine is larger than the male.

Husbandry

It is useful to have a working knowledge of the many terms peculiar to falconry (Figure 16.6) and of the considerable amount of specialist equipment (or 'furniture') used for falconry birds (Figures 16.7 and 16.8). This equipment should be individually fitted for each bird and carefully maintained. Failure to do so can result in severe injuries.

There are two basic systems for keeping raptors: tethered, or in aviaries.

- Tethered on blocks or perches is for flying birds. They should be taken off daily for exercise or demonstration flying to the lure, or for flying at quarry. Perches must be well maintained
- Aviaries are generally for breeding or 'exhibition' birds, or flying birds in the 'close season', though some birds may be 'flown from the aviary'.

Term	Definitions
Bate	To flap violently from perch or fist
Cast	1. Two or more birds flown together 2. To grab and hold for examination 3. To regurgitate a pellet
Cast off	To release from the fist
Casting	Indigestible part of the diet: hair, feathers, bone (in owls)
Cope	To trim beak or talons
Eyass	Young bird removed from the nest
Foot	To grab (prey or handler) with the talons
Fret-marks	Weak points in feather visible as a transverse line. Caused by metabolic, nutritional or behavioural stresses during the development of the feather
Imp	Process of repairing damaged feathers by splicing on another
Mantle	The act of spreading the wings to cover food
Rangle	Indigestible material (e.g. stones) sometimes ingested accidentally. Formerly given deliberately to clean out the crop
Rouse	Vigorous shaking of the feathers, usually just before flight
Stress-marks	*see* Fret-marks
Weather	To place outdoors

Figure 16.6 Glossary of falconry terms.

In both situations, shelter from inclement conditions should be provided. Further aspects of this subject are provided in the *Code of Welfare and Husbandry of Birds of Prey and Owls* from the British Field Sports Society and in two guidelines from the Federation of Zoological Gardens of Great Britain and Ireland: *Management Guidelines for the Welfare of Zoo Animals: Birds of Prey in Flying Demonstrations* and *Management Guidelines for the Welfare of Zoo Animals: Falconiformes*.

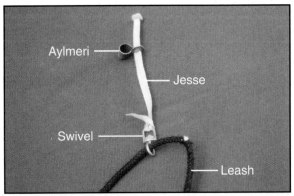

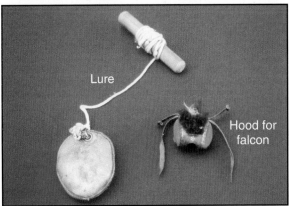

Figure 16.7 Falconry equipment.

Term	Definition/notes
Aylmeri	Leather anklet secured with a rivet or grommet
Bells	Attached to legs or tail to help to track bird
Bewit	Leather strap for attaching bells to the leg
Block	Solid perch with padded top (for falcons)
Bow perch	Semicircular bar with padded region for perching (for hawks, eagles or owls)
Cadge	Portable perch for carrying several birds together
Creance	Long line attached to jesses and used when training
Hood	Leather 'cap' used to cover the eyes and calm the bird (for falcons and sometimes hawks)
Jesse	Leather strap, passes through aylmeri (or directly round legs) to enable restraint
Leash	Attached to swivel, used to secure bird
Mews	Housing for tethered raptors
Mutes	Droppings
Swivel	Metal ringed device to link jesses to leash
Telemetry	Radio-tracking device attached to bird's tail when flown

Figure 16.8 Falconry equipment.

Diet

It is not possible to cover raptor nutrition fully here but there are certain principles:

- Raptors are 'whole carcass' feeders and so should be offered whole carcasses
  - Evisceration of carcasses will result in loss of essential nutrients
  - Feeding of muscle (e.g. beef) should be avoided, as it cannot provide balanced nutrition
  - The size of food item should reflect the size of bird eating it; for example, the kestrel *Falco tinnunculus* cannot cope with rabbit carcasses
  - It is wise to break long bones of rabbits and hares prior to feeding; if whole legs are swallowed they may cause an obstruction
- Where possible, the food offered should mimic the bird's natural diet; for example, kestrels or barn owls should be offered small rodents, larger owls should receive larger rodents, and the large eagles or vultures may be offered whole rabbit, hare or lamb carcasses
- No single food item will provide all the bird's nutritional requirements at all life stages; therefore a mixed diet should be fed
- Day-old chicks (DOCs) are the most common staple diet for most raptors and their value as a food item is considerable
  - Contrary to previous belief, DOCs have a good calcium:phosphorus ratio, good vitamin levels, and not excessive lipid levels
  - It should be noted that this applies only if the yolk sacs are not removed. An exception is when feeding merlins, which are prone to a fatty liver/kidney syndrome (Forbes and Cooper, 1993). This may be due to high lipid levels in the diet or may be due to high avidin levels in the yolk (Rees-Davies, 2000). It is wise, therefore, to feed merlins on deyolked DOCs plus immature rodent
- Vitamin supplementation should be unnecessary if a correct, well balanced diet is fed
  - Supplementation may even be counterproductive, as overdosage of one fat-soluble vitamin may lead to deficiency of another because of competitive absorption from the gut
  - Supplementation may, however, be appropriate at certain times; for example, the use of a high calcium/vitamin D_3 supplement prior to the breeding season
- Good quality food should be used
  - Carcasses should be fed fresh or properly thawed (and not refrozen)
  - Uneaten food should be removed daily
  - It is wise not to feed roadkill (even if found fresh) or shot game (even if head shot)
  - Feeding fresh pigeon should be avoided, as pigeons may carry many diseases. Freezing and subsequent thawing will eliminate some of these, but not all
- Water is essential. It is often stated that raptors do not drink but this is untrue, though their drinking may be infrequent. Birds of prey should always be offered clean, fresh water for bathing and drinking

- Some birds are messy feeders (especially on DOCs) and fail to clean themselves properly. It is important that food material is removed from under the talons, to avoid the development of skin necrosis and thence deeper infections.

For a comprehensive guide to this subject, see the excellent book *Raptor Nutrition* (Forbes and Flint, 2000).

Microchipping

Microchip implants should be inserted into the caudal third of the left pectoral muscle mass. The feathers should be parted and the site cleaned prior to implantation. Where necessary, bleeding should be stopped using digital pressure and the skin closed using tissue glue or a single suture. Anaesthesia is generally not required for this procedure but should be considered if the implanter is not confident or if the bird is very small.

Handling

It is impossible to examine a bird of prey without handling it.

- With raptors, the feet are more dangerous than the beak (though falcons may give a painful 'nip') and so it is essential to restrain the feet first
- If handling larger birds (eagles or vultures), the beak may also be capable of causing injury and these birds often require several handlers. In addition, vultures may vomit foul-smelling stomach contents when handled.

To examine a bird, it is 'cast'. If it is used to being hooded, the hood should be fitted first to reduce the bird's anxiety. Otherwise the bird can be taken into a dimly lit room. To cast a typical bird weighing approximately 1 kg (e.g. Harris' hawk):

1. Grasp the bird from behind with both hands, using a towel (*not* gloves). The thumbs should face toward the head.
2. Wrap the towel quickly around the body (taking care not to restrict breathing). Hold the wings in the towel by the thumbs and first two fingers of each hand (Figure 16.9a).
3. With your remaining fingers, grasp each leg as far down as possible to restrict movement (Figure 16.9b).
4. Place fingers between the bird's legs so that it cannot grab itself or damage its legs against each other. With smaller birds, one hand can hold the wings while the other holds the feet (Figure 16.9c). With larger birds, it is advisable to have several people helping.
5. If the bird is not hooded, part of the towel can be used to cover the eyes.

It is important to hold birds firmly so that they do not struggle and damage themselves. Once wrapped in a towel and secured, most birds do not struggle. As many falconers are very adept at handling their birds, it is often sensible to allow them to restrain their own bird.

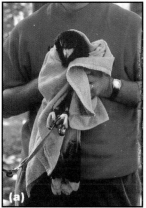
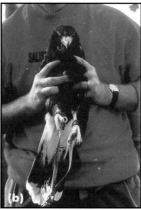
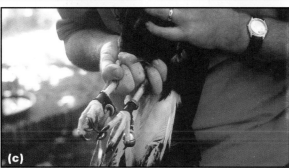

Figure 16.9 Casting. (a) Harris' hawk cast in a towel. (b) Towel removed: note position of fingers holding the legs. (c) Holding the feet: note the fingers between the legs.

Diagnostic approach

History

History taking is a very important aspect of the disease investigation and the following points should be covered.

- Species, age, sex (if known)
- When purchased or bred
- Other birds kept
- Disease history of this bird and others in collection
- Husbandry: aviary or tethered, flying bird or breeding only, when last flown (if at all)
- Diet:
  - What and how fed, and how much
  - Source – wild quarry (shot or caught?) or farmed
  - Supplements used
  - Is casting being fed?
- Weight:
  - What are the normal flying and moulting weights for this bird?
  - Is the weight being dropped deliberately at present (e.g. in training)?
  - Is the bird's weight higher or lower than would normally be expected at current level of feeding?
- Flying:
  - How keen is the bird to fly?
  - Is it tiring easily?
- Disease history: duration, recent injuries (no matter how minor), medications used or applied already
- Mutes: do they appear normal?
- Casting: when did the bird last cast and was it normal?

Physical examination

If at any stage the bird becomes very distressed or becomes very still, examination should be discontinued and the bird's condition reassessed. If necessary, the examination should be performed with supplemental oxygen to hand. If the bird cannot be examined without harming it, anaesthesia should be considered.

Head

- Beak and cere – damage, beak quality (signs of metabolic disturbance or poor diet)
- Nares – for discharge
- Eyes (Figures 16.10 and 16.11)
- Periorbital sinuses – distinguish periocular swelling from ocular disease
- Ears – for discharges or bleeding (post-trauma).

Eye reflexes
Hard to assess. Threat reflexes are often inapparent and because of the bird's conscious control of pupil size the pupillary light reflex is unreliable. A consensual light reflex may be apparent but this is often due to passage of light directly to the contralateral retina via the very thin bone separating the eyes.
Anterior segment
May be examined using routine direct or indirect ophthalmoscopy methods. Consideration should be paid to: • Eyelids and conjunctivae (e.g. swelling) • Nictitating membrane (e.g. trauma) • Cornea (e.g. ulcers, trauma) • Anterior chamber (presence of blood, pus, 'flare') (Figure 16.11) • Uvea (inflammation) • Lens (cataract, displacement). The nictitating membrane should be lifted to allow examination of the large lacrymal duct opening.
Drainage angle
May be visualized directly from the side in large owls.
Posterior segment
Examination presents problems as it is so difficult to dilate the pupil. Mammalian mydriatics are ineffective in birds, owing to the striated muscle in the avian iris. Topical vecuronium may induce mydriasis but should be used with great care. The most reliable method appears to be examination under anaesthesia. This is essential in all known or suspected cases of head trauma, as contre-coup injuries will result in bleeding from the delicate pecten. This will ultimately result in severe retinal damage and blindness unless prompt anti-inflammatory therapy is given. Without full binocular vision, birds will have difficulty hunting.

Figure 16.10 Ocular examination, an essential part of any clinical examination.

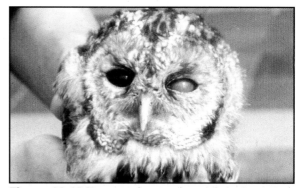

Figure 16.11 Hypopyon in a tawny owl *Strix aluco* (left eye).

Equipment
Syringe
Sterile saline
Appropriate antimicrobial (if being used in treatment)
Technique
For diagnostics
Use 20 ml sterile saline/kg bodyweight
1. Restrain bird and hold *upside-down*. The bird must be conscious.
2. Apply syringe tip (without needle) tightly against one naris and forcibly inject fluid. Water should appear from the other naris, from the choanal slit and sometimes from the conjunctivae.
3. Collect sample for culture and cytology as it exits from the choanal slit.
For treatment
The technique is the same except that an appropriate antimicrobial is added on the basis of culture and sensitivity testing. As a 'first-guess' choice, add enrofloxacin to the flush at a rate of 1 ml 2.5% per 20 ml water.
Underlying factors (e.g. irritant fumes, hypovitaminosis A) should not be forgotten but this technique performed every 2–3 days often results in cure of sinusitis without resort to systemic therapy.

Figure 16.12 Sinus flush, a useful technique in upper respiratory tract infection (nasal, sinus or periocular) for collecting samples and for treatment.

Sinus flushing may be performed for diagnosis or treatment (Figure 16.12).

Mouth

- Lesions (especially plaques) and *Capillaria* worms at the back of the mouth
- Choanal slit (Figure 16.13) – discharges, swelling in upper respiratory tract infections (URTI); take swabs from the rostral part in URTI
- Glottis – swelling, discharge, *Syngamus* worms.

Body condition

Assess by palpation of the pectoral muscle mass. Relate this to species, current weight (often done by

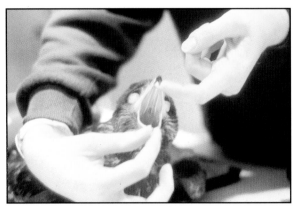

Figure 16.13 The choanal slit of a normal Harris' hawk. In upper respiratory tract infection samples may be taken from the rostral end for cytology and bacteriology.

the falconer, but should always be checked) and stage of training.

Skin and plumage

- Parasites
- Lesions
- Quality of feathering (including presence of 'fret' marks)
- Subcutaneous emphysema
- Uropygial gland.

Abdomen and crop

- Palpate abdomen for masses, etc.
- Palpate crop (not present in owls) for fluid filling, foreign bodies, etc.

Cloaca

Check for swellings or prolapse and for soiling of the surrounding feathers. Digital or auriscopic examination can be performed under anaesthesia, or when conscious for large, tractable birds.

Auscultation

Auscultate pectoral area (heart), dorsum between wings (lung sounds) and abdomen (air sac noise).

Limbs

Pectoral and pelvic limbs should be thoroughly examined with all joints flexed, extended and palpated. This part of the examination may need to be done under anaesthesia in order to assess shoulder and coxo-femoral joints fully.

Feet

Check for bumblefoot lesions, wounds, talon quality or damage and check thoroughly under equipment for skin trauma.

Sample collection

Blood

The preferred site for blood collection is the right jugular vein, which can be found and accessed easily in most species. In larger birds restraint may be difficult and either the bird should be anaesthetized or the brachial vein should be used. The medial metatarsal vein may also be used but working close to the feet may be risky in the conscious bird.

Samples for both haematological and biochemical analysis should usually be collected into lithium heparin tubes. Ideally a fresh blood smear should be made at the time of collection. Wherever possible, laboratories with specialized knowledge of raptors should be used. It is wise to consult with the laboratory prior to blood collection to determine their exact requirements. Normal ranges for haematology and biochemistry are given in Figure 16.14.

Parameter (units)	Northern goshawk	Peregrine	Harris' hawk	Golden eagle	European eagle owl
White blood cells (10^9/l)	6.26–16.0	3.5–11.0	4.8–10.0	6.0–15.0	3.5–12.1
Red blood cells (10^{12}/l)	2.15–3.07	2.90–4.00	2.63–3.50	1.8–3.1	1.65–2.35
PCV (%)	44–52	37–55	40–55	30–52	36–52
Haemoglobin (g/dl)	11.9–13.2	11.0–19.0	12.1–17.1	10.0–17.0	10.7–18
Heterophils (10^9/l)	3.41–9.97	1.5–8.5	2.3–6.71	4.0–12.0	2.2–9.23
Lymphocytes (10^9/l)	1.35–6.13	1.1–3.3	0.8–2.36	0.5–3.0	1.5–5.07
Monocytes (10^9/l)	0.0–0.66	0.0–0.60	0.2–1.49	0.0–0.5	0.0–0.48
Eosinophils (10^9/l)	0.0–0.33	0.0–0.30	0.0–0.75	0.0–0.4	0.0–0.48
Basophils (10^9/l)	0.0–0.50	0.0–0.60	0.0–1.5	0.0–0.3	0.0–0.35
Total protein (g/l)	25.0–37.0	27.0–40.0	31.0–45.7	25.0–40.0	30.1–34.5
Albumin (g/l)	9.0–15.0	8.5–16.0	13.9–17.0	10.0–16.0	11.1–13.5
Globulin (g/l)	16.0–26.0	17.0–25.0	21.0–29.4	22.0–26.0	18.7–22.4
Uric acid (μmol/l)	190–890	320–670	535–785	400–580	475–832
Calcium (mmol/l)	2.08–2.58	2.00–2.50	2.10–2.66	2.0–2.8	2.16–2.61
AST (IU/l)	40–134	50–110	160–348	< 250	<250
Creatine kinase (IU/l)	300–921	620–1200	224–650	< 500	<300
Bile acids (μmol/l)	< 80	< 80	< 80	< 80	<80
Zinc (μmol/l)	< 31.4	<31.4	< 31.4	< 31.4	<31.4

Figure 16.14 Normal haematological and biochemical data for some selected raptors. Data courtesy of J. Macdonald, Medlab, Tarporley, Cheshire, UK.

Common conditions

Common clinical signs and differential diagnoses are summarized in Figure 16.15. The list is by no means exhaustive, nor intended to be, but provides a guide to the more common conditions seen in captive birds of prey. A drug formulary for raptors is given at the end of this chapter.

Gastrointestinal disease

Crop stasis

If the crop has not emptied 6–8 hours after a feed, it should be seen as an emergency.

Fluids, antibiotics and metoclopramide (if foreign body has been ruled out) may be effective. Surgical emptying of the crop should be considered if an obstruction is suspected and when medical therapy is not effective.

Loose mutes

Mutes should be collected on paper for examination. Mutes produced while travelling or just after should not be used as they are often looser than normal. It should be noted that raptor mutes are normally looser and more voluminous than those of seed-fed cage birds; the faecal portion is not formed.

Polyuria should be distinguished from enteritis and physiological causes (e.g. prior to egg-laying):

- Is the bird drinking?
- Does it have access to water?
- Is the urine discoloured? (Green = biliverdinuria.)

Perform urinalysis (beware of faecal contamination), haematology/biochemistry analysis, radiography and blood lead/zinc estimation and, where indicated, organ biopsy.

Enteritis

This may be chronic (see ADR syndrome in Figure 16.15) or acute.

Acute enteritis is an emergency!

- Give fluids and warmth
- Perform parasitology, cloacal culture and sensitivity, faecal Gram stain, and haematology/biochemistry analysis.

Fitting (seizures) and neurological signs

Differentials include hypoglycaemia, hypocalcaemia, lead poisoning, vitamin B_1 deficiency, 'goshawk cramps' (aspergillosis), primary epilepsy (rare), meningitis and terminal state. Certain aspects of the history can give major clues to the diagnosis:

- Hypoglycaemia (during or just after exercise) – is the bird's weight low compared with normal flying weight?
- Hypocalcaemia (young growing bird, breeding female) – deficient diet?
- Lead poisoning: feeding shot quarry?
- Vitamin B_1 deficiency – deficient diet? Other causes ruled out?
- 'Goshawk cramps' (paresis or paralysis of legs only, no fitting) – rare in species other than goshawk.

Check whether the falconer has already given medication, and what the response was. During examination, note especially body condition and signs of trauma. Lead poisoning is implicated if the feet are gripping each other.

Fits need to be controlled fast!

Sign	Differential diagnoses	Primary tests	Secondary tests	Additional notes
Mouth/crop lesions	Trichomoniasis; candidiasis; bacterial infection; capillariasis; hypovitaminosis A; herpes virus; injury/burn	Wet mount/cytology of lesions Culture and sensitivity of lesions (after debridement) Thorough dietary history	Endoscopy of oesophagus and choanal slit Crop flush Haematology/biochemistry Biopsy	Accompanying signs include: head shaking, flicking food, dysphagia, regurgitation, acute/peracute death (Herpes virus)
Head shaking	See above; sinusitis/URTI (bacterial/fungal); otitis	As above (if mouth lesions) Sinus flush (cytology + culture/sensitivity) and/or choanal swab (cytology + culture/sensitivity) Aural examination + swab (cytology + culture/sensitivity) if discharge present Haematology	Endoscopy of choanal slit, ears, etc. Sinus radiography	
Respiratory disease	Distinguish between upper (nares + sinuses) and lower (trachea, syrinx, lungs and airsacs) respiratory tract disease			
Upper respiratory tract disease	See head shaking Also consider chlamydiosis if ocular signs present too	Choanal sampling/sinus flush (as head shaking), conjunctival smear for cytology if chlamydiosis suspected	As head shaking	Signs: ocular/nasal discharge, periorbital swelling, open-mouth breathing, head shake, sneezing, exercise intolerance, inspiratory effort
Lower respiratory tract disease	Bacterial/fungal infections; *Syngamus* (gapeworm) infection	Radiography (lateral + ventrodorsal body views) Haematology/biochemistry Endoscopy of trachea/airsacs Faecal parasitology Tracheal (deep) or airsac culture/sensitivity		Signs: change of voice (syringeal), inspiratory or expiratory (lungs/airsacs) effort, dyspnoea, exercise intolerance, weight loss, anorexia, vomition
ADR syndrome ('Ain't Doing Right')	See mouth/crop lesions; endoparasitism; aspergillosis; avian tuberculosis; enteritis (including crop/proventriculus infection); hepatic/renal disease	If mouth lesions, follow mouth/crop lesions Gross examination of mutes Haematology/biochemistry Radiography (lateral and ventrodorsal body views) Faecal parasitology + culture/sensitivity + acid-fast stain	Based on primary test results: barium study; endoscopy of coelomic cavity; renal/hepatic biopsy; proventricular flush for culture/sensitivity	Signs: loss of performance; weight loss; failure to gain weight; sometimes regurgitation, head flick
Regurgitation/vomition	Acute, 'sour crop' (foul-smelling crop/mouth): bacterial/fungal infections, foreign bodies – especially long bones; may be secondary to enteritis; trichomoniasis, capillariasis; lead poisoning; air sacculitis (see lower respiratory tract disease)	Crop wash (cytology, culture/sensitivity) Haematology/biochemistry Radiography Faecal parasitology (+ culture/sensitivity if enteritis present)		If mouth lesions, follow mouth/crop lesions If chronic, follow ADR syndrome If acute, treat as an emergency!

Figure 16.15 Common clinical signs in raptors.

- Take blood samples (haematology/biochemistry, lead)
- Immediately give treatment for most likely diagnosis based on history, etc.
- If unsuccessful, give glucose, calcium, sodium calcium edetate, and vitamin B_1 by injection
- If necessary, control fits with diazepam or under isoflurane anaesthesia until diagnosis made
- Perform radiography (for metal in gizzard).

Feather damage

Fret marks
Fret marks are damage lines on feathers due to dietary stress or metabolic stress at that stage of feather development.

- Many or all feathers affected

- Check dietary and disease history and check for endoparasites
- If problems are ongoing, perform haematology/biochemistry analysis and radiography
- The condition often reflects past problems and so there is no treatment other than to wait for the next moult
- Broken primaries, secondaries or tail feathers may be replaced by 'imping' a new feather on to the broken stump. Falconers should be encouraged to keep moulted feathers for future imping. If none of the bird's own feathers are available, feathers from other birds may be used but should be frozen for a period to reduce disease transmission.

Ectoparasites
Close examination should show the presence of ectoparasites, which may cause tatty feathers.

Feather chewing

This is often due to feather folliculitis: perform cytology and culture/sensitivity on feather pulp. Behavioural feather chewing may be seen in the Harris' hawk.

Aspergillosis

This is an all-too-common fungal disease of raptors. Certain species are especially prone, including the gyr *Falco rusticolus*, northern goshawk, golden eagle and snowy owl *Nyctea scandinavica*.

Various syndromes are seen, including lower respiratory disease, tracheal or syringeal obstruction (change of voice is practically pathognomonic for syringeal aspergilloma) and weight loss or ADR ('ain't doing right') syndrome. The disease process may be chronic (often where latent infection has been triggered by stress, such as training) or acute (often where the immune system has been overwhelmed by huge quantities of fungal spores). The prognosis is usually poor.

Diagnosis is by a combination of clinical examination and history, radiography, haematology, serum electrophoresis, endoscopy and tracheal/air sac culture (current serological tests available in the UK are of little value).

Individual aspergillomas should be removed surgically after stabilization of the bird, especially for the syringeal form; other forms must be managed medically. Therapy consists of antifungal drugs given orally or systemically and by nebulization or intratracheally. Therapy should continue for several weeks.

Prevention consists of avoiding inhalation of spores, particularly when young birds are in the nest. Rotting organic matter should be frequently removed from the birds' environment. Travelling boxes may also be a source of spores and should be cleaned and disinfected after each use (but note that cleaning immediately before use may even induce fungal spore release). Susceptible species may be given itraconazole at times of stress, e.g. training or travelling. Prophylactic dosing should be started 5–7 days *before* training, to allow effective tissue levels to be attained.

Bumblefoot

Bumblefoot is swelling of the plantar metatarsal pad complicated by secondary bacterial infection. It appears to be more common (and severe) in falcons but is now frequently seen in hawks, as well as occasionally in eagles, vultures and owls. This may reflect changing uses of birds in British falconry.

There are many suggested aetiologies, including injury, self-induced injury, incorrect perching, poor perch hygiene, excess perching weight and inactivity, Type III or IV hypersensitivity, hypovitaminosis A and cardiovascular changes. In general, *Staphylococcus* spp. are involved, though environmental organisms (such as *Escherichia coli* and *Proteus* spp.) and *Candida* spp. may be found.

The most important aspect of bumblefoot is that it is a two-footed problem. It is frequently seen in both feet but when it is unilateral the other ('good') leg should be thoroughly assessed for injury or lesions that may result in increased weight-bearing (and hence bumblefoot) in the contralateral limb.

Cooper (1978) proposed a classification of lesions:

- Type 1: a proliferative thickening or degenerative thinning of the epithelium (Figure 16.16a)
- Type 2: more extensive combination of acute inflammation and chronic reaction. Purulent material is usually present (Figure 16.16a)
- Type 3: generally a progression of Type 2 into the underlying tissues – bones, tendon sheaths, joints (Figure 16.16b). This type carries a very poor prognosis, and euthanasia should be considered.

In all cases the feet should be radiographed to assess underlying damage and, hence, prognosis. All lesions should be swabbed for culture and sensitivity (after curettage in Types 2 and 3). All cases should receive long-term antimicrobials based on culture and sensitivity test results. Prior to obtaining results, therapy may be commenced with clavulanate-potentiated amoxycillin or a combination of marbofloxacin and clindamycin.

Type 1 cases may not require surgery but the feet should be bandaged, using commercial bumblefoot pads or 'doughnut rings' of corn-dressing pads (Figure 16.16c). Dressings should be changed every 7–10 days. In unilateral cases, the unaffected foot should be dressed using a ball bandage to prevent development of lesions.

Food should be cut up, as the bird will be unable to tear for itself. Care should be taken not to include rings or equipment in dressings or to push rings up the leg, as constriction lesions may result. If the bird will not tolerate dressings, a padded bow perch may be used.

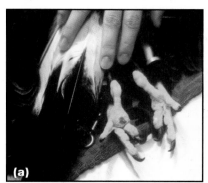
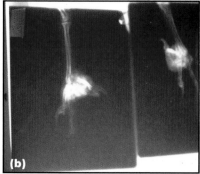
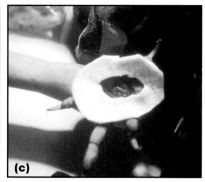

Figure 16.16 Bumblefoot. (a) Harris' hawk with Type 1 lesion (erythematous skin thinning) on the right foot and Type 2 lesion on the left foot. (b) Type 3 lesion in a Bateleur eagle. (c) 'Doughnut-ring' corn dressing being applied to a lesion on a Himalayan griffon vulture. The dressing is held on with cohesive bandage wrapped around the foot and between the digits.

More advanced cases require surgery to debride necrotic tissue. This should not be attempted without a thorough knowledge of the anatomy of the foot, as there is a risk of damaging important tendons and nerves (Harcourt-Brown, 1996, 2000). After debridement, swabs should be taken for culture. The wound may be flushed with antimicrobial solutions, or antibiotic-impregnated polymethylmethacrylate beads may be inserted (Remple and Forbes, 2000). Where possible, primary wound closure should be attempted. Where this is impossible, the wound may be left to granulate, although VetBioSIST (Cook, UK) appears to be useful in these situations (Chitty, 2000b). After surgery, feet are bandaged as described above.

Use of non-steroidal anti-inflammatory drugs is strongly recommended in all cases of bumblefoot.

Wing-tip oedema and necrosis syndrome (WTONS)

In this curious disease, blood flow to the wing tips appears to be reduced, resulting initially in oedema and then dry necrosis until the wing-tip and associated primary feathers are lost. It should be distinguished from 'blaine' (a traumatic carpitis), which is normally unilateral, centred on the carpus and warm to the touch.

The prognosis is good if the disease is caught early. Therapy involves broad-spectrum antibiosis and vascular stimulants (isoxsuprine orally and Preparation-H topically). All cases should be radiographed, because in the advanced stages erosive lesions may be seen developing in the second phalangeal bone. This is a poor prognostic sign, as is passage to dry necrosis.

The aetiology is still unknown but low ground temperatures may be involved. For prevention, no young raptor should be tethered within 45 cm of the ground (without supplying heat) in winter, nor should wet birds be left out at night in winter, whether tethered or in aviaries.

Squirrel bites

The typical squirrel bite is on the foot or leg, perhaps 2 mm long, and appears innocuous. It is therefore often left untreated other than staunching blood flow and initial cleaning. Unfortunately, these bites often introduce bacteria, and erosive infections commence. These may often not be apparent for a few weeks, by which time there may be osteomyelitis or tenosynovitis. Tendon rupture post-infection is not unknown. It is therefore recommended that squirrel bites should be seen as a matter of urgency, the wound thoroughly irrigated and antibiosis instigated – typically with a 14-day course of clavulanate-potentiated amoxycillin in the first instance.

Ectoparasites

The treatment of ectoparasites seen in raptors is summarized in Figure 16.17. Ticks are one of the very few indications for corticosteroids in raptors – general use should be avoided as they cause profound immunosuppression and a 'diabetic-like' syndrome. Other mites (e.g. *Cnemidocoptes* or *Dermanyssus* spp.) may occasionally be found. For a fuller overview of ectoparasites, see Chitty (2000a).

Endoparasites

Figure 16.18 summarizes the diagnosis of endoparasites seen in raptors. It is strongly recommended that a faecal sample be collected and submitted for parasitological examination twice a year. Drugs for treatment are given in Figure 16.20.

Supportive care

Emergency stabilization of the collapsed bird

1. *Before the bird arrives*: prepare a warmed chamber (approximately 25–30°C) and ensure that oxygen and fluids are available.
2. *Do not keep the bird waiting*: it should be seen at once, in a quiet room away from barking dogs and other stresses.
3. *Perform a brief examination* to find major injuries, lesions, etc.
   - Assess dehydration (brachial vein refill time can be useful: if more than 2 seconds, assume > 7% dehydration)
   - Stop blood loss (pressure, clamps, etc).

Parasite	Signs/significance	Treatment/control
Feather lice and mites	May result in feather damage Heavy infestation may be sign of ill-health	Piperonal powder or fipronil spray. Apply fipronil via a pad at base of neck, tail base and under each wing. *Do not soak* the bird (as per dogs)
Louse flies (hippoboscids or flat flies)	May cause anaemia in very young or very weak bird. Otherwise of little clinical significance but may act as vectors for important blood parasites, *Haemoproteus* spp. and *Leucocytozoon* spp.	Control as for feather lice and mites
Mosquitoes and gnats	May also act as vectors for blood parasites	Do not keep birds near insect breeding areas. If flown in high risk areas, apply fipronil spray to bare skin immediately before flying
Ticks	Severe, even fatal reactions to tick bites are seen. Typically massive haemorrhagic reaction centred on point of attachment, invariably on head. (Many birds also have ticks on rest of body without reaction.) Not known whether this is related to tick species, an infectious agent, or inappropriate immune reaction	Reaction: prompt use of fluid therapy, broad-spectrum antibiosis, and an i.m. injection of short-acting dexamethasone compound Control: Regular applications of fipronil (as above) Acaricidal spray may be applied to environment

Figure 16.17 Ectoparasites in raptors.

Class	Species	Signs	Diagnosis
Nematodes	*Capillaria*	White, necrotic mouth/crop lesions or enteric problems May see head flick or ADR syndrome and weight loss Rarely diarrhoea	Faecal flotation May visualize adults in pharynx or (via endoscopy) in crop or oesophagus
	Ascarids	Large numbers may cause gut impaction or rupture in young birds May cause weight loss or ADR syndrome	Faecal flotation
	Spiurid (stomach worm)	Inappetence, weight loss, ADR	Faecal flotation
	Syngamus (gapeworm)	Dyspnoea, cough	Faecal flotation or direct visualization and tracheal endoscopy
Cestodes and trematodes		Rarely of significance in the UK	
Coccidia	Especially *Caryospora*	Of great importance in falcons, especially merlin (*Falco columbarius*) May cause weight loss or ADR In severe cases results in haemorrhagic enteritis and death	Faecal flotation
Other gut protozoa	*Trichomonas*	Cause of white necrotic mouth and crop lesions ('frounce') Inappetence, dysphagia, head flick	Direct microscopy of (very) fresh wet preparation of lesions for motile protozoa
Blood parasites	*Haemoproteus Leucocytozoon Plasmodium*	Becoming more common Frequently collapsed and profoundly anaemic	Examination of blood smear Some birds may act as asymptomatic carriers so low numbers of parasites may not be significant

Figure 16.18 Endoparasites in raptors.

The aim at this stage is to assess prognosis; keep the examination brief and stress-free. In case of respiratory distress, supply oxygen by mask
4. *Give fluids* – preferably by intravenous bolus but if this causes too much distress, use the subcutaneous route (fluid plus hyaluronidase).
5. *Place in the warm chamber*, darken the area and observe every 10–15 minutes.

When the bird appears stronger, full clinical evaluation and sample collection may be carried out. If necessary this may be done under anaesthesia (if the bird is unable to cope with being handled when conscious).

Hospital equipment

Most of the equipment required for treating parrots will also suit raptors. Because the beaks of raptors are not as powerful as those of parrots, metal crop or stomach tubes are not essential and very useful tubes can be made from drip tubing or dog urinary catheters (ensure that the cut ends are smoothed off).

It is essential that hospitalized raptors do not damage wing or tail feathers, as this will reduce their flying ability until the next moult. They should be kept tethered in open areas or in kennels large enough that they do not strike the walls when bating or when being caught-up. When handling, the wings should be well restrained. To protect the tail, perching should be provided. A simple wooden block will suffice for short periods but it may be worth purchasing a travelling bow perch (for hawks) or a travelling block (for falcons). These are available from many makers of falconry equipment. If perching is not available, a tail guard can be made from X-ray film, stiff card or autoclave bags and secured at the tail base with tape.

If the practice does not hospitalize birds often, there is likely to be spoilage of food stocks. The problem can be reduced if the falconer is asked to bring a supply of the bird's normal food, which will also avoid diet change problems. Anorexic birds may be given a liquid diet by crop or stomach tube. In the short term, an amino-acid/electrolyte mixture may be used. For longer-term treatment, commercial meat-based diets may be used.

Drug administration

Intravenous
See the section on blood sampling above for intravenous access sites.

Intramuscular
Injection into the caudal third of the pectoral muscle masses is recommended. Injection into the leg muscles may be performed but is not advised when using nephrotoxic drugs, due to the presence of the renal portal blood flow (though fears about this may be overstated). Irritant substances may produce muscle damage that may be of great significance in the hunting bird. Irritant compounds (including enrofloxacin – concentrations > 2.5% should be avoided altogether – and some of the long-acting oxytetracycline preparations) should be used with care; if long-term administration is required it may be wise to use oral drugs, less irritant compounds, or drugs that need to be given less frequently.

Subcutaneous
This route may be used but is not popular, probably because of concerns over the rate of drug absorption.

Oral
This is an easy route in raptors. Liquid compounds may be given directly by stomach or crop tube (though this may cause stress). Tablets are easy to hide in food (e.g. in a chick head) and are usually taken readily.

Nebulization
This is useful in respiratory disease and allows use of drugs that may be toxic if given systemically (e.g. gentamycin, amphotericin-B).

Fluid therapy

Oral route
A crop or stomach tube is suitable for giving oral maintenance fluids or for medication of mildly debilitated birds. Many falconers are familiar with the technique (Figure 16.19) and often give fluids prior to presenting the bird to a veterinary surgeon. Isotonic solutions should be used, such as Hartmann's solution or various commercial products. Fluid should be given at a rate of 12 ml/kg bodyweight for diurnal birds and 8 ml/kg for owls (which have no crop).

Equipment
Tube – use either semi-rigid plastic tubing (made from drip tubing or dog urinary catheter) or commercial metal tubes
Technique
Two operators are required.
1. Restrain bird firmly.
2. Extend its neck fully and open the beak.
3. The glottis lies in the ventral midline: pass tube gently dorsolaterally. It may be palpated in the oesophagus or the tip may be seen in the crop.
4. Insert fluid.
To avoid regurgitation, warm fluid, inject slowly and do not exceed recommended volume (diurnal birds: 12 ml/kg; owls: 8 ml/kg). If there is resistance to passing the tube or if fluid appears in mouth, *stop*, withdraw tube and reassess.

Figure 16.19 Stomach and crop tubing.

Subcutaneous route
This method has long been disparaged as a technique, owing to the supposed slow uptake of fluid from this region, but in practice this does not always appear to be the case. Also, addition of hyaluronidase to the sterile fluids (at 150 units/l) greatly speeds absorption. This route is commonly used in collapsed birds where it is felt that excessive handling or anaesthesia would be inappropriate until the bird is further stabilized. Hartmann's (with hyaluronidase) is given at 20 ml/kg into the pre-crural fold. Typically this will be absorbed in approximately 15 minutes.

Intravenous route
This is the route of choice in the extremely debilitated bird or perioperatively. Either the right jugular or brachial vein may be catheterized. Fluids are then given either as a bolus (10 ml/kg/min – a useful technique if the bird is collapsed or at the start of surgery) or by continuous infusion using drip apparatus or a syringe pump. It may be tricky to maintain catheters in raptors in the long term.

Intraosseous route
Given the difficulties in maintaining intravenous catheters, this is the method of choice for continuing fluid therapy. Specialized intraosseous needles or spinal needles (or even hypodermic needles of an appropriate size) may be inserted into the distal ulna or proximal tibia. Pneumatized bones (e.g. humerus or femur) should *not* be used. A syringe pump or 'Flowline' apparatus must be used. Fluid is given at 10 ml/kg/h. The technique is simple but should be done in a sterile manner to avoid risk of osteomyelitis. Intraosseous needles appear to be well tolerated.

Anaesthesia

As with all species, pre-anaesthetic assessment is essential, though the high safety margin of isoflurane means that many of these assessments are now carried out under anaesthesia.

It is difficult to recommend any anaesthetic agent other than isoflurane. Halothane is risky, owing to its catecholamine sensitization of the myocardium, the simultaneous occurrence of respiratory and cardiac arrest in overdosage (isoflurane overdosage produces respiratory arrest before cardiac), and prolonged recovery (especially in sick birds) due to its significant degree of metabolism. Isoflurane also provides better analgesia. Where isoflurane is not available or practical (e.g. in the field) anaesthesia using medetomidine (200 µg/kg) and ketamine (10 mg/kg) may be used. Reversal of the medetomidine with an equal volume of atipamezole may be used. An accurate weight must be obtained first.

Anaesthesia should be induced by face mask using oxygen as the carrier gas. There appears to be no benefit in adding nitrous oxide.

- For short procedures, the bird can be maintained on a face mask
- For longer procedures, or where access to the head is required, an endotracheal tube should be placed and an appropriate circuit (e.g. Ayre's T-piece) used
- For ocular procedures, or those involving surgery of the head and neck, an air sac tube should be placed and anaesthesia maintained via this route.

During anaesthesia, heat should be supplied using a mat or a radiant heat source. Heart and respiratory rates should be monitored continuously. Pulse oximetry and ECG are also useful. At the end of the procedure, the bird should be lightly wrapped (to reduce flapping in recovery excitement) and placed in a warm quiet environment. Recovery is usually complete in a few minutes.

For a fuller description of anaesthesia of raptors and air sac tube placement, see Lawton (1996).

Drug formulary

Drug	Dose/route	Notes
Antibacterial agents		
Amoxycillin	150 mg/kg i.m. sid	*Must* use long-acting injection
Clavulanate-potentiated amoxycillin	150 mg/kg bid orally i.m.	
Clindamycin	100 mg/kg orally sid	Capsules may be used whole or opened for accurate dosing Dose may be halved if using with marbofloxacin
Enrofloxacin	15 mg/kg bid orally i.m.	Irritant injection (only use 2.5%) May cause vomition
Marbofloxacin	10 mg/kg sid orally i.m.	
Oxytetracycline	100 mg/kg sid i.m.	Long-acting injection May cause tissue necrosis
Piperacillin	100 mg/kg bid i.v., i.m.	
Potentiated sulphonamide	20–50 mg/kg bid orally	Do not use in dehydrated birds
Antifungal agents		
Amphotericin-B	1.5 mg/kg i.v. tid 5 mg/ml saline nebulize 15 min bid 1 mg/kg intra-tracheal bid	Aspergillosis Must hydrate when using systemically
Itraconazole	10 mg orally sid (prophylaxis) or bid (therapy)	Monitor liver function Excellent for aspergillosis
Nystatin	300,000 IU/kg bid orally 5 days	Not absorbed from gut Suitable for enteric fungal infections or topical use
Antiprotozoal agents		
Metronidazole	50 mg/kg sid orally	Trichomoniasis Useful for flushing wounds or bumblefoot lesions
Pyrimethamine	0.5 mg/kg bid orally 30 days	Leucocytozoonosis
Toltazuril	25 mg/kg orally once weekly × 3	
Endoparasiticides		
Fenbendazole	100 mg/kg orally once 20 mg/kg sid orally 5 days	Nematodes Capillaria
Ivermectin	200 µg/kg orally once	Nematodes
Praziquantel	5–10 mg/kg orally, s.c. once	Cestodes
Ectoparasiticides		
Ivermectin	200 µg/kg orally	Blood-sucking parasites
Fipronil		*Spray only. Do not soak*
Anti-inflammatory agents		
Dexamethasone	2–4 mg/kg sid i.m.	*Use with great care!* See text
Carprofen	5 mg/kg sid i.m., orally	
Meloxicam	0.1 mg/kg sid orally	= 2 drop/kg
Miscellaneous		
Metoclopramide	2 mg/kg bid i.v., i.m.	*Not* if gut obstruction suspected
Sodium calcium edetate	35 mg/kg bid i.m., i.v.	Lead/zinc toxicity If given i.m. then best diluted before use to reduce muscle necrosis
Diazepam	0.5–1 mg/kg i.v., i.m. bid–tid	To control fitting
Doxapram	10 mg/kg i.v.	Respiratory stimulant in anaesthetic overdosage
Isoxsuprine	½ pinch per kg bid	WTONS
Vitamin B_1	25 mg/kg i.m.	
Vitamin K_1	0.2–2.5 mg/kg sid i.m., orally	Anti-coagulant poisoning

Figure 16.20 Drug formulary for raptors.

References and further reading

Beynon PH, Forbes NA and Harcourt-Brown NH (1996) *Manual of Raptors, Pigeons and Waterfowl*. BSAVA Publications, Cheltenham

Chitty JR (2000a) Ectoparasites of raptors. In: *Proceedings of the British Veterinary Zoological Society Spring Meeting 2000*, pp. 30–31

Chitty JR (2000b) Use of VetBioSIST in Bumblefoot Management. In: *Proceedings of the Association of Avian Veterinarians Annual Conference & Expo 2000*, pp. 109–111

Cooper JE (1978) *Veterinary Aspects of Captive Birds of Prey*, 2nd edn. Standfast Press, London

Forbes NA and Cooper JE (1993) Fatty liver–kidney syndrome of merlins. In: *Raptor Biomedicine*, ed. PT Redig *et al.*, pp. 45–48. University of Minnesota Press, Minneapolis

Forbes NA and Flint C (2000) *Raptor Nutrition*. Honeybrook Farm Animal Foods, Evesham

Harcourt-Brown NH (1996) Foot and leg problems. In: *Manual of Raptors, Pigeons and Waterfowl*, ed. PH Beynon *et al.*, pp. 147–168. BSAVA Publications, Cheltenham

Harcourt-Brown NH (2000) *Birds of Prey: Anatomy, Radiology, and Clinical Conditions of the Pelvic Limb*. CD-ROM. Zoological Education Network, Lake Worth, Florida

Heidenreich M (1997) *Birds of Prey: Medicine and Management*. Blackwell Science, Oxford

Lawton MPC (1996) Anaesthesia. In: *Manual of Raptors, Pigeons and Waterfowl*, ed. PH Beynon *et al.*, pp. 79–88. BSAVA Publications, Cheltenham

Rees-Davies R (2000) Avian liver disease: etiology and pathogenesis. *Seminars in Avian & Exotic Pet Medicine* **9**(3), 115–125

Remple JD and Forbes NA (2000) Antibiotic-impregnated polymethylmethacrylate beads in the treatment of bumblefoot in raptors. In: *Raptor Biomedicine III, including Bibliography of Diseases of Birds of Prey*, ed. SJ Lumeij *et al.*, pp. 255–266. Zoological Education Network, Lake Worth, Florida

Useful addresses

Independent Bird Register, The White House Business Centre, Hatton Green, Hatton, Warwick CV35 7LA. Tel 07870 6088500; fax 01926 485006; email *jenny@ibr.org.uk*; www.ibr.org.uk Lost/found birds. Information resource. Publishes annual directory of useful addresses

Department of the Environment, Food and Rural Areas (DEFRA), Global Wildlife Division, Tollgate House, Houlton Street, Bristol BS2 9DJ

British Field Sports Society (BFSS), 59 Kennington Road, London SE1 7PZ

Federation of Zoological Gardens of Great Britain and Ireland, Zoological Gardens, Regents Park, London NW1 4RY

Acknowledgements

The author would like to thank Ashley Smith of the Hawk Conservancy and Jim Chick, Hawk Board Chairman for their help in compiling the data for Figure 16.3.

17

Reptile and amphibian anatomy and imaging

Sharon Redrobe and Roger J. Wilkinson

This chapter will focus upon the main aspects of reptile and amphibian anatomy relevant to the clinician and describe some aspects of diagnostic imaging techniques and interpretation.

Tortoises and turtles

Skeleton

Tortoises and turtles are characterized by possession of a shell. The domed carapace is connected to the ventral plastron by a bridge on either side. This 'bony box' is overlaid with keratinous scutes.

Juvenile tortoises up to one year old normally show a degree of shell flexibility. Adult pancake tortoises retain a flexible shell that allows them to crawl into rock cracks. Aquatic soft-shelled turtles have reduced ossification and leathery skin instead of scutes. Box turtles have a hinge that allows the front of the plastron to be drawn up against the carapace. African hinge-back tortoises achieve a similar effect with a hinged caudal plastron. Other species, including Mediterranean tortoises, may have a degree of plastral hinge.

The remainder of the skeleton is surprisingly conventional, although the pectoral and pelvic girdles are oriented vertically in order to buttress the shell. Large muscle masses run from the forelimb and pelvic bones to the plastron.

Digestive system

Tortoises lack teeth and rely upon the keratinous beak to cut food. The oesophagus runs down the left side of the neck to enter the gastric fundus on the left side of the coelomic cavity. The stomach lies transversely across the body, often apparently moulded into the caudal face of the liver. The pylorus empties into the duodenum on the right side. The arrangement of the pancreas varies with species but it can usually be found lying along the pyloric–duodenal junction. The spleen is a small ovoid organ that in some species is attached to the left end of the pancreas. In others it is separate and can be found next to the greater curvature of the stomach. The liver is large, incompletely divided into lobes and lies like a curtain across the coelomic cavity behind the heart and cranial to the stomach. The gall bladder is small and lies at the caudoventral border on the right side. The small intestine is relatively short and the caecum is also small. The colon is arranged into ascending, transverse and descending limbs, terminating in the proctodeum and thence the cloaca. Figure 17.1 shows a mid-sagittal section through a female tortoise.

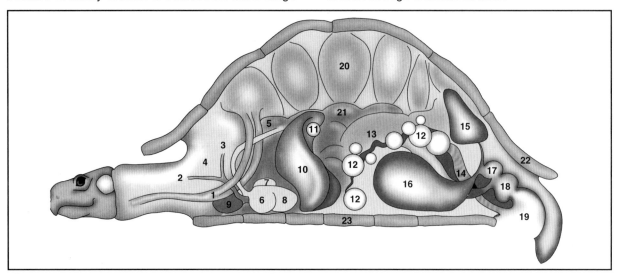

Figure 17.1 Female tortoise in mid-sagittal section. The gastrointestinal tract is incompletely shown. 1 = Tracheal bifurcation; 2 = Carotid artery; 3 = Subclavian artery; 4 = Thymus and cranial parathyroid gland; 5 = Aorta; 6 = Left atrium; 7 = Right atrium; 8 = Ventricle; 9 = Thyroid; 10 = Liver; 11 = Gall bladder in right lobe of liver; 12 = Ovarian follicles; 13 = Oviduct; 14 = Shell gland (caudal oviduct); 15 = Right kidney; 16 =Urinary bladder; 17 = Urodeum; 18 = Proctodeum; 19 = Cloaca; 20 = Lungs; 21 = Large intestine; 22 = Carapace; 23 = Plastron.

Respiratory system

The glottis is readily visualized in the caudal part of the tongue. The trachea is short and bifurcates almost immediately into the two mainstem bronchi that diverge laterally and are not obstructed when the head is withdrawn.

The lungs occupy the space beneath the dome of the carapace and are, in contrast to mammalian lungs, rather crude subdivided air sacs. The lungs lie dorsally and are separated from the rest of the viscera by a horizontal pleuroperitoneal membrane. There is no muscular diaphragm and no distinct thoracic and peritoneal cavities, but rather a single coelomic cavity. Ventilation is achieved through movements of the head, limbs and other voluntary muscles. Chelonians cannot cough.

Heart, blood vessels and thymus

Chelonian hearts have a single ventricle, which is functionally but not anatomically divided, and two atria. The heart lies horizontally, immediately above the plastron in the midline in front of the liver. Some pericardial fluid may be present, even in healthy animals. Two large carotid–subclavian arterial trunks run cranially and bifurcate at the caudal margin of the thyroid that sits in front of the heart.

A small thymus is present on each side between the carotid and subclavian arteries. These are associated with the cranial parathyroid glands. The caudal parathyroid glands lie adjacent to the aorta as it curves dorsally.

Urinary system

The kidneys lie outside the coelomic membrane beneath the carapace at the caudal margin of the lungs. The ureters run into the neck of the bladder and may thus empty either into the bladder that lies cranioventrally or into the urodeum caudally. This collecting chamber in turn communicates with the proctodeum and, through the cloaca, with the outside world. The bladder is large and very thin-walled. In many species it is bilobed. A small accessory bladder may also be present on either side at the bladder neck.

Reproductive system

Male

The testes are located immediately cranioventral to the kidneys. They fluctuate in size with season and exposure to females but are always considerably smaller than the kidneys. The erectile hemipene is normally housed in the proctodeum and is not involved in urination. Sperm is transferred to the female along a groove in the distended organ.

Female

In immature females the ovaries lie beneath the kidneys. With the onset of vitellogenesis, however, variable numbers of developing and regressing follicles come to occupy the space cranial to the bladder and further forward lateral to the intestinal tract and behind the liver. In pathological follicular stasis vast numbers of large follicles may fill the coelomic cavity. The upper part of the oviduct produces the egg white and the lower part ('shell gland'), which terminates in the cloaca, adds the calcified shell.

Radiography

Radiography can usefully be applied to examination of the skeletal system, lungs and gut of chelonians. Calcified eggs and uroliths can be located. Very little information will generally be gained concerning the kidneys, liver, heart, thyroid, pancreas or spleen.

X-ray machines capable of generating high milliampere exposures (300 mA) are optimal. Small units rely upon using a higher kVp to achieve an acceptable image. This is associated with loss of detail. For chelonian radiography, it is essential that the X-ray head can be rotated through 90 degrees to allow horizontal beam studies. For radiography of the head or limbs, non-screen film yields excellent results. Long exposure times are necessary and anaesthesia may be required.

Barium sulphate has been used in gastrointestinal studies. Five millilitres of a 30% solution administered by stomach tube is sufficient for adult Mediterranean tortoises. Gastric emptying may take 23–80 hours and total transit time 25–28 days (Holt, 1978). Transit may be faster, and more clinically useful, when using iodinated media (Meyer, 1998). Non-ionic iodine compounds (e.g. iohexol) are less toxic and less irritant should enterotomy follow. In Meyer's study, mean total transit times were 1.5–4 hours at 31°C and 3–8 hours at 21°C.

Non-ionic iodine-containing media are also appropriate for cystography. Double-contrast studies with air and contrast are useful for demonstrating eggs or calculi in the bladder.

Positioning of chelonians for radiography is described in Figure 17.2 and two radiographs shown in Figures 17.3 and 17.4.

View	Positioning	Uses
Dorsoventral	Sedation/anaesthesia unnecessary in vast majority. Ideally, limbs and head should be extended; can often be achieved by taping the caudal edge of the carapace to the cassette; patient will try to walk away from the tape whilst remaining *in situ*. Large, powerful species are restrained by placing cassette and patient inside a suitably sized box. Dorsal recumbency is stressful (lactic acidosis is common in sick chelonians), compromises respiration and complicates interpretation of results.	Particularly useful in the detection of eggs and foreign bodies and in assessment of mineralization of the pelvis. The lungs cannot be assessed.
Craniocaudal with horizontal beam (Figure 17.3)	Lateral or vertical orientation of the patient causes displacement of viscera. For horizontal beam studies the conscious patient can be immobilized by raising the legs above table level, using a beaker or tablet pot under the plastron.	Lung fields can be seen and compared.
Lateral with horizontal beam (Figure 17.4)	Use a plastral support as above. Ideally the patient should be imaged from both sides. The cassette is supported in a vertical position against the lateral aspect of the patient, using sandbags.	Two lung fields superimposed. Lateral view allows localization in two planes of lesions visible on craniocaudal or dorsoventral views.

Figure 17.2 Positioning for radiography in chelonians.

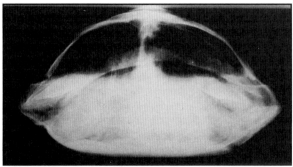

Figure 17.3 Horizontal beam craniocaudal radiograph of a chelonian with normal lung fields. (Photo: S. Redrobe.)

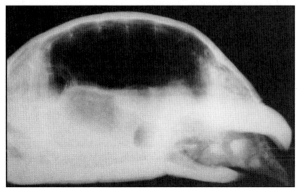

Figure 17.4 Horizontal beam lateral view radiograph of a chelonian. (Photo: S. Redrobe.)

Radiographic abnormalities

Skeleton
Figure 17.5 lists common radiographic findings in the skeletal system of chelonians.

Gastrointestinal system
Figure 17.6 lists common radiographic findings in the gastrointestinal system of chelonians.

Urinary and reproductive systems
Figure 17.7 lists common radiographic findings in the urinary and reproductive systems of chelonians.

Respiratory system
Pneumonia is common and may be unilateral or bilateral. Chronic lesions are often focal. Acute pneumonia is associated with patchy increase in density, usually concentrated ventrally. Focal lesions can be located for sampling using lateral and craniocaudal views.

Ultrasonography
Ultrasonography is a disproportionately important chelonian discipline, particularly in assessment of the heart, liver, kidneys and reproductive tract. Many animals can easily be sexed. Clinicopathological assessment of organ function is still in its infancy and many organs cannot be seen on radiographs.

To take advantage of the small scanning windows in most patients, a sector scanner with a small probe (ideally laterally flattened) is essential. Transducers of 7.5 MHz are ideal for most purposes in chelonians below 3 kg. A 5 MHz head may be required to image the liver and reproductive tract of animals over 1.5 kg. Powerful animals can damage a probe trapped between hindlimb and shell.

Metabolic bone disease	Common. Thin cortices, lucent bones. Pelvis and pectoral girdle most reliable.
Soft tissue calcification	Oversupplementation with vitamin D and/or calcium. Dystrophic calcification in inflammatory lesions, e.g. infectious granulomas.
Fractures	Uncommon except for carapacial trauma.
Septic arthritis	Common, especially in bacteraemic terrapins in dirty tanks. Lysis is the dominant sign, with little sclerosis. Surrounding soft tissue swelling. Shoulders and knees most often affected.
Articular gout	Quite common. Urate crystals are relatively radiopaque. Secondary osteoarthritis follows.

Figure 17.5 Common radiographic findings in the skeletal system of chelonians.

Helminthiasis	Common. Filling defects sometimes apparent on contrast radiography.
Foreign bodies	Very common, though presence does not prove obstruction. Rarely, lead ingestion can cause toxicity.
Obstruction	Common, especially when small individuals are housed on sand or fine gravel. Diagnosis can be assumed in a symptomatic animal when vast amounts of mineral are present in distended loops. Otherwise the passage of contrast media should be followed.

Figure 17.6 Common radiographic findings in the gastrointestinal system of chelonians.

Renal masses	Granulomas, pyogranulomas and neoplasms are visible when projecting into the caudal lung fields.
Uroliths	The bladder is extensive. Uroliths may be unexpectedly cranial or lateral. They may also be cloacal.
Follicular stasis	Increased area of soft tissue density in mid-coelom. Displacement of intestinal gas.
Calcified eggs	Do not assume that shelled eggs are necessarily an indication for intervention. Fractured eggs may be a cause or a sequel to dystocia. Abnormally thick-walled eggs are formed when passage through the oviduct is slowed. Abnormally positioned eggs may have escaped into the coelom. Eggs finding their way into the urinary bladder accumulate a rough margin of urates.

Figure 17.7 Common radiographic findings in the urinary and reproductive systems of chelonians.

Most chelonians can be scanned without sedation, particularly if cool and soporific. The assistance of a second person to hold the patient and retract one leg from the scanning site is very helpful. In animals with large enough scanning windows the probe is best applied directly to the skin via coupling gel. Where access is restricted, the site can be completely filled with gel and scanned through this. Alternatively a water-filled glove can be used as a stand-off (good for scanning eggs) or both probe and patient can be immersed in water. Non-waterproof probes should be wrapped in an examination sleeve.

Figures 17.8–17.10 illustrate acoustic windows in chelonians; ultrasound findings are listed in Figure 17.11.

View	Technique	Uses
Cervico-brachial	Retract ipsilateral forelimb. Struggling usually less if head not held. But access compromised if patient will not extend neck. Apply probe to junction of neck/forelimb. Angle beam parallel to plastron for important viscera.	Allows visualization of thyroid, heart, liver, gall bladder and stomach (Figure 17.9)
Pre-femoral	Retract ipsilateral hindlimb. Apply probe to prefemoral fossa. If carapace restricts access, fill fossa with gel or immerse in water. Angle dorsally for kidneys.	Allows visualization of bladder, gonads, oviduct and kidneys (Figure 17.10)
Transplastral	May be applicable to softshell turtles (*Trionyx*) and pancake tortoise *Malacochersus tornieri*.	

Figure 17.8 Acoustic windows in chelonians.

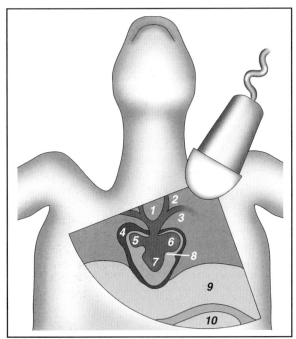

Figure 17.9 Ultrasonographic view of the cranial coelomic cavity in a tortoise via the cervico-brachial acoustic window. The important viscera are seen in the frontal plane immediately above the plastron. 1 = thyroid; 2 = carotid artery; 3 = subclavian artery; 4 = pericardial space (may contain fluid); 5 = right atrium; 6 = left atrium; 7 = ventricle; 8 = intensely echogenic atrio-ventricular valve; 9 = liver; 10 = stomach. Redrawn after McArthur and Wilkinson (in press) with the permission of Blackwell Science.

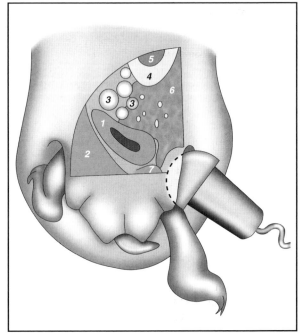

Figure 17.10 Ultrasonographic view of the caudal coelomic cavity in a female terrapin via the pre-femoral acoustic window. Due to shell anatomy, the plane of scanning is normally oblique rather than in the frontal plane. Thus, only one kidney is visualized at any one time. 1 = kidney; 2 = carapace; 3 = ovarian follicles; 4 = egg with calcified shell; 5 = yolk; 6 = urinary bladder containing hypoechoic urine and intensely echogenic urate crystals; 7 = leg musculature. Redrawn after McArthur and Wilkinson (in press) with the permission of Blackwell Science.

Thyroid	Homogeneous oval/drop-shaped organ cranial to heart and major vessels. Up to 14 mm diameter in adult Mediterranean tortoise (*Testudo*). May be enlarged in iodine deficiency. Neoplasia has been recorded.
Heart	In midline, above plastron. Single ventricle separated from 2 atria by echogenic valves. Gout and infectious lesions occur. Pericardial fluid may be normal; cytology required for diagnosis of pathological effusion. Atrial fractional shortening normally 30–50%.
Liver	Extends width of coelom behind heart. Homogeneous. Focal lesions caused by neoplasia or infection.
Gall bladder	Hypoechoic; 3–6 mm diameter on right side of liver.
Stomach	On left side caudal to liver. Best viewed when fluid-filled. Stomach tube if necessary.
Bladder	Difficult to distinguish from coelomic effusion. Intensely echoic small urate crystals are normal; larger calculi are not. Pathological presence of eggs has been reported.
Kidneys	Rounded tapering triangles. Normally homogeneous with thin hypoechoic medulla. Renal gout (echogenic mineralization) is common. Neoplasia and abscessation occur.
Testes	Rounded, homogeneous. Immediately cranioventral to kidneys. Much larger with access to females. Neoplasia reported.
Female reproductive tract	Developing follicles (spherical, homogeneous) may be found throughout coelom. Large numbers (>15) suggestive of follicular stasis. Usually concentrated cranial to bladder. Up to 25 mm at ovulation in common species. Non-calcified ova of this size may be visible within oviduct (fluid at poles). Shelled eggs are usually obvious. The hypoechoic albumen surrounds the yolk. Empty oviduct is visible as a pleated tube.

Figure 17.11 Ultrasound findings in chelonians.

Endoscopy

Endoscopy is an invaluable tool in chelonian medicine:

- The obstacle of the shell can be circumvented
- Because clinicopathological techniques are in their infancy, histopathology is disproportionately important. Endoscopy allows biopsies to be harvested from many organs.

Flexible endoscopes facilitate examination of the gastrointestinal system. However, rigid scopes give improved image clarity and, in addition to coelioscopy, can also be used to examine the upper gastrointestinal tract, cloaca, proctodeum, urodeum and bladder. Rod lens systems with a 30-degree oblique view are optimal. Facility for insufflation, irrigation and the passage of endoscopic instruments should be incorporated into the protective sheath. Flexible scissors, a flexible cup biopsy tool and an aspiration needle are the most important of these instruments. General anaesthesia is a requirement for all significant endoscopic examinations.

Coelioscopy is a surgical procedure. The endoscope should be sterilized, the surgeon should scrub and the entry site should be aseptically prepared and draped. Both left and right prefemoral fossae are suitable for access to coelomic organs. However, right-handed clinicians will usually find that a left-sided approach is most convenient. In this case, the patient should be positioned in right lateral recumbency with the left hindlimb taped back. Proper immobilization is important. A useful arrangement is to tape the animal to the side of a container filled with water at 30°C. A small skin incision is made at the centre of the fossa . Blunt haemostats are introduced through the subcutis to puncture the taught coelomic membrane. A distinct 'popping' sensation is usually apparent. Effort should be made to avoid the lungs dorsally and the bladder medially. Because of the rigid shell the coelom does not collapse and usually requires minimal insufflation. A small initial introduction of air is generally enough and avoids compromising ventilation. The lens can be cleaned by wiping it against viscera. Where biopsies

are taken, the serosa is best incised with scissors before harvesting with the biopsy tool. A single suture is usually sufficient to close the surgical skin wound.

Figure 17.12 list endoscopic findings in chelonians.

Lizards

Skeleton

Lizards possess a skull, vertebrae, ribs, pelvis, forelimb, hindlimb and tail. No sternum is present. There are generally five digits on each foot, arranged equally spaced. Chameleons have digits arranged into a pair and three digits to give an apposing grip for grasping branches.

The tail may be prehensile in some species, e.g. prehensile-tailed skink *Corucia zebrata*, or may act as a site of fat storage, e.g. leopard gecko *Eublepharis macularus*. Many species can shed the tail as a flight/fright response. This is known as autotomy and is particularly refined in geckos. The muscular spasm results in little bleeding but the shed tail is very active for a few minutes, which serves to distract the predator and enable the lizard to escape. Autotomy may occur in captivity as a result of direct trauma to the tail, e.g. handling by the tail or injecting into the tail, but may occur without direct contact as a result of a stress response. The tail will usually regenerate but the regrown tail is often of a different shade with smaller, less organized scales, and is stouter in geckos. The vertebrae of the regrown tail are usually cartilaginous rather than bony.

Skin, eyes and ears

Head ornamentation includes the three large rostral horns of the male Jackson's chameleon and the dewlap of the green iguana.

Lizards undergo ecdysis but shed pieces of skin rather than one contiguous slough. Geckos tend to eat their shed skin and so it is rarely found in the enclosure.

Lizards possess true eyelids. Chameleons are able to move their eyes independently, e.g. looking caudally as well as rostrally. Nocturnal lizards, such as the leopard gecko *Eublepharis macularus,* tend to have a vertical,

Liver	Usually the first organ encountered. Blunt edge extending caudally towards prefemoral fossa along body wall. Normally dark brown; may be yellow if lipidotic, in which case melanin pigment granules also become apparent. Biopsy easy, safe and useful.
Pleuroperitoneum	Dark, patterned underside of membrane forms roof of coelom.
Small intestine	Pale pink with superficial blood vessels. Inspect for intussusception or obstruction.
Large intestine	Larger diameter, thin-walled and with darker content.
Stomach	Large, smooth, pink structure in left cranial abdomen.
Pancreas	Best seen from the right side. Pale yellowish strip alongside duodenum.
Spleen	Discrete round organ in central cranial coelom. Often beneath small intestine. Biopsy easy and useful.
Bladder	Thin-walled and fluid-filled. Urate crystals may be visible in content. Cystocentesis relatively easy.
Kidney	Difficult to visualize at extreme caudodorsal limit of field of view. Dark brown. Ureter and blood vessels must be avoided at biopsy.
Ovary	Beneath kidneys in immature animals. Striking orange follicles of variable size occupy space in front of bladder. Vast numbers present in pathological follicular stasis. Oophoritis may also be a feature.
Testes	Globular, yellow-orange organs below kidney.
Heart	Identified by obvious beating. Beneath liver cranially. Pericardial effusions can be aspirated.

Figure 17.12 Endoscopic findings in chelonians.

slit-shaped iris, whereas diurnal lizards such as the green iguana *Iguana iguana*, have round iris fissures.

No external ear is present and the tympanic membrane is often visible. It is possible to look through the tympanic membranes of the leopard gecko from one side of the head to the other.

Alimentary tract

The alimentary tract consists of: mouth, oesophagus, stomach, small intestine, large intestine, colon, and (in some species) caecum.

Oral cavity

Teeth: Teeth are present in most species of lizard. Agamids, chameleons and tuataras are unique amongst the lizards in that they have acrodont dentition, i.e. simple laterally compressed triangular teeth ankylosed to the crest of the mandibles and maxillae, which are not continually replaced throughout life but are gradually worn down with age.

Tongue: The tongue of chameleons is retracted, like a sock, on to a bone at its base and ends in a sticky bud. When the tongue is propelled from the mouth, the bud captures the prey insect and the tongue is rapidly retracted into the mouth.

Digestive system

The stomach may be divided into cardiac, fundic and pyloric regions. The colon empties into the coprodeum of the cloaca. The liver occupies the full width of the coelom and touches the stomach and lungs, as no diaphragm is present. The liver may be pigmented in some species, e.g. chameleons, with no pathological significance. The gall bladder may be found within the lobes of the liver or located some distance away and connected by a long cystic duct. A bile duct empties its contents into the small intestine. Large coelomic fat pads are present in well fed lizards.

Respiratory system

The glottis is located at the base of the fleshy tongue on the floor of the mouth. The trachea bifurcates into mainstem bronchi that lead to two lungs of equal size. The lungs may terminate in a sac-like structure that does not take part in gaseous exchange.

Heart and blood vessels

The position of the heart is dependent upon the species of lizard. In iguanid lizards, the heart is at the thoracic inlet. The varanids (monitor lizards) have a more caudally positioned heart.

The heart consists of two atria, a left and right ventricle and a sinus venosus. The sinus venosus receives blood from the two anterior venae cavae, the posterior vena cava, the hepatic veins and the coronary vein. Both right and left aortic arches are present. A single pulmonary vein is present in most lizards.

Urinary system

The paired kidneys are usually confined within the pelvis. The kidneys empty into the urinary bladder via paired ureters. A urethra then empties the bladder into the urodeum of the cloaca. The bladder is large and may fill three-quarters of the coelom in lizards when full.

Reproductive system

The gonads are paired and attached to the vena cava on the left or the hepatic portal vein on the right. The gonad is separated from the vein by an adrenal gland on the left side, whereas the adrenal gland is on the opposite side of the vein on the right side. This has implications for gonadectomy, when the adrenal gland must be preserved; this is easier to preserve on the right side where the gland is not located within the mesovarium or mesorchium. The oviducts empty into the cloaca. The ductus deferens from each testis may join the ureter and enter the cloaca together or may remain separate. Paired erectile organs, hemipenes, are present in the male. Both sexes possess anal glands in the cranial tail.

Radiography

It is difficult to restrain lizards using mechanical restraint e.g. sandbags, ties. Small animals can be radiographed dorsoventrally through cardboard boxes or polythene bags. Some lizards will remain immobile if the head is covered with a small cloth.

The vagal–vagal response can be elicited in larger lizards (>200 g). Firm digital pressure is applied to both eyes for a few minutes. The animal will show a decreased heart rate and respiratory rate as the response occurs. The animal becomes immobile and may be positioned for radiography. This state will persist until noise or touch stimulates the animal.

The standard views are the dorsoventral (vertical beam) and lateral (horizontal beam) views. Positioning for radiography in lizards is illustrated in Figure 17.13.

View	Position	Uses
Dorsoventral	Sternal recumbency	Evaluation of skeletal density, abdominal masses
Lateral with horizontal beam (Figure 17.14)	Sternal recumbency. Position cassette as for lateral view in chelonians	The gastrointestinal tract is positioned on the ventral aspect of the coelom, allowing evaluation of the respiratory, cardiovascular and urogenital systems

Figure 17.13 Radiographic positioning for lizards.

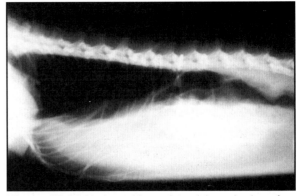

Figure 17.14 Horizontal beam lateral thoracic view of a green iguana. (Photo: S. Redrobe.)

Normal radiographic anatomy

The lungs are sac-like organs with no radiographic internal structure normally. A moderate amount of gas is normal within the gastrointestinal tract. The liver can rarely be distinguished from the intestines.

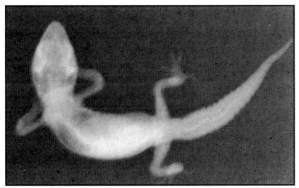

Figure 17.15 Dorsoventral radiograph of a leopard gecko *Eublepharis macularus* with severe nutritional hyperparathyroidism. Note the very poor skeletal density compared with the soft tissues. (Photo: S. Redrobe.)

Radiographic abnormalities

Skeleton

Poor skeletal density (Figure 17.15) is a common finding; if it is suspected, the voltage should be reduced. Normal lizards show similar bone/soft tissue contrast to mammals. Figure 17.16 lists common radiographic findings in the skeletal system of lizards.

Gastrointestinal system

Helminthiasis is common in lizards; filling defects are sometimes visible on contrast radiography. Foreign bodies are very common in pet iguanas but their presence does not prove obstruction. A diagnosis of obstruction can be assumed in a symptomatic animal when vast amounts of material are present in distended bowel loops or when the passage of contrast medium is impaired.

Urinary and reproductive systems

Figure 17.17 lists common radiographic findings in the urinary and reproductive systems of lizards and Figure 17.18 shows follicles and eggs in a green iguana.

Metabolic bone disease (Figure 17.15)	Common. Decreased bone opacity; decreased cortical thickness; angular deformities of the long bones; increase then decrease of the trabecular pattern as the disease progresses. Pathological fractures are common, especially of ribs and long bones. Recovered animals may retain angular deformities of long bones and may have an abnormal trabecular bone pattern.
Soft tissue calcification	Oversupplementation with vitamin D and/or calcium; renal failure; nutritionally induced hyperparathyroidism; or dystrophic calcification in inflammatory lesions, e.g. infectious granulomas. Affected tissues include subcutaneous tissues, kidneys, heart, aortic arch and oviducts.
Fractures	Long bone fractures differ radiographically between mammals and reptiles. More dependence is placed upon the callus formation for stabilization of the fracture in reptiles, hence the appearance of a fracture line in a functionally healed fracture. Radiographic changes associated with a healing fracture are only detected at 12–16 weeks.
Septic arthritis	Fairly common. Detected radiographically by soft tissue swelling in the affected area and osteolysis of the joint. Minimal new bone formation is present compared to mammals.
Articular gout	Urate crystals relatively radiopaque. Secondary osteoarthritis follows.

Figure 17.16 Common radiographic findings in the skeletal system of lizards.

Renal masses, nephromegaly	Enlarged kidneys protrude from the cranial pelvis. Colonic entrapment may present as excess gas in the distal colon and large amounts of faecal matter in the large intestine.
Uroliths	The bladder is extensive. Uroliths may be unexpectedly cranial or lateral. They may also be cloacal.
Follicular stasis (Figure 17.18a)	Increased area of soft tissue density in mid-coelom. Displacement of intestinal gas. Radiography of the abdomen will reveal multiple round soft tissue masses in the cranial abdomen. The caudal abdomen will show a loss of serosal detail due to fluid accumulation.
Calcified eggs (Figure 17.18b)	Dystocia is difficult to diagnose on radiographic findings alone. It is normal for the caudal coelomic cavity to be completely filled with 40–60 round soft tissue masses (follicles) or rounded, oblong structures that deform each other where they abut (eggs). The eggshell becomes more radiopaque the longer the eggs are retained. A diagnosis of dystocia is based upon history and clinical signs together with radiographic interpretation.

Figure 17.17 Common radiographic findings in the urinary and reproductive systems of lizards.

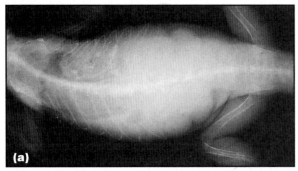
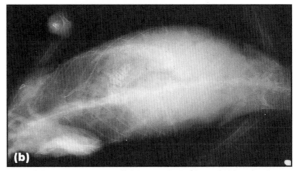

(a)

(b)

Figure 17.18 Dorsoventral radiographs of a green iguana, showing (a) multiple round follicles within the coelom, and (b) multiple shelled eggs within the coelom. (Photo: S. Redrobe.)

Respiratory system

Pneumonia is common but is difficult to detect radiographically unless it is severe. A fluid line may be observed on the horizontal beam lateral view.

Ultrasonography

Pet iguanas can often be scanned without sedation or anaesthesia. Less tractable animals require light general anaesthesia. The whole of the ventral surface of the animal can be scanned. Figure 17.19 shows an ultrasound image of a green iguana and Figure 17.20 lists ultrasound findings in lizards.

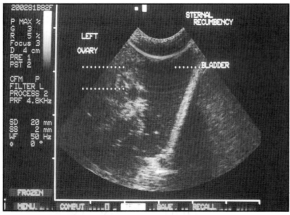

Figure 17.19 Ultrasound image of the ovary and bladder of a green iguana. (Photo: S. Redrobe.)

Endoscopy

Endoscopy is an invaluable tool in lizard medicine. Flexible endoscopes facilitate examination of the gastrointestinal system but their use is limited in captive pet lizards due to the small size of the lizard. Rigid scopes give improved image clarity and are invaluable in performing a coelioscopy. Rod lens systems with a 30-degree oblique view are optimal.

Endoscopy allows biopsies to be harvested from many organs. Facility for insufflation, irrigation and the passage of endoscopic instruments should be incorporated into the protective sheath. Flexible scissors, a flexible cup biopsy tool and an aspiration needle are the most important of these instruments. General anaesthesia is a requirement for all endoscopic examinations.

Coelioscopy is a surgical procedure requiring aseptic technique and general anaesthesia. The endoscope should be sterilized, the surgeon should scrub and the entry site should be aseptically prepared and draped. Access via a paramedian incision is suitable for access to most coelomic organs. Minimal insufflation is usually required to facilitate visualization in the coelomic cavity.

Figures 17.21 and 17.22 illustrate endoscopic findings in lizards.

Thyroid	Located anterior and dorsal to the heart, by the tracheal bifurcation. Single, bilobed or paired thyroid in different lizard species or within same species.
Parathyroid glands	Cranial pair at the bifurcation of the common carotid artery; caudal pair associated with the thymus. May be grossly enlarged in hyperparathyroidism; fibrotic parathyroids in chronic cases appear hyperechoic.
Heart	The thin myocardium in even large iguanas makes the interpretation of M mode images difficult. The atrioventricular valves and the hepatic vein leading from the liver to the sinus venosus can be imaged on the longitudinal view of the heart. The atria and ventricle can be imaged and measured.
Liver	Imaged from the flank, caudal to the elbow. Uniformly echogenic but less so than the fat pads. The anechoeic gall bladder is easily seen. Abscesses are discrete hyperechoic masses within the liver parenchyma. Hepatic lipidosis is imaged as a diffuse increase in echogenicity of the liver parenchyma. The portal vein and hepatic vein may be imaged, the portal vein being more echogenic.
Gall bladder	Fluid-filled organ near the liver.
Gastrointestinal tract	The thin-walled stomach of the herbivorous lizards is not easily seen. Gas is often present and obstructs the image. The large intestine can be detected and the large mucosal folds imaged.
Kidneys	Sited within the pelvis and can be imaged by placing the transducer just cranial to the pelvis and angling the transducer caudally. Enlarged kidneys are more easily imaged as they protrude from the pelvic area. Gout is detected as hyperechoic speckling. Neoplasia and abscessation may be detected as disruption to the normal architecture.
Testes	The testes are small oval structures in the dorsal abdomen. They are more hyperechoic than ovaries and have a homogeneous texture.
Female reproductive tract (Figure 17.19)	Ultrasonography is particularly useful for small ova difficult to see on radiography. Care must be taken to differentiate uncalcified eggs from bowel loops. This distinction is made by rotating the transducer through 90 degrees: the bowel appears as a tube whereas the follicles remain spherical. Eggs may be detected in the oviduct and the internal contents imaged. Ovaries may be detected, containing many small (<0.5 cm), round, hypoechoic areas (previtelline follicles). Large (up to 2.5 cm), round and more hyperechoic structures (vitelline follicles) develop later. Once ovulated, the spherical appearance is lost and the structures become ovoid. As the shell is deposited, the oval structure becomes increasingly hyperechoic.
Bladder (Figure 17.19)	Imaged readily, especially when full as it then occupies a large portion of the coelom. The anechoeic urine may have hyperechoic particles of urates floating within it. The fluid-filled bladder acts as an acoustic window through which to image the other organs.
Coelomic fat pads	Large coelomic fat pads in well-fed lizards may occupy a large area of the ventral coelom. The fat pads have a granular internal structure with hyperechoic septa.

Figure 17.20 Ultrasound findings in lizards.

Liver	Normally dark brown; may be yellow if lipidotic, in which case melanin pigment granules also become apparent.
Pleuroperitoneum	Dark, patterned underside of membrane forms roof of coelom.
Small intestine	Pale pink with superficial blood vessels. Inspect for intussusception or obstruction.
Large intestine	Larger diameter, thin-walled and with darker content.
Stomach	Large, smooth, pink structure in left cranial abdomen.
Spleen	Discrete round organ on greater curvature of stomach.
Bladder	Thin-walled and fluid-filled. Urate crystals may be visible in content.
Kidney	Difficult to visualize at extreme caudal coelom within pelvis if normal sized. Dark brown. Ureter and blood vessels must be avoided at biopsy.
Ovary (Figure 17.22)	Striking orange follicles of variable size occupy space in front of bladder. Vast numbers present in pathological follicular stasis.
Testes	Globular, cream-coloured organs attached to caudal vena cava.
Heart	Identified by obvious beating. Beneath liver cranially.

Figure 17.21 Endoscopic findings in lizards.

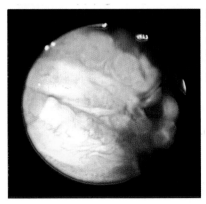

Figure 17.22 Endoscopic view of the ovary and oviduct of a green iguana. (Photo: S. Redrobe.)

Organ	Position along total length from rostrum to cloaca, expressed as % (Boidae)	Position expressed as cranial, middle or caudal third (Boidae)
Trachea	0–22	Cranial third
Heart	22–33	Cranial third
Lungs	33–45	Middle third
Air sac	45–65	Middle third
Liver	38–56	Middle third
Stomach	46–67	Middle third
Intestines	68–81	Caudal third
Right kidney	69–77	Caudal third
Left kidney	74–82	Caudal third
Colon and cloaca	81–100	Caudal third

Figure 17.23 The position of body organs in snakes.

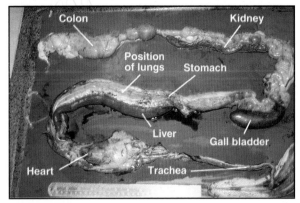

Figure 17.24 Postmortem specimen of a large boa constrictor divided into thirds to show relative organ positions. (Photo: S. Redrobe.)

Snakes

The topographical anatomy of snakes is similar to the general vertebrate organization. Because the body is long and thin, the organs are often ordered one or two at a time along the length. It is convenient to divide the snake into thirds along its length or to use percentages of snout–vent length when describing the positions of various organs (Figures 17.23 and 17.24).

Skeleton

The snake skull is more complex that the mammalian skull. The bones of the jaws are loosely connected to permit a wide gape so that prey can be swallowed whole. The bones of the 'nose' articulate with the cranium region to further increase the gape size. The halves of the lower jaw are connected by an elastic ligament that allows separation to further increase the opening of the mouth.

Each vertebra possesses a body, arch and spinous process. Numbers vary from 150 to over 400 and they are similar in shape. The vertebral bodies articulate as a convex/concave joint, with the cranial part being concave. The bodies of the tail vertebrae possess paired haemal processes on the ventral aspect, which house the coccygeal (caudal) artery and vein.

Paired ribs articulate with vertebrae beginning at the third vertebra, although some species also have ribs attached to the most cranial vertebrae. Snakes do not possess a sternum or costal cartilage. The ribs are fused to the vertebrae in the postcloacal region. The ribs function to protect the viscera and to propel the snake. Each rib ends in a rounded tip that contacts the inside of the ventral skin to transmit movement. The dasypeltid 'egg-eating snakes' possess ventral projections from the vertebral bodies that serve to break the egg as it passes down the oesophagus. Lateral spreading of the ribs produces the hood of the cobra.

Snakes do not possess a pectoral girdle and only some species possess a pelvic girdle. Cloacal spurs are present in some male snakes; these are remnants of the pelvic limb. Spurs are present in all male boa constrictors but also in some females (although they are generally smaller in females). Their presence is a reliable indicator of the male sex in sand boas (*Eryx* spp.) and the rosy boa *Lichanura trivirata* but are too variable in the Royal python *Python regius*.

Skin and external morphology

The skin is arranged into scales, each overlapping the next caudal scale. Small lateral and dorsal scales cover most of the body in a mosaic arrangement. Large single ventral scales extend to the cloaca, which opens as a transverse slit toward the caudal end of the body. Caudal to the cloaca the subcaudal ventral scales are paired. The postcloacal part of the snake is referred to as the tail.

Snakes do not possess eyelids, so the eyes are permanently open. A transparent scale, the spectacle or brille, protects the cornea. No external ear, auditory meatus or tympanic membrane is present though there is an inner ear and stapes.

Ecdysis

The tough, smooth, flexible skin does not grow to increase in size with the snake. The snake sheds its skin periodically in a process known as ecdysis. The germinative layer is active intermittently and therefore two separate layers may exist at the same time, producing an outer and inner epidermal layer. The deep part of the outer layer changes structure in the days prior to ecdysis, resulting in a cloudy appearance to the skin. The spectacle becomes opaque and the snake is often lethargic and inappetent at this stage. Approximately 5–8 days before ecdysis, the skin clears again as the outer epidermal layer breaks down. Ecdysis occurs after a further 4–7 days, immediately preceded by a slight dullness of colour.

Ecdysis begins at the lips. As the snake removes the skin it is turned inside out, although the final tail section may be slipped off right side out. The dermal layer contains the pigmentation of the skin and therefore the shed epidermal layer is transparent. Rattlesnakes do not shed the most caudal scales but retain them to form the rattle that therefore enlarges with successive moults.

Alimentary tract

Oral cavity

Teeth and fangs: Snakes are generally carnivorous, although some species feed predominantly on eggs. The teeth are arranged in rows facing caudally in the mouth and are produced continually. There may be teeth on both jaws or on one jaw or, in some species, no teeth at all. The loose connection between the bones of the jaws and skull enable the snake to pull food items into the mouth using first one side of the mouth and then the other. This action is often referred to as chewing, but it is merely movement of the food into the mouth and not maceration of the food as in mammals. Snakes appear to yawn after envenomation or ingestion of prey. This action allows repositioning of the skull and jawbones after separation.

Some snakes produce venom from special glands, which are not modified salivary glands as is often assumed. Enlarged teeth, called fangs, are involved in delivering the venom to the prey. The venom gland lies above the oral cavity, caudal to the eye and may extend down the body in some species.

The front-fanged snakes, e.g. vipers, possess venom ducts leading to the fangs. The fangs are hinged in the jaw and erected prior to envenomation. An enclosed channel in the tooth provides an efficient venom delivery injection system. Reserve fangs are arranged within the duct system so that if one set of fangs is broken off another set is immediately available for use.

Some snakes appear to spit out venom. In these species the venom is forced out of the fangs by muscular contraction of the venom glands. The venom serves to disable the victim to permit ease of capture and ingestion.

Tongue: The slender, forked tongue of snakes is housed in a sheath on the floor of the mouth. It is used as a tactile organ and to sample scent. Scent particles picked up by the flicking tongue are deposited into paired openings on the roof of the mouth. These openings communicate with the vomeronasal organ of Jacobson. Nerves from this organ connect to the olfactory area of the brain. The tongue may flick in and out through the labial notch even when the mouth is closed.

Salivary glands: The salivary glands produce copious amounts of fluid during the act of ingestion; little saliva is present in the mouth at other times.

Digestive system

The oesophagus is not distinct from the pharynx and oral cavity and is only differentiated from the tubular stomach by the glandular mucous membrane apparent in the stomach lining. The constriction of the pylorus at the distal end of the stomach opens into the small intestine, which is arranged in simple coils. The large intestine is a thin-walled straight tube by comparison. The Boidae possess a small caecum at the junction of the small and large intestine. The large intestine is separated from the cloaca by a membranous fold. Anal glands are positioned caudal to the cloacal external orifice and open into the cloaca.

Respiratory system

Paired nostrils are positioned on the dorsal aspect of the head, leading to the internal nares. There is no hard palate.

The larynx is prominent in the middle of the floor of the mouth. Complete tracheal rings and the larynx form the glottal tube that resists flattening when a large prey item is swallowed. The glottal tube continues the trachea proper, with complete and incomplete rings. The trachea bifurcates just caudal to the heart if two lungs are present. There is no diaphragm.

Most species of Boidae possess two lungs, although the right lung is usually larger. Colubridae and Viperidae possess only a vestigial left lung which may be completely absent in some species. In those species that possess only a right lung, a tracheal lung is often present. This is formed by a ballooning of the tracheal lining that lies parallel to the oesophagus and is a vascularized organ capable of gaseous exchange. The lung may terminate in a simple bag that does not take part in gaseous exchange.

Heart and blood vessels

The three-chambered heart is long and narrow. The single caudal vena cava and paired cranial venae cavae empty into the sinus venosus on the dorsal aspect of the heart. The right atrium and sinus venosus are difficult to distinguish externally but are separated internally by a sinoatrial valve. The single muscular ventricle communicates with the atria via paired atrio-ventricular valves. Blood leaves the ventricle through the semilunar valves of the right or left aortic arch or the pulmonary artery. The right aortic arch branches to form the bicarotid trunk then courses caudally to fuse with the left aortic arch in the dorsal midline. The small thyroid gland lies immediately cranial to the heart and is supplied by the smaller right common carotid. The left carotid supplies the head and cranial body. The (fused) dorsal aorta continues caudally along the ventral vertebral column to enter the haemal processes and becomes the caudal coccygeal vein in the tail.

Urinary system

The right kidney is positioned more cranially than the left. The paired ureters open into the cloaca. There is no urinary bladder.

Reproductive system

In the male, the testes are positioned cranial to the kidneys and are spindle shaped or oblong. The deferent duct opens into the cloaca. Twin penile structures called hemipenes are located within the tail caudal to the cloaca. The retracted hemipenes lie ventral to the anal sacs. When engorged they evert through the cloaca. Grooves extending from the deferent duct openings in the cloaca to the base of the hemipenes carry the spermatozoa. There is no urethra in the hemipenes.

In the female, the size and shape of the ovaries vary with the sexual cycle. They are positioned cranial to the kidneys and may possess many round ova. The paired pleated oviducts empty into the cloaca. Some species possess only a right oviduct.

Radiography

X-ray machines capable of generating high milliampere exposures (300 mA) are optimal for snakes. It is essential that the X-ray head can be rotated through 90 degrees to allow horizontal beam studies (Figures 17.25 and 17.26).

Conscious restraint using adhesive tape is often not satisfactory because of movement blur produced on the film. Radiolucent acrylic tubes are available to

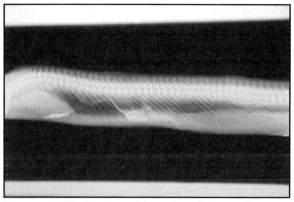

Figure 17.26 A horizontal beam lateral view radiograph of a normal snake. Note the position of the trachea and heart, and the lack of architecture within the lungs. (Photo: S. Redrobe.)

restrain sections of the snake for radiography. Snakes often require general anaesthesia for positioning.

The snake should be radiographed in sequential straight sections along its length. Radiographic markers placed along the length of the snake enable the accurate location of any radiographic findings.

Normal radiographic anatomy

The heart and liver are indistinct but are most discernible on the lateral view. There is a variable amount of ingesta and gas in the gastrointestinal tract. The right lung is positioned cranially, extending from the heart to just cranial to the right kidney. The left lung is much reduced and absent in some species. No internal structure of the lungs can be detected radiographically in the normal animal. The size of the liver can be estimated by assessing the displacement of other viscera.

Radiographic abnormalities

Skeleton

Healing fractured ribs show a greater periosteal reaction radiographically than in mammals and other reptiles. Exuberant new bone formation associated with the spine is a common finding and not always associated with lytic disease but may still be a sign of osteomyelitis. Skeletal remains from ingested prey may be confused with skeletal system pathology or soft tissue calcification. Figure 17.27 lists common radiographic findings in the skeletal system of snakes.

View	Positioning	Uses
Dorsoventral	Ventral recumbency, vertical beam	Spinal column, skull. Differentiation of location of lesions to left or right. Position of trachea, lungs
Lateral with horizontal beam (see Figure 17.26)	Ventral recumbency, horizontal beam. Position cassette as for chelonians	Position of trachea, heart, spinal column. Visualization of lungs, fluid lines

Figure 17.25 Positioning for radiography in snakes.

Soft tissue calcification	Oversupplementation with vitamin D and/or calcium. Dystrophic calcification in inflammatory lesions, e.g. infectious granulomas.
Fractures	Uncommon except for rib fractures.
Septic arthritis	Exuberant new bone formation and fusion associated with the spine, not always associated with lytic disease but may still be a sign of osteomyelitis.
Articular gout	Quite common. Urate crystals are relatively radiopaque. Secondary osteoarthritis follows

Figure 17.27 Common radiographic findings in the skeletal system of snakes.

Gastrointestinal system

It is difficult to identify masses of the liver, spleen, pancreas and kidney as distinct from the gastrointestinal tract on plain radiography. Contrast studies are valuable in the elucidation of gastrointestinal tract abnormalities, and to allow distinction between gastrointestinal tract and other soft tissue structures on the radiograph. Barium sulphate suspension is administered by gavage at 5 ml/kg. The immediate introduction of 45 ml/kg of air into the tube provides a double contrast study (Jackson and Sainsbury, 1992). Oesophageal folds, gastric rugae, the pyloric sphincter and duodenal villi may be identified 15 minutes following barium gavage. The administration of metoclopramide (2–5mg/kg) will reduce the gastrointestinal tract transit time from approximately 4–7 days to 20 hours.

Obstruction or constipation is a common finding in captive large snakes. Contrast studies are required to differentiate it from renal, gonadal or hepatic masses.

Urinary and reproductive systems

Granuloma, pyogranuloma and neoplasia present as masses in the area of the kidney. Multiple small masses noted in the area of the ovary may be follicular stasis. Eggs with shells or coiled fetal skeletons (in live bearers) may be noted.

Pulmonary and cardiovascular systems

Pneumonia is difficult to detect using radiography unless it is severe. A fluid line may be apparent on the horizontal beam lateral view.

In cardiomegaly, an enlarged cardiac silhouette and elevated trachea may be seen on the horizontal lateral view.

Pericardial gout is a potentially fatal sequel to dehydration and shows as radiopacity associated with the heart.

Ultrasonography

The small cross-sectional area and thin body wall of snakes means that high-resolution equipment is required in all but the largest patients. A 7.5–10 MHz sector transducer is generally used. In small snakes (100–250 g) a stand-off is required. This can be achieved by using a water-filled surgical glove placed between the transducer and the patient's skin. Alternatively, the patient is partially submerged in warm water and the transducer placed underwater at an appropriate distance from the animal to achieve the optimal image.

Tractable snakes may be scanned without the use of chemical restraint. Aggressive or highly mobile snakes require sedation or light general anaesthesia.

The snake is scanned across the ventral body wall methodically from a rostral to caudal direction using transverse and longitudinal scanning planes to enable all organs to be identified and noted as normal or abnormal. In larger snakes intercostal placement of the transducer may avoid the ribs interfering with the ultrasound picture but in smaller snakes acoustic shadows may 'stripe' the image. Figure 17.28 lists ultrasound findings in snakes.

Heart	Located by visualizing the beating organ beneath the scales. Sited ventrally in the caudal half of the front third of the snake. Atria, ventricles and atrioventricular valves may be visualized, depending on size. In snakes >300g, right and left aortic arches may be followed cranially to the common carotid artery. Pericardial fluid is rarely seen. Pericardial gout may be seen in debilitated, dehydrated snakes.
Liver	Caudal to the heart. Homogeneous. Focal lesions caused by infection or neoplasia. Lipidosis denoted by increased echogenicity.
Fat pads	Not readily identifiable in snakes of 'normal' weight. May fill whole abdominal area of a well fed or obese snake. More echogenic than liver, with hyperechoic septa within fat pads.
Gastrointestinal tract	The transducer is placed cranial to the mass and moved caudally. Masses within the body can be identified as arising from the tubular gastrointestinal tract or other, more solid, organs. The stomach wall is generally thin and poorly defined, unless abnormally thickened, e.g. in cryptococcidiosis.
Kidneys	Caudal to the gonads. Similar echotexture to the liver, being uniform throughout. Faecal pellets may be imaged within the large intestine in this area. Focal gout may occur. Neoplasia and abscessation may be seen.
Testes	Oval, hyperechoic structures caudal to the gall bladder/spleen/pancreas triad. Right testis positioned more cranially than the left. Testes have a uniform echotexture. In larger snakes the deferent duct may be seen as hyperechoic parallel lines originating from the testis.
Female reproductive tract	Shelled eggs are hyperechoic, dense spherical or oval structures caudal to the ovaries. Ultrasound beam may penetrate thin-walled or leathery eggs. The hypoechoic albumin is often positioned in one half of the egg with the more echogenic yolk occupying the other half. Moving fetuses may be observed in ovoviviparous snakes. Hyperechoic, homogeneous egg masses between fetuses are infertile eggs.
	Ovaries are difficult to locate in the non-cycling female when they may be only the size of the spleen. In sexually active, cycling females the ovaries may fill a large part of the coelom. Follicles on the ovary are spherical structures. Developing previtelline follicles are hypoechoic; mature vitelline follicles are hyperechoic.
Anal sac	Distal to the cloaca, hypo- or anechoic round or oval structure. Larger in most females than in males. Abscesses appear hyperechoic.
Hemipenes	Inverted hemipenes are located ventral to the anal sac and can be detected as a hyperechoic area. There is no equivalent structure in females.
Spleen, pancreas gall bladder	Triad serves as a useful landmark in the middle of the snout–vent length of the snake, caudal to the liver yet and cranial to the gonads and kidneys. Gall bladder is an anechoic focal area. Spleen is a small regular sphere slightly more hyperechoic than the liver and seen only in larger snakes. Pancreas is often indiscernible but may be seen as a less hyperechoic form in the group. In cases of anorexia, the gall bladder is often greatly enlarged, filling approximately one third of the diameter.

Figure 17.28 Ultrasound findings in snakes.

Endoscopy

Even small snakes can be endoscoped as the endoscope is usually narrower than the typical prey item. Flexible endoscopes facilitate examination of the gastrointestinal system. Rigid scopes give improved image clarity and, in addition to coelioscopy, can also be used to examine the upper gastrointestinal tract and cloaca. Rod lens systems with a 30-degree oblique view are optimal. General anaesthesia is a requirement for all significant endoscopic examinations.

Endoscopy allows biopsies to be harvested from many organs. Facility for insufflation, irrigation and the passage of endoscopic instruments should be incorporated into the protective sheath. Flexible scissors, a flexible cup biopsy tool and an aspiration needle are the most important of these instruments. Coelioscopy is a surgical procedure. The endoscope should be sterilized, the surgeon should scrub and the entry site should be aseptically prepared and draped. The coelomic cavity is small in snakes and visualization of the coelomic organs usually requires insufflation.

Figure 17.29 lists endoscopic findings in snakes.

Liver	Normally dark brown. May be yellow if lipidotic, in which case melanin pigment granules also become apparent. Biopsy is easy, safe and useful.
Pleuroperitoneum	Dark, patterned underside of membrane forms roof of coelom.
Small intestine	Pale pink with superficial blood vessels.
Large intestine	Larger diameter, thin-walled and with darker content.
Stomach	Large, smooth, pink structure.
Kidney	Dark brown. Ureter and blood vessels must be avoided at biopsy.
Ovary	Yellow follicles of variable size.
Testes	Globular, cream-coloured organs.
Heart	Identified by obvious beating.

Figure 17.29 Endoscopic findings in snakes.

Amphibians

Skeleton

Most adult amphibians have forelimbs, hindlimbs, a pelvis and a pectoral girdle. Newts and salamanders possess a tail; adult frogs and toads do not.

Skin and respiratory system

The epidermis and dermis are extremely thin. Even minor trauma can breach this barrier and become a source of systemic infection. Toxin-producing glands are present in some species and are stimulated by excitement or stress of the animal.

The lungs or skin are the primary site of respiration in terrestrial amphibians, whereas gills and skin are used in aquatic amphibians. There is no diaphragm. The glottis is readily visualized caudal to the tongue. The trachea is short and bifurcates into the two mainstem bronchi.

Alimentary tract

Some species have teeth that may inflict wounds on human handlers. The oesophagus enters the gastric fundus of the stomach. The stomach lies across the coelom. The pylorus empties into the duodenum. The liver is large and lies across the coelomic cavity behind the heart and cranial to the stomach. The colon terminates in the proctodeum and thence the cloaca.

Heart

Amphibian hearts have a single ventricle, which is functionally but not anatomically divided, and two atria.

Urinary system

Paired kidneys empty into ureters that run into the neck of the bladder. The bladder empties into the urodeum.

Reproductive system

Male

The testes are located cranioventral to the kidneys. There is no hemipene.

Female

The ovaries lie near the kidneys. With the onset of vitellogenesis, vast numbers of follicles may fill the coelomic cavity.

Radiography

Radiography can usefully be applied to examination of the skeletal system, lungs and gut of amphibians. Gastrointestinal tract foreign bodies and uroliths can be located. Very little information is generally gained concerning the kidneys, liver, heart, thyroid, pancreas or spleen.

Barium sulphate has been used in gastrointestinal studies. Non-ionic iodine compounds (e.g. iohexol) are less toxic and less irritant should enterotomy follow.

Dorsoventral and lateral views are possible (Figure 17.30).

Radiographic abnormalities

Skeleton

Metabolic bone disease is common and may be shown by thin cortices, lucent bones, spinal deformities or abdominal bloating. Soft tissue calcification may be caused by oversupplementation with vitamin D and/or calcium, or by dystrophic calcification in inflammatory

View	Technique	Advantages
Dorsoventral	Placement in plastic bag. Sedation or anaesthesia is required	This view is particularly useful in the detection of foreign bodies and in the assessment of mineralization of the skeleton.
Lateral with horizontal beam	Ideally the patient should be imaged from both sides. Position cassette as for chelonians	The two lung fields are superimposed. The lateral view allows localization in two planes of lesions visible on dorsoventral plate.

Figure 17.30 Radiographic positioning in amphibians.

lesions, e.g. infectious granulomas. Fractures are uncommon.

Gastrointestinal system

Foreign bodies and gastric impaction are very common and usually caused by ingesting too large a prey item or overfeeding by the owner. The presence of a foreign body does not prove obstruction. Rarely, lead ingestion can cause toxicity.

Urinary and reproductive systems

Renal and ovarian granulomas, pyogranulomas and neoplasms may be seen as masses projecting into the caudal lung fields.

Ultrasonography

As most patients are small, a sector scanner with a small probe (preferably laterally flattened) is essential. Transducers of 7.5 MHz are ideal for most purposes.

Most can be scanned without sedation. The probe is best applied directly to the skin via coupling gel. Where access is restricted, the site can be completely filled with gel and scanned through this. Alternatively both probe and patient can be immersed in water. Non-waterproof probes should be wrapped in an examination sleeve.

Figure 17.31 lists ultrasound findings in amphibians.

Heart	Lies in midline. Single ventricle separated from two atria by echogenic valves.
Liver	Extends width of coelom behind heart. Homogeneous. Focal lesions caused by neoplasia or infection.
Stomach	Caudal to liver. Best viewed when fluid-filled. Stomach tube if necessary.
Bladder	Difficult to distinguish from coelomic effusion.
Kidneys	Normally homogeneous with thin hypo-echoic medulla. Neoplasia and abscessation occur.
Testes	Rounded, homogeneous. Immediately cranioventral to kidneys. Much larger with access to females.
Female reproductive tract	Developing follicles (spherical, homogeneous) may be found throughout coelom.

Figure 17.31 Ultrasound findings in amphibians.

Endoscopy

Endoscopy is commonly used to remove gastric foreign bodies from captive amphibians.

Flexible endoscopes facilitate examination of the gastrointestinal system. However, rigid scopes give improved image clarity and, in addition to coelioscopy, can also be used to examine the upper gastrointestinal tract, cloaca, proctodeum, urodeum and bladder. Rod lens systems with a 30-degree oblique view are optimal. Facility for insufflation, irrigation and the passage of endoscopic instruments should be incorporated into the protective sheath. Flexible scissors, a flexible cup biopsy tool and an aspiration needle are the most important of these instruments.

General anaesthesia is a requirement for all significant endoscopic examinations. Coelioscopy is a surgical procedure. A small initial introduction of air is generally enough and avoids compromising ventilation.

Figure 17.32 lists endoscopic findings in amphibians.

Liver	Usually the first organ encountered. Blunt edge extending caudally Normally dark brown; may be yellow if lipidotic, in which case melanin pigment granules also become apparent.
Pleuroperitoneum	Dark, patterned underside of membrane forms roof of coelom.
Bladder	Thin-walled and fluid-filled. Cystocentesis is relatively easy.
Kidney	Difficult to visualize at extreme caudodorsal limit of field of view. Dark brown. Ureter and blood vessels must be avoided at biopsy.
Ovary	Follicles of variable size.
Testes	Globular, yellow–orange organs below kidney.
Heart	Identified by obvious beating.

Figure 17.32 Endoscopic findings in amphibians.

References and further reading

Brooks GH (1962) Resistance of the Ground Skink, *Lygosoma laterale*, to gamma radiation. *Herpetologica* **18**, 128–129

Frye FL (1991) *Biomedical and Surgical Aspects of Captive Reptile Husbandry, 2nd edition*. Krieger Publishing, Malabar, Florida

Gehrmann WH (1996) Evaluation of artificial lighting. In: *Reptile Medicine and Surgery*, ed. D Mader, pp.163–165. WB Saunders, Philadelphia

Holt PE (1978) Radiological studies of the alimentary tract in two Greek tortoises. *Veterinary Record* **103**(10),198–200

Jackson OF and Sainsbury AW (1992) Radiological and related investigations. In: *Manual of Reptiles*, ed. PH Beynon *et al.*, pp.63–72. BSAVA Publications, Cheltenham

Jacobson ER (1987) Reptiles. *Veterinary Clinics of North America: Small Animal Practice* **17**,1203–1225

Jacobson ER (1993) Snakes. *Veterinary Clinics of North America: Small Animal Practice* **23**, 1179–1212

Jacobson ER, Homer B and Adams W (1991) Endocarditis and congestive heart failure in a Burmese python (*Python molurus bivittatus*). *Journal of Zoo and Wildlife Medicine* **22**, 245

Kuchling G (1989) Assessment of ovarian follicles and oviductal eggs by ultrasound scanning in live fresh water turtles (*Chelodina oblonga*). *Herpetologica* **45**, 89–94

Lawton MPC and Cooper JE (1992) *Manual of Reptiles*. BSAVA Publications, Cheltenham

Love NE, Douglass JP, Lewbart G and Stoskopf M (1996) Radiographic and ultrasonographic evaluation of egg retention and peritonitis in two green iguanas (*Iguana iguana*). *Radiology and Ultrasound* **37**, 68–73

McArthur S and Wilkinson RJ (in press) *Medicine and Surgery of Tortoises and Turtles*. Blackwell Science, Oxford

Meyer J (1998) Gastrografin as a gastrointestinal contrast agent in the Greek tortoise *Testudo hermanni*. *Journal of Zoo and Wildlife Medicine* **29**, 183–189

Morris PJ and Alberts AC (1996) Determination of sex in white throated monitors (*Varanus albigularis*), Gila monsters (*Heloderma suspectum*) and beaded lizards (*H. horridum*) using 2 dimensional ultrasound imaging. *Journal of Zoo and Wildlife Medicine* **27**, 371–377

Pennick DG, Stewart JS, Paul-Murphy J and Pion P (1991) Ultrasonography of the Californian desert tortoise (*Xerobates agassizi*): anatomy and application. *Veterinary Radiography* **32**, 112–116

Redrobe S (1997) Aspects of ultrasonography of chelonia. *Proceedings of the Association of Reptile and Amphibian Veterinarians*, pp.127–130

Redrobe S (1997) Aspects of ultrasonography of lizards. *Proceedings of the Association of Reptile and Amphibian Veterinarians*, pp.179–182

Redrobe S (1997) Aspects of ultrasonography of snakes. *Proceedings of the Association of Reptile and Amphibian Veterinarians*, pp.183–186

Rubel GA, Isenburgel E and Wolvekamp P (1991) *Atlas of Diagnostic Radiology of Exotic Pets*. WB Saunders, Philadelphia

Russo EA (1987) Diagnosis and treatment of lumps and bumps in snakes. *Compendium on Continuing Education for Practising Veterinarians* **9**, 795–806

Sainsbury AW and Gili C (1991) Ultrasonographic anatomy and scanning technique of the coelomic organs of the Bosc monitor (*Varanus exanthematicus*). *Journal of Zoo and Wildlife Medicine* **22**, 421–433

Schildger BJ, Tenhu H, Kramer M, Casares, Gerwing M, Geyer B, Rubel A and Isenbugel E (1996) Ultraschalluntersuchung bei Reptilien. *Berlinische und Münchener Tierartztlichen Wochenschrift* **109**, 136-141 [in German]

Silverman S (1993) Diagnostic imaging of exotic pets. *Veterinary Clinics of North America: Small Animal Practice* **23**, 1287–1299

Silverman S and Janssen DL (1996) Diagnostic imaging. In: *Reptile Medicine and Surgery*, ed. D Mader, pp.258–264. WB Saunders, Philadelphia

Smith RN and Redrobe S (unpublished) *Notes on the anatomy of tortoises, snakes and fishes*. Department of Anatomy, University of Bristol, England.

Stoskopf MK (1989) Clinical imaging in zoological medicine: a review. *Journal of Zoo and Wildlife Medicine* **20,** 396–412

Zwart P, Cooper JE and Ippen R (1990) Pathology of the ovaries of Squamata with special emphasis on vitelline-protein induced ovaritis. *Verhandlung des 32nd Internationalen Symposiums uber Erkrankungen der Zoo und Wildtiere*. Akademie-Verlag, Berlin

18

Tortoises and turtles

Stuart D.J. McArthur, Roger J. Wilkinson and Michelle G. Barrows

Introduction

There are 12 families and approximately 257 species of Chelonia, most of them recognized by CITES as threatened or endangered. In the UK, the terrestrial chelonian is called a tortoise, a freshwater chelonian is a terrapin and a marine chelonian is a turtle. Figure 18.1 illustrates some commonly kept species.

Biology

Sexing

Most species are sexually dimorphic, though differences may not be obvious in juveniles.

- Males have a longer tail and a more distal vent than females
- The plastron of the male is concave
- Males of some aquatic species develop long claws on the forelimbs
- Females may be larger than males or have wider shells
- In the American box turtle *Terrapene*, males may have a red iris and females a yellow/brown iris.

Males have a single penis protruding from the floor of the cloaca and paired testes closely adherent to the kidneys. Females have paired ovaries suspended from the dorsal coelomic membrane containing numerous follicles. All species are oviparous.

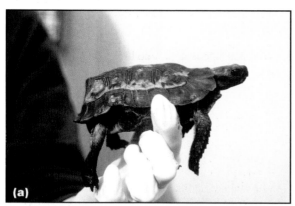
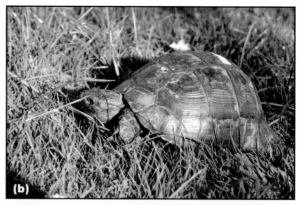
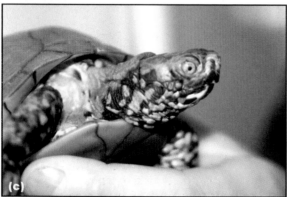
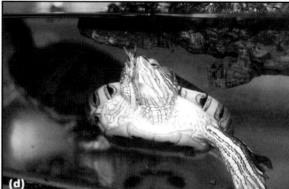

Figure 18.1 Some examples of captive chelonians: (a) African hinge-backed tortoise *Kinixys homeana*; (b) Greek tortoise *Testudo graeca*; (c) African box turtle *Terrapene carolina*;. (d) red-eared terrapin *Trachemys scripta elegans*. (a, b and d courtesy of S. Redrobe.)

Husbandry

Different chelonian species have widely differing nutritional and environmental requirements; details of species preferences may be found in Highfield (1996) and Ernst and Barbour (1989). It is vital that the practitioner has a good understanding of correct care in captivity. Incorrect husbandry is the most common cause of illness.

- Chelonians are best kept in small species-specific groups
- Overcrowding should be avoided and animals of differing sizes kept apart
- All should be regarded as potentially infectious. Individuals isolated or quarantined for several years cannot be guaranteed as free from infectious agents.

Housing

In winter, spring and autumn, all non-hibernating chelonians need a warm indoor area with appropriate heating, humidity and lighting. During summer months, some species cope well when maintained outdoors.

- Some tropical species are photophobic
- Photophilic species are best exposed to unfiltered sunlight whenever possible and additionally given access to a suitable ultraviolet light source.

Diet

The ideal diet mimics that eaten in the wild. There should be no reliance on only one or two items, nor are complete diets recommended as a major dietary constituent. All chelonians should have access to fresh water for drinking and bathing.

Herbivores

Herbivorous tortoises require vegetation that is high in fibre and calcium, and low in fat and protein. The diet should contain a Ca:P ratio of at least 1.5–2:1 (Scott, 1996). Natural foraging and feeding wild greens such as weeds, flowers and grasses will fulfil most requirements.

- Plant food should be washed to remove pesticides
- Poisonous plants (such as rhubarb, daffodils, potatoes, buttercup and yew) must not be fed
- Grocery greens complement a more natural diet but are generally higher in protein and lower in calcium, and may have an inverse Ca:P ratio
- Oxalates found in spinach, cabbage and beet greens bind calcium and may predispose to hypocalcaemia
- Goitrogens found in cabbage and kale may predispose to hypothyroidism.

Adult herbivores are normally fed daily and juveniles every other day.

Omnivores

Omnivorous species should be offered vegetable matter but they also take animal protein such as crickets, other adult insects, woodlice, mealworms, slugs, worms, 'pinky' mice, fish and small amounts of low-fat dog food.

- Insects should be gut-loaded and dusted with a high-calcium supplement
- Adult mice are nutritionally superior to 'pinkies'
- Whole fish are preferable to gutted fish
- Some species may prefer to be fed in water.

Aquatic species

Aquatic chelonians (turtles and terrapins) must be fed in water. Suitable dietary constituents include greens and fruit as for herbivorous tortoises, pondweed, pondfish pellets, insects, bloodworms, *Tubifex* worms, raw whole fish, prawns, 'pinky' and chopped adult mice, and small amounts of fresh meat. Low-fat dog food can be fed in small amounts but pellets are preferable to tinned food, as they cause less water pollution. The omnivorous red-eared slider *Trachemys scripta elegans* is primarily herbivorous as an adult.

Dietary supplementation

A supplementary calcium balancer/vitamin D powder should be offered.

Hibernation

Temperate-zone chelonians hibernate in winter and some species also aestivate in very hot weather. Tropical species should not be hibernated.

Mediterranean tortoises (*Testudo* spp.) are prepared for hibernation after the autumn equinox by being starved for 3–4 weeks.

- The hibernaculum should be at 2–9°C. A remote method of measuring temperature is advisable
- Fridges are suitable hibernacula if air is changed daily
- Insulated boxes and natural outdoor hibernation are less reliable
- Most unmanaged UK tortoises will hibernate for more than 5 months but a maximum of 3 months is advisable
- Animals not eating or urinating within a week of emerging from hibernation require intervention.

Handling and restraint

Access to the head is generally required during examination. The animal may retreat if approached from above or in front and so the approach should be from below and behind. A finger either side of the jaw will restrain the head if the animal weighs less than about 10 kg. The mouth may be opened with the other hand, while the restraining hand is rested on the cranial carapace to prevent retraction of the head.

If the animal has retreated, tilting it forward may encourage it to extend its forelimbs and head; or it may be lured 'out' with a favourite food. A blunt dental hook can be used carefully to draw out the head (Figure 18.2).

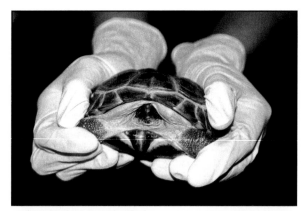

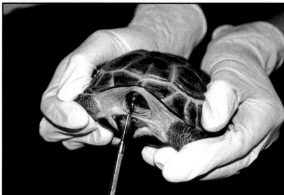

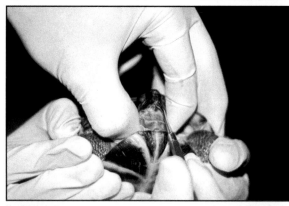

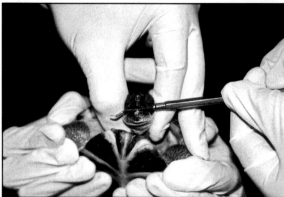

Figure 18.2 In small intractable species such as the Afghan or steppe tortoise *Testudo horsfieldi,* a blunt dental hook can be inserted under the upper jaw and the head gently drawn forwards and out. Care must be taken to avoid trauma from the probe. It is possible to fracture or pull off portions of the beak, or spear the roof of the mouth. Rotating the dental probe sidewise allows the beak to be opened, using the increasing width of the probe as a gag.

Protective clothing and appropriate techniques should be considered with aggressive species such as the common snapping turtle *Chelydra serpentina*. For example, the animal may be examined after it has already bitten and locked on to an object such as a towel. Aggressive animals may gape as a threat display to the clinician, enabling visual inspection.

Diagnostic approach

- Disinfect between patients or wear disposable gloves
- Treat all body secretions as potentially infectious.

History-taking (Figure 18.3) is disproportionately important in evaluating chelonian patients: physical examination is difficult and captive environmental conditions have special significance. Work-up of a case might include: history-taking; physical examination; haematology and blood biochemistry; faecal wet smear examination; radiography and ultrasonography; microscopy, cytology and microbial culture of exudates and lesions or aspirates; endoscopy; and exploratory surgery.

General
Date
Client identification
Animal identification or microchip number
Species (common and scientific names)
Sex and age
Reason for presentation
Keeper or establishment
Captive-bred or wild-caught
Duration
Previous ownership details
Disease history
Housing
Indoors, outdoors or both
Description (diagram useful)
Environment
How is heat provided?
Maximum, minimum and average day/night temperatures
How is humidity varied and monitored?
What lighting is provided?
What is the photoperiod and how is it managed?
Nutrition
Description of diet
Does food vary with season?
Any mineral or vitamin supplement offered?
How is food prepared?
Is water provided, changed and filtered?
Observations
Activity and appetite
How often are faeces passed?
How often is urine passed?
Reproductive data
Age at sexual maturity
When were eggs last laid?
Kept in isolation or as part of group?
Last contact with opposite sex?
Disease control
Quarantine programme? How long?
What disinfectants are used? Between groups or individuals?
When did this animal last meet a new chelonian?
Hibernation
Hibernated? When? How?
What post-hibernation management is offered?

Figure 18.3 History-taking.

Physical examination

A record of weight and body dimensions should be part of any individual health assessment. Length is best measured as straight carapace length (SCL). Figure 18.4 gives details for systematic examination.

Shell
Seam/scute quality, softness, pyramiding, ulceration, discharge, swelling, smell, colour, trauma
Limbs
• Surfaces, joint flexibility. Extend and compare opposite limbs. Abscess, oedema or swelling of the distal limbs? • If flesh limited and skin elasticity reduced, dehydration or emaciation possible • Nail overgrowth or excessive wear to feet
Skin
• Sloughing, shedding, parasites, swelling, oedema, abscess, granuloma, ulceration, exudate and malodour • Decreased skin elasticity may indicate dehydration • Jaundice (yellow/green skin pigmentation)
Head
Examine the tympanic membrane for swelling
Eye
• Examine conjunctivae, and eyelids should be examined for visual reflexes (menace and pupillary), swelling, discharge, corneal lesions, conjunctivitis, hyperplasia, cataract, intraocular haemorrhage, jaundice, foreign body. Compare both eyes. • Severe dehydration – eye sockets excessively recessed? • **NB** Ocular discharge is normal in some terrestrial species (e.g. red-foot/yellow-foot tortoises) but abnormal in others
Beak and jaw
• Instability, trauma, overgrowth? • Soft and flexible?
Oral cavity
• Mucous membrane colour (e.g. pallor, cyanosis or congestion), discharges? (Mucous membranes of oral cavity are normally pink.) Petechiation, ulceration, caseation and pharyngeal swelling all consistent with stomatitis • Ear abscesses associated with inspissated pus protruding into pharynx? • Submucosal swellings suggest gout, tumour or abscess formation
Nares
• Normally symmetrical and without discharge? • Cutaneous erosion, softness and depigmentation often occur with chronic upper respiratory tract discharge • Any discharge is abnormal
Ears
Check for swelling (e.g. abscess)
Cloaca
• Swelling, trauma, abnormal discharges, infection, myiasis and other parasitism? • Cloacal washes may be examined microscopically • Digital examination may allow assessment of gravidity, colonic and cloacal tone, cystic calculi and presence of space-occupying lesions
Other
Is the animal microchipped?

Figure 18.4 Systematic examination of a chelonian.

Sample collection

Blood

Skin disinfection should be undertaken. Jugular venepuncture (Figure 18.5) is advised where possible, as the sample is least likely to be lymph-diluted. An assistant should present the animal head first towards the veterinary surgeon. It may be easiest if the assistant holds back both of the forelegs.

1. Draw out the head into extension. Use a finger and thumb behind the occiput to restrain the neck and head.
2. Tip the chelonian into lateral recumbency, exposing the lateral neck.
3. Insert a needle (attached to a syringe) very superficially in a caudal-pointing direction, using a resting point on the extended head to keep everything steady. The jugular vein is sometimes visible as it extends caudally from the angle of the mandible. Occasionally the carotid artery is entered. It is acceptable to sample the carotid artery but adequate haemostasis after the needle is withdrawn should be ensured.
4. Following sampling from any vessel in the neck, apply pressure for several minutes in order to reduce post-sampling haematoma formation. (Post-sampling haematomas usually resolve over 2 weeks.)

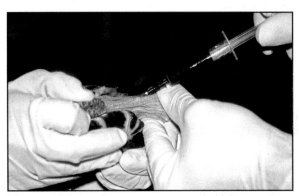

Figure 18.5 Jugular venepuncture and phlebotomy in *Testudo horsfieldi*.

If jugular venepuncture is impractical, the subcarapacial or subvertebral, cardiac and dorsal tail sites may be used (Figure 18.6).

Jugular venepuncture can be unsuitable for phlebotomy of large chelonians (>15 kg), or aggressive species such as snapping turtles, without chemical restraint.

Blood sampling protocol

1. Collect up to 3 ml blood/kg bodyweight.
2. Prepare several air-dried smears.
3. Preserve one lithium-heparinized sample for haematology.
4. Centrifuge a second lithium-heparinized sample, separate and store cooled immediately after collection, for biochemistry (alternatively use a spun lithium heparin gel tube).

Site	Comments
Dorsal venous sinus (dorsal coccygeal vein)	Unpredictably lymphodiluted, compromising diagnostic use. May damage the central nervous system if CSF encountered and disinfection is inadequate. NOT ROUTINELY ADVISED
Subcarapacial sinus ('subvertebral', USA)	Unpredictably lymphodiluted compromising diagnostic use NOT ROUTINELY ADVISED
Cardiac venepuncture	Only soft-shelled juveniles – if transplastronal needle insertion is used. During euthanasia, insert a lengthy needle between the neck and forelimb in the cranial inlet of the shell and direct caudoventrally

Figure 18.6 Alternative sites for blood sampling chelonians.

Normal biochemical data are summarized in Figure 18.7 and a suggested haematology profile for tortoises is given in Figure 18.8. Interpretation of haematological changes and the significance of changes in serum biochemistry values are summarized in Figures 18.9 and 18.10.

	Mediterranean tortoise *Testudo hermanni* [a]	Mediterranean tortoise *T. hermanni/ T. graeca* [b]
Total protein (g/l)	31–54	13–38
Albumin (g/l)		5–18
Calcium (mmol/l)	2.7–3.5	2.0–2.9
Phosphate (mmol/l)	1.7–3.3	0.45–1.7
Uric acid (μmol/l)	125–577	35–244
Creatinine (μmol/l)	<26	14–25
Aspartate aminotransferase (IU/l)	19–103	18–222
Lactate dehydrogenase (IU/l)	161–473	89–269
Gamma-glutamyl transferase (IU/l)	<10	0–1.0
Alkaline phosphatase (IU/l)	196–425	61–211
Potassium (mmol/l)	4.5–5.0	
Sodium (mmol/l)	130–144	
Chloride (mmol/l)	96–115	

Figure 18.7 Blood biochemistry values from apparently healthy captive chelonians. [a] Data from Göbel and Spörle (1992) – 17 captive animals, tail vein, season not stated. [b] Data from Harcourt-Brown (pers. comm.) – five captive *T. graeca*, seven *T. hermanni*, 6/12 female, tail vein, September.

Haematology, including differential white cell count and examination for haemoparasites
Total protein
Albumin
Calcium
Phosphate
Sodium
Potassium
Alkaline phosphatase
Lactate dehydrogenase
Aspartate aminotransferase
Creatinine kinase
Uric acid
Urea
Beta-hydroxybutyrate
Glucose

Figure 18.8 A suggested 'tortoise profile'. (Data from McArthur *et al.*, in preparation.)

Abnormality	Significance/Comments
Heterophilia	Seasonal (more in summer). Infection and inflammation. Absence does not rule out infectious disease
Heteropenia	Infection. Particularly viral
Eosinophilia	Seasonal (more in winter, especially if hibernating). Parasitism (particularly in non-mediterranean species). Sepsis
Lymphocytosis	Seasonal (more in summer). Females and young may have higher counts. Inflammation and healing. Parasitism. Leukaemia
Lymphopenia	Common in sick tortoises. Tail vein samples. Anorexia/malnutrition of any cause. Hibernation. Lymphoproliferative disease
Monocytosis	Acute or chronic infection e.g. stomatitis. Inflammation. Chronic renal failure
Azurophilia	Infection or inflammation
Basophilia	Intestinal parasitism. Haemoparasitism. High counts are normal in red-eared slider *Trachemys scripta,* snapping turtle *Chelydra serpentina* and possibly other species
Anaemia	Consider the possibility of lymphodilution of sample. PCV may be lower in females and juveniles. PCV varies with season. In healthy Mediterranean *Testudo* sp. haematocrit reaches a maximum at the end of hibernation. In sick tortoises with post-hibernation anorexia it is often low at this point despite clinicopathological evidence of dehydration. Poor nutritional and environmental conditions. Blood loss. Erythrolysis (autoimmune or haemoparasite-induced). Anaemia of chronic disease
Thrombocytopenia	In severe anaemia thrombocytes may be recruited into the erythrocyte pool

Figure 18.9 Interpretation of haematological changes in chelonians. (Data from McArthur *et al.*, in preparation.)

Parameter	Increase	Decrease	Comments
Albumin	Dehydration. Hibernation. Ovarian activity (March–July)	Lymphodilution. Anorexia. Malnutrition. Stomatitis. Intestinal parasitism and other enteropathies	
Calcium	May rise 200–400% in females in breeding season: 4–6.5 mmol/l (exceptionally up to 11) typical March–July. Over-supplementation with calcium or vitamin D. Sample lipaemia	Deficiencies of Vitamin D, UV light or dietary calcium	
Phosphate	Sample haemolysis. Immature animals. Nutritional secondary hyperparathyroidism. Not an obvious feature of renal disease	Anorexia	Normal range in Mediterranean species <1.7 mmol/l
Uric acid	Sample lipaemia. Excess dietary protein. Intrinsic renal failure (uric acid >1000 µmol/l)	Lymphodilution. Hepatic disease	Normal levels do not exclude the possibility of renal pathology
Urea	Dehydration plus protein catabolism or excess dietary protein		Marked seasonal variation (highest at end of hibernation)
Aspartate aminotransferase	After injections in healthy animals. Wide variety of diseases		Significant amounts in liver, kidney and heart (but not skeletal) muscle
Creatine (phospho-) kinase	After injections in healthy animals		Present in skeletal and heart muscle
Lactate dehydrogenase	Sample haemolysis. Traumatic venepuncture. Tissue damage		Present in liver, kidney, skeletal and heart muscle, with smaller amounts in gut
Alkaline phosphatase	Metabolic bone disease. Immatures. Follicular stasis		
Glucose	Post-hibernation	Hepatopathy. Anorexia. Malnutrition. Septicaemia	Marked seasonal variations. Post-hibernation surge does not occur in depleted animals, important in post-hibernation anorexia. Most chronically sick patients have April–May glucose 3–6 mmol/l. Acutely ill animals in spring may still have normal concentrations
Beta-hydroxybutyrate	Low food intake: plasma levels 0.4–0.75 mmol/l in times of significant food but increase to 2.0 mmol/l after 2 months of drought		May be a useful measure of health status in animals with unknown history. Objective measure of energy balance
Potassium	Sample haemolysis. Renal failure	Anorexia. Enteritis	
Sodium	High water loss (e.g diarrhoea). Reduced water intake		Considerable seasonal variation (lowest in late spring)

Figure 18.10 Significance of changes in serum biochemistry values in chelonians.

'Normal' and 'abnormal' values given by laboratories must be treated with caution. For many species there are no reference data. Massive seasonal changes in normal haematology and biochemistry values are possible. Post-hibernation values are relatively hyperuricaemic, uraemic and leucopenic (Lawrence and Hawkey, 1986). Mature females are seasonally hyperalbuminaemic and hypercalcaemic (summer).

Faecal examination

Faecal examination involves wet smear, flotation and sedimentation. Faeces normally contain 'parasite-like' plant elements, yeasts and fungi (herbivores) or parasites and parasite eggs of prey species (carnivores).

Urinalysis

- Normal pH in the urine of herbivores and omnivores is 8.0–8.5

- Post-hibernation, or after prolonged anorexia, it is often 5.0–6.0
- Urine specific gravity 1.003–1.017, depending on water availability, but cannot be used as an indicator of renal function
- Green staining indicates biliverdinuria consistent with hepatopathy or haemolysis.

Diagnostic imaging

Diagnostic imaging techniques include ultrasonography, endoscopy, radiography and MRI/computed tomography. All have great diagnostic potential and are covered in Chapter 17.

Common conditions

Figure 18.11 summarizes a problem-solving approach to chelonian medicine.

Disease	Aetiology	Clinical signs	Diagnosis	Treatment
Anorexia	Any acute or chronic disease, e.g. gastrointestinal, hepatic, renal, intraocular, CNS. Inappropriate environment or food. Maladaptation. Social disruption. Psychological or behavioural	Multiple and varied depending upon the likely cause	Full examination. Case history. Faecal examination. Blood biochemistry/haematology. Urinalysis. Cytology. Microbiology. Ultrasonography. Radiography. Endoscopy. MRI	Optimize husbandry and nutrition. Treat primary disease
Beak deformities	Lack of abrasive substrate. Accelerated growth (protein excess). Metabolic bone disease. Hypovitaminosis A. Other metabolic disease	Beak deformities	Assess nutrition and husbandry. Blood biochemistry	Correct cause. Trim beak with a high-speed burr or abrasive disc
Cloacal organ prolapse	General debility. Neurological. Coelomic space-occupying lesion or cause of straining. Metabolic disease. Obesity. Excessive libido. Infection	A structure prolapsed through the cloacal opening	Digital and visual examination. Endoscopy. Histopathology. Blood biochemistry. Radiography	Reduce and retain with purse string suture. Remove if heavily infected or necrotic. Correct cause
Cystic calculi	Dehydration (especially if uricotelic). Acidosis/alkalosis. Hepatopathy. Unsuitable mineral balance in diet or water source may predispose	May be none. Dysuria/anuria. Posterior paresis. Increased weight. Coelomic enlargement. Straining. Dystocia	Radiography (DV). Ultrasonography. Exploratory coeliotomy. Cloacal endoscopy. Calculi should be differentiated from ectopic eggs	Correct underlying cause. Attempt dissolution. Coeliotomy and removal. Lithotripsy
Diarrhoea	Inappropriate diet. Food intolerance. Intussusception. Parasitism. Enteritis/colitis. Septicaemia. Toxaemia. Yeast overgrowth. Deranged gut flora. Inappropriate environment. stress. Excessive fruit/sugar in the diet. Metabolic disease. Infection	Varies with cause. Soft faeces may be normal in summer if fluid intake is good	Faecal examination. Blood biochemistry. Haematology	High-fibre diet. Fluids. Possibly potassium supplementation. Probiotics (e.g. faeces from a healthy colony mate). Antiparasitic agents. Antifungals
Dystocia	Inability to exhibit nesting behaviour: inadequate site; competition; aggression; excessive stocking. Inappropriate environment. Maternal or fetal morphological and developmental abnormalities. Mechanical obstruction. Infection. Systemic illness	May be none in early stages. Abnormal posture. Hindlimb paresis. Anorexia. Lethargy. Continuous or repetitive straining. Malodorous cloacal discharge. Involuntary elimination of urine	Presenting signs. Case history. Weight. Ballottement. Cloacal examination. Radiography. Ultrasonography. Laparoscopy. Blood parameters	Provide suitable nesting area. Medical induction (calcium supplementation and oxytocin injections). Surgical removal of eggs
Ear infections	Infection ascending Eustachian tube; may disseminate and predispose to septicaemia. Poor hygiene. Immunosuppression may predispose	Swelling of one or both tympanic scales. Asymmetry of the head	Lesions are pathognomonic. Microbiology	Usually surgical. Appropriate antimicrobials postoperatively. Always check the pharyngeal exit points of the Eustachian tubes of both sides
Ectoparasites	Fly strike often secondary to trauma or infection. Ticks more likely if recently imported	The presence of maggots or ticks	Observation of parasites	Manual removal of parasites. Removal of underlying disease or predispositions. Amitraz (Petney and Knight, 1988)
Endoparasites	Coccidians. Amoebae. *Cryptosporidium*. Flagellates, Ciliates. Ascarids. *Proatractis*. Oxyurids (pinworms). Trematode flukes. Yeast	Often none. Debility and enteric signs. Regurgitation and/or diarrhoea possible	Faecal examination. Identification of organisms, larvae or eggs	Appropriate antiparasitic agent. Oxyurids, amoebae, ciliates, trichomonads, coccidians and flagellates may not require treatment. Cryptosporidia, *Protractis* and ascarids justify specific treatment
Follicular stasis	A failure of induced ovulation?	Isolated females. Anorexia. Hind limb paresis. Increased weight. Absence of faeces	Diagnosis of exclusion. Serial utrasonography. Coelomic endoscopy. Haematology. Blood biochemistry. Exploratory coeliotomy	Ovariectomy. Contact with male. Proligestone
Frost damage	Hibernation in sub-zero temperatures. Poor monitoring and protection during hibernation	Blindness. Intraocular haemorrhage. Circling or inactivity. Distal limbs may become swollen	History. Signs	Long-term nursing. Recovery less likely with multifocal neurological dysfunction. Sight damage may respond to Vitamin A supplementation (Lawton and Stokes, 1989)
Gout	Tophi secondary to hyperuricaemia of dehydration. Renal failure. Excessive access to protein. Tophi may occur in areas of inflammation	Deposition of urate (tophi) in joints, peri/myocardium, liver, renal cortex, spleen, brain, gonads, oral mucosa	History of chronic dehydration or inappropriate diet. Catabolism/negative energy balance. Radiography. Histopathology	Active fluid therapy. Allopurinol (15 mg/kg daily). AVOID medications increasing renal excretion of uric acid (e.g. Probenecid). Consider euthanasia

Figure 18.11 A problem-solving approach to chelonian medicine. (continues) ▶

Disease	Aetiology	Clinical signs	Diagnosis	Treatment
Heat damage	Unable to escape from heat source	Distressed. Profound oro-oculonasal discharge. Carapace/plastron burns and necrosis. Posterior paresis	History. Clinical signs	Bathing in cool water. Oral or parenteral cooled fluids. Analgesia, antimicrobials, fluid therapy, nutritional support and wound care should be considered
Hepatic disease	Infectious agents. Migrating parasites. Inflammatory disease. Toxins. Nutritional disease. Neoplasia	Weight loss or gain. Anorexia. Malaise. Inactivity. Biliverdinuria. Jaundice	Blood biochemistry. Haematology. Radiography. Ultrasonography. Endoscopy. Cytology of coelomic fluid. Biopsy. Microbiology. Histopathology	Fluid and nutritional support. Antimicrobials. Viral hepatitis requires barrier nursing
Hepatic lipidosis (The liver is a major fat body; hepatic lipidosis is a relative phenomenon and must be interpreted in relation to season and possible disease)	Follicular stasis. Hypothyroidism. Diabetes. Unsuitable diet. Bacterial and fungal toxins. Disrupted lipid metabolism. Starvation. Prolonged hibernation periods. Anorexia. Viral disease. Excessive PTH	Malaise. Inactivity. Anorexia. Debility	Liver biopsy. Histopathology	Treat primary disease. Nutritional support. Rehydration and electrolyte replacement. Amino acid supplementation. Treatment is often prolonged but even severely debilitated animals may improve given many months of care
Hypervitaminosis A	Vitamin A by injection has a high risk of iatrogenic hypervitaminosis A	Epidermal detachment. Blisters on skin of proximal limbs, revealing a moist exposed dermis. Changes to internal organs may also occur	History of inappropriate parenteral Vitamin A. Liver assay	Prevent further vitamin A administration. Supportive care. Lesion care. Severe cases may require euthanasia
Hypothyroidism and hypoiodinism	Diets low in iodine or high in vegetable thiocyanates (e.g. greens, cabbage, brassicas, mustard seed, turnips). Giant species appear predisposed, though smaller terrestrial species also affected	Goitre. Malaise. Inactivity. Anorexia. Debility. Subclinical disease may be common	Dietary history. Histopathology of thyroid tissue. (September T4 values 10–25 nmol/l in *Testudo* sp.; Harcourt-Brown, pers. comm.)	Dietary correction. Iodine supplementation. Thyroid supplementation
Hypovitaminosis A		Non-specific. Blepharitis. Conjunctivitis. Rhinitis. Lower respiratory tract disease. Cutaneous abnormalities. General decline	Dietary history. Clinical signs. Histopathology of tissue biopsies. Vitamin A assays of liver or blood	Supplement with oral vitamin A products. Omnivorous species can be fed liver weekly. Oral dosing with natural sources of carotene, preformed Vitamin A, or both, is safer than the use of injections
Intestinal impaction or obstruction	Ingestion of sand, gravel or other indigestible bedding. Intussusception. Volvulus. Neoplasia	Anorexia. Straining. Regurgitation of fluids and food	Plain/contrast radiography. Ultrasonography. Endoscopy	Hydration. Mineral oil/water enemas and laxatives. Foreign body removal: endoscopic; transplastron coeliotomy
Lower respiratory tract infections	Viruses, bacteria, fungi or mixed. Standards of nutrition and husbandry may be poor	Abnormal posture. Inspiratory and/or expiratory dyspnoea. Inactivity. Anorexia. Lethargy. Increased or abnormal respiratory sounds. Increased respiratory rate, especially at rest. Concurrent disease	Radiography. Haematology. Blood biochemistry. Microbiology. Cytology. Serology. Transtracheal, percutaneous or transcarapacial lung wash. Tracheal endoscopy. Lung/lesion biopsy. Virus isolation. Electron microscopy	Supportive care. Nutritional and fluid support. Isolation of affected individuals. Antibacterial/antifungal/antiviral agents. Nebulization. Direct application of treatment to lung tissue through transcarapacial route
Metabolic bone disease (nutritional secondary hyperparathyroidism)	Dietary deficiency of calcium and suitable Vitamin D. Diet with unsuitable Ca : P ratio. Lack of exposure to UV light. Disruption of Vitamin D metabolism	Soft shell. Muscular weakness. Cloacal prolapse. Osteomalacia. Osteoporosis. Rickets. Fibrous osteodystrophy. Lateral flattening of the pelvis. Parrot beak. Pyramiding of scutes and alterations in carapace conformation of juveniles. Egg retention in gravid females. Secondary nephropathy if chronically hyperparathyroid	History. Blood biochemistry. Radiography	Correct diet and environment. Improve UVB light. Parenteral calcium. Supplement Vitamin D₃. Calcitonin injections may prove suitable with further research
Posterior paresis	Herpesvirus or other infections. Pesticides. Hypocalcaemia. Osteoporosis of spine/vertebrae. Heat or frost damage. Gravidity. Renomegaly. Cystic calculi. Toxicosis	Posterior paresis	Blood biochemistry. Diagnostic imaging. Histopathology of nervous tissue from biopsy or at postmortem	Remove underlying cause. Long-term convalescence. Consider euthanasia if poor response to long-term treatment
Renal failure	Dehydration. Infections. Hyperparathyroidism? Iatrogenic (e.g. aminoglycoside therapy)	Malaise. Inactivity. Anorexia. Debility. Anuria. Polyuria (uncommon). Generalized oedema in terminal renal disease	Blood biochemistry. Renal biopsy and histopathology. Gout may be apparent on ultrasonography. Renal function tests are not yet available	Fluid therapy. Appropriate antimicrobials. Allopurinol. Treatment for gout and hyperparathyroidism

Figure 18.11 continued A problem-solving approach to chelonian medicine. (continues) ▶

Disease	Aetiology	Clinical signs	Diagnosis	Treatment
Septicaemia	Infections. Poor husbandry	Acute debility. Erythematous plastron. Petechial haemorrhages on mucous membranes. Sudden death. Localized infections may be apparent	Blood culture necessary for definitive diagnosis. Contaminants hard to distinguish. Disseminated infection suggests previous septicaemia. Postmortem findings. Presumptive diagnosis from response to treatment	Appropriate antimicrobials (intravenous, intraosseous or intramuscular). Supportive fluid therapy. Nutritional support. Environmental support
Sight problems	Keratitis or keratoconjunctivitis. Corneal trauma, scar tissue or lipidosis. Hibernation/frost damage. Excessive UV light. Hypovitaminosis A. Hepatoencephalopathy. Gout. Viral CNS infection	Poor visual reflexes. Failure to stop when presented with solid objects or dangerous drops	All inactive or anorexic animals deserve an ocular examination	Remove predispositions. Improve husbandry and nutrition. Establish long-term rehabilitation protocol. Low-dose oral Vitamin A supplementation (Lawton and Stokes, 1989)
Stomatitis	Viral aetiology, especially if an outbreak. Other infections. Immunosuppression. Metabolic disease. Hibernating recently fed animals. Infection of penetration injuries from food items. Local irritation	Oedematous swelling of the ventral neck. Yellow diptheroid membrane on the mucosa of the tongue, oropharynx and nasopharynx. Dysphagia. Hypersalivation. Occasionally dyspnoea. Occasionally nasal discharge	History. Clinical signs. Cytology. Histopathology. Immunohistochemistry. Electron microscopy. Virus isolation. Serology. PCR. Transmission studies	Barrier nursing. Oesophagostomy tube. Clean mouths and debride daily (povidone–iodine). Hospitalization and supportive care may be required for weeks or months. Acyclovir 80–200 mg/ml may be beneficial if herpesvirus related and treated early (blood levels should be monitored). Antibacterials and antifungals to prevent secondary infections
Upper respiratory tract infections	Viruses, bacteria, fungi, chlamydiae, mycoplasmas or mixed. Poor husbandry	Nasal discharge (serous, sanguineous or purulent). Abnormal posture. Inactivity. Anorexia. Lethargy. Ocular discharge. Oral discharge. Increased or abnormal respiratory sounds. Concurrent disease	History of exposure to chelonians carrying an infectious agent. Microbiology. Endoscopy. Biopsy. Cytology. Histopathology. Electron microscopy. Virus isolation	Appropriate antimicrobial, potentially antimycoplasmal or antiviral agents. Improve standards of husbandry and nutrition. Supportive nursing. Isolate affected individuals

Figure 18.11 continued A problem-solving approach to chelonian medicine.

Post-hibernation anorexia (PHA)

Aetiological aspects of post-hibernation anorexia include:

- Failure to observe that a confined animal is no longer in hibernation
- Failure to hydrate the animal suitably before and after hibernation
- Failure to feed the animal suitably before and after hibernation
- Failure to provide suitable heat and light before and after hibernation
- An excessively long period of hibernation
- Disease or trauma acquired during the hibernation period (e.g. frost damage and rat bites)
- The culmination of chronic undetected disease noticed in the post-hibernation period.

Animals experiencing inactivity or anorexia in the post-hibernation period should undergo a comprehensive examination. The history should be reviewed for predisposing adverse husbandry.

Zoonoses

Salmonellosis is the most important reptilian zoonosis.

- The main group at risk from salmonellosis is children (because of unsanitary habits when handling reptiles)

- Pregnant women, children younger than 5 years of age and persons with impaired immune system function (e.g. with AIDS or on immunosuppressive therapy) should not have contact with reptiles
- Disposable gloves are essential when performing faecal flotation and smear examinations
- All keepers of chelonians should be advised to practise high standards of hygiene in order to reduce the possibility of contracting salmonellosis from their pet.

Other zoonotic organisms reported in captive chelonians include *Mycobacterium* spp., *Campylobacter fetus*, *Yersina pseudoturberculosis*, *Vibrio cholerae*, *Chlamydia psittaci*, *Dermatophilus congolensis*, *Borrelia burgdorferi*, *Leptospira* spp., *Listeria monocytogenes*, *Flavobacterium meningosepticum*, *Erysipelothrix rhusiopathiae* and *Coxiella burnetti* (Schmidt and Fletcher, 1983; Harvey and Greenwood, 1985; Divers, 1998b; Macdonald, 1998; Blahak, 2000).

Supportive care

Hospitalization vivaria

An appropriate treatment vivarium is essential when managing any chronically ill chelonian case (Figure 18.12). Vivaria should be constructed from non-porous, non-abrasive, disinfectable materials with

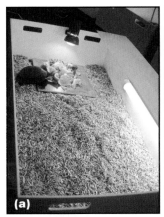
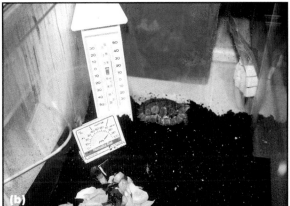
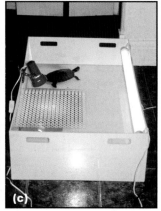

Figure 18.12 (a,b) Hospitalization vivaria for terrestrial chelonians. Vivaria contain maximum/minimum thermometers and humidity gauges. (c) Hospitalization vivarium for a semi-aquatic chelonian.

sealed joints and edges. Cat and dog cages are unsuitable unless exceptional circumstances (such as patient size) necessitate their conversion. For most semi-aquatic chelonians, a plastic or glass tank with a haul-out area is suitable. Where the animals are kept out of water, regular misting is advisable. In humid environments, plastic mats limit ground contact where excreta may predispose to plastral infections.

Drug administration

Routes for drug administration are summarized in Figure 18.13. The sites used for blood sampling (jugular, subcarapacial, subvertebral, cardiac and dorsal) are also available for intravenous injection. Injection into the jugular may be indicated in administration of some medications, such as anaesthetic agents, fluids or antibiotics.

Fluid therapy and nutritional support

In most chelonians, dehydration is impossible to assess until it has become well established. Most unwell chelonians benefit from oral fluids. Potassium deficits can be safely replaced. The ideal solution for many chelonians is unknown: no objective data are available.

- Fluids should be warmed to optimum temperature before administration

- Fluids equivalent to 1–3% of bodyweight can be safely administered to potentially dehydrated chelonians during initial stabilization by any combination of routes
- Proprietary nutritional support products (Critical Care Formula, Vetark UK) are routinely used by the authors, complemented by liquidized vegetables

Oral methods

Nutritional support or oral fluid therapy can be given by:

- Hand feeding (with syringe where needed): this can be performed by keepers
- Stomach tube (gavage) (Figure 18.14): excellent for short-term nursing
- Oesophagostomy tube (Figure 18.15): the method of choice for stabilizing patients with upper digestive tract disease, handling stress or long-term debility that requires repeated enteric medication, nutrition or fluids. The tubes are generally well tolerated. Most animals are unaware of their tube and will happily eat around it.

Suitable tubes include Jackson cat catheters, dog urethral catheters and nasogastric feeding tubes cut to a plastron length with the female mount preserved. Semi-aquatic specimens also tolerate such tubes, which

Route	Comments
Oral	Gastrointestinal transit times vary widely and may make absorption unreliable. Oral route difficult in large strong species. Gastrointestinal infections and infestations are most logically treated orally
Per cloaca/colon	Cloacal dosing with fenbendazole is relatively easy even in uncooperative species
Antibiotic-impregnated PMMA beads	Implantation of beads is most applicable to the treatment of osteomyelitis or septic arthritis
Intrapneumonic	A catheter is surgically positioned within a focal lung lesion via a drilled hole in the carapace and then secured with tissue glue
Intravenous, intraosseous or intracoelomic injections	Intravenous injections are technically challenging. Intraosseous drug administration is almost equivalent to intravenous therapy. Relatively large volumes of fluids can be given with minimum stress into the coelomic cavity of most chelonians
Intramuscular injection	Ideal for many medications. The volume of fluid that can be given is limited
Subcutaneous injection	Unsuited to fluid therapy. Potential irritancy should be considered

Figure 18.13 Routes for drug administration in chelonians.

1. Before passing a stomach tube, always ensure that it is filled with liquid and not air.
2. Mark the tube to half the plastron length.
3. Lubricate the tube – it should slip in gently; force should be avoided.
4. The trachea is avoided by running the tube dorsally along the roof of the mouth and pharynx.
5. Fluids should not exceed 5% of bodyweight (in ml) per day, given in divided doses.

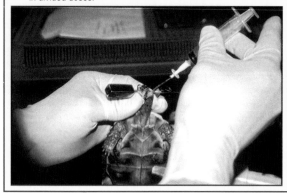

Figure 18.14 Oral gavage for fluid and nutritional support.

1. Extract the head.
2. Insert long-handled crocodile forceps orally into the oesophagus, with the neck held in extension.
3. Push the forceps laterally to protrude out in the mid to distal third of the oesophageal region.
4. Use a scalpel to cut down over the protruding tips of the forceps and push the tips through the oesophageal wall and skin. Local analgesia should be considered for the area of skin where an incision is made.
5. If the dorsal and ventral jugular veins, carotid artery or lymphatic vessels are visible, avoid them. In the unlikely event of hitting one of the above vessels, apply temporary pressure to a swab or plug of cotton wool or place a haemostatic mattress suture.
6. Use the forceps to pick up the end of the tube and draw it in through the skin, up the oesophagus and out of the mouth by withdrawing the forceps.
7. Reverse the grip on the tube and take it back down the oesophagus until it is in the region of the stomach. This is easy to feel if gentle (pre-measuring the tube is helpful).
8. Put a finger suture around the tube and anchor it to the skin of the neck, or withdraw the tube a little, stick on a tape butterfly and put two mattress sutures through the tape and skin of neck to anchor it.
9. Take up the other end of the tube and apply a small strip of tape to the tube and nuchal scute of the carapace. Adequate nuchal scute anchorage generally prevents self-removal. Continue taping with more strips.
10. Always flush the tube with water after use or it will block.

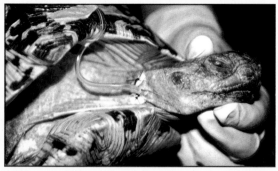

Figure 18.15 Oesophagostomy tube placement.

are easily anchored by placing a blob of superglue or epoxy on the taping sites. These animals may require reduced water exposure.

Non-enteral fluid therapy

- Bathing: tortoises can be bathed in shallow warm water once or twice daily for 10 minutes. In severely hyperuricaemic patients, fluids may be actively flushed into the cloaca and bladder, removing lower urinary tract toxic excretion products and facilitating lower urinary tract fluid absorption
- Intravenous fluids: only suited to severely debilitated chelonians requiring emergency treatment or anaesthetized animals, as jugular cut down is required
- Intracoelomic fluids (Figure 18.16): up to 3% bodyweight can be given through a surgically prepared site in the prefemoral fossa, but care must be taken to avoid trauma to the bladder or compression of the respiratory space
- Epicoelomic fluids (Figure 18.17): injection through the cranial plastronal inlet immediately dorsal to the plastron and below/into the pectoral muscles
- Intraosseous fluids (Figure 18.18): a needle is inserted into the bone between the carapace and plastron, into the carapace itself or into the tibia and then attached to a syringe driver.

Figure 18.19 lists fluids for parenteral administration.

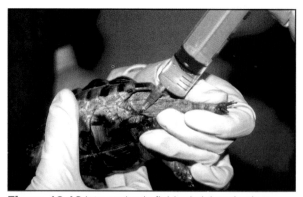

Figure 18.16 Intracoelomic fluid administration in a Mediterranean tortoise.

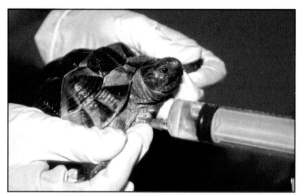

Figure 18.17 Epicoelomic fluid administration in a Mediterranean tortoise.

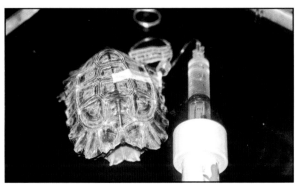

Figure 18.18 Intraosseous fluid administration in the cog-wheel turtle *Heosemys spinosa*.

Indication	Fluid of choice
Hypertonic dehydration (water deficiency)	0.18% NaCl/4% glucose or 5% glucose
Isotonic or hypotonic dehydration (water deficiency plus chronic anorexia)	1:1 mixture of 5% dextrose and Ringer's solution
To achieve diuresis	0.18% NaCl/ 4% glucose or 5% glucose
Blood loss	0.9% (normal) saline or whole blood
Septic shock	0.9% (normal) saline or Ringer's solution
Hyperkalaemia	5% glucose
Mixed water and electrolyte loss (diarrhoea)	Ringer's solution

Figure 18.19 Fluids for parenteral administration to chelonians.

Anaesthesia

Anaesthesia is usually well tolerated, even in debilitated chelonians. Pre-anaesthetic stabilization is advised where possible. General anaesthesia normally involves the use of an injectable agent followed either by incremental top-up or by maintenance using a volatile agent (Figure 18.20). In either case, assisted ventilation is necessary and the animal should be intubated.

Intubation

After appropriate induction, items such as a shortened urethral catheter, plastic giving-set tubing, plastic intravenous cannula or an uncuffed endotracheal tube can be used (Figure 18.21).

1. Pull the tongue forward with protected forceps.
2. Insert the tube through the rima glottides, found centrally two-thirds of the way down the tongue.

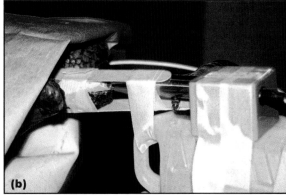

Figure 18.21 (a) Endotracheal intubation and tube fixation. (b) Stabilization of anaesthetic circuits using tape, tongue depressors and heat bottles, automatic ventilation and oesophageal pulse oximetry.

Agent	Dose	Comments
Injectable		
Propofol	5–14 mg/kg i.v. or intraosseous (i.o.); 15–30 mg/kg i.o. (Fonda, 1999)	Typical induction times in chelonians less than a minute unless perivascular injection occurs. Recovery in reptiles typically 25–40 minutes
Alphaxalone/alphadolone	9–12 mg/kg i.v. suggested	Induction after i.v. injection 30 seconds. Anaesthesia generally smooth and uneventful. Recovery tends to occur reliably 10–20 minutes post injection. Repeat doses for maintenance result in predictable extension of anaesthesia
Ketamine	5–30 mg/kg alone or with other agents such as midazolam (Bienzle *et al.*, 1992) may facilitate intubation and further induction/maintenance with volatile agents. 75 µg/kg medetomidine plus 7.5 mg/kg ketamine i.v. have been successful (Lock *et al.*, 1998; Norton *et al.*, 1998)	Reversal of combination with atipamezole at 100–380 µg/kg (4 x dose of medetomidine) associated with mild vomiting
Volatile		
Halothane	2–3% for maintenance (Butler *et al.*, 1984)	
Isoflurane	1.5–4% for maintenance (Bennett, 1995)	

Figure 18.20 Anaesthetic agents for chelonians.

3. Use ordinary connectors to link endotracheal tubes to a circuit such as an Ayres T-piece.
4. Apply intermittent positive pressure ventilation (IPPV).

Ventilation

Two to six breaths per minute can be used during manual (Ayres T-piece or a human facial resuscitation bag) or automatic ventilation. Care should be taken to avoid over-inflation.

Analgesia

Analgesic agents are summarized in Figure 18.22. Adequate renal function should be ascertained prior to the use of non-steroidal anti-inflammatory drugs.

Agent	Anecdotal doses
Butorphanol	0.05–0.4 mg/kg i.m. 20 minutes before anaesthesia (Bennett, 1998)
Buprenorphine	0.01 mg/kg i.m. as a postoperative analgesic (Malley, 1997)
Carprofen	2–4 mg/kg i.m., i.v., s.c. or orally – initial dose. Follow with 1–2 mg/kg every 24–72 hours (S. Divers, pers.comm. 2000)

Figure 18.22 Analgesic agents for chelonians. Doses are anecdotal.

Common surgical procedures

It is possible to give only an outline of common surgical procedures here. It is unwise to undertake elective surgery prior to imminent hibernation, as anabolic process will be limited. All the procedures listed warrant general anaesthesia and analgesics. Common surgical procedures are outlined in Figure 18.23 and illustrated in Figures 18.24 and 18.25.

Suture materials

Metal and nylon haemoclips and monofilament suture materials are appropriate to reptilian surgery; catgut and braided materials should be avoided as anecdotal evidence suggests they may provoke chronic inflammatory reactions or harbour infectious agents. Skin sutures may be removed after 4–6 weeks.

Coeliotomy

The coelomic cavity is surgically entered either through the plastron or through the pre-femoral fossa. A pre-femoral soft tissue approach appears relatively straightforward, as little hardware is required, but access and the procedures possible are limited. Closure is described in Figure 18.23.

Surgery	Procedure/Comments
Ear abscess curettage	1. Open the tympanic scute around its ventral circumference (3 to 9 o'clock). 2. Remove the contents of the middle ear (usually inspissated pus). Use one or more hypodermic needles to pierce the lesion and lever it out. 3. Check the other ear. The condition is often bilateral. 4. Check the exit of the Eustachian tube in the pharynx for further infection. 5. Consider culture and sensitivity testing. 6. Flush the Eustachian tube after the middle ear has been surgically cleaned. 7. The incision is generally left open, allowing further flushing as necessary.
Limb amputation and bead implantation	High amputations minimize stump trauma. Preserve a flap of skin in order to reconstruct and protect the surgical site from further contact trauma. Other treatment options for septic arthritis or osteomyelitis include the use of implanted antibiotic-impregnated beads.
Eye enucleation	The eye is removed along with the lid margins. Dead space is closed and the skin sutured with sheathed nylon or a monofilament material.
Cloacal organ prolapse	A recent prolapse should be cleaned, lubricated and reduced. A temporary purse string suture can be used to retain the structure. A chronically prolapsed structure that has become necrotic or heavily infected may be best removed. Rectum, uterine horn, penis, portions of the bladder and cloaca itself may be involved. The penis is the most commonly removed structure. Postoperative care is minimal but checks should be made for possible infection. The tortoise will be infertile. Urination and behaviour are unaffected.
Shell trauma	Devascularized or heavily infected fragments of carapace or plastron must be discarded. Treat infected lesions with dressings. Do not cover with fibreglass.
Transplastron coeliotomy	Entry: 1. Open shell using a burr or cutting disc attached to a high-speed drill with a flexible extension and foot switch. 2. Cut through the plastron at an angle. This makes the inner aspect of the flap smaller than the outer. Once replaced, the flap will not fall into the tortoise and can be easily fixed back in place. The flap can either be cut on four sides and removed or cut on three sides and reflected back on the fourth through a scored hinge. 3. Mark the coeliotomy site on the plastron. Prepare the plastron aseptically. The size and location of the entry flap should take into account underlying structures such as the bladder, pelvic musculature, pectoral musculature and heart, which should be avoided unless the surgery specifically requires access to them. Where possible the large paired coelomic blood vessels are preserved. Closure: 1. Repose the coelomic membrane and suture. 2. Reflect the plastron flap back into position. 3. Fix layered glass fibre sheets over the flap site using an epoxy mixture. 4. The tortoise either remains in dorsal recumbency until the fibreglass holds the flap, or the flap is supported until the resin is hard. Bandaging the flap and applying resin until coelomic drainage ceases has also been successful

Figure 18.23 Common surgical procedures.

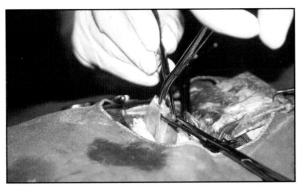

Figure 18.24 Removal of an obstructive foreign body (bone), through a transplastron coeliotomy.

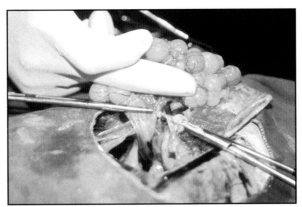

Figure 18.25 Ovariectomy through a transplastron coeliotomy (follicular stasis).

Microchipping

Current regulations restricting the trade of captive-bred species on CITES schedules specify that parents and offspring of most species of chelonians captive-bred in the UK should now be marked by the insertion of a passive microchip prior to being sold. A CITES permit identifying the animal by species, age, microchip number and its origin should accompany the animal during the sale. The small size of juvenile chelonians means that in certain circumstances (e.g. where the animal is less than 10 cm in length) the chip should accompany the animal and some other form of identification (e.g. a photograph or photocopy image of the plastron) be used instead, until the required size is reached.

- The microchip is probably best placed in the dorsal subcutaneous tissues of the left hindlimb, though other conventions have been suggested (the British Veterinary Zoological Society is a good source of up-to-date information)
- Tissue glue may be used to close down the site
- The site should be carefully followed up for signs of haemorrhage or infection
- It is unwise to microchip prior to hibernation.

Euthanasia

Injectable agents for euthanasia may result in unexpected recovery, because the chelonian brain survives periods of prolonged anoxia (Lutz and Manuel, 1999). Intracoelomic injection is not advised, as the time to death may be unnecessarily prolonged compared with intravenous injection.

The preferred technique for euthanasia is:

1. Intramuscular injection of ketamine at 100–200 mg/kg
2. Intravenous injection of 200 mg/kg pentobarbitone solution
3. Pith the animal to destroy the brainstem.

The insertion of a dental spike or needle into the brain through the foramen magnum or the roof of the mouth will achieve pithing and is always advised.

Drug formulary

It should be noted that there are unpredictable species differences in drug metabolism in chelonians. For species other than Mediterranean tortoises, further information should be sought (e.g. McArthur and Wilkinson, in preparation). With the exception of enrofloxacin, none of the drugs in the formulary is licensed for use in reptiles in the UK and much of the information is anecdotal or derived from a small number of cases. Whilst the authors believe the use of these agents to be justifiable, they cannot accept any responsibility for adverse reactions. Owners should be asked to sign a consent form for the use of an unlicensed product in each case.

Drug	Dose	Indication
Acyclovir	80 mg/kg orally sid	Herpesvirus infection
Allopurinol	20–50 mg/kg orally sid	Gout, hyperuricaemia
Amikacin	5 mg/kg i.m. every 48 h	Antibiotic with efficacy against Gram-negative bacteria and anaerobes
Ampicillin	50 mg/kg i.m. bid	Antibiotic with poor efficacy against Gram-negative bacteria
Butorphanol	0.4 mg/kg i.m. once	Analgesic
Calcium	10 mg/kg i.m. sid	Induction of oviposition
Carbenicillin	400 mg/kg i.m. every 48 h	Antibiotic with efficacy against Gram-negative bacteria
Carprofen	4 mg/kg s.c. once	Analgesic
Ceftazidime	20 mg/kg i.m. every 72 h	Antibiotic with efficacy against Gram-negative bacteria and anaerobes
Clarithromycin	15 mg/kg orally every 48 h	Antibiotic with efficacy against *Pasteurella*
Doxycycline	50 mg/kg i.m. initially, then 25 mg/kg sid	Antibiotic, antimalarial

Figure 18.26 Drug formulary for chelonians. (continues) ▶

Drug	Dose	Indication
Enrofloxacin	10 mg/kg sid s.c. or i.m.	Antibiotic with efficacy against Gram-negative bacteria
Fenbendazole	50 mg/kg orally on days 1, 21	Anthelmintic (nematodes)
Fluconazole	1 mg/kg orally sid	Antifungal (yeasts)
Ketoconazole	20 mg/kg orally sid	Antifungal (broad spectrum)
Metronidazole	50 mg/kg orally sid or 100 mg/kg on days 1, 14	Antibiotic with efficacy against anaerobes, antiprotozoal
Oxfendazole	65 mg/kg orally on days 1, 14	Anthelmintic (nematodes)
Oxytocin[a]	1–10 IU/kg i.m. x 1–3	Induction of oviposition
Piperacillin	100 mg/kg i.m. every 48 h	Antibiotic
Praziquantel	10 mg/kg orally, i.m. once	Anthelmintic (cestodes)
Proligestone	20 mg/kg s.c. once or more	Follicular stasis
Sulpha-dimethoxime	50 mg/kg orally every day for 7 days	Coccidiosis
Vitamin A	2000 IU/kg s.c. weekly	Hypovitaminosis A
Vitamin D_3	4 IU/kg orally sid	Metabolic bone disease

Figure 18.26 continued Drug formulary for chelonians.

a More effective with concurrent administration of a beta-blocker (e.g. propranolol).

References and further reading

Bennett RA (1995) Reptile anaesthesia. In: *Kirk's Current Veterinary Therapy XII*, pp. 1349–1353. WB Saunders, Philadelphia

Bennett RA (1998) Anaesthesia and analgesia. In: *Seminars in Avian and Exotic Medicine*, **7**(1), 30–40

Bienzle D, Boyd CJ, Valverde A and Smith DA (1992) Sedative effects of ketamine and midazolam in snapping turtles. *Journal of Zoo Animal Medicine* **23**, 201–204

Blahak S (2000) Infectious diseases in reptiles with special reference to zoonoses. *Der praktische Tierartz* **81**, 113–126

Butler PJ, Milsom WK and Wolkes AJ (1984) Respiratory, cardiovascular and metabolic adjustments during steady state swimming in the green sea turtle. *Journal of Comparative Physiology (B)* **154**, 167–174

Divers SJ (1998a) The diagnosis and treatment of lower respiratory tract disease in tortoises with particular regard to intrapneumonic therapy. *Proceedings of the Association of Reptile and Avian Veterinarians 1998*, pp. 95–98

Divers SJ (1998b) Two cases of reptile mycobacteriosis. *Proceedings of the Association of Reptile and Avian Veterinarians 1998*, pp. 133–138

Ernst C and Barbour R (1989) *Turtles of the World*. Smithsonian Institution Press, Washington DC

Fonda D (1999) Intraosseous anaesthesia with propofol in Red-eared Sliders *Trachemys scripta elegans*. *Proceedings of the Association of Veterinary Anaesthetists of the European Society of Laboratory Animal Medicine*, Newcastle 1999

Göbel T and Spörle H (1992) Blutentnahmetechnik und Serumnormalwerte wichtige Parameter bei der Griechischen Landschilkroete (*Testudo hermanni hermanni*). *Tieraertzliche Praxis* **20**, 231–234

Harvey S and Greenwood JR (1985) Isolation of *Campylobacter fetus* from a pet turtle. *Journal of Clinical Microbiology* **21**, 260

Highfield AC (1996) *Practical Encyclopaedia of Keeping and Breeding Tortoises and Freshwater Turtles*. Carapace Press, The Tortoise Trust, London

Lawrence K and Hawkey C (1986) Seasonal variations in haematological data from Mediterranean tortoises (*Testudo graeca* and *Testudo hermanni*) in captivity. *Research in Veterinary Science* **40**, 225–230

Lawton MPC and Stokes LC (1989) Post hibernation blindness in tortoises. In: *Third International Colloquium on the Pathology of Reptiles and Amphibians*, Orlando, Florida, pp. 97–98

Lock BA, Heard DJ and Dennis P (1998) Preliminary evaluation of medetomidine/ketamine combinations for immobilisation and reversal with atipamezole in three tortoise species. *Bulletin of ARAV* **8**(4), 6–9

Lutz PL and Manuel L (1999) Maintenance of adenosine A1 receptor function during long term anoxia in the turtle brain. *American Journal of Physiology* **276**(RICP45), R633–R636

MacDonald J (1998) An investigation into the oral flora of UK captive *Testudo* sp., with special regard to the prevalence of *Yersinia enterocolitica*. BVZS Autumn meeting (Nov 1998), Zoological Society of London

Malley AD (1997) Reptile anesthesia and the practicing veterinary surgeon. *In Practice* **19**, 351–370

McArthur SDJ, Wilkinson RJ and Innis C (in preparation) *Medicine and Surgery of Tortoises and Turtles*. Blackwell Science, Oxford

Norton TM, Spratt J, Behler J and Hernandez K (1998) Medetomidine and ketamine anaesthesia with atipamezole reversal in private free ranging tortoises *Goperus polyphemus*. *Proceedings of the Association of Reptile and Avian Veterinarians, Kansas City 1988*, pp. 25–27

Petney TN and Knight MM (1988) Treatment of ticks on tortoises using Amitraz. *Journal of the South African Veterinary Association* **59**(4), 206

Schmidt RE and Fletcher KC (1983) Non O-Group 1 *Vibrio cholerae* infection in a Desert Tortoise (*Gopherus berlanderi*). *Journal of Wildlife Disease* **19**, 358–359

Scott PW (1996) *Nutritional Diseases in Reptile Medicine and Surgery*. BVZS Proceedings 1996

Zwart P (1992) Urogenital system. In: *Manual of Reptiles*, ed. PH Beynon *et al.*, pp. 117–127. BSAVA Publications, Cheltenham

19

Lizards

Darryl Heard, Greg Fleming, Brad Lock and Elliott Jacobson

Introduction

The order Squamata contains approximately 7150 species, of which almost two-thirds are lizards and amphisbaenids (Pough *et al.,* 1998).

Biology

Although diversity would appear to make it difficult to generalize about husbandry and medicine, most common pet lizards are from a few families and share similar biology (Figures 19.1 and 19.2).

Family	Common name	No. genera	No. species	Comments
Agamidae	Agamas, flying dragons	45	300	Moderately sized to large. Diurnal. Primarily terrestrial. Scales often modified to form extensive crests, frills or spines.
Chamaeleonidae	Chameleons	4–6	130	Extensive development of casques, horns and crests. Able to change colour. Feet zygodactylus. Tails prehensile in arboreal species. Elongate tongues. Independently mobile eyes. Laterally compressed bodies. Exclusively diurnal and primarily insectivorous.
Iguanidae	Iguanas	8	34	Moderately sized to large. Terrestrial, rock-dwelling or arboreal. Primarily herbivores as adults, consuming leaves, fruits and flowers.
Phrynosomatidae	Horned, spiny and fence lizards	10	125	Broad range of morphological and ecological types.
Polychrotidae	Anoles	11	> 440	Diverse group. Many have brightly coloured dewlaps.
Corytophanidae	Basilisks	3	9	Well developed head crests and casques. *Basiliscus* spp. known to run on water.
Eublepharidae	Geckos	5	25	Most terrestrial. Lack subdigital setae for climbing. Have eyelids. Most inhabit arid or subhumid environments.
Gekkonidae	Geckos	82	870	Eyes covered by immovable spectacle. Range from deserts to tropical rainforest. Usually nocturnal. Arboreal or terrestrial. Many very vocal. In some, calcium carbonate stored in expansions of endolymphatic system on the neck.
Teiidae	Teiids, whiptails, caiman lizards, tegus	9	105	Moderately large. Usually active and diurnal. Diverse range of habitats. Caiman lizard *Dracaena* is primarily arboreal and has large molariform teeth for crushing snails.
Lacertidae	Wall and sand lizards	29	215	Small to moderately sized. Active. Terrestrial or rock-dwelling. Primarily insectivorous; some partially herbivorous.
Xantusiidae	Desert night lizards	3	17	
Scincidae	Skinks	100	1090	Most have smooth, shiny cycloid scales underlain by osteoderms. Diverse habitat, diet and size range. Most diurnal. Short legs.
Gerrhosauridae	Plated lizards	6	30	Scales in transverse rows with underlying osteoderms. Prominent lateral fold along body. Small to large. Terrestrial.
Varanidae	Monitor lizards	1	40	Small to very large. Active. Fast-moving foragers. Primarily insectivorous or carnivorous, some piscivorous and carrion-eaters.
Helodermatidae	Beaded lizard, gila monster	1	2	Stout lizards. Short, blunt tails for fat storage. Venomous. Carnivorous. Terrestrial or arboreal. Diurnal or nocturnal.

Figure 19.1 Lizard families. (Data from Rogner, 1997; Pough *et al.*, 1998.)

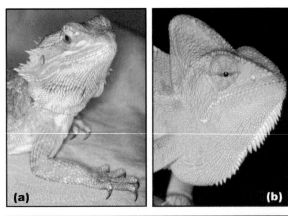

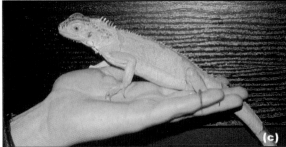

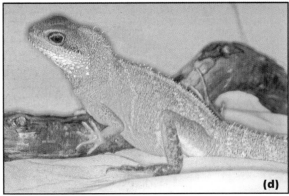

Figure 19.2 Some commonly kept lizards. (a) The bearded dragon *Pogona barbata* is a dryland agamid lizard from Australia. They are recommended as pets because they are easily socialized and relatively simple to maintain. (b) Veiled chameleon *Chamaeleo calyptratus*. (c) A juvenile green iguana *Iguana iguana*. (Courtesy of S. Redrobe.) (d) Chinese water dragon *Physignattus cocincinus*.

Sexing

Sex determination is frequently requested and is important for differentiating gender-related medical problems.

Secondary sexual characteristics

Accuracy depends on the species, the characteristic and experience. Secondary sexual characteristics are usually not developed in juveniles.

- In Jackson's, Johnston's and some other chameleons the males have cephalic horns, while females do not
- Male lizards, including green iguanas and gila monsters, usually have more robust bodies and heads than females, but the difference is often subtle

- Many male iguanids and gekkonids possess highly developed femoral and/or pre-anal pores
- Hemipenes often increase the size of the male's tail distal to the cloaca; this is especially apparent in many geckos.

Cloacal probe

The lizard is restrained, and a smooth, blunt instrument inserted into the inverted hemipenes on either side of the cloaca. The probe is gently manoeuvred until it enters the hemipenile pocket in the tail base. The insertion depth in males is species-dependent. In females the probe will have no, or very limited, penetration. Probing is of limited value in monitors and green iguanas, because of the blind diverticula present in females, but it appears more reliable in island iguanas (*Cyclura* spp.).

Eversion of the hemipenes

Manual eversion or 'popping' is accomplished by rolling a thumb firmly up the tail base towards the cloaca. The pressure exerted forces the hemipenes, if present, to evert from the cloaca. Care is needed to prevent injury.

Hydrostatic eversion uses isotonic saline injected into the tail at the caudal extent of where the hemipenis would be located. Fluid is instilled until the hemipenis has everted or resistance is felt at the plunger. For humane reasons, and to achieve adequate relaxation, this procedure is performed under anaesthesia. A blind diverticulum can be mistaken for a hemipenis, especially in neonates and monitor lizards; the hemipenis is usually more ornate and has a red sulcus running the length of the organ, as compared to just a red tip to the blind diverticulum.

Imaging

- Ultrasonography has limited value for sex determination, depending on operator expertise. The ovaries in sexually active female lizards are easiest to detect. Immature and acyclic females are indistinguishable from males, in the authors' experience
- Radiography is useful for adult monitors with mineralized hemibacula within the hemipenes
- Endoscopy is very accurate and can be used to sex most age classes of lizards. A flank incision is made with the anaesthetized animal in lateral recumbency. The gonad is visualized directly. Intracoelomic insufflation of room air or carbon dioxide is essential.

Husbandry

A critical evaluation of environment and nutrition is an essential component of the history. The veterinary surgeon should be aware of appropriate husbandry for the commonly kept species. The list of further reading at the end of this chapter includes many good texts; information is also readily available through the Internet and from local herpetological societies.

Housing

Ecological considerations

Captive husbandry is based upon knowledge of the ecosystems in which lizards live in the wild. Lizards inhabit a wide diversity of ecological niches, from arid desert to tropical rainforest, and from subterranean to high arboreal. The first step in determining environmental requirements is species identification. There is often more than one common name for a species, which may also be applied to a variety of dissimilar species. Therefore, it is recommended that the scientific name be used. Once identified, it is often possible to determine the environment the lizard comes from, its diet and some basic ecology. This information is then used to determine the type of captive habitat (vivarium) required (Figure 19.3).

Behavioural requirements

Most lizards are distressed and/or adversely affected by close contact with humans. Although this may decrease with time in some species, others will never adapt. Consequently, most lizards require some area to hide and/or flee from handlers. It is sometimes very difficult to assess whether a lizard is adversely affected by close contact. Chameleons, for example, become immobile rather than fleeing. Inappropriate housing and stress can result in the ultimate demise of these animals through 'stress' and immunocompromise.

Care must be taken when housing two or more animals or species together because of aggression and predation. Territoriality is dependent upon species, sex, age, season, health and nutritional status. Lizards housed together as juveniles may 'suddenly' turn on each other as adults. A large male lizard may dominate other males during the breeding season. Females will also establish a hierachy and/or defend preferred nesting sites. Some skinks are highly defensive of their young, providing parental care similar to that of mammals. If it is necessary to house animals together, providing multiple areas for hiding, feeding, drinking, basking and reproduction can minimize aggression and injury.

Size and design

Size requirement varies with species, size, age, sex and season. The enclosure should be as large as possible within space and monetary constraints. Minimally, sufficient space should be provided to allow the animal to stretch lengthwise and turn without touching the sides of its enclosure. Additionally, the cage should be of a sufficient size to allow for the provision of a thermal gradient (see below), shelter, and feeding and watering sites.

Terrestrial lizards require more floor area than height. Enclosures for arboreal species are either tall or are placed on an elevated shelf. Aquatic species require access to both water and basking areas. Care must be taken when assigning a lizard to a particular cage design since some species may require a combination of requirements. For example, the caiman lizard is both arboreal and semi-aquatic.

Cages should be built of materials that are impervious to liquids (including disinfectants), do not rot or corrode, and can be readily cleaned. It should be possible to view all areas of the inside of the cage to make it easy to check the occupants regularly, without having to move the furnishings. Entry into the cage should be easy and uncomplicated so animals cannot escape. Adequate airflow should be provided using ventilation panels or air-exchangers. Chameleons (and other small arboreal lizards) can be housed in fine gauge wire cages constructed around potted plants.

Substrates

Silica sand should be avoided as it is abrasive and may cause skin and eye irritation. Substrates such as ground corncob, walnut shells and wood shavings, should also be avoided as they may be ingested and cause gastro-intestinal blockage.

Heating

Lizards are poikilothermic, utilizing external heat sources to regulate body temperature. This heat is preferably provided in a gradient across the vivarium using light bulbs, ceramic heaters and/or cage heat tapes. Two heat forms should be provided: one that determines the background ambient temperature (e.g. heat tape); and a basking light. All heating devices should be protected to prevent direct contact and thermal injury. 'Hot rocks' should be avoided as they frequently malfunction and may produce contact burns.

Habitat/lifestyle	Examples	Temperature and heating	Humidity (%)
Tropical	Green iguana, green tree monitor, Jackson's chameleon	Day: 27–29°C Night: 24°C	80–100
Desert	Bearded dragon, Gould's monitor	Day: 29–32°C Basking: 38–49°C Night: 27°C	30–40
Temperate	Blue-tongued skink	Day: 27–32°C Night: 21–27°C	30–60
Arboreal	Green iguana, Jackson's chameleon	Air heating	n/a
Terrestrial	Blue-tongued skink, leopard gecko	Air and floor heating	n/a
Semi-aquatic	Basilisk, caiman lizard, Nile monitor	Water, air and floor heating	n/a

Figure 19.3 Classification system for determining captive habitat requirements for some commonly kept lizards. Classifications can be combined (e.g. green iguana). This is an approximation and it is recommended that reference be made to more detailed husbandry books (e.g. Rogner, 1997) for more detailed information on species requirements. n/a = not applicable.

Light
All lizards should be provided with a cycle of light and dark. A 12h:12h cycle is optimal for most non-reproductive and tropical species, though some species require changes in daylength, simulating seasons, for spermatogenesis. The temperature of the enclosure should cycle with the light cycle.

Most lizards require ultraviolet light of appropriate wavelength to synthesize vitamin D.

Humidity
Tropical species require humidity approaching 100%, attained by frequent misting and the use of live plants and large water containers. Desert species require an ambient humidity of around 30–40%, though many live in microenvironments (e.g. burrows, crevices, caves) that have a higher humidity. Inappropriately high humidity may result in blister disease or dermatitis, while dysecdysis may occur at low humidity.

Water
Predominantly aquatic species are maintained in aquaria, with continuous filtration and water quality control similar to that for fish. Some lizards, e.g. chameleons, do not recognize water bowls as a source of water, requiring either frequent misting of vegetation or a drip system from which the animal can drink. The latter is readily constructed from a used intravenous fluid bag and infusion set. Desert-adapted species have lower water requirements (20 ml/kg/day) than wetland/rainforest species (60 ml/kg/day) and may be able to attain their water requirements from their diet.

Hygiene
All objects intended for the vivarium should be cleaned in a dilute bleach solution (1:10) and/or placed in a freezer to remove unwanted insects and parasites. Many lizards defaecate in their water bowls, necessitating that water sources are changed, cleaned and scrubbed with disinfectant daily to prevent proliferation of potentially pathogenic bacteria.

Diet
The vast majority of lizards prey on arthropods, including insects (e.g. crickets, mealworms). Some, e.g. monitors, eat vertebrates; a few lizards are herbivores. Dietary preference may vary with age, size and time of year. Species from temperate climates may not eat during winter. Gravid females may not eat for several weeks close to parturition.

Whole animal prey is preferably fed killed to avoid injury to the lizard. If it is essential to feed live prey items (see Chapter 24: Legislation), the size and number should be appropriate for the species. Carnivores should be fed either whole prey items or a diet with a balanced Ca:P ratio. Food for insectivores should be dusted with a supplement and/or fed on a supplement before being offered. Diets for herbivores, based on vegetables and fruits, usually require vitamin and mineral supplementation. Several commercial companies offer balanced diets for common species, but much research is still required to determine the nutrient requirements of many lizards. Feeding should be observed to ensure that the lizard is not ingesting substrate with the food. This can also be avoided by placing the lizard in a clean plastic tub for feeding.

Handling
Small lizards can be examined in a clear container. If presented in a cloth bag, they should be restrained through the bag before opening it. Grasping the fore- and hindlimbs laterally against the thorax and the tail base, respectively, holds medium to large lizards (Figure 19.4). Care must be taken not to restrict respiratory movement. Wrapping the animal in a towel facilitates handling; placing a towel over its head to restrict vision often has a calming effect.

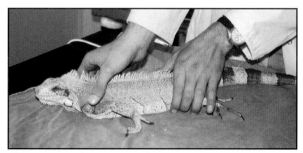

Figure 19.4 Grasping the fore- and hindlimbs laterally against the thorax and the tail base, respectively, holds medium to large lizards. (Courtesy of S. Redrobe.)

Tiletamine/zolazepam combinations (4–8 mg/kg i.m.) can be used to facilitate handling of large lizards. The main disadvantage of this combination is prolonged recovery, with residual sedation lasting as long as 24–48 hours. Lizards are more likely than other reptiles to suffer from inhalant anaesthetic overdosage because of the relative efficiency of their respiratory system.

Some lizards (i.e. iguanids) can be immobilized for short periods of time, sufficient for radiography, by gently pressing down on the eyes from above. This response has been ascribed to inducing the ocular vasovagal response (Lawton, 1997), although there is no research to document this in iguanas. The effect can be prolonged by placing wads of cotton wool over the eyes, secured in place by self-adhesive elasticized bandage. The animals will revive spontaneously in response to either loud noises or positional changes.

Given the opportunity, iguanids, monitors and tegus can inflict severe wounds with their powerful tails, claws and teeth. The gila monster and beaded lizard are venomous and often appear deceptively sluggish. The tokay gecko is large and aggressive with a powerful bite. Some geckos have very delicate skin that will tear upon restraint and these animals should only be examined in an enclosure or under anaesthesia. Chameleons become stressed by physical restraint and should be placed on a small branch for examination. Never grasp a lizard by the tail; most species can perform autotomy, shedding the tail in an attempt to escape.

Diagnostic approach

Physical examination

Examination is begun from a distance by observing the animal's activity, behaviour and posture. A lizard in a new environment will usually explore; monitors may show increased tongue flicking. Abnormal body posture and ambulation may suggest musculoskeletal and/or neurological disease. Tremors or muscle fasciculation are often a sign of hypocalcaemia secondary to metabolic bone disease and/or renal disease.

Physical examination is systematic and must include the oral cavity. Anaesthesia may be indicated in large lizards for a safe and complete examination.

Skin

The skin is examined for parasites and evidence of trauma caused by fighting, mating or burns. Lumps, bumps and discoloration may indicate infection or neoplasia. Haemorrhage into the scales may be due to septicaemia/bacteraemia. Shedding or ecdysis occurs in stages and retained skin (dry and brown) must be differentiated from normal (flexible and transparent) shedding. Skin retention often occurs around the digits and the tail and can cause ischaemic necrosis. Extensive skin folds, skin tenting and eyes sunken into the orbits are evidence of dehydration, while prominent pelvic bones often indicate cachexia.

Head

The mouth can be opened with a soft blunt spatula or by applying gentle downward pressure on the dewlap. A complete oral examination should be performed, looking for signs of trauma, infection (stomatitis), neoplasia and the oral extent of any rostral lesions.

The eyes, nostrils and tympanic membranes should be free from debris and discharge. The tympanic membranes can be transilluminated in some small species. Some species of iguanid and agamid excrete salt from specialized nasal glands and may have a white, dried material around the nares and or on the glass front of the enclosure. Rostral trauma, due to rubbing on cage wire or from repeated attempts to escape from the owner, is common.

Body

The head, body and limbs should be palpated for masses. Focal soft-tissue masses are usually abscesses or cutaneous parasites, while more diffuse swellings around the long bones or mandible more likely represent metabolic bone disease (MBD) or cellulitis. Iguanas with MBD will often have soft mandibles and maxillae that are easily depressed on palpation.

Placing a wet paper towel between the body wall and the diaphragm of a stethoscope enhances auscultation of the lungs and heart.

Gentle palpation of the coelomic body cavity can be performed for evidence of cystic calculi, faecoliths, enlarged kidneys (renal disease), impactions, retained eggs or ova, and coelomic masses. Palpation is facilitated by anaesthesia to relax the abdominal muscles and prevent struggling.

The cloaca should be free from faecal staining. Digital palpation can often be rewarding for evidence of cloacal masses or renomegaly.

Sample collection

Blood

Blood volume is approximately 5–8% of total bodyweight, and 10% of the blood volume may be withdrawn safely. The anticoagulant of choice is lithium–heparin; a small amount is drawn into the syringe, sufficient to coat the syringe and needle. Calcium–EDTA is preferable for haematological examination, although it may lyse cells. Blood samples for bacteriological culture are collected aseptically and placed in paediatric blood culture bottles for submission.

Blood collection sites are summarized in Figure 19.5. Haematological reference ranges are summarized in Carpenter *et al.* (2000). Blood is most easily

Site	Technique	Comments
Ventral coccygeal vein (ventral midline of the vertebral bodies of the coccygeal vertebrae; often protected by haemal arches)	Restrain lizard in dorsal recumbency or leave in sternal recumbency. Placing the tail over the edge of a table will facilitate access, or tail is dorsoflexed. Ventral approach: Insert needle on midline, at 45–90 degrees to skin, and sufficiently posterior to the cloaca to avoid the hemipenes and the scent glands. Advance the needle slowly until either blood is aspirated or contact is made with the ventral aspect of the vertebral body. If the needle hits the vertebrae, it is backed off until blood flow is attained. Lateral: Insert needle, at an angle of 45 degrees, between the transverse spinous process and the ventral tail, directed slightly dorsomedially.	Preferred site for venepuncture
Ventral abdominal vein (large subcutaneous vessel in the midline of the abdominal wall)	Insert needle cranially, at an acute angle to the skin and in the midline of the abdomen, caudal to the umbilicus.	Potential for puncture of bowel, haemorrhage and large haematoma formation. Can be used in debilitated patients for catheterization following a cut-down and surgical exposure
Cardiac puncture	Place lizard in a supine position. Cardiac location may vary from within the thoracic girdle to almost mid-abdomen (monitor lizards). Use a Doppler flow probe to determine site accurately. Blood is obtained via the thoracic inlet just above the symphysis of the clavicles.	Not recommended except in terminal patients because of hazards to animal

Figure 19.5 Blood collection sites.

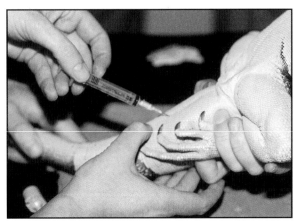

Figure 19.6 Blood sampling from an iguana. (Courtesy of S. Redrobe.)

collected from the ventral coccygeal vein (Figure 19.6). In some animals, it may also be collected from the ventral abdominal vein. Needle (23–27 gauge) and syringe (1–3 ml) selection is based on lizard size.

Lung/tracheal lavage

A tracheal wash is performed when there is evidence of lower respiratory disease; it is facilitated by general anaesthesia. The lizard is intubated with a sterile endotracheal tube and a sterile catheter passed down its lumen until resistance is encountered. Alternatively, the catheter is pre-measured depending upon the site to be sampled (trachea, bronchus, or lung). Sterile saline (1–5 ml/kg) is then infused and aspirated several times. The liquid sample is decanted into a sterile tube for submission for cytological examination and bacterial culture as indicated. Cytological examination should include a fresh wet mount to detect parasitic protozoans, larvae and eggs.

Gastric lavage

Gastric lavage is indicated when upper gastrointestinal disease is suspected. In large lizards anaesthesia may be required. Alternatively, lizards are allowed to bite down on a tape roll and the tube passed through the open mouth. Metal gavage tubes can be used without a mouth gag. The distance to the stomach is pre-measured, approximately half the way from the snout to the vent, and marked on the tube for accurate placement. Application of sterile lubricant will assist in passing the tube. Once the tube is in place, sterile warm saline is injected and aspirated a few times to obtain a sample. The collected sample is submitted for cytological and parasitological examination, and culture as indicated. A cytological sample should be acid-fast stained to facilitate detection of *Cryptosporidium* spp.

Colonic lavage

Colonic washes are used to obtain intestinal faecal samples. The lizard is restrained manually and a soft red rubber catheter (8–12 French), lubricated with water-soluble gel, inserted into the cloaca. Forcing the catheter may result in a perforation of the cloaca or rectum. Sterile saline (1% of bodyweight) is infused and aspirated several times. It is usual for only 25–50% of the infused saline to be recovered. The resulting sample is submitted for cytological and parasitological examination, and culture as indicated.

Diagnostic techniques

Faecal analysis

A fresh faecal sample (<24 hours) may be collected by the owner, placed in a double plastic bag (or film canister), and kept in the refrigerator until it can be brought to the clinic for evaluation. Alternatively, a cloacal/colonic wash is used (see above). Routine faecal evaluation should include:

- A wet mount (for motile flagellates)
- A sediment mount (for cestode, trematode, protozoal or nematode eggs)
- Flotation (for nematode eggs)
- Sample mixed with eosin (for *Entamoeba* cysts)
- Gram staining (to evaluate bacteria)
- Cytological stains (for inflammatory and neoplastic cells).

Blood culture

Blood culture for aerobic and anaerobic bacteria is useful when screening for suspected bacterial infection. A recent study (Hanel *et al.,* 1999) demonstrated that many healthy lizards, particularly carnivores, are normally blood culture-positive for *Clostridium* spp. The significance of this is unknown but it makes clinical interpretation of blood culture results confusing.

Common conditions

The diversity of lizards suggests that many diseases remain unrecognized and undescribed. This is reflected in the new infectious agents described each year and should make the veterinary surgeon alert to the unexpected. Disease is usually multifactorial and it is often difficult to determine a specific cause, particularly in chronically ill animals. Unfortunately, ill reptiles are often in the chronic stages of disease when presented because of their ability to mask signs, their inherent resilience and owner ignorance.

Disease processes tend to progress slowly in reptiles. Healing and resolution of disease can take weeks, and it may take several weeks to determine a prognosis. To avoid owner frustration, it is important to make clear the time that may be involved. Successful resolution is often dependent on basic nursing care, such as maintaining an appropriate environmental temperature and providing nutrition and hydration through gavage feeding.

Many reptile owners have multiple animals. It is important, therefore, to differentiate a herd health problem from an individual pet problem. For example, the owner of a large gecko collection, who is losing animals from a chronic wasting disease, would benefit more from the information gained from the necropsy of representative animals than treatment of an individual animal showing clinical signs.

Viral infections

Examples of viruses isolated from lizards are given in Figure 19.7. Viral infection should be suspected: if an animal fails to respond to antimicrobial therapy; if tissue samples reveal possible intracellular inclusions; if multiple animals are involved; if there is a high mortality; and when all other causes have been ruled out. Viruses may also act multifactorially with other agents and poor husbandry to produce disease.

Bacterial infections

The occurrence of bacterial infections in captive lizards is variable between families; for example, they are common in green iguanas, monitors and chameleons, but sporadic in bearded dragons. Primary infections can often be attributed to a compromised immune system as a consequence of inappropriate husbandry leading to stress. Malnutrition will also compromise the host and allow secondary bacterial infections.

While both Gram-positive and Gram-negative bacteria have been implicated, Gram-negatives seem to be most often involved. The most common bacteria isolated from lesions are *Aeromonas hydrophila*, *Serratia marcescens*, *Corynebacterium*, *Pseudomonas*, *Salmonella*, *Proteus* and *Edwardsiella*. A newly described *Neisseria* has been isolated from the oral cavity and bite wounds of iguanas (Plowman *et al.*, 1987). Anaerobic bacteria of the genera *Bacteroides*, *Fusobacterium*, *Clostridium* and *Peptostreptococcus* may be underdiagnosed.

There has been much publicity about green iguanas and salmonellosis. *Salmonella* can be shed intermittently by healthy reptiles and presents a major zoonotic concern (Draper *et al.*, 1981; Barten, 1993). Owners of iguanas and other reptiles should be very aware of this problem and use appropriate hygiene to curtail infection. Detection of *Salmonella* is made difficult by the low sensitivity of bacterial culture; consequently, it is recommended that all lizards be considered potential reservoirs.

Skin infections caused by *Dermatophilus* have been reported in chameleons (Jacobson, 1990; Origgi *et al.*, 1999). This genus is unique in forming filamentous structures that segment transversely and longitudinally. The lesions are seen as raised brown multifocal encrustations.

Infections of joints are common in iguanas and chameleons, with the interphalangeal joints the most affected. Fractures, penetrating wounds, nail bed injury and haematogenous spread from localized or systemic infections can result in arthritis. In iguanas, husbandry conditions often contribute to septic arthritis as inappropriate caging or relocation can induce an iguana to dig at its cage in attempts to escape. Correction of underlying problems is essential.

Antimicrobial treatment is based on knowledge of probable bacteria, culture and sensitivity and/or evaluation of Gram-stained samples. Commonly used antibiotics (amikacin, enrofloxacin, trimethoprim–sulphonamides) are usually ineffective against

Virus	Lizard species	Clinical and pathological signs	References
Poxviridae	Flap-necked chameleon *Chamaeleo dilepis*	Intracytoplasmic inclusions within circulating monocytes	Jacobson and Telford, 1990
Iridoviridae (lizard erythrocyte virus)	Flap-necked chameleon, Fischer's chameleon *Bradypodion fischeri*	Intraerythroctic inclusions	Telford and Jacobson, 1993
Adenoviridae	Jackson's chameleon *C. jacksoni*	Anorexia and death. Proliferation of the mucosal epithelial lining of the oesophagus and trachea. Eosinophilic intranuclear inclusions within oesophageal and tracheal epithelial cells	Jacobson and Gardiner, 1990
	Dragons *Pogona barbatus*, *P. vitticeps* and *P. henrylawsoni*	Intranuclear inclusions in hepatocytes and enterocytes in the small intestine	Julian and Durham, 1985; Frye *et al.*, 1994; Jacobson *et al.*, 1996
Dependoviridae	Neonate bearded dragons *P. vitticeps*	Intranuclear inclusions in hepatocytes and small intestinal enterocytes. Two different sized particles visualized by electron microscopy. Larger particles consistent with an adenovirus; smaller particles consistent with Dependovirus.	Jacobson *et al.*, 1996
Herpesviridae	Green iguana	Recovered from the liver, spleen, kidney, heart, and lung of apparently normal green iguanas. Cytopathic effects and intranuclear eosinophilic inclusions observed in iguana cell cultures incubated at 30°C and 36°C. Despite in-vitro cytopathic effects, pathogenicity inconclusive based upon in-vivo transmission studies. While it has been suggested that a form of lymphocytic leukaemia may be related to herpes virus infection in green iguanas, a causal relationship has not been demonstrated	Clark and Karson, 1972; Frye *et al.*, 1977; Frye, 1995
Reovirus	Green Iguana	Anorexia. Virus isolated from multiple organs. Prevalence and pathogenicity?	Blahak, 1994
Paramyxoviridae	Caiman lizard *Dracaena guianensis*	Mass die-off shortly after importation of animals from Peru. Anorexia, weight loss, ± dyspnoea. Proliferative pneumonia. Tissue inclusions. Virus isolated from lungs and other tissues	Jacobson *et al.*, 2000

Figure 19.7 Viruses identified in lizards.

anaerobic bacteria. Metronidazole is a useful adjunct to antimicrobial therapy when anaerobic bacteria are a possibility.

Fungal infections

Relatively few fungi have been identified in lizards. In green iguanas, a necrotizing pneumonia associated with branching septate hyphae resembling *Aspergillus* was seen on histopathological examination (Migaki *et al.,* 1984) and candidiasis has been associated with stomatitis (Rosenthal and Mader, 1996). An iguana with a fistulous tract leading from one nare was found to have numerous fungal granulomas in the lung and viscera, combined with mycotic osteomyelitis of the nasal septum (Jacobson, 1993). Mycotic enteritis has been diagnosed in a chameleon (Shalev *et al.,* 1977).

Parasites

Parasites are common in imported lizards. In the wild, parasites usually produce minimal injury to the host but they become a problem when lizards are placed in high stress situations, malnourished and exposed to other infectious agents. Whereas wild lizards may range over great distances, being exposed to different environmental conditions, captive lizards live in the same enclosure throughout their lives and may be re-exposed to internal or external parasites (mites) on a daily basis such that the parasite may overwhelm its host. Enclosure hygiene is an important part of parasite control.

External parasites

Mites and ticks are common on freshly imported lizards. In addition to causing external problems, they may also be vectors for viral, rickettsial and filarial pathogens. The snake mite *Ophionyssus natricis* is more common on snakes but in mixed lizard and snake collections it may cause a lacklustre appearance and dermatitis and shedding problems. Red mites, known as 'chiggers', inhabit skin folds around the legs, eyes, tympanic recesses and ear openings, and may cause areas of blackened discoloration (Harvey-Clark, 1995). Ticks usually inhabit hard-to-reach areas such as the gular skin fold under the chin, tympanic recesses, cloacal folds and skin folds around the limbs. Treatment of tick and mite infestations may be accomplished with ivermectin. For mites the environment must also be treated, as the female mite lays eggs in crevices of cage furniture. New cage furniture, such as mosses or tree limbs, should be disinfected and placed in a freezer for 24–48 hours to kill any free-living mites. Ticks may be removed with tweezers or haemostats.

Internal parasites

Protozoans have been identified in the gastrointestinal and circulatory systems of lizards. Most are non-pathogenic. Ciliates may cause subspectacular infections in geckos. *Entamoeba invadens* is carried by turtles and crocodilians and can be contracted by lizards through ingestion of cysts from faecal material of affected hosts. Infection results in anorexia, dehydration and wasting, due to gastritis and colitis resulting from the reproduction of the parasite in the gastrointestinal tract; the organism may spread to the liver and kidneys (Lane and Mader, 1996). Herbivorous lizards seem to be less susceptible than carnivores.

Coccidians have been reported in lizards but are poorly understood due to their complicated life cycles. The most frequently reported genera are *Isospora* and *Caryospora.* Coccidiosis is the most commonly reported parasitic disease of bearded dragons, with *I. amphiboluri* identified as the causative agent (McAllister *et al.,* 1995). Clinical signs include mild anorexia, diarrhoea, regurgitation, dehydration and haemorrhagic enteritis. Monitor lizards have also been known to be infected with *Eimeria* and *Klassia.* Systemic microsporidiosis has been reported in an inland bearded dragon (Jacobson *et al.,* 1998).

Cryptosporidium spp. have been identified as a cause of chronic wasting in several lizard species (Lane and Mader, 1996; Coke and Tristan, 1998).

Haemoparasitic protozoans are often identified on routine blood screening, and most are transmitted through insect vectors. They are not fully understood and are rarely implicated in clinical disease. Tapeworms are common in lizards with a diet of fish and amphibians, which they use as intermediate hosts. Clinical disease is rare.

Nematodes are common in the digestive system of lizards. Oxyurids have been reported in the colon of bearded dragons and iguanas. Although clinical signs of anorexia, regurgitation, obstruction and bloat have been attributed, infections are usually non-pathogenic.

Filarial disease has been reported in green iguanas and in chameleons but its importance is unknown. the worms are transmitted by arthropod vectors. Microfilaria enter the circulatory system and may result in oedema, necrosis or thrombosis and vessel blockage.

Pentastomids are primitive arthropods that inhabit the lungs and trachea of reptiles. Three genera are known to infect lizards: *Elenia, Sambonia* (both monitor lizards only) and *Raillietiella.* Adults inhabit the lungs where females deposit fully embryonated eggs. The eggs are carried out of the lungs by the ciliary lining and are then swallowed and passed in the faeces. Most infections are asymptomatic. However, immunocompromised lizards may incur pulmonary damage and secondary bacterial infection. Ivermectin at 200 µg/kg s.c. for 10 days followed by surgical removal of dead adults has been used with minimal success.

Nutritional disease

Nutritional requirements in captivity are mostly unknown; diets are based on extrapolation from mammals and those few lizard species in which studies have been performed. Requirements in captivity vary from those in the wild because of different activity levels and reproductive states. Disease also alters requirements and may affect digestion and absorption directly or indirectly.

The most common nutritional disease is metabolic bone disease (see below). Hypovitaminosis E has been incriminated as an alternative cause of muscle tremors, as well as flaccid paralysis in extreme cases. It may be due to feeding herbivorous diets low in vitamin E.

Hypovitaminosis A has been described in chameleons due to inadequate ingestion of pre-formed vitamin A (Ferguson *et al.*, 1996). Clinical signs include respiratory infections, ocular problems, neurological dysfunction, dysecdysis, spinal kinking and increased formation of hemipenal plugs. Treatment relies on parenteral administration of vitamin A palmitate and adequate dietary intake (>37.5 IU/day) (Ferguson *et al.*, 1996; Stahl, 1997).

Hypothiaminosis is usually seen in animals fed frozen thawed fish. Freezing and improper thawing decrease thiamine and increase thiaminase activity. Herbivorous lizards can develop hypothiaminosis if fed plants that contain phytothiaminase. Clinical signs are generally non-specific and include muscle tremors, incoordination, muscle weakness, torticollis, seizure activity, abnormal posture, jaw gaping and dysphagia. Treatment involves oral or subcutaneous supplementation of thiamine. The diet should also be altered to provide herbivores with alternative plant material and adding supplemental thiamine to frozen fish.

Biotin is a B vitamin that is available in almost all foods. Only those lizards fed a diet consisting wholly of raw unfertilized eggs, e.g. beaded lizards and gila monsters, are deficient. Raw egg whites contain avidin, which has anti-biotin activity, while fertilized eggs have some embryonic tissue that contains biotin. Treatment consists of changing the diet or supplementing the diet with vitamin B complex orally or by injection.

Oversupplementation with vitamins and minerals may be just as hazardous as deficiency. Toxicosis is more likely with parenteral than oral administration. Particular care must be taken when administering vitamins A and D, and selenium.

Obesity is a problem in some captive lizards, especially monitors. Low environmental temperatures decrease metabolic rate and caloric requirement. This is compounded by decreased activity in small enclosures and feeding fatty foods. Obesity predisposes to the development of fatty liver and, through increased antioxidant requirement, hypovitaminosis E.

Neoplasia

Lizards are susceptible to neoplasia, with tumours of all major body systems being reported.

Gastrointestinal disease

Stomatitis is relatively common. Predisposing factors include immunosuppression, inappropriate diet and, possibly, underlying metabolic bone disease. The acrodont teeth (not rooted but simply attached to the surface of the mandibular and maxillary bones) of many species of lizard also appear to predispose to periodontal disease (McCracken and Birch, 1994). Clinical signs include altered gingival colour, malodour, anorexia, inability to use the tongue, oral discharge, discoloured teeth, swelling and bleeding. Oral abscesses and/or osteomyelitis may follow chronic severe stomatitis.

Gastritis and/or enteritis may be due to bacteria, viruses and/or endoparasites. The main clinical sign is chronic debilitation and cachexia, and occasionally regurgitation. Diarrhoea may also be present. Foreign body ingestion is common in lizards and is occasionally associated with obstruction. Obstruction due to a foreign body, intussusception and/or intestinal torsion may be associated with anorexia, occasionally regurgitation/vomiting, wasting and/or abdominal distension. Renomegaly secondary to renal disease may cause colonic obstruction. Intussusception, intestinal torsion and rectal prolapse may be sequelae of endoparasitism and gastroenteritis.

Respiratory disease

Respiratory disease may present with the non-specific clinical signs of depression, anorexia and moderate weight loss. With severe disease, signs include altered mucosal colour, dyspnoea, glottal discharge and open-mouthed breathing. Signs of respiratory disease are an indication for a tracheal wash. Possible causes of respiratory disease include bacterial, parasitic, viral and fungal infections.

Musculoskeletal disease

The main problem in lizards is metabolic bone disease (MBD). MBD (Figure 19.8) refers to a variety of conditions that result from dietary imbalances of calcium and phosphorus and/or from a lack of appropriate wavelengths of light. MBD is also known as fibrous osteodystrophy or nutritional secondary hyperparathyroidism. It is very common in small to mid-sized, juvenile iguanas and chameleons. A common factor in iguanas is

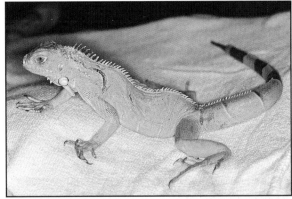

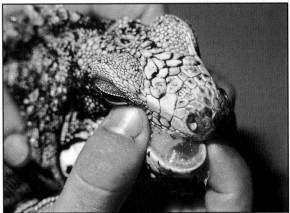

Figure 19.8 Clinical signs of severe metabolic bone disease in green iguanas include spinal deformities and associated paresis/paralysis and malleability of the jaws ('rubber jaw').

inadequate exposure to ultraviolet light, primarily of the UVB wavelength range of 290–315 nm, necessary for the presumed synthesis of vitamin D_3 (1,25-dihydroxycholecalciferol). It is also necessary for the animal to achieve its preferred optimal temperature for some part of the day to activate the enzymes necessary for the synthesis of vitamin D_3. Preliminary data indicate that vitamin D_3 is not absorbed from the gastrointestinal tract of green iguanas in significant amounts (Bernard *et al.*, 1991).

MBD can also result from an inversion of the desired dietary Ca:P ratio of 1–2:1 (Bernard *et al.*, 1991). Inadequate calcium intake alone can contribute. Renal disease and primary hyperparathyroidism are also potential causes. MBD results in deposition of fibrous tissue in and around bone, especially in the long bones and mandible. A swollen or rubbery appearance and feel of the mandible, and alterations in posture, are early signs (Figure 19.8). As the mandible loses density, it can be pulled caudally by the constant tension of the musculature, resulting in brachygnathism. Swelling around the femur and pathological fractures of the long bones are common as the condition progresses. Secondary effects may include joint infections, common in iguanas and chameleons.

Urinary tract disease

Renal disease is most commonly identified in adult green iguanas (Divers, 1997). Clinical signs are non-specific and include anorexia, dehydration, abdominal distension due to ascites, weight loss, weakness and muscle fasciculation. Renal disease may include renomegaly, which can cause colonic obstruction and constipation. Enlarged kidneys may be palpated in the caudal coelomic cavity, extending forward from the pelvis. They may also be visualized by radiography and ultrasonography. Enlarged kidneys should be differentiated from the fat bodies that are also present in the caudal coelomic cavity.

Uric acid is the primary nitrogenous metabolic product of protein metabolism. Although it is excreted by the kidneys, it is secreted into the renal tubules and does not reflect glomerular filtration rate (GFR). Hence, an animal may have extensive renal dysfunction, including markedly decreased GFR, yet have normal blood uric acid levels. In lizards, renal dysfunction is most often reflected in a decreased Ca:P ratio (<1.0). Gravid females can have markedly high blood levels of these electrolytes, but the ratio should still be >1.0. Creatine, but not creatinine, levels are elevated early on. Hypokalaemia is less common and usually seen in the latter stages of disease. The animal may also be acidotic, as reflected in low total carbon dioxide levels. Microscopic inspection of a urine sample obtained by cystocentesis may reveal blood, inflammatory cells or renal casts indicative of active infection and acute disease. Kidney biopsies can be obtained from within the caudal coelomic cavity or from behind the back legs.

Renal disease is treated using the same principles as for mammals. The observed muscle fasciculation is probably due to low circulating levels of ionized calcium. However, care must be taken when treating with calcium to do so only when phosphorus levels have been reduced, possibly with the use of oral phosphate binders. This is done to reduce the likelihood of tissue mineralization.

Cystic calculi are common in adult iguanas. Their causes are probably multifactorial and may be linked with water deprivation and subsequent dehydration. Clinical signs are variable and have included lethargy, depression, anorexia, constipation and hindlimb paresis. Most cystic calculi in reptiles are composed of urate salts; calcium urate stones are radiodense and so visible on radiographs while ammonium urate stones are best diagnosed by palpation. Treatment involves surgical removal (see below) and antibiotics.

Reproductive disorders

Most lizards lay eggs but some, including skinks and gila monsters, bear live young. Several populations of *Lacerta* and *Cnemidophorus* are entirely female and reproduce by parthenogenesis (Pough *et al.*, 1998).

Most reproductive problems are recognized in females, particularly green iguanas and chameleons. In egg retention (dystocia), the female fails to pass some or all the shelled eggs from the reproductive tract. In obstructive dystocia the ova are unable to pass due to their malformation or to anatomical abnormalities. In non-obstructive dystocia the female fails to lay due to lack of suitable nesting sites, stress, or abnormal hormonal stimulation. Surgical management of dystocia is indicated when medical management and/or husbandry changes have failed, when there is evidence of a physical obstruction, or if the owner wants to prevent reproductive problems or eggs being produced.

Follicular stasis refers to normal yolk formation without subsequent ovulation. The failure to ovulate is probably related to the solitary status of many pet iguanas and the absence of a suitable breeding environment. Female iguanas normally experience prolonged follicular development. The presence of large pre-ovulatory follicles is an indication for ovariosalpingectomy to prevent future reproductive cycling. However, treatment may not be necessary in most iguanas as they may either be entering a normal phase of reproduction or resorb the follicles.

Skin disease

Subcutaneous masses/swellings are common in green iguanas and chameleons. While bacteria are most often recovered from abscesses, other possible causes are fungi, foreign bodies, neoplasia and metazoan parasites. Subcutaneous abscesses are frequent and may be caused by a single bacterial species or a mixed infection (Figure 19.9). In chameleons, abscesses in the angle of the jaw, oral cavity, periorbital tissue and joint spaces are common. Orbital and oral abscesses are also common in green iguanas. Agents isolated from the abscesses of iguanas include *Neisseria iguanae*, *Corynebacterium*, *Morganella morgani*, *Salmonella marina*, *Serratia marcescens*, *Micrococcus* and *Fusobacterium necrophorum*. Bite-wound inoculation of bacteria is probably an important source of infection.

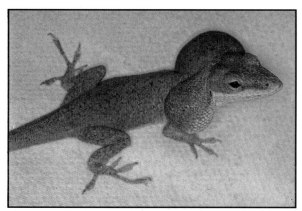

Figure 19.9 A green anole with bilateral neck abscesses secondary to conspecific bite wounds.

Neurological disease

Neurological disease can result from a variety of causes, including trauma, nutritional deficiencies, neoplastic and degenerative conditions, infection and toxicity. Observation of the patient prior to restraint is important for observation of mental status, degree of alertness and presence of any abnormal postures. Stimulation of movement can reveal abnormalities in ambulation. Other signs include head tilt or turn, opisthotonus, ataxia, circling and seizure activity.

Reflexes that are useful to evaluate neurological status include the righting reflex, foot withdrawal, tail or vent stimulation, and the panniculus reflex. Lizards placed on their backs should lift their heads first then roll the rest of the body to a normal position fairly rapidly at normal temperatures. Stimulation by pressure or pain (from a needle) on a leg, tail or vent will cause a withdrawal of the limb, the tail will twitch and the vent will wink (open and close). The panniculus response is used to localize spinal lesions. Pushing against the lateral muscula-ture or using a needle to stimulate the skin along the lateral margins of the body causes a normal lizard to push back against palpation and to twitch the skin in response to a needle. Where there is a spinal cord injury the animal will not push back against palpation and the twitching is present cranial but not caudal to the lesion. Because muscular movement and nerve conduction velocity are tem-perature-dependent, all neurological evaluations should be conducted at an appropriate temperature for the particular species.

Electromyography is generally difficult to interpret, as nerve conduction velocity varies with ambient tem-perature; normal velocity for a given temperature and species is usually not known. If a normal conspecific is available as a control, a large difference between the two might support a diagnosis of a conduction distur-bance. Plain radiographs are useful in cases of spinal or skull fractures. Magnetic resonance imaging is most useful for soft tissue causes of a neuropathy such as tumours or other masses. Computed tomography is most useful in diagnosing bony causes of neurological disease. A myelogram can be performed in green iguanas and other large lizards to further localize spinal lesions (Divers, 2000).

Behavioural problems

Male green iguanas may become aggressive towards their owners or cagemates. In one study involving 16 adult males, castration performed before the onset of the breeding season significantly reduced offensive aggression (Lock, pers. comm.). Castration during the breeding season did not have a significant effect on aggressive behaviour. Defensive aggres-sion remained intact. When performed in immature iguanas castration may prevent the development of aggressive behaviours, though scientific studies to support this are lacking.

Supportive care

Injection sites

Intramuscular injections are given into either the proximal fore- or hindlimb. Very little of the venous return from the hindlegs passes via the renal portal system through the kidneys. Intravenous injections of non-irritant solutions are administered into either the ventral coccygeal or abdominal veins, or through an intraosseous catheter (see below).

Thermoregulation

Since lizards are poikilothermic, control of environ-mental and, hence, body temperature is an important adjunct to supportive care. Determination of cloacal temperature is used as a guide to thermoregulatory management. Debilitated and/or moribund lizards are unable to thermoregulate and may remain on hot surfaces even when significant burns occur. Hospital-ized lizards should be maintained within their pre-ferred optimum body temperature range for at least a portion of the day. Some authors recommend the use of full-spectrum lamps for patients hospitalized more than a few days.

Fluid therapy

Daily weight measurement and recording is an important guide to water loss or gain. When in doubt, fluids should be provided either orally or parenterally. Small patient size makes venous and intraosseous catheterization difficult.

The authors prefer 20–24 gauge over-the-needle catheters for venous catheterization. Catheters can be placed in either the ventral abdominal or cephalic vein after making a skin incision and blunt dissection to expose the vessel. The cephalic vein passes diago-nally across the forelimb.

Intraosseous catheterization requires spinal nee-dles (18–22 gauge) to prevent a bony core blocking the catheter. In very small lizards a small (25–27 gauge) hypodermic needle is used. The needle length is approximately one third to half the length of the bone into which the needle is to be placed. Intraosseous catheterization sites include the distal femur, proximal tibia and proximal humerus. The most easily access-ible is the distal femur.

Subcutaneous administration of fluids is not appropriate for correction of deficits. Fluid absorption is minimal because subcutaneous tissues are poorly vascularized, and peripheral vasoconstriction is the usual response to dehydration and hypotension. Hypertonic dextrose solutions administered subcutaneously will exacerbate dehydration and fluid deficits.

Balanced electrolyte solutions, e.g. 0.9% NaCl or lactated Ringer's, are used for routine fluid administration. Some authors avoid lactated Ringer's solution in reptiles because of the prolonged half-life of lactate (Prezant and Jarchow, 1997) and advocate a 50:50 combination of 5% dextrose and a non-lactated multiple electrolyte solution. Blood glucose levels in reptiles range from 30 to 100 mg/dl or higher, depending on species. Isotonic dextrose solution (5%) or combinations are indicated when hypoglycaemia is present or expected.

A general guideline to fluid selection is:

- For 5–10% of blood volume lost, use balanced electrolyte solution at three times the volume of the estimated blood loss
- For 10–20% loss, use plasma expanders
- For 20–30% loss, use whole blood transfusion. Blood is preferably collected into heparinized syringes or acid citrate phosphate dextrose anticoagulant and transfusions are confined to the same species.

Small-volume syringe infusors are essential for accurate fluid infusion in small patients. They allow a continuous infusion that is preferable to bolus injection. The rate of fluid infusion is dependent on hydration status, daily fluid requirement, severity of haemorrhage, type of fluid to be infused, and the presence or absence of underlying renal or cardiac disease.

Nutritional support

Nutritional support is an important component of any supportive care plan and the authors recommend an aggressive approach. Daily bodyweight measurement is an important diagnostic guide to nutritional status. Body condition is best evaluated by examining the pelvic area and tail. Cachexia will be observed as an increased ability to visualize the bones of the pelvis and the tail. The eyes and muscles of the head may also appear sunken.

Nutritional support is provided through a feeding tube or oesophageal tube. The placement of an oesophageal catheter facilitates feeding of long-term hospitalized patients and/or anorectic animals maintained at home. It also minimizes handling of aggressive lizards and/or animals that become stressed with handling (i.e. chameleons). The procedure is described later.

The volume of food administered and its frequency is determined by the species and condition of the animal. Animals that have been anorectic for prolonged periods should initially be given an isotonic electrolyte solution containing glucose. If the animal appears to tolerate this, additional food material can be added to the solution. The formulation of the material is dependent on normal diet. For example, insectivores may be given puréed mealworms and crickets or a liquid gruel made from moist cat food. Carnivores can also be given such a gruel, while herbivores can be fed a vegetable purée. Several commercial reptile diets are available and can be puréed for oral administration. Stomach volume is approximately 5–15 ml/kg – this can be adjusted depending upon the presence of reflux. Care must be taken to ensure normal peristalsis and gastric emptying, which is assessed by observing defecation and/or contrast fluoroscopy.

Anaesthesia

Reptile anaesthesia has recently been reviewed by Heard (2001). Lizards may be induced with an inhalant anaesthetic (preferably isoflurane in oxygen), administered into a plastic bag, induction chamber or mask. Breath-holding is not as large a problem as some authors suggest. Gently running fingers along the chest wall will often elicit respiration and facilitate anaesthetic uptake. Some lizards may be intubated awake.

The preferred injectable induction agent is propofol (3–5 mg/kg) administered into the ventral coccygeal vein. This dose is lower than that recommended by previous authors but is usually sufficient for intubation. Maximum effect may not be observed for 2–5 minutes after injection. This lower dose also appears to be associated with less apnoea.

Endotracheal intubation (Figure 19.10) is used in medium to large lizards to facilitate administration of inhalant anaesthesia and to provide assisted ventilation. The glottis is a slit-like opening between the arytenoid cartilages and located at the base of the tongue on the floor of the oral cavity. It is closed except during exhalation and inspiration. Relaxation of the jaw muscles and direct application of local anaesthetic (2% lignocaine (lidocaine) injection or lignocaine gel) to the glottis facilitates intubation. Gentle ventral traction on the lower jaw will cause the mouth to open. Alternatively, aggressive lizards will often open their mouths in response to gentle tapping on the rostrum. In small to

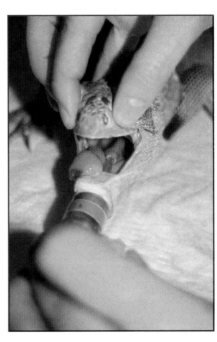

Figure 19.10
An iguana intubated for anaesthesia. (Courtesy of S. Redrobe.)

medium lizards, a rubber cooking spatula is inserted into the mouth to open it. Once open, the mouth is prevented from closing with a mouth gag. If the glottis is closed, it is necessary to wait for it to open or to use the bevel of the lubricated ET tube to gently force it open. The trachea of chameleons is very short and flexible. In small reptiles, attaching the animal's head, ET tube and breathing system to a tongue depressor reduces the possibility of the tube's being twisted or removed.

Lizards are ventilated once or twice per minute. Unless contraindicated by severe respiratory dysfunction, the animal is ventilated with room air once the procedure is complete to hasten recovery.

Common surgical procedures

General principles and instruments

Aseptic technique is as important as it is for 'higher' vertebrates. Clear plastic adhesive drapes are used to improve visualization for anaesthetic monitoring. Electrosurgical units are useful for haemostasis of blood vessels within the coelomic cavity. Surgery is facilitated by binocular magnification loupes of 2.5–5.0×. Haemostatic clips and appliers are used to control haemorrhage in deep recesses or near vital structures where ligation would be difficult or could result in damage to major vessels. Small curettes and cerumen loops aid in removal of caseous and inspissated pus from abscesses. Sterile cotton-tipped applicators are used for manipulation of delicate tissue and to absorb fluid. Absorbable gelatin sponge is used in small patients to control haemorrhage from unidentified blood vessels.

The phases of wound healing are similar to those seen in mammals but spread over a longer time. Skin sutures are left in place for 4–8 weeks. Many factors are thought to affect wound healing. It has been suggested that ecdysis promotes wound healing and some surgeons prefer to remove sutures after an ecdysis when wound strength may be increased. Environmental temperatures at the high end of the optimum range promote healing. Cranial-to-caudal wounds heal more quickly than dorsal-to-ventral wounds. Open wounds heal well by second intention, with a low incidence of infection.

Oesophageal catheterization

The tube is placed under general anaesthesia.

1. Pass a haemostat through the mouth into the oesophagus.
2. Make an incision over the tip of the haemostat and pull it through the skin using blunt force.
3. Grasp a sterile feeding tube with the haemostat and pull it into the oesophagus and back out of the mouth.
4. Redirect the tip of the catheter back down the mouth into the oesophagus and through into the stomach.
5. Advance the catheter to the marked pre-measured length, approximated by measuring from behind the last rib and/or mid-abdomen, or until resistance is felt.

6. Attach the tube to the neck with a 'finger-trap' suture and tape it along the back of the animal in a position where it cannot be dislodged.

The catheter should be flushed with water after every feeding to ensure patency, and is maintained until the animal is eating normally and maintaining bodyweight.

Coeliotomy

A midline or paramedian approach is used for exploratory surgery. Equivalent exposure to the coelomic cavity is obtained by both paramedian and ventral midline approaches. The paramedian approach minimizes the risk of damaging the large ventral abdominal vein, located between the umbilical depression and the pubic bone. A ventral midline approach can also be used (Figure 19.11), provided care is taken to avoid damage to this vessel. Ligation of the ventral abdominal vein appears to have no adverse effects.

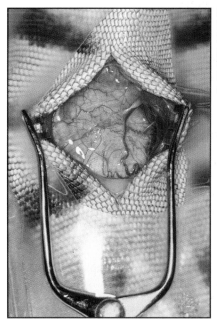

Figure 19.11 Mid-abdominal incision in a green iguana for removal of a large cystic calculus.

Incisions are made in the soft pliable skin between scales if possible. However, most lizards have small scales and it is not possible to make an incision between them. In laterally compressed species such as chameleons, a flank incision is initiated just caudal to the last rib on one side of the body and extended by following the curve of the rib.

Closure is accomplished in two layers. The body wall and coelomic membrane are closed in a single layer, using a simple continuous pattern with a synthetic absorbable material on a fine atraumatic needle. The muscle of the body wall is thin and must be handled gently to avoid tearing. Closing the body wall achieves apposition of the skin that tends to invert in most lizard species. Skin closure is performed using a non-absorbable material in an everting pattern (e.g. horizontal mattress) or skin staples.

Female reproductive tract surgery

Ovariectomy or ovariosalpingohysterectomy is performed as part of the treatment for dystocia, yolk coelomitis or salpingitis, or for prevention of future reproduction or reproductive problems. A short operative time is critical, and in a severely debilitated patient ovariectomy alone is adequate as the oviducts will atrophy. Unilateral ovariosalpingohysterectomy (removal of one side of the reproductive tract) will preserve reproductive viability.

The normal anatomy of the lizard reproductive tract is described in Chapter 17. In iguanas the right ovary is closely associated with the right caudal vena cava. The left ovary has the left adrenal gland interposed between the ovary and the left vena cava. The ovary is suspended from the caval veins by a ligament. This ligament is very short when the ovary is inactive, making removal more challenging, but is stretched out and contains many large blood vessels when reproductively active or during preovulatory follicular stasis. The oviducts and shell glands are relatively small, until they receive the ova, as are the associated blood vessels.

The reproductive tract is mobile within the coelom and the oviduct, ovary and shell gland are readily accessible through a single coeliotomy approach. The normal oviduct is thin-walled and transparent but the wall becomes thickened and often friable when salpingitis is present, making closure difficult. Biopsy specimens and cultures of the reproductive tract or ovaries should be made for diagnostic purposes and to aid in postoperative management.

Ovariectomy

In pre-ovulatory follicular stasis:

1. Identify and gently elevate the large, grape-like, yellow pre-ovulatory follicles.
2. Identify the individual large vessels in the ovarian ligament. Apply two haemostatic clips or ligatures and transect the vessel between them.
3. Once all the vessels are ligated, transect the remaining ligamentous attachments and remove the ovary.
4. Repeat the procedure on the contralateral ovary.

In the quiescent state:

1. Grasp the right ovary by its ligamentous attachment and elevate it using microsurgical forceps.
2. Place haemostatic clips between the ovary and the right vena cava. Generally, in small to medium iguanas, two clips are used: one in a cranial-to-caudal direction and one in a caudal-to-cranial direction.
3. Transect the ovarian ligament on the ovarian side of the clips and remove the ovary.
4. Note that the left adrenal gland lies between the ovary and the left caval vein in the suspensory ligament. Remove the left ovary in a similar manner but with the haemoclips applied between the ovary and the left adrenal gland. Take care not to damage the adrenal gland.

Oviduct removal

1. After the ovaries are removed, identify the oviducts.
2. Clip or coagulate (bipolar cautery) the small vessels supplying the oviducts and shell glands.
3. Transect the dorsal oviduct ligament. Dissection is initiated at the infundibulum, progressing caudally until the junction between the uterus and the cloaca is reached.
4. Apply one or two haemostatic clips or ligatures at the base of each shell gland and transect the tissue distal to the ligatures or clips.

In post-ovulatory eggbinding, where the ova have been released from the ovaries, these are relatively small and obscured by the large egg-filled oviducts.

1. Exteriorize the oviducts, allowing visualization and isolation of the blood vessels supplying the oviducts and uterus. These vessels are generally engorged and numerous.
2. Isolate each vessel, ligate with two haemostatic clips or ligatures, and transect. This process is begun at the infundibulum and continued caudally until each individual shell gland can be ligated or clipped at the cloaca and transected.
3. Following removal of the oviducts, the ovaries are identified and removed using a technique similar to that described above for removal of quiescent ovaries.

Salpingotomy

Where reproductive viability must be preserved, a salpingotomy is performed. After the underlying problem causing the dystocia is addressed, the prognosis for reproductive viability is good.

1. Once the oviduct and uterus are identified, make an incision over an egg/fetus approximately the length of the egg or fetus. If the incision is too small the oviduct will tear as the egg/fetus is manipulated through it. Generally three to six eggs/fetuses can be manipulated through a single incision.
2. Inject warmed saline or lubricating jelly to separate the oviduct wall from the egg/fetus and provide lubrication for manipulation. Remove the first egg/fetus through the salpingotomy incision (generally easy).
3. Manipulate eggs/fetuses cranial and caudal to the incision towards the incision and remove.
4. After removal of all the eggs/fetuses, close the salpingotomy incision with a simple continuous pattern using a fine (6-0 to 8-0) monofilament synthetic absorbable material on a fine atraumatic needle. This can be oversewn with an inverting pattern but this is generally not necessary.

Male reproductive tract surgery

Castration

The approach is through a paramedian coeliotomy. Visualization of the gonads is accomplished by retraction of the viscera to the left or right side of the coelomic cavity. The right testicle (Figure 19.12) is more tightly

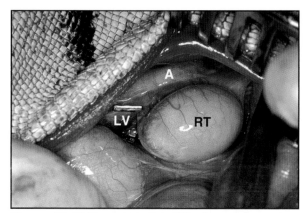

Figure 19.12 The right testicle (RT) of an adult green iguana as seen through a mid-abdominal surgical incision. Note the close proximity of the large vein (blue, LV) and adrenal gland (A).

adhered to the right vena cava by its short vascular mesorchium and the right adrenal gland is located on the opposite side of the vessel. The left testicle is more loosely associated with the left vena cava and has the left adrenal gland interposed between the testicle and the vessel. The adrenals are elongated, granular glands easily distinguished from the rounded smooth testicles. The testicles are less mobile than the ovaries, making surgical manipulation more difficult. During the breeding season the testicles may be markedly enlarged, reducing the space between the testicle and the vena cava, and making castration even more challenging. Castration in immature iguanas is less difficult due to the small size of the gonad (often only one haemoclip required) and the less well developed blood supply to the testicles.

1. Gently elevate the right testicle at either pole and apply a haemostatic clip between the testicle and the vena cava.
2. Use microsurgical scissors to cut the tissue distal to the clip and elevate the testicle further.
3. Apply another haemostatic clip cranially or caudally to the first and transect the tissue distal to the clip. Continue the procedure until the testicle is removed.
4. Remove the left testicle following application of haemostatic clips between the testicle and the adrenal gland.

Note: If the vessels supplying the testicle are not completely occluded, considerable haemorrhage can occur, especially during the breeding season. This haemorrhage can be controlled by digital pressure or the application of absorbable materials to the affected area. If the vena cava is damaged, one or two haemostatic clips can be applied longitudinally along the defect.

Prolapsed hemipenis
Prolapse of the penis (paraphimosis) is a common problem. Causes include: excitement or stress, with subsequent trauma to the exposed hemipenis by cagemates or substrate; injury due to traction, pulling or forced separation during copulation; damage to and

swelling of the penis secondary to probing for sex determination; infection; inflammation; neurological deficits involving the retractor penis muscles or vent sphincter; and impaction of the cloaca with urates. The prolapsed organ is often oedematous due to passive congestion caused by venous engorgement and may have lacerations from cagemates or the substrate. Secondary infections and necrosis due to exposure of the prolapsed organ are also concerns. The prolapsed tissue is often covered with inflammatory exudate.

1. Under sedation or anesthesia, clean and lubricate the prolapsed organ and remove any lacerations.
2. Replace the tissue in the appropriate location (into the tail or cranial cloaca). A moistened cotton-tipped applicator is often helpful in reducing the prolapse. If the prolapse is too large to reduce, cold compresses or hygroscopic fluids such as glycerine or concentrated sugar solutions may help reduce tissue oedema. Additionally, incising the vent laterally on one or both sides may enlarge the vent opening.
3. Once the prolapse is reduced, place a purse string or one or two transverse sutures in the vent. The transverse suture pattern has the advantage of allowing defecation and urination. In larger lizards the opening at the caudal margin of the cloaca from which the affected hemipenis protrudes can be closed after the prolapsed organ is reduced. This has the advantage of preserving the normal anatomy and function of the cloaca.
4. Remove the suture after 2 weeks.

Penile amputation
If severe damage, infection or necrosis is present, or in cases of recurring penis or hemipenis prolapse, amputation can be performed without compromising the ability to urinate. In lizards amputation of one hemipenis will still allow reproductive viability.

1. Place mattress sutures in viable healthy tissue at the base of the prolapse to control haemorrhage.
2. Amputate the organ distal to the sutures.
3. Suture the mucosa of the stump in a simple continuous pattern using an absorbable synthetic material.
4. Replace the stump into the cloaca. Instil antibiotic ointment into the cloaca or administer systemic antibiotics if infection is present.

Cystotomy
The urinary bladder of normal lizards is thin and transparent but calculi and subsequent cystitis can make the bladder wall quite thick. The bladder is highly mobile in the coelomic cavity, making cystotomy a relatively simple procedure. The bladder should be isolated and a pair of stay sutures placed at the cranial and caudal margins of the planned incision. Initiation of the incision should be in a relatively avascular portion of the bladder. A two-layer inverting closure is recommended. Following closure of the incision, the coelomic cavity should be irrigated.

Gastrointestinal tract surgery

The basic principles are similar to those for mammals and for other reptiles. Surgical intervention is indicated for removal of foreign bodies, obstruction, intestinal impaction and the resolution of intussusception. Gastrointestinal procedures that have been performed successfully in reptiles include foreign body removal, resection and anastomosis, and anastomosis for colorectal atresia.

The intestine is quite thin, especially in smaller lizards, requiring the use of fine suture material and atraumatic needles. The gastrointestinal tract is generally mobile, though the extent varies between species. If possible, the affected portion of bowel should be exteriorized; if this is not possible, it should be isolated with gauze sponges to prevent contamination of the coelomic cavity. Following closure of the incision copious irrigation should be performed.

Colopexy

Prolapse of the colon can occur secondary to tenesmus; diagnosis and treatment of the primary cause is needed to prevent recurrence. Colopexy can help maintain the reduced colon while the primary problem is tackled.

1. Approach the coelomic cavity through a left paramedian incision and identify the descending colon. It is helpful to place one or two cotton-tipped applicators into the colon through the cloaca to help in identification.
2. Apply traction to the colon to reduce the prolapse. While applying traction to the colon, sutures are placed from one side of the body wall, full thickness through the colon wall, then through the other side of the body wall.
3. Once the prolapse is reduced, the coeliotomy is closed, incorporating the colon in the body wall closure. Synthetic absorbable sutures on an atraumatic needle are placed in a simple interrupted pattern. The colon heals into the body wall, creating permanent adhesion.

Digit/limb amputation

When a phalanx or entire digit is to be amputated, the incision is planned and initiated to allow skin closure to be flush with the metacarpal or metatarsal portion of the foot.

In most animals it is recommended that limbs are amputated as proximally as possible, to prevent trauma to the stump. Normal reptile skin is tough and resistant to trauma but scar tissue is delicate and easily damaged. Because lizards generally hold their bodies close to the ground, even a short stump can be useful.

To obtain a functional stump, the skin is incised to create a flap on the ventral surface that can be pulled over the stump and sutured in place dorsally. The end of the bone is padded with viable soft tissue and the flap sutured in place. This places normal viable skin in contact with the substrate and places the incision/scar tissue dorsally and laterally. Entire limb amputation is best accomplished at the scapulohumeral or coxofemoral joints. Muscles should be transected as distally as possible to allow for adequate coverage of the site.

Tail amputation

In lizards with disease or trauma of the distal tail, autotomy may be performed in order to remove the distal segment and allow regeneration. This procedure is accomplished under general anaesthesia. The skin is first incised and then the tail is grasped proximal to the lesion and firmly bent and twisted, allowing the tail to fracture through a fracture plane. The tail is twisted until it disarticulates, exposing muscle, tendon and vertebrae. Bleeding is generally minimal, but a bandage may be applied to the stump to keep it clean. Within a few days a scab will form over the end of the tail and the regeneration process will begin. Prognosis for regeneration diminishes as the tail is amputated more proximally.

Fracture management

Fractures in lizards are usually the result of trauma or MBD and are rarely open or comminuted. Although studies are lacking, it appears that healing of fractures occurs more slowly in lizards than in mammals and birds, with most traumatic fractures healing in 6–8 weeks. Fractures secondary to MBD heal in 3–4 weeks following correction of hypocalcaemia. General orthopaedic principles of rigid alignment and stabilization, with minimal disruption of callus and soft tissue, apply. Most fractures heal without surgical intervention, though with varying degrees of mal-union.

External coaptation

Splints and other bandages are commonly used. Most fractures secondary to MBD lend themselves well to external coaptation. Pathological fractures that occur after the bone has lost approximately one-third of its calcium content do not lend themselves to internal fixation because the bone is too soft to support implants. Most pathological fractures have minimal displacement. Where displacement is significant, an intramedullary pin may be inserted to provide axial alignment; however, external coaptation is also utilized as the stability provided by the pin is inadequate in soft bone. General anaesthesia is recommended for application of external coaptation. All forms of external coaptation need to be monitored on a regular basis for evidence of swelling, slipping, vascular compromise or other problems that may require splint replacement.

Fixation

Most methods of internal fracture fixation have been used successfully in lizards. The principles are similar to those for mammals. Intramedullary pins and orthopaedic wire are inexpensive and provide axial as well as bending stability. The more horizontal orientation of the limbs in lizards makes insertion of pins into the humerus and femur more difficult than in mammals. It is recommended that pins be placed retrograde through the trochanteric fossa of the femur or the greater tubercle of the humerus and seated into the distal segment. Countersinking the pin will minimize damage to surrounding structures. Steinman pins, Kirschner wires and small spinal needles are useful as pins in small patients.

External skeletal fixation (ESF) provides fracture stability without interfering with joint function and may be applied even in small lizards. ESF devices are placed in a cranial-to-caudal plane because of the horizontal orientation of the limbs. Biphasic ESF devices are most commonly used and incorporate Kirschner wires, spinal needles or hypodermic needles as fixation pins, with an acrylic polymer or other rigid material for the connecting system. The apparatus is versatile and lightweight. There are no reports of using bone plates in lizards but, with the availability of small cuttable plates and fingerplates which accept screws as small as 1.5 mm in diameter, bone plating could be used in larger lizards with healthy bone cortices.

Drug formulary

An abbreviated formulary is given in Figure 19.13. An excellent literature-based formulary for exotic practice has recently been compiled by Carpenter *et al.* (2000).

References and further reading

Allen ME and Oftedal OT (1994) The nutrition of carnivorous reptiles. In: *Captive Management and Conservation of Amphibians and Reptiles*, ed. JB Murphy *et al.*, pp. 71–82. Society for the Study of Amphibians and Reptiles
Baer DJ (1994) The nutrition of herbivorous reptiles. In: *Captive Management and Conservation of Amphibians and Reptiles*, ed. JB Murphy *et al.*, pp. 83–90. Society for the Study of Amphibians and Reptiles
Barten S (1993) The medical care of iguanas and other common pet lizards. *Veterinary Clinics of North America: Small Animal Practice* **23**, 1213–1249
Bartlett RD and Bartlett P (1997) *Lizard Care from A to Z.* Barron's Educational Series Inc., Hauppage, New York
Bernard J, Oftedal OT, Barboza PS *et al.* (1991) The response of vitamin-D deficient green iguanas (*Iguana iguana*) to artificial ultraviolet light. In: *Proceedings of the American Association of Zoo Veterinarians*, pp. 147–150
Blahak S (1994) Isolations of new paramyxo- and adenoviruses from snakes and a reovirus from an iguana. In: *Second World Congress of Herpetology*, pp. 29–30
Boyer TH (1998) *Reptiles – A Guide for Practitioners.* AAHA Press, Lakewood, Colorado
Carpenter JW *et al.* (2000) *Exotic Animal Formulary, 2nd edn.* WB Saunders, Philadelphia
Clark H and Karson D (1972) Iguana virus, a herpes-like virus isolated

Drug	Dose	Comments
Antiparasitic agents		
Albendazole	50–75 mg/kg orally	Nematodes, trematodes and cestodes
Fenbendazole	50–100 mg/kg orally, repeat in 2 weeks or 25–40 mg/kg orally, every day for 3–5 treatments	Nematodes. Repeated low dose without placement in food recommended
Ivermectin	0.2–0.4 mg/kg orally, s.c., i.m., repeat in 2 weeks or 5–10 mg/l of water, topical spray every 4–5 days for up to 4 weeks for ectoparasites	Nematodes (not spray), ticks and mites. Always use test animal when administering to multiple animals of unfamiliar species. Low therapeutic index
Levamisole	10–50 mg/kg s.c., i.m., repeat in 2 weeks	
Mebendazole	20–25 mg/kg orally	
Metronidazole	50–100 mg/kg orally, repeat in 2 weeks	Antiprotozoal
Oxfendazole	68 mg/kg orally, repeat in 2 weeks	Nematodes
Praziquantel	8 mg/kg i.m., s.c., repeat in 2 weeks	Cestodes (flukes at higher dosages?)
Sulphadimethoxine	50 mg/kg orally a day for 3–5 days, then every other day	Coccidia
Thiabendazole	50 mg/kg orally, repeat in 2 weeks	Nematodes
Antimicrobial agents		
Amikacin	5 mg/kg i.m. then 2.5 mg/kg every 3 days	Safest of the available aminoglycosides. Ensure animal well hydrated. Aerobic Gram-negative bacteria
Ampicillin	3–6 mg/kg s.c., i.m. sid	Gram-positive aerobic and some anaerobic bacteria
Carbenicillin	200–400 mg/kg i.m. sid	
Ceftazidime	20 mg/kg i.m., i.v. every 3 days	Gram-negative and Gram-positive aerobic and some anaerobic bacteria
Enrofloxacin	5–10 mg/kg orally, s.c., i.m. sid	Gram-negative bacteria. Tissue necrosis common at injection site
Metronidazole	20 mg/kg orally every 1–2 days	Anaerobic bacteria
Oxytetracycline	10–20 mg/kg i.m. every 2–4 days	Gram-negative and Gram-positive aerobic bacteria, *Chlamydia*. Tissue damage at injection site
Trimethoprim/sulphadiazine	20–30 mg/kg orally sid for 2 days, then every other day	Gram-negative aerobic bacteria
Tylosin	25 mg/kg i.m. sid	Mycoplasma
Miscellaneous		
Calcium gluconate	100–200 mg/kg i.v., s.c., i.m., as indicated	Hypocalcaemic tetany
Vitamin A palmitate	2000 IU/30 g orally once, repeat in 7 days	Chameleons

Figure 19.13 Drug formulary for lizards.

from cultured cells of a lizard, *Iguana iguana*. *Infection and Immunity* **5**, 559–569

Coke RL and Tristan TE (1998) *Cryptosporidium* infection in a colony of leopard geckos, *Eublepharis macularius*. In: *Proceedings of the Annual Meeting of the Association or Reptilian and Amphibian Veterinarians*, Kansas City, pp. 157–163

De Lisle HF (1996) *The Natural History of Monitor Lizards*. Krieger Publishing Company, Malabar, Florida

De Vosjoli P (1993) *The General Care and Maintenance of Prehensile-Tailed Skinks*. Advanced Vivarium Systems Inc., Lakeside, California

De Vosjoli P and Mailloux R (1993) *The General Care and Maintenance of Bearded Dragons*. Advanced Vivarium Systems Inc., Lakeside, California

Divers SJ (1997) Clinician's approach to renal disease in lizards. In: *Proceedings of the Annual Meeting of the Association of Reptilian and Amphibian Veterinarians, Houston, Texas*, pp. 5–11

Divers SJ (2000) Spinal osteomyelitis in a green iguana, *Iguana iguana*: cerebrospinal fluid and myelogram diagnosis. In: *Proceedings of the Annual Meeting of the Association of Reptilian and Amphibian Veterinarians, Reno, Nevada*, pp. 77–80

Draper C, Walker R and Lawler H (1981) Patterns of oral bacterial infection in captive snakes. *Journal of the American Veterinary Medical Association* **179**, 1223–1226

Ferguson GW, Jones JR, Gehrmann WH *et al.* (1996) Indoor husbandry of the panther chameleon *Chameleo (furcifer) pardalis*: Effects of dietary vitamins A and D and ultraviolet irradiation on pathology and life history traits. *Zoo Biology* **15**, 279–299

Frye F (1995) *Iguana iguana: Guide for Successful Captive Care*. Krieger Publishing Company, Malabar, Florida

Frye FL, Munn RK, Gardner M, Barten SL and Hadfy LB (1994) Adenovirus-like hepatitis in a group of related Rankin's dragon lizards (*Pogona henrylawsoni*). *Journal of Zoo and Wildlife Medicine* **25**, 167–171

Frye F, Oshiro L, Dutra F and Carney J (1977) Herpesvirus-like infection in two pacific pond turtles. *Journal of the American Veterinary Medical Association* **171**, 882–884

Hanel R, Heard DJ, Ellis GA and Nguyen A (1999) Isolation of *Clostridium* spp. from the blood of captive lizards: real or pseudobacteremia? *Bulletin of the Association of Reptilian and Amphibian Veterinarians* **9**, 4–8

Harvey-Clark CJ (1995) Common dermatologic problems in pet reptilia. *Seminars in Avian and Exotic Pet Medicine* **4**, 205–219

Heard DJ (2001). Reptile anesthesia. *Veterinary Clinics of North America: Exotic Practice* **4**, 83–118

Henkel F-W and Schmidt W (1995) *Geckoes – Biology, Husbandry, and Reproduction*. Krieger Publishing Company, Malabar, Florida.

Jacobson ER (1990) Diseases of the integumentary system of reptiles. In: *Small Animal Dermatology*, ed. Nesbitt G and Ackerman L, pp. 225–239. Veterinary Learning Systems, New Jersey

Jacobson ER and Gardiner CH (1990) Adeno-like virus in esophageal and tracheal mucosa of a Jackson's chameleon. *Veterinary Pathology* **27**, 210–212

Jacobson ER and Telford SR (1990) *Chlamydia* and poxvirus infection of monocytes in a flap-necked chameleon. *Journal of Wildlife Disease* **26**, 572–577

Jacobson ER (1993) Diseases and medical problems in iguanid lizards. In: *Proceedings of the Southern Regional Conference of the American Association of Zoological Parks and Aquariums*, pp. 260–267

Jacobson ER, Green DE, Undeen AH, Cranfield M and Vaughan KL (1998) Systemic microsporidiosis in inland bearded dragons, *Pogona vitticeps*. *Journal of Zoo and Wildlife Medicine* **29**, 315–323

Jacobson ER, Kopit W, Kennedy FA and Funk RS (1996) Coinfection of a bearded dragon, *Pogona vitticeps*, with adenovirus- and dependovirus-like viruses. *Veterinary Pathology* **33**, 343–346

Jacobson ER, Origgi F, Pessier AP *et al.* (2001) Paramyxovirus-like infection in caiman lizards, *Draecena guianensis*. In: *Proceedings of the Annual Meeting of the Association of Reptilian and Amphibian Veterinarians*, pp. 59–60

Julian AF and Durham PJK (1985) Adenoviral hepatitis in a female bearded dragon (*Amphibolurus barbatus*). *New Zealand Veterinary Journal* **30**, 59–60

King D and Green B (1999) *Monitors – The Biology of Varanid Lizards*. Krieger Publishing Company, Malabar, Florida

Lane TJ and Mader DR (1996) Parasitology. In: *Reptile Medicine and Surgery*, ed. DR Mader, pp. 185–203. WB Saunders, Philadelphia

Lawton MPC (1997) Hands free, non-chemical restraint of iguanidae for radiography. In: *Proceedings of the Annual Meeting of the Association of Reptilian and Amphibian Veterinarians, Houston, Texas*, pp. 1–3

Martin J and Wolfe A (1992) *Masters of Disguise – A Natural History of Chameleons*. Facts On File, Oxford, England

Mattison C (1987) *The Care of Reptiles and Amphibians in Captivity*, 2*nd* edn. Blandford Press, London

McAllister CT, Upton SJ, Jacobson ER and Kopit W (1995) A description of *Isospora amphiboluri* (Apicomplexa: Eimeriidae) from the inland bearded dragon, *Pogona vitticeps* (Sauria: Agamidae). *Journal of Parasitology* **8**, 281–284

McCracken H and Birch C (1994) Periodontal disease in lizards. A review of numerous cases. In: *The Proceedings of the Annual Meeting of the American Association of Zoo Veterinarians*, pp. 108–115

Migaki G, Jacobson E and Casey H (1984) Fungal diseases in reptiles. In: *Diseases of Reptiles and Amphibians*, ed. Hoff G *et al.*, pp 183–204. Plenum Press, New York

Necas P (1999) *Chameleons – Nature's Hidden Jewels*. Krieger Publishing Company, Malabar, Florida

Origgi F, Roccabianca P and Gelmetti D (1999) *Dermatophilus* in *Furcifer (Chamaeleo) pardalis*. *Bulletin of the Association of Reptilian and Amphibian Veterinarians* **9**, 9–11

Plowman C, Montali R, Phillips L, Schlater L and Lowenstine L (1987) Septicemia and chronic abscesses in iguanas (*Cyclura cornuta* and *Iguana iguana*) associated with a *Neisseria* species. *Journal of Zoo Animal Medicine* **18**, 86–93

Pough FH, Andrews RM, Cadle JE *et al.* (1998) *Herpetology*, Prentice Hall, Upper Saddle River, New Jersey

Prezant RM and Jarchow JL (1997) Lactated fluid use in reptiles: Is there a better solution? In: *Proceedings of the Annual Meeting of the Association of Reptilian and Amphibian Veterinarians*, Houston, p. 83

Rogner M (1997) *Lizards. Volumes 1 & 2*. Krieger Publishing Company, Malabar, Florida

Rosenthal K and Mader DR (1996) Microbiology. In: *Reptile Medicine and Surgery*, ed. DR Mader, pp. 117–125. WB Saunders, Philadelphia

Shalev M, Murphy JC and Fox JG (1977) Mycotic enteritis in a chameleon and a brief review of phycomycoses of animals. *Journal of the American Veterinary Medical Association* **171**, 872–875

Stahl SJ (1997) Captive management, breeding, and common medical problems of the veiled chameleon (*Chamaeleo calyptratus*). In: *Proceedings of the Annual Meeting of the Association of Reptilian and Amphibian Veterinarians*, Houston, pp. 29–40

Telford S and Jacobson ER (1993) Lizard erythrocytic virus in East African chameleons. *Journal of Wildlife Disease* **29**, 57–63

Thomas CL *et al.* (1996) Swollen eyelid associated with *Foleyella* sp infection in a chameleon. *Journal of the American Veterinary Medical Association* **209**, 972–973

Warwick C, Frye FL and Murphy JB (1995) *Health and Welfare of Captive Reptiles*. Chapman & Hall, London

Wissman M and Parsons B (1993) Dermatophytosis of green iguanas (*Iguana iguana*). *Journal of Small Exotic Animal Medicine* **2**, 137–140

20

Snakes

Paul Raiti

Introduction

There are approximately 2400 species of snake. The majority that are presented to veterinary surgeons belong to the families Boidae and Colubridae (Figures 20.1 and 20.2).

Biology

Sexing

Sexual dimorphism occurs among snakes but external physical differences are more obvious when conspecific members of each sex are examined together. Male Boidae generally have larger pelvic spurs than females, used for tactile stimulation during copulation (Figure 20.3). All male snakes possess comparatively longer tails than females, because the hemipenes are retracted inside the tail.

The most accurate method of gender identification is a technique known as 'probing', which is performed by gently inserting an appropriately sized blunted steel instrument into the base of the tail. Females can be probed to a depth of approximately 2–6 ventral scales; males can be probed to a depth of 7–15 ventral scales.

Husbandry

Housing

As a general rule, snakes should be housed individually.

Family	Typical species	Family characteristics
Boidae (boas and pythons)	*Boa constrictor,* Rainbow boa *Epicrates cenchria* Royal python *Python regius* Green tree python *Morelia viridis* Blood python *P. curtus* Burmese python *P. molurus*	Primitive snakes, thought to have evolved from lizards. Vestigial limbs called pelvic spurs (clawlike structures near base of tail). Two lungs. Diminutive caecum. Linearly arranged depressions parallel to one or both lips (heat-sensitive organs enhancing ability to detect endothermic prey). Boas have undivided ventral tail scales and are viviparous (bear live young). Pythons have divided ventral tail scales and are oviparous (lay eggs).
Colubridae	Corn snake *Elaphae guttata* Kingsnake *Lampropeltis getulus* Garter snakes *Thamnophis* spp. Gopher snake *Pituophis melanoleucus*	Considered modern in evolutionary terms. Right lung only. No caecum or pelvic spurs. Venomous colubrids include the rear-fanged mangrove snake *Boiga dendrophila* and the hog-nosed snake *Heterodon nasicus.*

Figure 20.1 Commonly kept pet snakes.

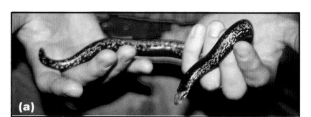

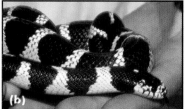

Figure 20.2 A boid and a colubrid. (a) Sand boa *Eryx* sp. (b) Kingsnake *Lampropeltis getulus.* Courtesy of S. Redrobe.

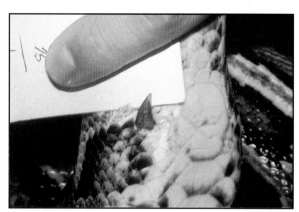

Figure 20.3 Pelvic spurs in a Burmese python (*Python molurus bivittatus*).

- Cage size should be adequate to permit normal behaviour for the particular species. As a rule of thumb, the diagonal of the enclosure should approximate the length of the snake
- Enclosures must be escape-proof and provide adequate ventilation
- Glass or plastic aquaria are adequate for most colubrids and smaller boids. Secure lids such as screen tops fastened with clamps work well
- Wooden cages should be well sealed with polyurethane to prevent deterioration and mould formation.

Environmental temperature

Despite being classified as poikilotherms, snakes have a preferred optimal temperature zone (POTZ) – a range of temperatures in which physiological processes such as immunogenics, digestion and reproduction occur.

- Most tropical snakes can be maintained between 25 and 30°C
- Temperate snakes can be kept between 22 and 26°C.

The high end of these ranges is provided by heat sources such as heating pads or incandescent lights. The core temperatures of larger snakes, such as boa constrictors and Burmese pythons, are best attained by regulating the room temperature to approximately 26°C and then providing focal hot spots. Night-time temperature drops of 2–5°C are recommended.

Enclosure design

Design can be broadly categorized into types that provide housing for fossorial (burrowing), ground-dwelling (Figure 20.4), semi-aquatic or arboreal species.

Fossorial, ground-dwelling and semi-aquatic species: Substrate or bedding material should be non-toxic if ingested, easy to remove from the cage, and resistant to microbial colonization.

- Burrowing snakes such as sand boas (*Eryx* spp.) that are found in dry desert habitats should be provided with several inches of fine-grain sand
- Newspaper or wood shavings (excluding cedar) are appropriate for ground-dwelling snakes such as boa constrictors, ball pythons and most colubrids
- Other ground-dwelling boids that require higher humidity levels, such as the rubber boa *Charina bottae*, rainbow boa and viper boa *Candoia asper*, should be provided with a shallow bowl containing moistened sphagnum moss
- Semi-aquatic colubrids such as garter snakes and water snakes (*Natrix* spp. and *Nerodia* spp.) should be kept on a dry substrate similar to ground-dwelling snakes but must have a relatively large water bowl.

Arboreal species: Arboreal snakes, such as green tree pythons and the emerald tree boa *Corallus caninus,* require climbing fixtures such as tree limbs, arranged horizontally at various levels. Higher humidity requirements are satisfied by a combination of sphagnum or peat moss as a substrate, live plants and daily misting. Appropriate ventilation (screen top and a fan that circulates room air) is important to counter the potentially deleterious effects of stagnant humid air.

Water bowls and hide boxes

All snakes should be provided with a shallow water bowl. Most species, with the exception of arboreal snakes, periodically like to spend time immersed in water, especially prior to ecdysis (shedding). Bowls

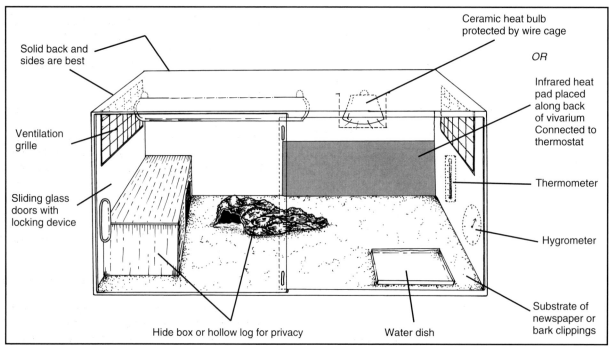

Figure 20.4 A vivarium suitable for a ground-dwelling snake.

should be replenished with fresh water every 48 hours and disinfected once a week with a suitable solution, such as chlorhexidine.

Snakes should also be provided with a shelter (hide box), which provides security and decreases stress. Snakes that have no place to hide commonly abrade the perinasal tissues, leading to infection and subsequent shedding problems.

Ecdysis

Throughout their lives, all snakes periodically shed the entire epidermis. This process is controlled by the thyroid gland and occurs more frequently in juveniles than in adults. Approximately 2 weeks prior to shedding, lymph-like fluid is produced between the old and new layers of skin. The snake takes on an opaque hue which is most visible over the eyes (Figure 20.5). Maintaining higher levels of humidity is critical in permitting removal of the epidermis. The shed skin should be a complete cast of the snake.

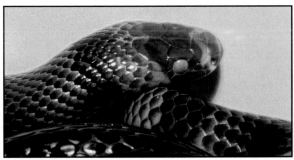

Figure 20.5 Normal pre-shedding appearance in a Honduran milksnake *Lampropeltis triangulum hondurensis*. Note the cloudy spectacle.

Diet

As a group, snakes consume a wide variety of prey, including mammals, reptiles, amphibians, eggs, fish, molluscs, earthworms and insects.

- Most captive snakes eat rodents such as mice or rats
- Water snakes are fed live fish to prevent deficiencies
- Rabbits and chickens are fed to the larger constricting snakes.

Snakes are susceptible to potentially life-threatening rodent bites during the shedding process, when it is normal for them to be anorexic (Figure 20.6). To prevent injuries and to decrease the risk of parasite

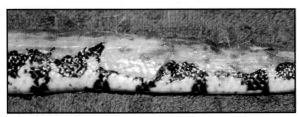

Figure 20.6 Massive desleeving injury to a boa constrictor (*Boa constrictor*) from a mouse that had been left with the snake during the night. The boa was anorexic because it was shedding.

transfer from rodents, it is recommended that thawed or pre-killed laboratory-raised animals should be offered. It should be noted that UK legislation may prohibit the feeding of live vertebrate prey.

Boids have a slower metabolism than colubrids. As boids reach adulthood, the frequency of feedings should gradually decrease to one meal every 2–4 weeks.

Quarantine

To maintain the long-term health of any reptile collection, it is imperative to place all new acquisitions in quarantine.

- A separate room with a closed door is strongly recommended
- There should be no sharing of cage furniture, prey items or even room air with the established collection
- Gloves should be worn during any physical contact with the quarantined snakes
- Snakes should be quarantined for a minimum of 4 months before being added to the main collection. During that time they should be stressed as little as possible and treated for parasitism, abscesses, etc.
- Haematology and plasma biochemical analysis should be performed on wild-caught snakes
- Wild-caught snakes should begin to eat regularly during the quarantine period.

Captive breeding

All snakes require a period of physiological rest for the maintenance of long-term health. This usually occurs during changes in climatic conditions such as decreases in temperature, rainfall and daylight hours. During this period, which may last several months, there is a 'priming' effect upon the reproductive system. As the breeding season approaches, the hypothalamus–pituitary–gonadal axis is activated.

- In captivity, this cycle is mimicked by decreasing ambient temperatures for 2–3 months
- Temperate snakes tolerate temperatures of 10–15°C; tropical snakes are cooled to 20–24°C
- Prior to this, the reptiles are fasted for 1 month to empty the gastrointestinal tract
- Food is withheld but water is provided during the cooling period
- The animals should be checked weekly for any signs of illness, such as dehydration or dyspnoea
- Water bowls should be cleaned and replenished with fresh water weekly.

At the end of the dormancy stage the temperatures are gradually increased. Feeding resumes intensely, particularly in females. The snakes are then paired for breeding.

- Male snakes possess two hemipenes, located in the base of the tail
- During copulation, one of the organs is everted and inserted into the female's cloaca
- Ovulation occurs several weeks later, usually preceded by shedding

- The caudal half of the female's body subsequently begins to swell as the fertilized ova develop
- After the next shed, egg laying or parturition occurs.

Viviparous snakes require basking spots of relatively higher temperature during pregnancy. Similarly, eggs need to be incubated at relatively stable temperatures that depend on the particular species. Pythons, which practise maternal brooding of the eggs, are capable of raising their body temperatures to 32°C to ensure proper development of the embryos.

Handling and restraint

Most snakes presented to the veterinary surgeon are relatively docile but newly acquired wild-caught animals tend to be more resistant to handling. Species such as tree boas, green tree pythons and reticulated pythons are more likely to bite as soon as visual contact is made.

Each snake should be enclosed in an escape-proof container, such as a cloth bag tied with a knot. The bag should be within a secure box.

- Any snake more than 1.5 m long (particularly boas and pythons) should be handled by two people
- The snake is approached from behind its head and grasped gently but firmly just caudal to the jaws (Figure 20.7)
- When lifted, the body should be supported (Figure 20.7)
- Larger uncooperative pythons (Burmese, blood and reticulated) may require the use of chemical restraint in order to perform a detailed examination and diagnostic tests
- It is not uncommon for frightened snakes to expel the contents of the cloaca and musk glands.

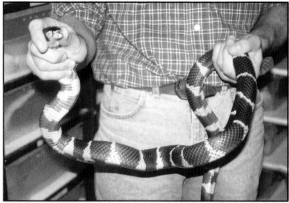

Figure 20.7 Holding a kingsnake with two hands. (Courtesy of S. Redrobe.)

Venomous snakes should only be handled by those competent in snake handling. Antivenin should be available and Health and Safety legislation adhered to. Examination is performed more safely under anaesthesia.

Diagnostic approach

Initially, the snake should be weighed and a thorough case history obtained. The underlying causes of most diseases can be readily identified by obtaining a detailed history. Suggested husbandry modifications should be discussed, followed by physical examination.

Physical examination

Observing the snake prior to handling enables the clinician to evaluate general appearance, state of nutrition and posture.

- When lifted, the snake should demonstrate good muscle tone and mental awareness
- There should be no retained pieces of epidermis on the body
- Loose skin folds and prominent ribs are consistent with dehydration and malnourishment
- The ventral scales should be checked for discoloration, swelling or ulcerations
- Indentations lateral to the dorsal spinous processes are due to fractured ribs; this is occasionally seen in wild-caught snakes
- The vent should be clean and free of any matted excretions
- Most snakes will actively flick the tongue when handled.

After assessing the snake's overall condition, the clinician may continue the examination in a more detailed fashion, commencing with the head.

- The mouth is opened by gently inserting a rubber spatula or an avian steel speculum between the jaws
- The oral membranes are usually pale pink
- The gingivae are checked for swelling, haemorrhage, exudate, loose teeth, etc.
- The teeth are curved, needle-like projections sheathed in the gums
- The glottis is on the floor of the oral cavity and opens to its maximum extent during inhalation (Figure 20.8). There should not be any exudate in the glottis

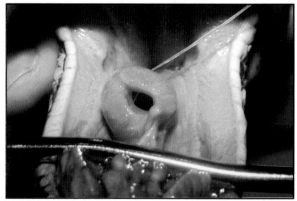

Figure 20.8 Normal oral cavity in a Burmese python. The glottis is open during inhalation and the gingivae are a pale pink.

- The lingual sheath is under the glottis
- The cranial portion of the oesophagus begins at the back of the oral cavity and can be pigmented with melanin
- Each eye is covered by a single scale called the spectacle. Beneath the spectacle lies the cornea. Both structures are separated by the subspectacle space, which contains fluid produced by the nasolacrimal apparatus
- Nocturnal snakes have vertical pupils; diurnal snakes have round pupils. Pupillary responses can be assessed using a bright light source.

Tractable snakes are palpated by using the index finger or thumb to press between the ventral processes of the ribs, beginning at the neck and continuing to the tail.

- The first palpable mass is the three-chambered heart, located in the cranial quarter of the body. Its contractions are visible except in large or obese snakes
- The stomach is at the midway point of the body and is usually not palpable unless the snake has recently eaten or there is significant pathology present
- The gall bladder, which lies just caudal to the stomach, is sometimes palpable when there is biliary stasis secondary to anorexia or active inflammation of the hepatobiliary system
- Developing ova, in the caudal third of the body, can sometimes be palpated similar to 'marbles on a string'
- The kidneys are elongated and located in the caudal quarter of the body
- Pathological swelling of the caudal third of the snake's body may be due to constipation, renomegaly, or retained products of conception
- The reproductive, urinary and gastrointestinal tracts empty into the cloaca. The vent is the orifice through which products of all three tracts pass externally
- The tail extends beyond the vent. Clinically significant structures contained within the tail are the paired musk glands, paired hemipenes (lateral to the musk glands) and the tail vein. Pathological swelling of the base of the tail is due to infections of the musk glands or inspissated semen.

Sample collection

Blood

The indications for blood collection are the same as for domestic animals.

- Sedation may be necessary with larger or intractable specimens
- Syringes should be pre-heparinized prior to venepuncture, due to the length of time it may require to obtain an adequate volume of sample
- For most laboratories a minimum of 0.2–0.4 ml of whole blood is adequate for haematology and plasma biochemical analysis but it is advisable to check with the laboratory in advance

- The maximum volume of blood that can be safely taken from a reptile is calculated by using the formula: weight (g) × 1% = ml blood.

The preferred method for blood collection is cardiocentesis. A bloodflow Doppler is sometimes required to locate the heart, particularly in bulky snakes such as the larger boids.

- After disinfection of the skin with isopropyl alcohol, a 25 or 22 gauge needle attached to a tuberculin or 3 ml syringe is inserted at an angle of 45 degrees into the ventricle, and gentle aspiration is performed (Figure 20.9)
- With each contraction of the ventricle, blood enters the syringe
- If pericardial fluid is aspirated, the needle is withdrawn and venepuncture is performed again, using a new pre-heparinized syringe.

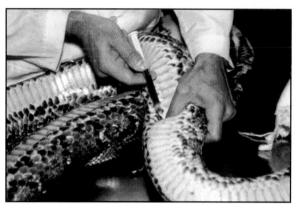

Figure 20.9 Cardiocentesis in a sedated Burmese python. (Courtesy of William Cermak.)

The coccygeal vein (tail vein) can be utilized in larger snakes (but restraint and obtaining an adequate volume of blood can be problematical):

- The site is on the ventral midline of the proximal third of the tail
- The needle is inserted at an angle of 45 degrees until it comes into contact with the vertebrae
- It is then withdrawn 1–2 mm and gentle aspiration is performed.

Normal haematological and biochemical values are summarized in Figure 20.10.

Pulmonary wash

Harvesting cellular material from the lower respiratory tract for cytology, parasitology and bacterial culture and sensitivity is important for diagnostic and therapeutic reasons. Frequently, sedation is not required in debilitated snakes. Appropriately sized sterile feeding or urethral catheters work well:

1. Pass the catheter through the glottis.
2. Instil sterile saline (5–10 ml/kg) into the lung.
3. Massage the snake's body to assist in loosening any pulmonary exudates.
4. Aspirate.

Parameter	Range
Haematology	
RBC (10^6/mm³)	0.4–2.5
WBC (10^6/mm³)	6.7–8.1
Haemoglobin (g/dl)	5.2–12
Haematocrit (PCV) (l/l)	0.16–0.45
Biochemistry	
Total protein (g/l)	29–80
Uric acid (µmol/l)	60–600
Urea (mmol/l)	0.17–1.87
Creatinine (µmol/l)	10–45
Glucose (mmol/l)	0.5–6
Calcium (mmol/l)	2.5–5.5
Phosphorus (mmol/l)	0.9–1.85
Lactate dehydrogenase (IU/l)	30–600
Gamma glutamyltransferase (IU/l)	0–15
Alkaline phosphatase (IU/l)	80–45
Aspartate aminotransferase (IU/l)	5–35
Alanine aminotransferase (IU/l)	260
Triglycerides (µmol/l)	0.6–2
Cholesterol (mmol/l)	1.3–3.6

Figure 20.10 Haematological and plasma biochemical values for snakes.

Diagnostic techniques

Faecal analysis
Cloacal excretions are usually a mixture of faeces and urates. Faecal material is brown and is semi-formed to solid in consistency. Direct smears mixed with saline should be examined immediately for the presence of protozoans. A portion of faeces is suspended in a hypertonic solution (such as zinc sulphate), centrifuged and examined for parasitic ova and motile larvae.

If a faecal specimen is not available, a colonic wash can be performed:

1. Infuse sterile saline (approximately 10–20 ml/kg) into the cloaca by inserting a ball-tipped feeding needle through the vent.
2. Massage the coelomic cavity.
3. Aspirate.

Urinalysis
There are significant differences between reptilian and mammalian urine. In snakes, uric acid is the principal product of protein catabolism. Precipitates of uric acid are normally passed as hard concretions. Reptilian kidneys lack loops of Henle, which means that they consistently produce urine with a specific gravity of 1.002–1.010, regardless of hydration status. The pH ranges from 6 to 7.

Snakes do not possess urinary bladders; urine is stored in the ureters and cloaca, where it mixes with faeces. Evaluation of urine sediment should be interpreted in light of this fact.

Biopsy techniques

- Sedation and local anaesthesia are necessary for biopsies of the skin and oral mucosa

- General anaesthesia is required for internal tissue sampling
- Multiple tissue samples are always preferable to single biopsies
- Normal tissue should be included with abnormal tissue
- It is usually preferable to remove a solitary mass and then perform a biopsy on it (excisional biopsy), rather than simply harvesting a small tissue sample (incisional biopsy).

At the time of biopsy, the clinician should be prepared to perform additional techniques such as touch impression smears and bacterial culture and sensitivity. Tissues for histopathology, electron microscopy and immunohistochemistry can be placed in 10% buffered formalin.

Skin biopsy: When performing skin biopsies, disinfection of the skin is done with isopropyl alcohol. It is preferable not to obtain biopsies of the integument while the snake is undergoing ecdysis. A number 11 scalpel blade is used to make a circumferential full-thickness incision in the interscalar skin, incorporating several normal and abnormal scales. Because the skin inverts when incised, an everting technique such as a horizontal mattress pattern is used for closure.

Ultrasound guidance: Ultrasonography is helpful in identifying organs and lesions for biopsy. Ultrasound-guided biopsy permits penetration and harvesting of targeted tissues while avoiding vasculature. Spring-loaded biopsy instruments work well, particularly in larger boids. The author prefers an 18 gauge needle with a sample notch of 1.7 cm. The depth of penetration is 22 mm and so care must be taken to ensure that the tissue to be sampled has sufficient thickness.

Endoscopy: This is an excellent tool for examinination and biopsy of the gastrointestinal and respiratory tracts. Biopsy by laparotomy is the most common method of tissue sampling of organs such as the liver, kidneys and intracoelomic masses. Because of the unique linear anatomy of snakes, laparotomy incisions are made directly above the targeted biopsy site.

1. After standard disinfection of the skin with alcohol and betadine, make an incision between the first and second rows of lateral scales.
2. Penetrate the muscle layer and coelomic membranes bluntly, using forceps.
3. Close the coelom by suturing the thin musculature with absorbable material such as polyglycolic acid.
4. Remove non-absorbable skin sutures after approximately 4 weeks.

Common conditions

Common disease problems are summarized in Figure 20.11.

Disease	Causes	Clinical signs	Diagnosis	Treatment
Constipation and cloacal prolapse	Overfeeding. Obstructive causes. Neurogenic. Idiopathic	Tenesmus. Enlarged caudal part of body. Prolapsed tissue	Clinical signs. Palpation. Radiology	Cholinergics. Enemas. Colopexy
Dermatitis (blister disease)	Poor husbandry with secondary bacterial infection. Sepsis	Vesicles. Necrosis of scales	History. Physical examination. Cytology and culture/sensitivity tests from lesions	Correct husbandry problems. Topical and systemic antibiotics. Maintain hydration status
Dysecdysis and retained spectacle	Dehydration. Lack of abrasive surfaces in cage. Mites and ticks. Systemic disease	Retained patches of epidermis	Physical examination	Identify underlying cause. Soak in shallow water for several hours
Dystocia	Lack of appropriate nest box. Use of subadult or geriatric breeders. Uterine infections. Obstructive causes. Idiopathic	Excessive cruising in cage. Bulge(s) just cranial to vent. May be asymptomatic	Check normal gestation time for species of snake. Only a portion of eggs or neonates have passed within prior 24 hours. Radiography. Ultrasonography	Check hydration. Provide nesting box. Administer calcium or oxytocin. Ovacentesis. Surgery
Enteritis	Parasites. Bacterial, fungal or viral infections. Neoplasia	Diarrhoea, sometimes with blood	Faecal examination. Endoscopy and biopsy	Appropriate drugs
Musk gland adenitis	Poor husbandry. Trauma. Idiopathic. Neoplasia	Swollen tail base, sometimes with a fistula	Physical examination. Culture and sensitivity tests. Biopsy	Flush gland. Topical and systemic antibiotics
Neurological disease	Trauma. Hypothiaminosis. Inflammatory bowel disease (IBD). Iatrogenic drug overdose. Organophosphate toxicity. Sepsis	Ataxia. Tremors. Lack of righting reflex. Anisocoria. Opisthotonus. Coma	History. Physical examination. Haematology. Plasma biochemistry. Liver or kidney biopsy for IBD	Treat underlying cause if identified. Support with parenteral fluids. Diazepam for seizures
Pneumonia	Stress. Hypothermia. Poor ventilation. Bacterial, viral, fungal, parasitic, secondary to stomatitis	Dyspnoea. Puffy throat. Oral exudate	Physical examination. Radiography. Cytology, culture and sensitivity tests on exudate	Increase temperature. Antibiotics. Parenteral fluids. Bronchodilators
Prolapsed hemipenis	Excessive breeding attempts. Usually idiopathic	Protrusion of copulatory organ from vent	Physical examination	Surgery, either by placing organ back into sulcus, or amputation
Regurgitation	Improper cage temperature. Dehydration. Excessive handling of snake after it has eaten. Parasites. Viral infection. Neoplasia. Obstruction	Regurgitation of partially digested food several days after eating	History. Faecal examination. Radiography. Endoscopy. Biopsy	Based on underlying cause
Renal disease (gout)	Ambient temperature too cold. Chronic dehydration. Overfeeding. Bacterial infection. Misuse of aminoglycosides	Anorexia. Dehydration. Sometimes swollen caudal third of body due to renomegaly	Haematology. Plasma biochemistry. Renal biopsy	Parenteral fluids. Vitamins. Allopurinol. Anabolic steroids. Antibiotics. Increase cage temperature
Stomatitis	Trauma. Cage temperature too cold. Bacterial infection. Neoplasia. Gout	Gingivitis. Oral abscesses. Swollen jaw	Direct smears for cytology. Radiography to rule out osteomyelitis. Culture and sensitivity tests. Biopsy	Parenteral fluids. Oral debridement. Topical and systemic antibiotics
Subspectacle abscess	Ascending infection from oral cavity. Sepsis. Idiopathic	Hypopyon. Swollen globe	Physical examination	Surgical drainage of subspectacle space
Thermal burns	Overexposure to heat sources	First-, second- or third-degree burns	History. Physical examination	Parenteral fluids. Topical and systemic antibiotics

Figure 20.11 Common disease problems in snakes.

Viral infections

The most common viral diseases of snakes are inclusion body disease (IBD) and paramyxovirus infection.

Inclusion body disease

IBD is caused by a retrovirus and primarily affects boids, though it has also been isolated from colubrids. The virus produces different clinical syndromes depending upon the strain of the virus and type of snake affected (Schumacher, 1996). In boas it causes regurgitation – usually within a few days after feeding. Affected snakes may slowly waste away or die acutely. After several months the symptoms may progress to an encephalopathy characterized by strabismus, head tilt, tremors, paralysis and opisthotonus (Figure 20.12).

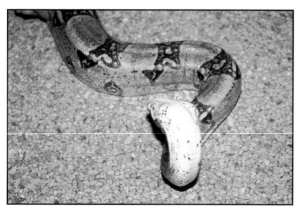

Figure 20.12 Opisthotonus (head tilt) in a boa constrictor with inclusion body disease.

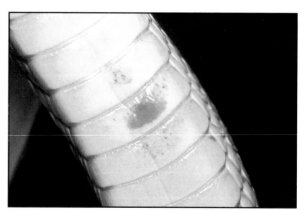

Figure 20.13 Ecchymoses of the ventral scales in a Trans-Pecos ratsnake *Elaphe subocularis.*

In pythons, the disease runs a much more acute course characterized primarily by similar neurological symptoms followed by death. Boas, particularly South American species, are considered to be the natural reservoirs. Horizontal transmission is suspected to occur by blood-sucking arthropods such as the snake mite. Vertical transmission also occurs.

Diagnosis of IBD is based on histopathological identification of eosinophilic intracytoplasmic inclusions in tissues stained with haematoxylin and eosin. Biopsies of the liver, pancreas or kidney are the best sources for demonstrating viral inclusions.

There is no effective treatment. Once the virus has been diagnosed in a collection, each snake should have biopsies taken and be culled if positive. In addition, the group should be prevented from reproducing and 'closed' to the addition of any snakes.

Paramyxovirus infection

Paramyxovirus affects the respiratory and central nervous systems and has been isolated from viperids, colubrids and boids. Signs range from flaccid paralysis and dyspnoea to sudden death without symptoms. A presumptive antemortem diagnosis is done by measuring haemagglutination inhibition titres (Schumacher, 1996). An increase of at least 2-fold in titres measured 2 weeks after resting titres is highly suggestive of paramyxovirus disease.

Bacterial infections

The majority of bacteria identified from infections in captive snakes are Gram-negative aerobic microorganisms, including *Pseudomonas, Aeromonas, Klebsiella, Escherichia coli* and *Salmonella.* Examples of anaerobic bacteria are *Clostridium* and *Bacteroides.* Occasionally, Gram-positive bacteria such as coagulase-positive staphylococci are also identified. Most of these bacteria are opportunistic pathogens: they are part of the body's normal flora that can cause disease during periods of immunosuppression. Sepsis occurs from haematogenous invasion from the integument, respiratory, gastrointestinal or lower urogenital tracts. The presence of petechiae or ecchymoses strongly suggests septicaemia (Figure 20.13).

Treatment

Bacterial diseases should be treated based upon results of culture and sensitivity testing. Bactericidal drugs are preferred to bacteriostatics. Important points to consider when choosing an antibiotic are: penetrability of the targeted lesion; route of administration; maintenance of adequate hydration; and recommended temperature during antibiotic administration. If bacterial culturing and sensitivity cannot be performed, it is prudent to choose a combination of antibiotics that will provide activity against Gram-negative, Gram-positive, aerobic and anaerobic bacteria. The Formulary at the end of the chapter summarizes drug dosages.

Zoonoses

Snakes with salmonellosis should be considered permanent carriers. Mycobacteriosis has occasionally been identified in snakes; lesions affect primarily the integument, gastrointestinal and respiratory tracts. Soil and stagnant water are the most common sources. Snakes with zoonotic diseases should be humanely euthanased with a barbituric acid derivative administered by the intracardiac route.

Fungal infections

Fungal dermatitis is the most common manifestation of mycotic disease in snakes. Grossly, the lesions appear as discrete areas of wrinkled scales that are often raised and discoloured. Frequently, the ventral scales are affected since they come in contact with contaminated substrates.

Many fungal organisms are normal inhabitants of the intestinal tract (e.g. *Geotrichum, Rhizopus, Candida* and *Trichosporon;* Raiti, 1998). The combination of immunosuppression and unhygienic husbandry practices permits establishment and proliferation of these organisms on the integument and mucous membranes of the gastrointestinal and respiratory tracts. Injuries from rodent bites can also become contaminated with mycotic organisms.

Biopsy of suspicious lesions and subsequent identification by culture is recommended. Treatment consists of a combination of topical and systemic antifungal drugs.

Parasites

Ectoparasites

The most common external parasite of snakes is the snake mite *Ophionyssus natricis*. Poor husbandry and an inadequate quarantine period of new acquisitions permit these haematophagous arthropods to reach very high populations before they are detected. Adult mites are black and nocturnal. The most common sites are at the edges of the spectacles and in the skin fold perpendicular to the chin. Besides dysecdysis, mites cause anaemia and transmit bacteria (aeromonads).

Treatment for snake mite must be long term and includes eradication of mites both on the host and in the environment. The author has used ivermectin topically and parenterally with success. Ivermectin for injection can be diluted with propylene glycol as a 10% solution to facilitate volume calculations in smaller snakes. It is essential that therapy is continued for 8 weeks, due to the life cycle of the mites (DeNardo and Wozniak, 1997). The enclosure, water bowls and hide boxes should be washed with a 1% sodium hypochlorite solution.

Ticks of the genera *Amblyomma* and *Aponomma* commonly infest wild-caught snakes, particularly those of African origin. Ticks are capable of causing dysecdysis and anaemia and of transmitting rickettsial diseases. Treatment is with injectable ivermectin followed by removal of the ticks with forceps several hours later.

Endoparasites

Nematodes and flagellates are the most prevalent intestinal parasites seen in snakes.

Helminths: The hookworm *Kalicephalus* is the most common nematode and causes anorexia, weight loss and enteritis. These strongyles have a direct life cycle and are capable of extensive tissue migration. Infection occurs through ingestion of embryonated ova or transcutaneous penetration by larvae. Subcutaneous nodules can contain thousands of larvae.

Ascarids, such as *Ophidascaris*, are not as pathogenic as strongyles but can cause intermittent regurgitation and weight loss.

The snake lungworm *Rhabdias* causes lower respiratory tract disease that is often complicated by a secondary bacterial pneumonia. Ova are detected when a pulmonary wash is performed.

Nematode microfilariae have been identified in snakes and cause blockage of capillaries.

Trematodes (flukes and tapeworms) require one or more intermediate hosts, such as molluscs, fish or amphibians. Flukes inhabit the hepatobiliary system and cause cachexia and diarrhoea. The operculated ova are seen on faecal examinations primarily in wild-caught snakes. Adult tapeworms primarily inhabit the intestinal tract. Tapeworm larvae are capable of extensive tissue migration. *Spirometra* larvae commonly produce subcutaneous swellings and can be extracted after incising the skin.

Protozoa: Flagellates such as *Trichomonas* are commonly found in small numbers of clinically normal snakes. One type of flagellate, *Monocercomonas*, has been associated with nephritis and salpingitis. Large numbers of flagellates are commonly seen with nematodes during faecal examinations. They should be eliminated with an appropriate antiprotozoal drug such as metronidazole.

Entamoeba invadens probably has a commensal relationship in reptilian herbivores such as tortoises. In the intestine these parasites subsist on plant carbohydrates. In snakes, amoebas burrow into the intestinal lining and cause haemorrhagic enteritis with associated high morbidity and mortality (Frank, 1984). They can also invade the bile duct and cause cholangiohepatitis. Quadrinucleated cysts or the motile trophozoites are visible upon direct faecal examination. Metronidazole is the treatment of choice.

Coccidiosis causes anorexia, weight loss and diarrhoea. Oocysts are readily identified on faecal flotations. *Eimeria* (four sporocyts) and *Isospora* (two sporocysts) are commonly seen in colubrids. *Caryospora* (single sporocyst) is approximately one-half the size of other coccidia and is more common in boids. The author has had better success eradicating coccidiosis using injectable sulpha drugs rather than the oral forms.

The coccidian parasite *Cryptosporidium serpentis* produces two syndromes in snakes (Schumacher, 1996). The first is an acute form characterized by regurgitation within a few days after eating. The parasite colonizes the gastric crypts, causing an intense inflammatory reaction. Hypertrophy of the stomach is so severe that frequently a midbody swelling becomes apparent. The chronic form is characterized by a gradual wasting away of the affected snake without regurgitation. The parasite spreads by ingestion of infective oocysts by the host. Diagnosis is by identifying the oocysts from gastric washes, biopsy of the gastric mucosa, or a fluorescent antibody test performed on the faeces. Oocysts stain red with acid-fast reagents. Affected snakes should be permanently isolated from the main collection. Paromamycin has shown promise in preventing oocyst shedding but has not been proved to cause eradication of the parasite.

Pentastomids: These are primitive arthropods with a zoonotic potential. Snakes acquire this parasite after ingesting an infected rodent. The larvae migrate to the lungs, where adults either attach to the pulmonary epithelium or remain motile, sometimes migrating to air sacs. The ova, with four claw-like appendages, are identified in the faeces or pulmonary exudate. Treatment can be attempted by surgical removal. Ivermectin has reportedly been used effectively in a tokay gecko (Micinilio, 1996).

Gastrointestinal disease

Stomatitis (mouth rot)

Bacterial infections of the oral cavity (Figure 20.14) are common. Local infection due to trauma from rodents or the snake rubbing its rostrum against abrasive surfaces are the most common causes. Chronic stressors such as suboptimal ambient temperature play a role, especially in larger boas and pythons. Sometimes stomatitis is secondary to a primary systemic process such as sepsis, renal failure, viral disease or neoplasia.

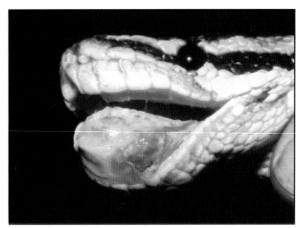

Figure 20.14 A large granuloma of the oral cavity in a royal python with necrotic stomatitis.

Haematology and plasma biochemical analysis should be performed in addition to direct smears of the infected gingivae for cytology and bacterial culture and sensitivity testing. If cellulitis is present, radiography should be used to rule out osteomyelitis. Treatment consists of sedation, debridement, topical antibiotic therapy if possible, parenteral fluids and systemic antibiotics.

Regurgitation
Regurgitation is the effortless expulsion of partially digested food. In snakes this problem usually occurs within 1–3 days after consumption of a meal. The most common causes are improper ambient temperature, consumption of too large a meal or excessive handling of the snake shortly after eating.

- If a snake is being kept too warm or too cool, decomposition of ingesta occurs faster than the digestive process, leading to regurgitation
- Snakes that require high humidity levels are prone to regurgitation when they become dehydrated
- The consumption of an exceptionally large meal can overtax gastric function, leading to regurgitation. Emerald tree boas are particularly prone to this problem
- Less common causes are ingestion of foreign bodies and consumption of prey items such as spoiled rodents that were not kept at the proper freezing temperature.

The most common infectious causes are parasites (cryptosporidia, nematodes), viruses (IBD), ulcers and neoplasia. Endoscopy, gastric biopsy, faecal analysis, culture and sensitivity testing are diagnostic.

Enteritis
Parasitism is the leading cause of enteritis in snakes (see above). Treatment with parenteral fluids and appropriate parasiticides is often dramatic but long-term treatment for 4–6 weeks and retesting of stools every 6 months is necessary to ensure parasite eradication.

Enteritis can also be associated with renal and hepatic diseases and with infiltrative bowel disease (parasitic migration, lymphoma).

Disruption of normal enteric flora through the misuse of antibiotics has been incriminated as a cause of fungal overgrowth and subsequent diarrhoea (Raiti, 1998). When an overwhelming number of fungal hyphae is seen on direct faecal smears, it may be prudent to administer a fungicidal drug that is not absorbed from the gut, such as nystatin.

Bacterial disease is an uncommon cause of diarrhoea in snakes. Bacterial culturing of faeces can be performed when other causes have been ruled out.

Intussusception is a potential consequence of enteritis. It should be suspected when a soft tissue mass is palpated in the caudal half of juvenile snakes that carry high parasite burdens.

Constipation and cloacal prolapse
The most common causes of constipation and cloacal prolapse are overfeeding and associated tenesmus. Green tree pythons and emerald tree boas are particularly prone to these conditions due to their slow metabolic rate. Chronic dehydration is also a contributing factor. Ingested substrates can become entangled in rodent hair and form a trichobezoar. Obstructions due to granulomas, retained ova and neoplasia are less common causes. Treatment of non-obstructive constipation is by administering a cholinergic (e.g. metaclopramide or cisapride) and soaking the snake in water for 24 hours to stimulate peristalsis. Enemas can be coupled with massaging of the colonic contents. Occasionally, surgical removal of the obstruction is necessary.

Prolapse of the cloaca can also be neurological in origin. Snakes with congenital defects such as scoliosis can have a colonic neuropathy resulting in megacolon and subsequent prolapse (Figure 20.15). Surgical repair is described later and illustrated in Figure 20.15.

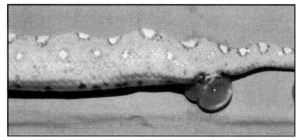

Figure 20.15 Cloacal prolapse in a juvenile green tree python. Note the scoliosis, which had caused motor paralysis of the distal colon and cloaca.

Nutritional disease

Obesity
Obesity (Figure 20.16), due to a combination of hyperalimentation and lack of exercise, is probably the most prevalent nutritional disease in snakes. It is best to compare captive animals with photographs of wild specimens. Obesity predisposes snakes to constipation, dystocia, atherosclerosis, hepatic lipidosis and liver failure. Treatment consists of gradually reducing the intake of calories and the use of drugs to treat liver failure (e.g. vitamins, antibiotics, parenteral fluids and steroids).

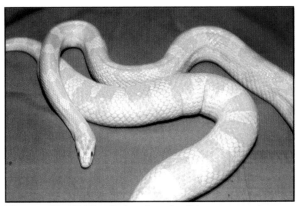

Figure 20.16 Obesity in a female albino corn snake. Note the excessive skin folds on the caudal half of the body due to fat deposits.

Hypothiaminosis

Vitamin B₁ deficiency is seen in piscivores such as garter and water snakes that are fed primarily frozen fish, or fish that have very high levels of thiaminase (such as sardines and whitefish). Freezing inactivates thiamine, which is necessary for proper functioning of the central nervous system. Unless the diet is supplemented with thiamine, or fish with high thiaminase levels are boiled, cerebrocortical degeneration and subsequent necrosis result. Symptoms consist of tremors, paralysis and loss of the righting reflex. In the acute stages, response to treatment with injections of thiamine is often dramatic.

Ocular disease

Subspectacle abscess

Accumulation of purulent exudate between the spectacle and cornea can be due to sepsis or an ascending infection from the oral cavity. The globe is not swollen unless a panophthalmitis develops or there is a blockage of the nasolacrimal duct. Grossly the eye appears distinctly opaque. Occasionally a fluid line is visible. Treatment consists of lancing and removing a small piece of the spectacle at the ventral portion of the eye while the snake is anaesthetized. Parenteral antibiotics based upon bacterial culture and sensitivity are administered for approximately 3 weeks. It may also be necessary to flush the subspectacular space with saline solution, which is infused through the surgical window. Healing should be completed after the next shed.

Respiratory disease

Pneumonia

The major symptom of lower respiratory tract disease (LRTD) is dyspnoea, characterized by open-mouth breathing. A frothy or purulent exudate may be visualized in the glottis. Bacterial disease is the most common cause of LRTD but parasites (lungworms, pentastomids) and viruses (paramyxovirus) have also been identified. Stress and hypothermia are common causes of immunosuppression.

Pulmonary wash or endoscopy to harvest material for cytology and bacterial culture and sensitivity is recommended. Most of the bacteria isolated are *Pseudomonas*, *Aeromonas*, *Klebsiella* and *Escherichia coli*. Radiographs demonstrate pulmonary infiltrates in the dependent portions of the lungs. Treatment consists of parenteral fluids, antibiotics and maintaining the ambient temperature at the upper level of the snake's POTZ to stimulate the immune system.

Urogenital disease

Gout

Uric acid is produced in the liver and excreted by the renal tubules. Renal failure is the most common cause of gout in reptiles. When blood levels of uric acid reach saturation point, uric acid crystals precipitate within the mucous membranes, pericardial sac, myocardium, liver (Figure 20.17) and kidneys. Frequently, there is a diffuse swollen appearance to the caudal fourth of the snakes's body due to bilateral renomegaly. The oral cavity should be examined for tophicaseous deposits. Affected snakes are anorexic and dehydrated. The causes of renal disease are a combination of one or more of the following: suboptimal ambient temperature, chronic dehydration, infectious diseases, or overdosing with nephrotoxic drugs such as aminoglycosides.

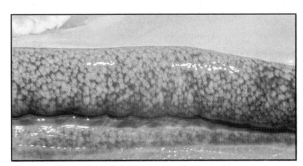

Figure 20.17 Massive deposits of uric acid crystals in the liver of a green tree python that had died due to renal failure.

Haematology and plasma biochemistry commonly demonstrate haemoconcentration, increased total solids, leucocytosis, hypocalcaemia, hyperphosphataemia and hyperuricaemia; however, it is normal for snakes to have postprandial elevations of uric acid for 5–7 days (Zwart, 1992). Renal biopsy gives valuable information as to aetiology, treatment options and prognostics. Treatment consists of intracoelomic fluids, allopurinol, vitamins, anabolic steroids and antibiotics.

Dystocia

Dystocia may be non-obstructive or obstructive. Non-obstructive dystocia is more common and is usually seen in snakes that are gravid for the first time. Frequently, the cause of uterine inertia is idiopathic; however, several factors have been incriminated – such as breeding animals of suboptimal size, lack of appropriate nesting sites, obesity, and the use of geriatric breeders. Hypocalcaemia is not considered a significant cause of uterine inertia in snakes.

Non-obstructive causes of dystocia in viviparous snakes are embryonic death due to suboptimal basking temperatures, and uterine infections. Obstructive causes are abnormally large eggs, compressive injuries to the spine, coelomic granulomas, and retained products of conception from previous breedings.

Treatment of the non-obstructive form consists of supplying an appropriate nesting site and administration of oxytocin. Response to oxytocin is quite variable, because vasotocin is the naturally occurring reproductive neuropeptide found in reptiles. Eggs that have not passed within 24 hours after the first egg has been deposited are not viable, due to hypoxia.

Decompression of the distal egg(s) by transcutaneous aspiration followed by oxytocin administration (Figure 20.18a) significantly increases the likelihood of oviposition. If the eggs still have not passed after 24 hours, gentle manipulation of each egg toward the vent is attempted while the snake is anaesthetized with isoflurane. Each egg is then grasped with forceps and extracted (Figure 20.18b). If this is not possible, the retained eggs must be removed surgically (see below).

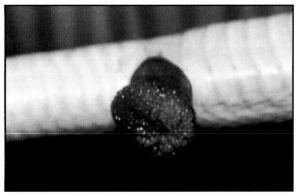

Figure 20.19 Prolapsed hemipenis in an albino kingsnake. This tissue is viable and should be kept moist until surgical repair.

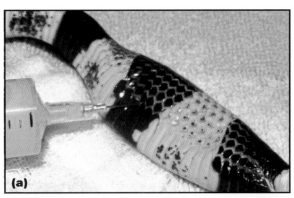
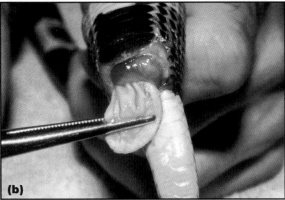

Figure 20.18 (a) Transcutaneous ovacentesis to collapse an egg in a grey-banded kingsnake *Lampropeltis alterna*. (b) The collapsed egg is removed from the anaesthetized snake using grasping forceps.

Prolapsed hemipenis

This condition (Figure 20.19) occurs during multiple breeding attempts by the male snake. If the hemipenis appears normal it can be placed back into the sulcus while the snake is anaesthetized with isoflurane. A purse-string suture holds it in place. The suture should

not be removed for at least 1 month. If the hemipenis is engorged with blood it can sometimes be decompressed by aspiration before an attempt is made to replace it into the tail. If the organ is infected or necrotic, it should be amputated at its base. The snake will still be capable of breeding.

Skin disease

Dermatitis (blister disease)

Bacterial infections of the skin are associated with poor husbandry. Prolonged contact with urine and faeces in a humid environment is conducive to bacterial multiplication and subsequent invasion of the dermis. Initially, lesions appear as vesicles on the ventral scales. Eventually the blisters rupture, exposing tissue which subsequently becomes necrotic (Figure 20.20). Death can occur due to sepsis. Fluid from the vesicles should be examined for strongyle larvae and bacterial culture and sensitivity tests should be performed.

Treatment consists of rehydration with parenteral fluids, and the use of topical and systemic antibiotics. Resolution can take weeks to months. Increased shedding frequency during the recuperative process is to be expected, as this promotes healing.

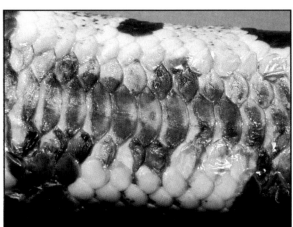

Figure 20.20 Ventral dermatitis (blister disease) in a royal python. The vesicles have ruptured and there is extensive necrosis of the skin.

Dysecdysis and retained spectacles

The most common cause of abnormal shedding, in which retained pieces of dried epidermis adhere to the affected snake's body, is suboptimal ambient humidity. Other causes of dysecdysis are mites, ticks and systemic disease.

Soaking the snake in a shallow water bath for several hours usually solves the problem. It is recommended that the owner check the sloughed skin to make sure that the spectacles and nasal plugs have been shed. If not, when husbandry problems have been corrected and humidity levels are increased, both layers of spectacles will be removed during the next shed.

Thermal burns

Most burns (Figure 20.21) occur on the ventral scales due to snakes resting on heating stones. Occasionally, burns are seen on the dorsum of the body from overhead heating fixtures. Treatment consists of topical antibiotics such as silvadiazine, protective bandages, parenteral fluids and systemic antibiotics. Increased shedding frequency contributes to the healing process. Scars eventually become pigmented with melanin. Healing can take 6–8 months.

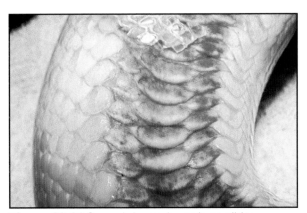

Figure 20.21 Second-degree burns in an albino Burmese python.

Musk gland adenitis

Infections of the musk gland(s) produce a swelling at the base of the tail. Eventually, ulceration of the gland occurs, seen as a cavity filled with necrotic debris. Treatment consists of debridement, bacterial culture and sensitivity, and topical/parenteral antibiotics. This condition is more common in snakes that are kept in unhygienic enclosures where the substrate supports a large bacterial population.

Neurological disease

The most common causes of neurological disease in snakes are inappropriate use of miticides, IBD, trauma, drug overdose, thiaminase toxicity, sepsis, hypothermia (hibernating boids at too low a temperature), incorrect incubation temperatures during embryonic development, and parasitic migration. Symptoms include tremors, lack of righting reflex, anisocoria, ataxia, paralysis and opisthotonus. The diagnosis rests heavily upon the case history, appropriate diagnostics and

response to treatment. Most neurological diseases carry a guarded prognosis at best. Early treatment of thiamine deficiency and organophosphate toxicity offer the most promising results. Supportive treatment should include parenteral fluids.

Toxicoses

The most common toxicities seen in clinical practice are due to overdosing with acaricides and therapeutic drugs. The use of organophosphates to treat mites is particularly dangerous to snakes. Impregnated strips containing dichlorvos have caused the most problems. Symptoms are due to overstimulation of nicotinic cholinergic sites causing muscle fasciculations, tremors, spasms and muscular paralysis. Death is due to respiratory failure. Treatment consists of atropine, parenteral fluids and diazepam (if seizures occur).

Overdosing with ivermectin or metronidazole causes ataxia, tremors and paralysis. Treatment consists of nutritive support and parenteral fluids. Permanent head tilt and strabismus have been seen associated with ivermectin toxicosis. Due to their neuroblocking mechanism, it is prudent not to administer aminoglycosides concurrently with sedatives or general anaesthetics.

Neoplasia

A wide variety of neoplasms have been identified in snakes. Most affect the integument, digestive tract and lymphoreticular systems. Carcinomas and sarcomas are the most common malignant neoplasms of the integument and internal organs. Lymphoma is the most common malignancy of the haematopoietic system. Sometimes lymphoblasts are identified in the haemogram of affected snakes, denoting leukaemia. Neoplasia should be included in the differentials when any mass or enlarged organ is identified. Examination of needle aspirates or tissue biopsies provides the diagnosis.

Congenital defects

Improper incubation temperatures and inbreeding are the most common causes of congenital defects in snakes. Temperatures that are too warm or too cold commonly cause snakes to be born with scoliosis and neurological dysfunctions such as loss of the righting reflex and ataxia. Less common abnormalities are external herniations, anophthalmia and bicephalus.

Supportive care

Injection sites

Most injections are administered intramuscularly in the heavy longissimus muscles located parallel to the spine. The subcutaneous route may also be used but some drugs, such as enrofloxacin and ketamine, are irritating and capable of causing sterile abscesses. There is also slower absorption, which can affect the drug's distribution and onset of action. The preferred sites for intravenous injections are intracardiac or the coccygeal vein.

Fluid therapy

Parenteral fluids are usually administered intracoelomically or subcutaneously:

- Intracoelomic injections are performed in the caudal fourth of the body. The needle is inserted between the first two rows of lateral scales just dorsal to the ventral scales and is then directed cranially at an angle of 30 degrees to the long axis of the body. Fluids should be warmed prior to administration
- Subcutaneous administration of fluids is performed lateral to either side of the dorsal spinous processes. When done correctly, the fluids can be seen moving in a cranial direction under the skin.

Sedation, anaesthesia and analgesia

Sedation

Propofol, an ultra short-acting anaesthetic, is ideal for techniques such as radiography, skin biopsy, pulmonary wash and abscess debridement; it can also be used to facilitate intubation and induction with gas anaesthesia. Dissociative sedatives such as ketamine or tiletamine and zolazepam can be used if propofol cannot be administered (Figure 20.22).

Anaesthesia

Preparation of snakes prior to anaesthesia should include a thorough history, physical examination, accurate weighing and haematology and plasma biochemical analysis. During anaesthesia, physiological stabilization is achieved by providing adequate hydration, correct body temperature and effective pulmonary gas exchange. Figure 20.23 lists sedatives, analgesics and anaesthetic agents for use in snakes.

- A parasympatholytic such as glycopyrrolate decreases respiratory secretions and blocks vagal induced bradycardia. Glycopyrrolate is safer than atropine (particularly in small snakes) as it does not cross the blood–brain barrier
- Injectable pre-anaesthetics such as propofol or the dissociative sedatives may be used to facilitate intubation and induction
- It is safer to sedate debilitated snakes via mask induction with isoflurane. The veterinary surgeon must use appropriate clinical judgement. Isoflurane is considered the gaseous anaesthetic of choice because of its rapid induction and recovery. It does not sensitize the myocardium to circulating catecholamines and provides excellent muscle relaxation
- A surgical plane of anaesthesia is determined by the lack of various reflexes such as the righting reflex, tail pinch withdrawal reflex and tongue retraction reflex
- Maintaining the snake's core temperature at 28°C is critical during and after any procedure requiring sedation or anaesthesia. Circulating warm water pads and radiant heat sources are extremely useful in preventing hypothermia
- Cardiac monitoring with the use of electrocardiology, bloodflow Doppler or pulse oximetry is strongly recommended. The normal pulse should be in the range of 20–40 beats per minute, depending on the size of the snake (smaller specimens have faster cardiac rates). Positive pressure ventilation is recommended at the rate of one breath every 15 seconds.

Analgesia

The use of analgesics (see Figure 20.23) should be a component of every surgical procedure ranging from topical debridement to laparotomy. Signs of acute pain in snakes are excessive writhing movements or motor rigidity.

	Propofol	Dissociatives (Tiletamine, ketamine)
Administration	i.v., intracardiac	i.m.
Advantages and uses	For techniques lasting <20 min Rapid induction and recovery times	Induction time 30–45 min Increase heart rate and blood pressure
Disadvantages	Causes bradycardia Apnoea	Long recovery time (up to several hours, depending on dose)

Figure 20.22 Choices for sedation.

Drug	Dose	Comments
Butorphanol tartrate	0.5–1.0 mg/kg i.m., i.v. one to two times daily	Analgesic
Carprofen	1–5 mg/kg i.m., i.v., orally, once daily	Analgesic
Diazepam	5 mg/kg i.m.	To control seizures
Doxapram HCL	5–10 mg/kg i.v., i.m.	Respiratory stimulant
Epinephrine	0.02 mg/kg intracardiac or i.v.	Cardiac stimulant
Flunixin meglumine	0.1–0.5 mg/kg i.m. once or twice daily	Analgesic
Glycopyrrolate	0.01 mg/kg i.m. 30 minutes prior to anaesthesia	Parasympatholytic
Isoflurane	Induction 3–4%; maintenance 1–3%	Gas anaesthetic
Ketamine HCL	10–30 mg/kg i.m.	Sedative
Lignocaine (lidocaine) 2%	Infiltration s.c.	Local anaesthetic
Medetomidine	100 µg/kg i.m. plus 5 mg/kg ketamine HCL i.m.; reverse with atipamezole at 5 × medetomidine dose	Anaesthetic
Propofol	5–10 mg/kg i.v., intracardiac	Short-acting anaesthetic
Tiletamine and zolazepam HCL	5 mg/kg i.m.	Sedative

Figure 20.23 Analgesics, sedatives and anaesthetics for use in snakes.

Common surgical procedures

Repair of cloacal prolapse

To repair the prolapse (Figure 20.24), while the snake is under general anaesthesia:

1. Use a blunt probe to replace the prolapsed tissue gently, making sure that the telescoped portion has been completely reduced (Figure 20.24b).
2. Place external colopexy sutures at the junction of the ventral and lateral scales.
3. After penetrating the skin, the suture needle is permitted to bounce off the probe before it is pushed back out through the skin.
4. Place several sutures bilaterally, using an absorbable material such as polyglycolic acid. These sutures are removed approximately 2 months later.

Salpingotomy

Retained eggs may require surgical removal (Figure 20.25).

1. Make an incision between the ventral and lateral scale rows over the retained egg(s).
2. Exteriorize the portion of the oviduct with eggs and incise the oviduct.
3. After removing the first egg, remove any remaining eggs through the same incision.
4. If necessary, perform the same procedure with the second oviduct.
5. Close the oviduct with simple interrupted sutures using 5-0 polyglycolic acid.
6. Suture the skin with an everting pattern. Suture removal is in 4–6 weeks.

The snake should be allowed to rest for a year before being bred again.

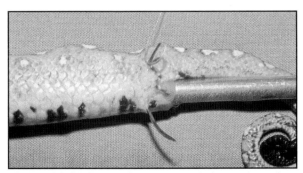

Figure 20.24 Repair of the prolapsed cloaca shown in Figure 20.15. A bilateral colopexy is being performed after insertion of a probe to reduce the prolapsed tissue.

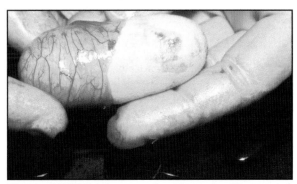

Figure 20.25 Salpingotomy in a kingsnake. (Courtesy of William Cermak).

Drug formulary

Drug	Dose	Comments
Antimicrobials		
Amikacin	2.5–5 mg/kg i.m. every 3 days Ball python: 3.48 mg/kg i.m. once and then every 4 to 5 days	25°C
Ampicillin	3–6 mg/kg s.c., i.m. daily	26°C
Carbenicillin	200–400 mg/kg i.m. daily	30°C
Ceftazadime	20 mg i.m. every 3rd day	30°C
Cefuroxime	100 mg/kg i.m. every 2nd day	30°C
Cephalothin	40–80 mg/kg i.m. every 2nd day	30°C
Clotrimazole	Apply topically	PBT; antifungal
Dimetridazole	40 mg/kg orally every 5th day	30°C
Enrofloxacin	5 mg/kg i.m. daily	27°C
Gentamicin	2.5 mg/kg s.c. every 3rd day	24°C
Itraconazole	23.5 mg/kg orally daily	PBT; systemic antifungal
Ketoconazole	25 mg/kg orally daily	PBT; systemic antifungal
Metronidazole	20 mg/kg orally every 2nd day	PBT
Nystatin	100,000 IU/kg orally daily for 7 days	PBT; enteric fungal overgrowth
Piperacillin	100 mg/kg i.m. every 2nd day	28°C
Sulphadiazine cream	Apply topically daily	PBT

Figure 20.26 Drug formulary for snakes. (continues) ▶

Drug	Dose	Comments
Antiparasitic agents		
Fenbendazole	100 mg/kg orally every 2 weeks until negative	Nematodes, cestodes
Ivermectin	200 µg/kg i.m. every 2 weeks until negative	Nematodes
	5 mg/l water sprayed topically once weekly on snakes and enclosure for 8 weeks concurrent with 200 µg/kg i.m. every 2 weeks for 8 weeks	Mites
	200 µg/kg i.m. once followed by manual removal 24 hours later	Ticks
Levamisole HCL	10 mg/kg i.m. every 2 weeks until negative	Nematodes, microfilariae
Metronidazole	100 mg/kg orally every 2 weeks until negative	Flagellated protozoans, amoebas
	50 mg/kg orally daily for 4 weeks	Amoebas
Paromamycin	300–350 mg/kg orally every other day for 3 weeks; then every fifth day for 3 months	*Cryptosporidium* (long-term cure not proven)
Praziquantel	10 mg/kg orally or i.m. every 2 weeks	Cestodes, trematodes
Quinacrine	20–100 mg/kg orally every 2nd day for 2–3 weeks	Haemic protozoans
Sulphadimethoxine	90 mg/kg orally first dose; 45 mg/kg orally daily for 1 week	Coccidians
Trimethoprim and sulphamethoxazole	30 mg/kg orally or i.m. and every other day until negative	Coccidians
Thiabendazole	50 mg/kg orally every 2 weeks until negative	Nematodes
Miscellaneous		
Allopurinol	20 mg/kg orally	Treatment of gout (decreases uric acid levels)
Aminophylline	10 mg/kg i.m.	Bronchodilator
Atropine sulphate	0.1–0.2 mg/kg once daily	Organophosphate toxicity
Barium sulphate suspension	5 ml/kg orally	GIT contrast study
Calcium lactate	10–25 mg/kg i.m.	Hypocalcaemia
Cimetidine	5 mg/kg i.m. twice daily	Gastritis, decreases P levels due to renal disease
Cisapride	1 mg/kg orally once daily	Stimulates gastric motility
Dexamethasone	1 mg/kg i.m. once daily	Anti-inflammatory
Epogen	1 mg/kg once weekly	Bone marrow stimulant (anaemia)
Lactated Ringer's solution	10–25 ml/kg intracoelomic, s.c., once or twice daily	Corrects dehydration
Metoclopramide	0.05 mg/kg orally once daily	Stimulates gastric motility
Oxytocin	20–40 IU/kg i.m., i.v., once or twice daily	Uterine stimulant
Stanozolol	5 mg/kg i.m., orally, once weekly	Anabolic steroid
Vitamin B complex	0.5 ml/kg i.m. every 2nd day	Appetite stimulant
Vitamin B$_1$ (thiamine)	25 mg/kg i.m. once daily	Thiaminase toxicity
Vitamin K	0.5 mg/kg i.m. once daily	Liver disease, warfarin toxicity

Figure 20.26 continued Drug formulary for snakes.

References and further reading

Bennett RA (1996) Anesthesia. In: *Reptile Medicine and Surgery*, ed. DR Mader, pp. 241–247. WB Saunders, Philadelphia

Bennett RA (1996) Neurology. In: *Reptile Medicine and Surgery*, ed. DR Mader, pp. 141–147. WB Saunders, Philadelphia

Boyer TH (1987) Snakes. In: *Essentials of Reptiles: A Guide for Practitioners*. AAHA Press, Lakewood, Colorado

Brown CW and Martain RA (1991) Dystocia in snakes. In: *The Compendium Collection: Exotic Animal Medicine in Practice*, ed. DE Johnston, pp. 86–92. Veterinary Learning Systems, Trenton, NJ

Cooper JE (1994) Biopsy techniques. *Seminars in Avian and Exotic Pet Medicine: Endoscopic and Imaging Techniques*, 3, 161–165

Cranfield MR and Graczyk TK (1996) Cryptosporidiosis. In: *Reptile Medicine and Surgery*, ed. DR Mader, pp. 359–363. WB Saunders, Philadelphia

DeNardo D and Wozniak EJ (1997) Understanding the snake mite and current therapies for control. *Proceedings of the Association of Reptilian and Amphibian Veterinarians*, Houston, Texas, 137–147

Frank W (1984) Non-hemoparasitic protozoans. In: *Diseases of Amphibians and Reptiles*, eds GL Hoff, FL Frye and ER Jacobson, pp. 259–384. Plenum Press, New York

Frye FL (1981) Parasitology. In: *Biomedical and Surgical Aspects of Captive Reptile Husbandry*, ed. FL Frye, pp. 305–312. Krieger Publishing Co. Inc., Malabar, Florida

Frye FL (1994) Ultrasonic doppler blood flow detection in small exotic animal medicine. *Seminars in Avian and Exotic Pet Medicine: Endoscopic and Imaging Techniques* 3, 133–139

Funk RS (2000) A formulary for lizards, snakes, and crocodilians. *Veterinary Clinics of North America: Exotic Animal Practice* 3(1), 333

Lawton MPC (1991) Reptiles, Part Two: Lizards and snakes. In: *Manual of Exotic Pets*, ed. PH Beynon and JE Cooper, pp. 244–260. BSAVA, Cheltenham

Mattison C (1990) *A–Z of Snake Keeping*. Sterling Publishing Co. Inc., New York

Micinilio J (1996) Ivermectin for the treatment of pentastomids in a tokay gecko (*Gekko gecko*). *Bulletin of the Association of Reptilian and Amphibian Veterinarians* 6(2), 4

Raiti P (1998) Use of nystatin to reduce suspected overgrowth of enteric fungal organisms in a diamond python (*Morelia spilota spilota*) and two honduran milksnakes (*Lampropeltis triangulum hondurensis*). *Bulletin of the Association of Reptilian and Amphibian Veterinarians* 8(1), 4

Schumacher J (1996) Viral diseases. In: *Reptile Medicine and Surgery*, ed. DR Mader, pp. 224–234. WB Saunders, Philadelphia

Zwart P (1992) Urogenital system. In: *Manual of Reptiles*, ed. PH Beynon *et al.*, pp. 117–127. BSAVA, Cheltenham

21

Amphibians

David L. Williams

Introduction

The class Amphibia contains around 4500 species. Amphibians live in habitats ranging from tropical rainforest to subarctic tundra and they vary from being entirely aquatic to existing in arid grasslands. A wide variety of amphibians is kept successfully in captivity for a variety of reasons: as pet or display species kept by individuals or in zoological collections, as species for laboratory research and in captive breeding programmes. This last category stands out as particularly important, given the international decline in amphibian species (Stebbins, 1995).

It is important that captive amphibians such as cane toads, *Xenopus* or American bullfrogs are not released into the wild where they could establish colonies.

Die-offs of local populations are relatively common, and veterinary surgeons may be confronted with requests to investigate large numbers of dead frogs in the UK with signs of 'red leg' (see below) (Cunningham *et al.,* 1995).

Amphibians evolved from primitive fish around 350 million years ago and were the first animals to venture from water on to dry land. They can be divided into three orders:

- Anura or Salientia (tailless adult forms comprising frogs and toads)
- Urodela or Caudata (tailed adult forms comprising the salamanders, newts and sirens)
- Apoda or Gymnophiona (legless burrowing species comprising the caecilians).

Biology

The biological features of most importance in dealing with amphibians are:

- Poikilothermia (ectothermia): as with reptiles, amphibians rely on heat from the environment for body warmth. Keeping the animal within its preferred temperature range is important for health in captivity. The preferred temperature varies widely between different species and so understanding the requirements of a particular animal is paramount.
- Hydration: the thin non-keratinized amphibian skin is permeable and highly liable to desiccation, requiring a moist environment. Ensuring that the correct level of hydration is maintained is essential for health.

- Reproduction: in many amphibian species eggs are laid in water and fertilized externally. Aquatic larvae metamorphose into adults which, in most cases, live in terrestrial habitats, returning to the water to lay eggs. In some frogs and the plethodontid salamanders, the eggs are laid in moist terrestrial sites, the larval stages develop in the egg and the young emerge fully formed. This direct development circumvents the free-living larval stage. Some amphibians are viviparous, giving birth to fully metamorphosed young, which have been nourished during their larval stages through oviductal secretions in the mother, although no direct placental attachment occurs. Several amphibians are ovoviviparous, with developing eggs carried in the oviducts, stomach, skin pouches or even the mouth, without gaining any apparent nutritional support from the adult.

Commonly kept amphibians

African clawed toads

The African clawed toad *Xenopus laevis* is commonly kept as a laboratory animal and its care is relatively straightforward. An aquarium is required, with water at 20–26°C to a depth of 10–20 cm. *Xenopus* require two meals a week, consisting of worms, fish or pieces of meat. Mating can be induced by injection of human chorionic gonadotrophin. *Xenopus* tadpoles are unusual in that they will feed on suspended food particles.

Fire-bellied toads

Fire-bellied toads (*Bombina* spp.) come in a variety of beautiful colours. The different species have very different requirements. The fire-bellied toad *B. bombina* is predominantly aquatic and requires at least as much water in the vivarium as dry land, whereas the oriental fire-bellied toad *B. orientalis* may be kept in a terrestrial environment with damp moss in most of the vivarium. The oriental species breeds readily whereas *B. bombina* is, for reasons unknown, difficult to breed in captivity.

Ceratophrys and *Pyxicephalus* toads

These two unrelated toads from South America (*Ceratophrys*; Figure 21.1a) and Africa (*Pyxicephalus*) are large horned toads with voracious appetites. They ambush prey and so a deep layer of leaf mould and

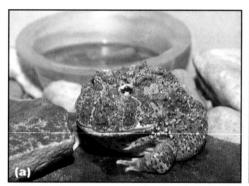
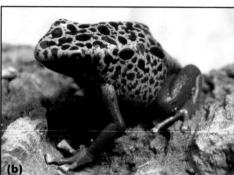

Figure 21.1 Two examples of anurans. (a) *Ceratophrys* toad in an inappropriate captive environment, dry with no leaf litter for burrowing. (b) Blue arrow poison frog *Dendrobates azureus*. (Courtesy of T. Skelton.)

moss (between 23°C and 30°C) is ideal for burrowing. They are excellent individuals for captive breeding. They are aggressive to other amphibians and should be kept alone or with like-sized members of the same species if breeding is attempted, which is generally achieved with chorionic gonadotrophin.

True toads

The family Bufonidae includes the European common toad *Bufo bufo*, which habituates well to captivity provided the temperature does not exceed 23°C. A breeding pair and the offspring can easily be accommodated in a 100 litre vivarium. The North American marine toad *B. marinus* can grow to more than 20 cm in length. Some imported animals do not adapt well to captivity; many develop Cowan's maladaptation syndrome and die. The term maladaptation was used by Cowan (1968) to describe the demise of reptiles through inadequate mirroring by the captive environment of the natural surroundings enjoyed by the species in the wild. The same is without doubt true of amphibians, although some attribute much of this to parasite burdens in captive animals. Those that do survive are well suited to captivity although the vivarium must be large, with deep leaf litter and a high level of humidity provided by regular spraying. The problems associated with accidental or purposeful release of this species into the wild in several parts of the world show how important it is that pet animals should be rigorously prevented from escaping.

True frogs

The bullfrog *Rana catesbeina* prefers a large vivarium, ideally in a secure greenhouse. The bullfrog lives at a wide range of temperatures and grows best between 20 and 25°C. The leopard frog *R. pipiens* is native to North America and similarly grows well at lower temperatures. It has been widely used in laboratory research and is easy to maintain. The European common frog *R. temporaria* inhabits temperate climes and often hibernates during the winter.

Poison arrow frogs

The poison arrow frogs *(Dendrobates* spp.; Figure 21.1b) are exceptionally colourful animals from Central and South America and possess a virulent poison in their skin. The poison is only dangerous if ingested or introduced into the bloodstream but, even so, dispos-

able gloves should be worn when handling these animals. The preferred environmental temperature of this species is between 28 and 32°C.

Tree frogs

Tree frogs *(Hyla* spp.) comprise a large family, which are mostly arboreal, with disc-like distal protuberances on each digit, facilitating climbing. Their main prey are flies, which can readily be bred in captivity. A commonly kept member of this family is White's tree frog *(Litoria caerulea)*, a placid species that thrives in captivity. The species grows well at 26–28°C, although it can withstand lower ambient temperatures.

Axolotls

The Mexican salamander or axolotl *Ambystoma mexicanum* is a classic example of neoteny, being an adult with an unmetamorphosed larval form. Captive examples of this species are common, having been widely used in laboratory research, although in its native habitat of mountain lakes it has become sufficiently scarce to be listed as an endangered species. Axolotls can be kept between 10 and 25°C, although in cooler waters their feathery gills become reduced in size and function. The axolotl can be bred in captivity with reasonable ease.

Salamanders

The tiger salamander *Ambystoma tigrinum* is a characteristic member of the Ambystomidae. This stocky individual adapts well to captivity once it has overcome its initial timidity. It grows well between 15 and 25°C, the preferred temperature reflecting its place of origin, which can be across a wide range of North America. An enclosure mimicking its natural environment is preferred.

Husbandry

Housing

Apart from totally aquatic species such as the African clawed toad *Xenopus laevis* and the axolotl *Ambystoma mexicanum*, most amphibians require a vivarium with a terrestrial area and some shallow water. Adequate cover is required to provide hiding places.

A gradation of temperature across the vivarium, from moist enclosed areas to drier open spaces, allows the animal to manipulate its environment. This helps to reduce the occurrence of the non-specific maladaptation syndrome seen often in lower vertebrates in captivity.

Utraviolet light is required by many captive amphibians for correct calcium homeostasis, though exact UV level requirements are unknown. Excessive irradiation can lead to dermal burns or cataracts.

Different species require different environments, depending on their normal behaviour in the wild: many frogs and toads are terrestrial and several prefer a substrate in which they can lie partly exposed. Thus vivaria furnished with deep leaf litter are ideal. All amphibians require water, and in a captive state the same concerns about water quality, circulation and hygiene should be kept in mind as for aquarium fish. Pond or rainwater should be used in preference to tap water. Other amphibians such as the tree frogs are arboreal and require branches with foliage at a suitable height for climbing. There has been little research on the behavioural requirements of amphibians and whether enrichment of the environment is appropriate. Nevertheless it can be assumed that an enclosure close to the native environment is to be pretend to an inappropriate setting.

Diet

Generally, adult amphibians are carnivores and should be fed a variety of invertebrates. Larger species such as bullfrogs and cane toads can be voracious and will eat newborn mice. Invertebrates may contain little calcium, and metabolic bone disease can be a problem in amphibians. Low calcium levels can result from invertebrates such as mealworms and crickets being housed on bran and not being fed adequately. Vitamin and calcium supplements should be given to, and with, the invertebrates, which should be fed on fruit and table scraps. Smaller amphibian species can be fed cricket nymphs or ants, which form a substantial proportion of the diet of tropical species in the wild. Tadpoles may take meat in small portions, but many graze off the natural microflora on pond weed when small.

Captive breeding

Almost all amphibians need to return to water to breed. Anurans, with few exceptions, fertilize their eggs externally, with males ejaculating on the eggs extruded from females. Salamanders, however, fertilize their eggs internally, with females taking sperm packets or spermatophores into their vents after the males have deposited them on the substrate. Anurans are highly vocal during their courtship whereas urodeles are not. The males clasp the females during mating, a process known as amplexus. Visual cues are important in sexually dimorphic species such as the Old World newts (*Trituris* spp.) where the males have colourful markings on their enlarged dorsal fin and broad tail. Female receptivity is induced by male courtship glands on the chin (mental glands) or side of the head (genial glands). Many amphibian species are seasonal breeders, although amount of rainfall is a key factor in initiating breeding behaviour in some (Duelmann and Trueb, 1986; Stebbins, 1995).

Handling and restraint

The handling of amphibians can be difficult and potentially hazardous for both handler and animal for several reasons: the mucus covering and relative fragility of the skin, the ease of transepidermal absorption of topically applied chemicals and the propensity of some species to discharge noxious toxins. Before catching the animal, hands should be wetted but not washed with soap or detergent. Ideally, wetted powder-free plastic gloves should be used when restraining an amphibian. Small amphibians can be caught by using a palming technique, catching in the cup of the hand either against the side of the cage or aquarium. Larger species can be caught by holding the head between the first two fingers as it crosses the palm, with the thumb gently restraining the neck. In this way the forward straining movement of the animal attempting to escape will only press it further into the handler's grip. Other methods of restraint include capture in fine nylon nets, but care must be taken to avoid trauma.

Amphibians should be transported in cooled, waterproof, adequately ventilated containers, with damp vegetation or sponge in the bottom, except for immature forms and entirely aquatic species such as *Xenopus* or the axolotl, which require immersion in water.

Diagnostic approach

Clinical examination and history taking

First the species being presented should be identified, especially where owners are unsure of their pet's identity or its requirements in captivity.

A detailed history should be taken. This should concentrate on environmental conditions such as temperature, temperature fluctuations (both daily and over longer periods), humidity, housing, water quality, frequency of water changes and any changes in environment concurrent with or preceding the development of the animal's disease. A record sheet is useful. This can be filled in either by the veterinary surgeon or by the owner while sitting in the waiting room, ensuring that the history is taken in a methodical and complete manner. The owner should be made aware of the importance of record keeping, making note of the animal's activity, when food was offered and when it was eaten.

If possible, the amphibian should be brought to the clinic in its normal environment rather than in a holding or transport container. This allows the veterinary surgeon to examine the environment and suggest improvements if required.

The animal should first be examined in its environment. Many amphibians exhibit considerable changes in behaviour and physical characteristics after handling, such as excessive skin secretions. Similarly, a true respiratory rate can be estimated only in the resting undisturbed animal.

Physical examination

Once the animal has been handled, a thorough examination should be undertaken, starting with the head, including the eyes, nostrils and mouth. Careful examination of the skin is important to look for abrasions or areas of hyperaemia, ulceration or nodule formation, together with subcutaneous fluid or gas. Bacteriological or mycological sampling can often be valuable, as can microscopic examination of wet preparations from skin lesions stained with Giemsa or Gram stains, and looking for flagellates with dark-field illumination. Similarly, examination of the cloaca should, where possible, be followed by collection of faeces or a wet preparation. In this way a good clinical database can be built up for that individual animal and, even when the animal is apparently normal, act as a baseline against which to evaluate samples from diseased animals of the same species.

Diagnostic tests and techniques

Blood sampling

Blood samples can be easily taken, either by direct cardiac puncture or by venepuncture from the central ventral abdominal vein. A cardiocentesis is best performed with the animal in dorsal recumbency, using a 25 gauge needle directed under the xiphoid process at a 10–20 degree angle to the ventral part of the body. A haematocrit, red and white blood cell counts and a differential count should be obtained. These will differ substantially between species and sexes and at different times of the year; a normal sample from an unaffected member of the same species should be obtained for comparison. This is particularly important given the paucity of data on blood values in amphibians. A blood culture can be useful when septicaemia may be involved.

Centesis of the dorsal lymph sac can also yield useful samples for culture and cytology. The animal should be held upside down briefly, to allow the lymph to drain caudally. Fluid is removed using a 25 G needle inserted at a slight angle to the skin surface, in the dorsal midline, with the bevel facing downwards.

Radiography

Radiography can be useful for assessing bone density or for identifying foreign bodies or gastrointestinal obstruction. In such cases, a 1:10 dilution of contrast medium can be used for a contrast gastrogram. Dental non-screen film gives excellent detail in these small animals.

Common conditions

Viral disease

The Lucke tumour herpesvirus is the only viral cause of disease in amphibians to have been intensively studied and well characterized. The virus causes renal adenocarcinomas in leopard frogs but is unlikely to be encountered in veterinary practice.

Other viruses include a group of iridoviruses known as tadpole oedema virus, which give rise to subcutaneous oedema, haemorrhages and cutaneous necrosis in frogs, particularly, as their name suggests, in tadpoles.

Amphibians are also affected by arboviruses, but their pathogenicity is unknown at present.

Bacterial disease

'Red leg'

Generalized bacterial disease manifesting as reddening of the skin was first described in wild amphibians over 100 years ago. It is common in captive amphibians kept at high density in a less than optimally hygienic environment. Gram-negative organisms such as *Aeromonas*, *Pseudomonas*, *Citrobacter*, *Salmonella*, *Flavobacterium* and *Chlamydia* may cause disease, ranging from localized infection of traumatized skin to septicaemia manifesting as 'red leg.'

Clinical signs may involve no more than skin hyperaemia (Figure 21.2a) or may include petechiation, ecchymoses and frank ulceration (Figure 21.2b). Systemic signs often include anorexia but may also involve ascites and generalized subcutaneous oedema. In chronic infections, ocular or CNS involvement may also occur, with ocular inflammation or neurological signs of incoordination, spasms or vomiting. Such signs show that the condition is not merely a dermal condition but rather a generalized infection with septicaemia, which manifests predominantly as redness of the skin, giving the name red leg.

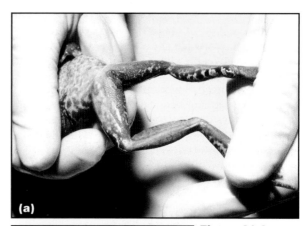

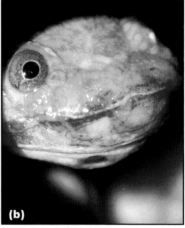

Figure 21.2
(a) Skin hyperaemia may be the only sign of Gram-negative septicaemia. Note the recommended wetted plastic gloves. (Courtesy of A. Cunningham.)
(b) Frank ulceration in other areas may also occur in so-called 'red leg'.

The isolation of *Aeromonas* or another Gram-negative organism from lesions does not confirm that the bacterium is the causative agent; *Aeromonas* is a common commensal organism, both on the skin and in the gastrointestinal tract and an occasional pathogen. Thus, any traumatic skin lesion may be colonized by a small number of these bacteria. Finding a profuse growth of this organism alone associated with red skin lesions, or findings at postmortem examination of hepatomegaly with a dark red swollen hepatic parenchyma and occasionally necrotic foci in other viscera, are sufficient to give a diagnosis of the disease.

Immunosuppression may occur if animals are kept at too low a temperature and may predispose to overwhelming infection by organisms such as *Aeromonas*, resulting in red leg. Also, poor tank hygiene may yield a high local growth of bacteria in the environment that overwhelms even a functional immune system.

Dead wild amphibians may be brought to a veterinary surgeon by members of the public distressed by large scale die-offs of animals with redness of the caudal limbs. It should be explained that this is a condition caused by Gram-negative septicaemia and unlikely to be related to human intervention. Culture of the skin surface as well as heart blood can help confirm the diagnosis; *Aeromonas hydrophila* is the most commonly associated organism, although other bacteria can be involved. In affected captive groups the individuals responsible should be isolated. Swabs should be taken from the skin surface of these animals for antibiotic culture and sensitivity, and culture of a lymph sac sample obtained by centesis is advised. Appropriate antibiotics should be given initially by subcutaneous or intramuscular injection in the clinic followed by oral administration at home. For in-contact animals, prophylactic administration of antibiotics is probably best attempted through a medicated bath (see below).

Oral administration of antibacterials may cause dysenterobiosis, whereby the normal flora of the intestinal tract becomes significantly altered. For this reason, injectable agents may be preferable, despite the difficulty of using them. Topical administration through a medicated bath might be best in such cases. Alternatively the concurrent use of a probiotic may be advisable, although there are few or no data on the efficacy of probiotic use in preventing or alleviating antibiotic-induced dysenterobiosis in amphibians.

Mycobacterial disease

Mycobacterial infections are not uncommon in amphibians, caused by water-borne atypical mycobacterial species such as *Mycoplasma marinum*, *M. xenopi* and *M. fortuitum*. The infections cause skin nodules (Figure 21.3) or ulcerations, although such lesions are not confined to mycobacterial agents. With severe disease the animal is unable to regulate its transcutaneous water balance and cutaneous respiration may be affected. Animals will die relatively quickly unless supplemental oxygen is provided in gaseous form or dissolved in the water. Severe internal granulomatous disease may occur, manifesting as gradual weight loss with anorexia. Diagnosis is by demonstration of mycobacteria; given the difficulty in sampling and culturing these organisms, a skin biopsy sample showing acid-fast organisms is usually preferable to culture techniques, although the latter can allow determination of antimycobacterial sensitivities. Although the literature suggests treatment with amikacin or enrofloxacin, the author has not found these to be particularly effective. Mycobacteriosis is not particularly infective to other in-contact amphibians, but it is zoonotic and can give rise to a persistent granuloma formation, 'aquarist's nodule'. For this reason euthanasia of affected animals is recommended here.

Fungal disease

Localized and systemic fungal infections are reasonably common in amphibians, resulting mainly in focal skin clouding, discoloration and ulceration. The three particularly important diseases are *Saprolegnia* infection in aquatic amphibians, phycomycosis and chromomycosis in anurans. Diagnosis is by skin biopsy and identification of fungal hyphae or sporulating bodies.

Saprolegnia causes grey-white mycelial mats on the skin surface with underlying tissue necrosis and is reasonably pathognomonic in appearance. *Ichthosporidia* occurs in amphibians less commonly than in fish but has a similar appearance: small white nodules indicative of granulomata in the skin and also throughout internal organs at postmortem examination.

Chromomycosis is a chronic debilitating disease characterized by skin ulceration and chronic weight loss indicating systemic involvement (Figure 21.4). Given that the causative organisms are conidia-forming

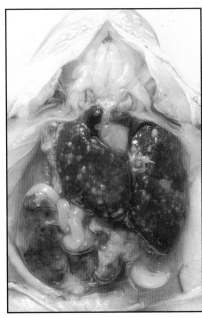

Figure 21.4 Fungal disease may involve the viscera, with systemic signs. (Courtesy of JE Cooper and the Edward Elkan Memorial Collection.)

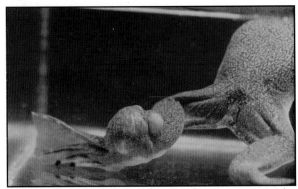

Figure 21.3 Skin nodule on the hindleg of an African clawed toad caused by mycobacterial infection. (Courtesy of JE Cooper and the Edward Elkan Memorial Collection.)

pigmented fungi, the characteristic finding on post-mortem examination from histopathological samples or from skin scrapings are pigmented hyphae and spores, hence the name chromomycosis. Phycomycosis, however, is caused by non-pigmented fungi related to *Mucor*, giving white visceral masses seen at post-mortem examination. Systemic infection results in non-specific signs such as anorexia, inactivity and weight loss. Both chromomycosis and phycomycosis are potentially zoonotic diseases and thus, while treatment with antifungal agents such as amphotericin B or nystatin might be successful in limiting disease, euthanasia is probably the most appropriate choice.

With any fungal disease, precipitating factors are important in the development of the condition; a careful evaluation of husbandry is therefore essential in dealing with any such disease. It may be that individual animals become clinically affected only if they are immunosuppressed or otherwise physiologically compromised. Given this possibility it is worthwhile obtaining a blood sample to give a full haemogram to show if there is a neutropenia or lymphopenia.

As some animals may be predisposed to clinical signs of infection, affected animals should be isolated to avoid transmission of disease. Many fungi are zoonotic, so gloves should be worn when handling affected animals. Aquarist's nodule can occur in people exposed to fish infected by atypical mycobacteria, or a much more serious mycobacterial infection can supervene in immunosuppressed individuals, such as those undergoing chemotherapy or infected by HIV.

Parasitic disease

Amphibians are affected by a wide range of parasites: protozoans such as *Entamoeba;* nematodes such as *Rhabdias* and *Capillaria;* cestodes; trematodes; leeches; and mites, e.g. the chigger mites of the genus *Hannemania*, present as subcutaneous larval forms.

External protozoans can be found on the skin and gills of aquatic amphibians, and in many cases traditional remedies such as copper sulphate or sodium chloride baths can be invaluable. Visceral protozoal infections, such as those caused by *Entamoeba ranarum* and various coccidial species, can be more pathogenic and more difficult to treat. Parasites such as gastrointestinal flagellates may be quite normal commensals in a healthy animal and may only cause problems after overwhelming infection in an already sick animal. *E. ranarum* does, however, cause hepatic and gastrointestinal haemorrhage and necrosis and affected animals should be treated with metronidazole. Complete control is difficult owing to the protozoan's direct lifecycle and the infective cysts produced. The host animals may need to be culled and the environment meticulously sterilized to control the problem.

Differentiating the normal gastrointestinal nematode burden in a healthy amphibian from a pathogenic load can be difficult. Animals found to have nematode eggs on a routine faecal examination should be treated with fenbendazole and then placed in a newly cleaned environment to avoid re-infection. The lungworm *Rhabdias* is a major pathogen, with a free-living larval form that penetrates the skin before reaching the lungs, causing substantial systemic problems when infestations are large. The best treatment for this often resistant organism is probably ivermectin, although the narrow range between an efficacious therapeutic dose and a toxic one means that fenbendazole or levamisole may be the best initial treatment.

Pseudocapillaroides xenopii is a nematode that causes dermal ulceration, haemorrhage and often septicaemia in the *Xenopus* toad. Diagnosis is by microscopic examination of skin biopsy samples or skin scrapings. Anthelminthic treatment together with physical removal of desquamating infected skin and improved tank hygiene is important in curing this infestation. Several trematodes and cestodes do occur in the wild, but their need for intermediate hosts often renders them non-pathogenic or at the least self-limiting in captivity. Gastrointestinal blockage by a heavy cestode burden can be an exception, and treatment is required. Parasiticides used in fish can generally be used in amphibians, although a wide variety are available to treat different infestations.

Nutritional disease

As with reptiles, nutritional bone disease can be a major problem in captive amphibians. Deformed bones with poor bone density on radiography and particularly poorly calcified cortices and pathological fractures are signs of calcium deficiency, although the swollen limbs of reptiles do not seem such a noticeable feature of metabolic bone disease in amphibians. In severe chronic cases inanition, generalized weakness and death occur. Metabolic bone disease can also occur with a lack of ultraviolet irradiation in captive amphibians, and signs of the disease should alert the veterinary surgeon to enquire about the age of any ultraviolet bulb used (most bulbs reduce their ultraviolet emissions substantially after about 6 months) as well as the diet.

Vitamin A deficiency or excess is not regularly seen in amphibians although clearly could occur with dietary deficiency or over supplementation. Deficiency in vitamin B_1 is much more common as amphibians are often fed fish and the thiaminase contained in many species can reduce the levels of thiamine in the amphibian to nil. Neurological signs include weakness, ataxia and paralysis. Treatment is by injection of vitamin B_1 and supplementation with 25 mg of thiamine per kilogram of fish. Vitamin E deficiency occurs when feed stuff is old or improperly stored resulting in ataxia with muscular degeneration. Iodine deficiency prevents metamorphosis in tadpoles, and dietary supplementation is necessary, although the exact dietary requirements are at present unclear. Oxalate toxicity usually occurs with overfeeding of spinach, and tadpoles are particularly prone to renal calculi as a result. This illustrates the importance of feeding a balanced and varied diet.

Environment-related disease

Apart from disease related to low temperature or inappropriate humidity, two other conditions related to the environment should be noted: gas bubble disease and trauma to the skin.

Gas bubble disease

Gas bubble disease of amphibians results from over-aeration of water. This yields a supersaturated solution, producing gas bubbles on and in the animal's skin, with erythema, petechiation or subcutaneous emphysema in severe acute cases and skin necrosis in severe chronic causes. Bubble formation in the gut or lymph sac may occur. The cause of the supersaturation should be dealt with, and affected animals should receive supportive care.

Skin trauma

Chemicals such as ammonia or other detergents severely affect the skin of many amphibians. Rapid and prolonged irrigation with cold water of a neutral pH is essential in affected animals. Several cases arise because of incomplete rinsing of vivaria after cleaning with detergents.

Physical trauma can adversely affect the amphibian skin, and abrasions should be irrigated with 2% sodium chloride or 0.1% cetrimide. Prophylactic systemic antibiosis is sensible only in such conditions. Lacerations should be sutured with 4/0–6/0 vicryl. Animals should be kept in a bath of dilute saline until healing has occurred to prevent concurrent infection.

Ocular disease

The most common ocular disease in amphibians is lipid keratopathy (Carpenter *et al.*, 1986). Dense white corneal opacities are seen, often with corneal thickening (Figure 21.5). Histopathology shows cholesterol deposition and associated foamy macrophages. Biochemical evaluation demonstrates deposition of cholesterol ester in the cornea and liver (Carpenter *et al.*, 1986; Russell *et al.* 1990), with corneal changes being associated with more generalized xanthomatosis. Although the cause is unknown, the predominance of disease among females and the development of massive eggs in several affected individuals suggests that the excessive mobilization of lipid associated with egg production is responsible. Dietary fat may be important in the disease as in some reported cases frogs had been fed newborn mice containing high levels of maternally derived milk lipids, though other animals with the disease had been fed on mealworms and crickets. A simple nutritional origin is thus unlikely, but diet should be taken into account when taking the history of affected animals.

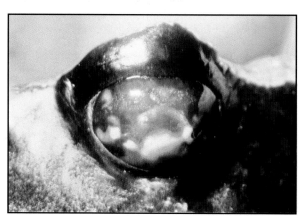

Figure 21.5 Corneal lipidosis in a horned toad.

Other ocular lesions include uveitis, which is often associated with septicaemia. In the same way that skin reddening is a sign of generalized Gram-negative infection, the eye may also be a target organ, with inflammation associated with the vascular plexus of the iris. Other ocular conditions have been noted but are generally single spontaneous cases from corneal ulceration to glaucoma.

Tympany and anasarca

Osmoregulation is critical to amphibians, which is not surprising considering that they depend so intimately on the hydration of their environment. Abnormalities in water regulation can lead to abnormal uptake of water or the formation of gas within the coelomic cavity, thus leading to the accumulation of lymph fluid in the dorsal lymph sacs or in the coelom, leading to anasarca. Aspiration of the fluid gives temporary relief but, as with dropsy in fish, the fluid rapidly returns. Long-term amelioration is difficult. It may be that there is infection with Gram-negative organisms and thus systemic antibiosis with a drug such as enrofloxacin may be appropriate.

Neoplasia

The only well studied neoplasm of amphibians is renal adenocarcinoma associated with the Lucke herpesvirus. Other neoplasms occur spontaneously, and most reports in the literature concern single cases. Most involve the integument and may be related to environmental contamination with carcinogenic agents. As so many infectious and parasitic agents cause dermal nodules (see Figure 21.3), biopsy is mandatory in the evaluation and diagnosis of such lesions.

Anaesthesia and analgesia

The anaesthesia of amphibians involves many of the same techniques and drugs as that of fish. Tricaine methane sulphonate (MS-222, Sandoz) or benzocaine has been used for many years, but recently phenoxyethanol has been more widely suggested. MS-222 is used at a dilution of 1:2500 in sterile water. Benzocaine is used at the same dilution but its insolubility in water means that a concentrated solution in acetone is preferred, to be added to a larger volume of water obtaining the dilution of 1:2500 at the time of anaesthesia. Intramuscular ketamine has been used at 50 mg/kg, or halothane or isoflurane can be bubbled through the water in which the amphibian is held.

The plane of anaesthesia can be maintained or changed by applying either water containing anaesthetic (Figure 21.6) or normal water to the skin of the amphibian throughout the procedure.

The use of isoflurane mixed with K–Y gel has been reported, although this has the disadvantage over isoflurane used as a gaseous agent in mammals of lack of rapid recovery as the agent is not lost through respiration, and the amount absorbed is

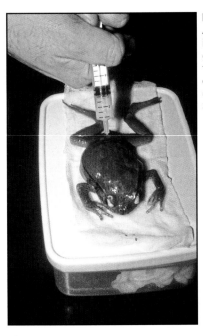

Figure 21.6
Anaesthesia using isoflurane in K–Y gel syringed on to the dorsal surface of the animal. (Courtesy of S. Redrobe.)

difficult to quantify. The author has had problems with slow recovery of frogs after two or more anaesthetics using this technique within a few days. Nevertheless the technique is easy, with a small amount of isoflurane-containing K–Y gel applied to the skin of the amphibian and then wiped away when a suitable plane of anaesthesia has been reached. Although cooling can reduce the movement of amphibians, it has no analgesic effects and should not be used for anaesthesia.

Whatever anaesthetic techniques and agents are used, anaesthetized animals should be carefully monitored (Figure 21.7); an aquatic amphibian anaesthetized in MS-222 or benzocaine solution should be continually observed to ensure that its nostrils are not submerged. An amphibian, once anaesthetized, can be laid on a damp towel for surgery.

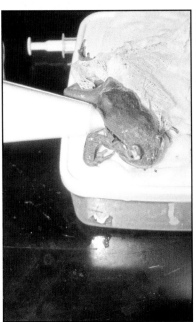

Figure 21.7
Monitoring anaesthesia with a Doppler ultrasound probe. A similar system can be used to determine heart rate in any amphibian. (Courtesy of S. Redrobe.)

Supportive care

Several measures, although not directly therapeutic, can improve an amphibian's chance of recovery. Obviously optimal hygiene and correct temperature, humidity, lighting and diet are essential in a hospital environment, but ill animals have several additional requirements.

Fluid and electrolyte balance

Fluid and electrolyte balance are often disturbed in ill amphibians, and bathing in a hypertonic electrolyte solution to remove excess fluid may be invaluable; Crawshaw (1998) advocated bathing either in a bath with 0.5% salt or in Ringer's solution. Ill terrestrial amphibians tend to lose more water than healthy ones and become dehydrated; water baths and increased humidity reduce this. Bathing in Ringer's solution with an osmolarity of 200 mOsm/l normalises plasma osmolarity.

Temperature

Sick amphibians have higher metabolic rates than healthy ones; increasing the ambient temperature prevents excess heat loss, and encouraging feeding (or stomach tubing if necessary) ensures that sufficient nutrients are present to fuel this increased metabolism. Lower vertebrates often manifest a behavioural pyrexia, moving to an area where the temperature is higher than their preferred norm; such an area should be provided in one part of the vivarium.

Supplemental oxygen

Amphibians in shock have reduced tissue perfusion and thus lower transdermal oxygen uptake. Supplemental oxygen can be given by increasing ambient oxygen levels or by oxygenating the water in the vivarium.

Administration of drugs

Oral route

Given the small size of most amphibians dealt with by veterinary surgeons, the accurate dosing of drugs is important. Good restraint ensures that dosing is precise and causes as little stress as possible to the animal. Giving drugs orally is considered optimal for most agents. The mouth should be opened with a thin piece of plastic such as a pen top or a small plastic drinks' stirrer. A microlitre pipette with a disposable plastic tip is the best way of administering a small volume of drug; volumes as low as 10 µl can be dispensed.

Topical route

The topical route can be used to give drugs to amphibians, given the permeable nature of their skin. Small amounts of drug may be applied directly to the skin, but there is always the chance of irritation from undiluted drugs. This is particularly the case when using intravenous preparations, which often contain benzyl alcohol as a carrier. If the animal shows signs of obvious agitation or excessive mucus production the drug should be removed by copious irrigation with cold chlorine-free water. Ophthalmic ointments are not recommended for topical use as they often contain high concentrations of drug and may cause overdosage. Petroleum-based ointments are occlusive and cause local irritation.

Medicated baths
A medicated bath can be invaluable for giving drugs to sick amphibians, but the amount of drug absorbed is unclear. Such a route is excellent for application of drugs to aquatic organisms such as *Xenopus* or for rehydration. Temperature and pH should be monitored: a pH of between 7.2 and 7.4 is ideal for most cases. Amphibians should be medicated in a small bath in a plastic smooth-sided container. They should be monitored continually while in the bath; a weak amphibian can easily drown.

Injections
Although subcutaneous or intramuscular injections can be used to medicate amphibians, there are several potential problems. Using chlorhexidine gluconate on a bacteriology swab to sterilize the injection site can cause irritation; povidone–iodine should not be used because of its harmful effects even in diluted form. Subcutaneous injections can be difficult because of the lack of abundant skin folds in amphibians.

Intramuscular injections are easier and should probably be given in the forelimb; the venous drainage of the hindlimb may compromise the kidney through the route of the renal portal system, which is present in all amphibians (Holtz, 1999). Recent research, however, suggests that this system has little effect on drug kinetics or toxicity, except with nephrotoxic agents such as gentamicin, which are not recommended anyway. Indeed hindlimb musculature is more pronounced in amphibians, rendering injection into this site easier than in the forelimb. Intravenous injections are possible but difficult. The ventral central abdominal vein may be used but its wall is fragile and liable to extravascular escape of drug.

Intracoelomic injection can be useful for the administration of larger volumes of fluid, especially during rehydration. The animal should be held in dorsal recumbency and the needle directed so as not to puncture any abdominal viscera. The injected fluid should be at or slightly above the animal's own temperature. Drugs can be injected into the dorsal lymph sacs of anurans, providing a rapid method of systemic drug administration; thus intraosseous fluid therapy, although possible, is usually not required.

Pharmacotherapeutics
Pharmacotherapeutic data on amphibians are lacking. Veterinary surgeons are therefore forced to extrapolate from data obtained for fish or reptiles. These values are likely to be significantly different for amphibians especially where drug absorption, distribution and excretion are concerned. Because of this uncertainty, drugs intended for a group of amphibians should

be tried on one or two animals from the group first. These sentinel animals should be monitored for 24 hours. Veterinary surgeons who do medicate large groups of amphibians should be encouraged to publish their results, especially if detailed drug levels are known. This would allow some definitive pharmacokinetic evaluations to be undertaken.

The wide range of amphibian sizes renders metabolic scaling important to define the dose rate for a specific size of amphibian, especially when doses are being extrapolated from much larger reptilian species. Most published dose rates are, however, still given in standard milligrams per kilogram, and so the drugs detailed in Figure 21.8 are given in this manner. Nevertheless, higher dose rates should be given for smaller animals and those with higher preferred body temperatures. For with poikilothermic species such as amphibians, the temperature at which the animal is maintained during treatment has a significant effect on the metabolism and excretion of the drug. This is increasingly being recognized in reptiles, with dose rates given in the context of a specific environmental temperature. This is less so with amphibians, and treated animals should be kept within their optimum temperature.

Common surgical procedures

The variety and complexity of surgical procedures attempted on amphibians is only limited by the surgeon's expertise and enterprise. Biopsies are readily performed and diagnostically rewarding. Exploratory laparotomies can be performed but the central midline ventral abdominal artery must not be perforated.

Foreign bodies
Gastrotomy is regularly performed because several captive amphibians ingest items that cause gastrointestinal blockage. The objects can be removed by endoscopy as the expansive oral cavity of most amphibians facilitates such a procedure, yet the stomach wall is thin and liable to perforation. Gastrointestinal blockage may cause gastric dilation with compromise of lung function, a true emergency. Medical treatment with a laxative can be useful for intestinal foreign bodies but in severe gastric impaction surgery is necessary.

Euthanasia

The preferred method of euthanasia in amphibians is an overdose of barbiturate anaesthetic by intravenous or intracoelomic injection. An alternative is a waterbath with an overdose of anaesthetic such as MS-222 or benzocaine. Although cervical dislocation and pithing by a needle inserted into the foramen magnum is practised in some research laboratories and can be highly effective, it requires considerable practice and is thus not advised where the simpler injectable technique is possible.

Drug formulary

Drug	Treatment	Comments/References
Antibacterials		
Amikacin	5 mg/kg s.c., i.m., i.c. sid	Minimum of seven treatments (Raphael, 1993)
Carbenicillin	200 mg/kg s.c., i.m., i.c. sid	Crawshaw, 1992
Ceftazidine	20 mg/kg i.m. every 48 hours	Walker and Whitaker, 2000
Ciprofloxacin	Bath 5 mg/l for 6–8 hours sid	Minimum of seven treatments; recommended for treatment of large numbers of animals
Enrofloxacin	5–10 mg/kg s.c., i.m., i.c., orally sid	Minimum of seven treatments (Lecher and Papich, 1994)
Gentamicin	2–4 mg/kg i.m. every 72 hours Bath 1.5 mg/l for 1 hour daily	For *A. hydrophila* (Jacobson *et al.*, 1991)
Metronidazole	10 mg/kg orally sid 50 mg/kg orally sid for 3 days for anaerobes 100–150 mg/kg orally every 14 days for amoebic infections	Poynton and Whittaker, 1994 Walker and Whittaker, 2000 Walker and Whittaker, 2000
Trimethoprim/ sulphadiazine	15–20 mg/kg i.m. every 48 hours for 5–7 treatments	
Antifungals		
Amphotericin B	1 mg/kg i.c. sid for 15–30 treatments	Walker and Whittaker, 2000
Fluconazole	60 mg/kg orally sid for seven treatments	Walker and Whittaker, 2000
Itraconazole	2 mg/kg orally sid for 14–28 treatments	Wright and Whitaker, 2000
Ketoconazole	10 mg/kg orally sid 10–20 mg/kg orally sid for 14–28 treatments	Crawshaw, 1992 Wright, 1996
Malachite green	Bath 0.2 mg/l for 1 hour daily	Saprolegniasis (Wright, 1996)
Sodium chloride	Bath 4–6 g/l for 72 hours Bath 10–25 g/l for 5–30 minutes	Crawshaw, 1992 For saprolegniasis (Wright, 1996)
Antiparasitics		
Fenbendazole	100 mg/kg orally every 14 days for two treatments	Nematodiasis
Levamisole	10 mg/kg i.c., i.m. every 14 days for two treatments	Nematodiasis (Raphael, 1993); *Rhabdias* infection (Jacobson *et al.*, 1991)
Ivermectin	0.2 mg/kg orally every 14 days for two treatments or s.c. once	Crawshaw 1993 but note comment in text
Bunamide HCl	50 mg/kg orally every 14 days for two treatments	Cestodiasis (Jacobsen *et al.*, 1991)
Niclosamide	150 mg/kg orally every 14 days for two treatments	Cestodiasis (Jacobsen *et al.*, 1991)

Figure 21.8 Drug formulary for amphibians.

References and further reading

Brooks DE, Jacobson ER, Wolf ED, Clubb S and Gaskin JM (1983) Panophthalmitis and otitis interna in fire-bellied toads. *Journal of the American Veterinary Medical Association* **183,** 1198–1201

Carpenter JL, Bachrach A Jr, Albert DM, Vainisi SJ and Goldstein MA (1986) Xanthomatous keratitis, disseminated xanthomatosis and atherosclerosis in Cuban tree frogs, *Veterinary Pathology* **23,** 337–339

Cowan DF (1968) Diseases of captive reptiles. *Journal of the American Veterinary Medical Association* **153,** 311–312

Crawshaw G (1993) Amphibian medicine. In: *Current Veterinary Therapy XI: Small Animal Practice*, ed. RW Kirk and JD Bonogura, p. 140. WB Saunders, Philadelphia

Crawshaw G (1998) Amphibian emergency and critical care. *Veterinary Clinics of North America: Exotic Animal Practice* **1,** 207

Cunningham AA, Langton TES *et al.* (1995) Investigations into unusual mortalities of the common frog in Britain. *Proceedings, 5th International Colloquium on the Pathology of Reptiles and Amphibians* 19–27

Duellmen WE and Trueb L (1994) *Biology of Amphibians.* Johns Hopkins University Press, Baltimore

Emerson and H. Norris C (1905) 'Red-leg', an infectious disease of frogs. *Journal of Experimental Medicine* **7,** 32–58

Holtz P (1999) The reptilian renal protal system; influence on therapy. In: *Zoo and Wild Animal Medicine, Current Therapy, IV*, ed. M Fowler and E Miller, p. 249. WB Saunders, Philadelphia

Jacobsen E, Kolias G and Peters L (1991) Dosages for antibiotics and parasiticides used in exotic animals. In: *Exotic Animal Medicine in Practice Vol 1*, ed. D Johnston, p. 202. Veterinary Learning Systems, Trenton, New Jersey

Raphael B (1993) Amphibians. *Veterinary Clinics of North America: Small Animal Practice* **23,** 1271–1286

Russell FH (1898) An epidemic septicaemic disease among frogs due to the *Bacillus hydrophilus fuscus. Journal of the American Medical Association* **30,** 1442

Russell WC, Edwards DL, Stair EL and Hubner DC (1990) Corneal lipidosis, disseminated xanthomatosis and hypercholesterolaemia in cuban tree frogs (*Osteopilus septentrionalis*). *Journal of Zoo and Wildlife Medicine* **21,** 99–104

Stebbins RC (1995) Declining amphibians. In: *Amphibians: a Natural History*, ed. RC Stebbins and NW Cohen. Princeton University Press, New Jersey

Walker IDF and Whitaker BR (2000) Amphibian therapeutics. *Veterinary Clinics of North America: Exotic Animal Practice* **3,** 239–255

Wright K (1996) Amphibian medicine. In: *Reptile Medicine and Surgery*, ed. DR Mader. WB Saunders, Philadelphia

Wright KM and Whitaker BR (2000) *Amphibian Medicine and Captive Husbandry.* Krieger Publishing, Malabar

Acknowledgements

Both Dr Andrew Cunningham and Professor John E. Cooper have been instrumental in my interest in amphibians. Figure 21.2a was provided by Dr Cunningham while Figures 21.3 and 21.4 are from the Edward Elkan Memorial Collection of Lower Vertebrate Pathology, courtesy of Professor Cooper who coordinates the collection.

22

Ornamental fish

Bruce Maclean

Introduction

Fish keeping is a popular hobby and there is a huge variety of species (more than 20,000) about which the veterinary surgeon might be consulted. By far the most likely to be seen are koi *Cyprinus carpio* and goldfish *Carassius auratus* (Figure 22.1), possibly in a mixed pond with other coldwater fish such as orfe and tench. This chapter is based largely on dealing with these species, but is generally applicable to all pet ornamental fish. More detailed and specific veterinary information on various species and groups can be found in Stoskopf (1993) and the *BSAVA Manual of Ornamental Fish* and there is a wide variety of books dealing with the specific husbandry requirements of individual species.

It should be noted that in the UK fish are not covered by the Veterinary Surgeons Act, but the Protection of Animals Act and the Medicines Act do apply.

Biology

Figure 22.2 shows the simplified anatomy of a fish. A full discussion of fish biology is not possible here but a few points of clinical relevance must be made:

Skin

- Consists of epidermal cells, scales in most species, covered by a layer of mucus
- Scales are embedded in the dermis and covered by a layer of the epidermis; thus loss of scales will almost always damage the skin, leading to osmotic balance problems in that area (as do burns or ulceration in mammals)
- Mucus is an important protective part of the skin. This layer may be thickened by irritation (e.g. from parasites or chemicals in the water). While this is a defensive reaction, it can protect ectoparasites from water-based antiparasitic treatments.

Gills

- The main gaseous exchange surfaces of fish and a major site of nitrogenous waste excretion and of control of fluid balance
- Usually delicate and protected by gill-covering plates (opercula). Any irritation tends to result in hyperplasia, leading to compromised function and predisposing to necrosis and secondary infection
- Basically consist of series of arches, from which delicate filaments extend
- Targeted by some parasites (e.g. gill flukes).

Internal organs

- Broadly similar to mammals in structure and function, though usually simpler
- No diaphragm present
- Swim-bladder present in some fish; essentially a gas-filled bag, it helps to maintain the fish's buoyancy
- Kidneys are along the spine (above swim-bladder in koi).

Because fish are poikilothermic ('cold-blooded'), they are far more susceptible to changes in their external environment than are mammals. Water temperature will significantly affect their immune status and drug metabolism.

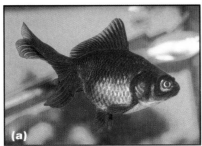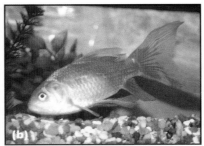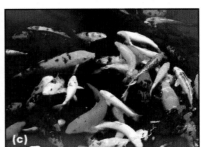

Figure 22.1 Some commonly kept fish: (a) black molly; (b) goldfish; (c) mixed koi. Courtesy of S. Redrobe.

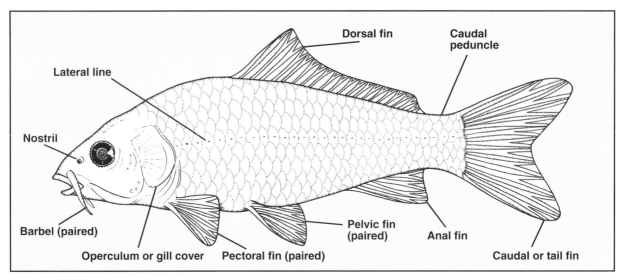

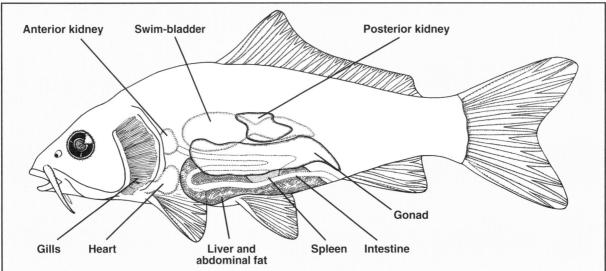

Figure 22.2 External and internal anatomy of a fish. (Reproduced from the *BSAVA Manual of Ornamental Fish, 2nd edition*, edited by William Wildgoose.)

Husbandry

Systems

Ornamental fish are maintained in a wide variety of systems, from individual goldfish in small tanks to large, possibly intensive systems in facilities dealing with hundreds of individuals (Figure 22.3). Systems are concerned with methods for keeping the water in ideal conditions for the fish. The golden rule is that stress to the fish, whether from inappropriate environmental conditions or disturbance, should be minimized.

Features employed in trying to keep water quality optimal include some form of filter, which may have one or all of the following mechanical, biological, chemical or ultraviolet components. The water may be treated before use, by filtration or chemical chelation, and for tropical fish the addition of various salts may be required. Heating may be used (generally in indoor tanks) and there are many readily available heaters and heater/thermostats.

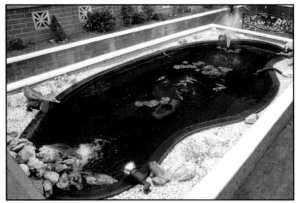

Figure 22.3 A large preformed fibreglass pond suitable for goldfish and small koi. (© W.H. Wildgoose.)

Water quality

An essential facet of fish keeping is maintaining water quality (Figure 22.4). If this is appropriate, even delicate fish should have few health problems. If water

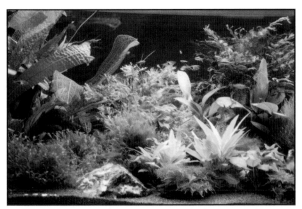

Figure 22.4 Showpiece tropical freshwater aquarium. These are often heavily stocked with a variety of fish species and plants to simulate a natural environment. Regular maintenance and efficient filtration systems are required to ensure good water quality. (© W.H. Wildgoose.)

quality is poor, even robust fish are likely to suffer greatly. The prime aim in water quality maintenance, and the prime reason for all the filters used in aquatic systems, is control of ammonia and nitrite, the main toxic products of the fish's metabolism.

Most fish excrete mainly ammonia, which is broken down largely by bacterial action to nitrites and thence to nitrates, which may be taken up by plants or converted to nitrogen. Further nitrogenous waste may come from uneaten food or other organic contaminants.

- Ammonia is at the most toxic end of the process, with toxicity roughly decreasing through the various stages from nitrite (still toxic) to nitrate (relatively low toxicity)
- Ammonia is most toxic in water of high pH (in which it is less dissociated, NH_3 being more toxic than NH_4^+)
- Actual toxic levels will vary in different water conditions (notably pH), from species to species, and from fish to fish. Test kits generally give guidance in their literature. More detail is given in Butcher (1992) and Wildgoose (in press) but any ammonia level above 1 ppm (part per million, mg/l) indicates pollution. With levels above 2 ppm, fairly urgent water changes or treatments are necessary
- Bacteria (mainly *Nitrosomonas* and *Nitrobacter*) are necessary for this process. Biological filters try to provide a large surface area for the growth of such bacteria. The population of bacteria takes time to build up (sometimes months), which means that rapidly stocking a new pond or tank, or drastically changing the stocking density, can cause major problems before the filter adapts.

Diet

Ornamental fish are generally fed on commercial complete diets, possibly supplemented by live foods (whether deliberately in a tank or naturally in a pond). As a result, dietary deficiencies are uncommon. Commercial diets are usually pellets or flakes.

- Fish should be fed no more than they will eat immediately, twice a day – there should be no uneaten food after a few minutes. This minimizes problems of water pollution, as well as allowing monitoring of whether the fish are feeding
- Live foods may be useful for variety, or even to help relieve constipation, but there are dangers of parasite or disease transmission; for example, deformed or sick cheap feeder fish are potentially a source of fish tuberculosis.

Handling and transport

Stress

For many fish, the stress of being caught can be considerable and can precipitate collapse and death. This should always be considered and discussed with the client. Most fish will not suffer unduly if caught quickly and with minimum fuss, but if they show any signs of distress (such as gasping or loss of balance) it is usually wise to stop all attempts to catch them; they should be allowed to settle down again. Persisting in trying to catch them may prove fatal and it is questionable whether the potential benefits outweigh the risks.

Once caught, most fish settle quickly if not further manipulated. They should be rapidly transferred to an observation container or at least held in the water with the net around them, but not closely so.

Netting

Damage to the fish's protective layers (mucus, skin, scales), fins and appendages must be minimized. For this reason the net mesh should be as fine as possible. Figure 22.5 shows damage to a catfish caused by netting.

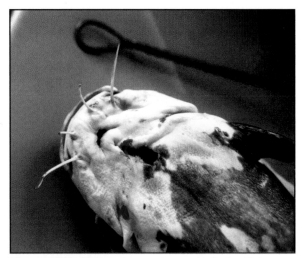

Figure 22.5 Netting damage to a red-tailed catfish (*Phractocephalus hemioliopterus*).

Particular care must be taken with fish that have sensory 'tentacles' (e.g. many catfish and other ornamental species such as arawanas). The risk of damage to these appendages can be high and must be considered when assessing whether the benefits of restraining the fish in this way are worth the potential problems.

Such fish are usually best sedated in their tank or pond. Where catching is to be attempted, it may be advisable to obtain the owner's signed consent that they are willing to accept the risks.

Transport

It is often beneficial to visit the premises, particularly where more than one fish is affected or if the fish is in a garden pond. Time or financial considerations on the owner's part may preclude this and so the practice should be able to give advice on transport of the affected fish to the surgery.

For short distances, the best carrier is a sealed container filled to the brim with water. This will not allow any gas exchange with air, but over short distances this is not usually a problem. The water cannot swish around, which minimizes trauma to the fish. Failing this, the standard carrier is a strong polythene bag, preferably double (from a local aquatics shop), approximately half filled with water and the rest with as much air as possible before the bag is sealed. For long journeys, oxygen rather than air might be advisable. The bag should be well cushioned and placed in a container such as a polystyrene box or bucket in case the bag splits. Ideally, the fish should be starved for 24 hours before a long journey and kept in the dark during transport.

Physical handling

To minimize damage to the fish, wet surgical gloves should be worn or the hands should be thoroughly wet before handling.

The risk of zoonoses does exist, notably fish tuberculosis, which can cause nodular disease in humans. Any open wounds on the hands should be covered and the hands and arms should be washed after handling in standard antibacterial wash such as chlorhexidine or povidone–iodine.

First aid advice

Prior to seeing the fish, certain first aid measures might be advised.

Water change

In any acute-onset condition, it is usually best to recommend that the owner change as much of the water (up to 50%) as feasible. To reduce the shock to the fish, the water being added should conform as closely as possible to the water already occupied by the fish in terms of temperature and composition. This might make water changes impractical, particularly for sensitive tropical species with highly specific requirements, but should be attempted. Aerated tap water up to 50% will generally be tolerated by goldfish and koi if necessary, but tropical or marine species need appropriately treated water.

Water temperature

For coldwater fish in particular, raising the temperature of the fish may help but this should be carried out gradually (e.g. by moving the container to a warmer room or area, or adding a heater – *NOT* by pouring in hotter water). If it involves catching the fish, this may not be worth the stress it will cause.

Diagnostic approach

Clinical history

A large area of concern in the investigation of any fish problem is the environment and husbandry of the fish. Good local aquarium centres may be invaluable in assessing the filter system and in providing equipment if pond drainage or major hospital enclosure is necessary.

It is useful to have a checklist or history sheet such as the example in Figure 22.6. The main relevant features of the form (which can be used for tanks as well as ponds) are considered in Figure 22.7.

Pond environment sheet for	
Species	
Date	
Pond shape/dimension	

Contents

Lining	
Substrate	
Furnishings	
Live plants	
Occupants	

Water

Volume	
Source	
Pretreatment(s)	
Changes	
Quality monitoring	
Routine treatment(s)	

Filtration

Type	
Duration of operation	
Cleaning/treatments	

Heating & Lighting

Supply source	Hours of use

Photoperiod	
Temperature (day)	
Temperature (night)	

Feeding

Foodstuff(s)	
Frequency & amount	
Supplements used	

Cleaning and disinfection

Frequency	
Disinfectant(s)	

Figure 22.6 Example of a pond environment sheet.

Pond lining	Unlikely to be a source of problems in itself, but improperly treated concrete could be leaching toxins into the water (in a fresh pond), or a leaking butyl liner may allow leaching of contaminants from the soil. Has the level been dropping unexpectedly?
Substrate	A thick layer of decaying material is conducive to bacterial growth and pollution. Less likely to be a problem in tanks, but improperly sourced gravel or sand may leach toxins. Disturbance (if the tank or pond has recently been cleaned) may release high concentration of toxins
Furnishings	Check for any sharp projections, also for metal objects that might be spreading heavy metals into the water
Plants	A well planted pond or tank may have problems with low oxygen levels in early morning
Occupants	Are all the species compatible with each other? Are shoaling fish in sufficient numbers to avoid stress? Are sex mixes appropriate (many male fish can be aggressively territorial)?
Water	Quality and pretreatments are discussed elsewhere
Filter types	It is helpful to have some knowledge of different filter types and the role of various sections in them. Water quality will generally indicate whether the filter is efficient
Heating and lighting	Should be appropriate for the species
Season and weather	For outside ponds, season and weather or temperature may be important. The immune response of fish is very dependent on temperature.

Figure 22.7 Summary of environmental factors of import to a clinical history.

The normal principles of history taking apply. Subjects should include any management changes, new fish additions and the pattern of the problem; for example, a sudden-onset 100% morbidity is more likely to be caused by toxins than by infection. Any previous owner-administered treatments (of which there may be many, especially amongst koi keepers) should be taken into account. This is especially important if they have mixed their own treatments from base chemicals: it only takes a small calculation error, or an out-of-date chemical, for there to be highly toxic levels of commonly used chemicals in the water.

Water quality testing

The main water parameters for diagnostic consideration are the nitrogenous waste products (ammonia, nitrite and nitrate); simple test kits are readily available. Most kits rely on subjective assessment of colour changes but are generally accurate enough for clinical work. Sample validity is important. Water in a restricted space, such as a transport bag, will be rapidly polluted by the fish (to the level of death within a few hours in the case of well fed fish in a small bag) and should not be sampled. If an owner has just changed some of the pond or tank water, a sample taken at that point may be misleadingly normal.

The relative parameters give a rough guide to timescales: where ammonia is high and nitrite relatively low, a recent problem is likely (1–2 weeks); moderate levels of both suggest a timescale of 2–3 weeks; and low ammonia/high nitrite indicates a longer timescale.

Multitest kits often include water acidity (pH) with the nitrogenous waste parameters. The pH value can be vital for tropical fish but is unlikely to be a problem for coldwater fish such as koi and goldfish.

Oxygen is another useful parameter. Oxygen levels should be tested when they are lowest, i.e. just before the sun comes up or the lights go on for planted tanks or ponds (because during the night the plants, as well as the fish, use up oxygen).

Other parameters may be important, particularly water hardness, and salinity and copper levels (in marine systems). Many specific toxins can be tested for (consult the laboratory) but, without a specific idea, a general search for possible water toxins could test for many and still not pick up the one that is causing the problem.

Observation

Fish should be observed initially with as little manipulation as possible (another reason why home visits are preferable for collections):

- Some parasites, such as anchor worms or fish lice in coldwater fish, or intestinal worms protruding from the cloaca in tropical fish, may be apparent on visual examination
- External lesions and changes should be noted but it is necessary to know what is normal (some tropical species have remarkable normal adornments)
- Behaviour should be noted:
  - Any flashing/flicking (darting around, intermittently exposing the generally paler underside) or rubbing (on substrate or any hand objects)
  - Whether a fish is swimming separately from the main group (in sociable fish)
  - Whether a fish is able to swim normally and maintain balance and water position
  - Whether fish are concentrating around areas of maximum oxygenation (usually where the water surface is disturbed).

Physical examination

Physical examination is somewhat more limited than in mammals in terms of the information it can provide. It may be useful but the potential benefits must be weighed against the risks of stress associated with handling.

If the fish is already confined in a restricted space, gentle patience should allow a reasonable physical examination. External lesions or internal swellings can be palpated and further assessed. Scrapings, needle biopsies and centesis can be carried out. Small fish may be simply viewed from all angles in a clear container.

Laboratory investigations

'Skin scrapes'

'Skin scrapes' are recommended from all fish patients. Skin parasites may or may not be a differential for the problem under consideration, but the parasite load can give an indication of the fish's general condition. These 'skin scrapes' are actually mucus scrapes. The mucus is scraped gently off the fish and assessed under the microscope immediately, as many parasites soon become distorted and unrecognizable. Anything bigger than a bacterium and that moves in a purposeful manner when viewed at ×100 magnification is of interest. Figure 22.8 shows the 'fish louse' Argulus.

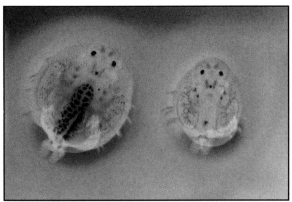

Figure 22.8 The crustacean parasite Argulus is commonly called the fish louse. Adults can measure up to 7 mm in length: the parasite on the right is a juvenile, which has less distinct body markings. (© W.H. Wildgoose.)

Gill scrapes

Gill scrapes are recommended in most cases. The fish should usually be anaesthetized or sedated. As with 'skin scrapes', mucus is gently scraped off the gills and immediately examined under the microscope.

Microbiological investigations

It is difficult to obtain a valid microbiological sample from a live fish, since the water is likely to be full of various bacteria that are potentially pathogenic. The situation should be discussed with the laboratory (which should be experienced in dealing with fish samples). At the very least a sample is needed from deep within a lesion, with centesis of material or swabbing from a deep ulcer only after significant scraping of material from the surface. It is also advisable to submit smears, to check for acid-fast organisms.

Postmortem examination

Fish tend to autolyse very quickly after death and thus need to be examined as soon as possible; more than a few hours will almost certainly mean that very little pathological information can be gleaned from internal examination. For this reason, it is often necessary for the veterinary surgeon to carry out an initial postmortem examination and collect samples. The laboratory should be consulted for advice on sampling but the general steps are as follows.

- Take an early kidney swab if microbiological testing is required
- Obtain samples from at least liver, kidney, heart and intestines (plus brain if feasible and if CNS signs were present) in formalin or formal/saline for histopathology
- Possibly keep tissues or the carcass frozen for further analysis.

Other investigation techniques

Investigations such as radiography (Figure 22.9), ultrasound, endoscopy, blood sampling (Figure 22.10), MRI and CT scanning may be useful in appropriate circumstances. Some ingenuity may be required in obtaining the images, and the problem of lack of normal values can make results difficult to interpret.

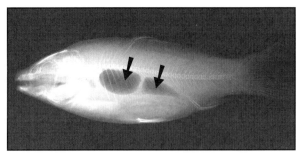

Figure 22.9 A lateral radiograph of a normal koi. Radiography of fish can provide information about lesions affecting the bony skeleton and swim-bladder (arrowed). This species has a bilobed swim-bladder. (© W.H. Wildgoose.)

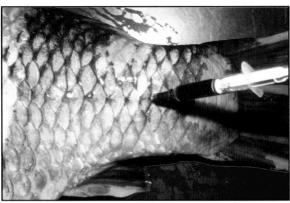

Figure 22.10 Taking a blood sample from the caudal vein of a koi. A long needle is inserted just below the lateral line and enters the vein, which is found immediately beneath the vertebral bodies. This route can also be used to administer drugs intravenously. (© W.H. Wildgoose.)

Common conditions

Common presenting signs and differentials are summarized in Figure 22.11, along with comments on approach, investigation and treatment where appropriate. The majority of fish health problems can be traced to underlying stress, so in any group problem water quality or toxins should always be considered.

Presenting sign	Causes	Comments
Mortality		
Individual		Thorough general approach necessary
Multiple, peracute (24–48 h)	Water quality/toxins – especially if high mortality/morbidity	History important in defining possible toxins
	Other	Infection possible, especially if recent introductions. General approach
Multiple, acute or chronic (days–months)	Toxins	History important. An underlying water quality/toxin problem, or other stress, is likely, even if infection or parasitic infestations are present
	Infection	May be present but usually requires an underlying problem
	Parasites	Few ectoparasites cause mortalities – gill flukes are the major ones. Some internal parasites can cause mortalities
	Other	General approach
Behavioural changes		
Gasping at surface; crowding at water inlets	Gill problems (see text)	
	Low oxygen	Worse in early morning. Worse in big fish. Associated with heavily planted ponds or some toxins (e.g. formaldehyde)
	Anaemia	Similar investigation to more familiar small animals, in theory
Flashing underside, rubbing on handy projections	Ectoparasites	Skin scrapes
	Water-borne irritant	
Lethargy, inappetence, separating from group	Almost any illness	General approach
Abnormal posture or swimming angle	Terminal	Very ill fish may swim abnormally (usually on their sides or belly up)
	Central nervous disease	Possible differentials as for more familiar animals; protozoal infection a major possibility. In the absence of diagnostics, try corticosteroids, potentiated sulphonamides, thiamine
	Swimbladder problem	Direct (e.g. infection/inflammation) or indirect through pressure on the swimbladder (e.g. from intracoelomic mass). Radiography and other investigations; therapeutic trials (anti-inflammatories, antibiotics)
	Toxins	Various; note particularly organophosphates
Skin/surface changes		
Excess mucus (essentially skin irritation)	Water irritants	Try to find cause
	Ectoparasites	Skin scrapes
Loss/change of colour	Debility	General approach
	Diet	For brightly coloured fish, 'colour feeding' (i.e. provision of pigments or precursors in the diet) may be necessary
	Excess mucus	See above
Lumps	Viruses (?)	'Candle wax' lesions – carp pox or lymphocystis (which will generally spontaneously regress but recur). Not a problem unless at a vital site, in which case surgery may be required
	Parasitic cysts	Any size – may be myxosporidians, trematodes or nematodes
	Ichthyophthirius ('Ich')	Pinhead white spots
	True tumours	Surgical removal if causing a problem
Visible parasites	*Argulus* (fish louse) (approx 5 mm diameter, oval, translucent with visible internal organs; see Figure 22.8)	Difficult to treat. Organophosphates reportedly effective. Draining and drying out the pond, plus manual removal, will eliminate
	Lernaea (anchor worms) (1–3 cm long, red, thin, attached to any part of body)	as *Argulus*
	Leeches (dark brown, usually 1–5 cm long, attached to any part of body)	To a certain extent natural, but large numbers can cause problems. Treatment as *Argulus*
	Intestinal nematodes, e.g. *Camallanus* (red, thread-like, protruding from vent)	Mainly in tropical fish. Treatment is levamisole in water
Haemorrhage/ulcer	Bacterial infection	Usually also underlying cause (see text)
	Protozoal infection	Particularly in tropical fish, e.g. *Hexamita* 'hole in the head' disease. Treat with antiprotozoal such as metronidazole
'Cotton-wool' growth	Fungi	Almost certainly secondary – dig for an underlying problem. Also beware confusion with stringy mucus. Treat with proprietary antifungal
Fin changes		
Ragged/damage	Trauma	Treatment involves supportive care and prevention of infection
	Ectoparasites	Skin scrapes
	Bacterial infection	See ulcers
Haemorrhages	As skin haemorrhage	

Figure 22.11 Common presenting signs and major differentials. (continues) ▶

Presenting sign	Causes	Comments
Eye changes		
Corneal opacity	Trauma	Check for possible cause. Treat to prevent infection
	Infection	Diagnosis difficult; therapeutic trial or surgery options if suspected
	Water quality problem	Testing and correcting are necessary
	Nutritional	Unlikely if complete diet; possibly add vitamins to food
	Parasitic flukes	Little specific treatment; cleaning out pond/tank may reduce intermediate stages
Exophthalmos	Oedema	See 'Dropsy' in text
	Orbital infection	Bacterial (bear in mind mycobacterial), fungal or parasitic. Biopsy and/or surgery might be indicated
	Orbital tumour	Biopsy and/or surgery indicated
General		
Coelomic swelling ('dropsy')	Coelomic fluid	See 'Dropsy' in text
	Constipation	Especially in goldfish or others fed purely flaked food. Try live foods or oral liquid paraffin
	Internal mass	Tumour/granuloma/abscess
	Egg binding	Difficult to treat and diagnose. Try raised temperature
Anorexia	Unable to eat	Check mouth for lesions, etc . May be overgrown beak (common in puffer fish)
	Uninterested in food	Thorough general approach

Figure 22.11 continued Common presenting signs and major differentials.

Gill problems

Gills are relatively delicate structures and are vital to the fish's health. Any problems in the gills are likely to have severe detrimental effects on health. Three major problems commonly affect gills: waterborne toxins and irritants; parasites; and infection (Figure 22.12).

- Gill flukes (*Dactylogyrus* spp.) are one of the parasites most likely to cause significant health problems in pond fish. They are also one of the more difficult ectoparasites to treat successfully. Diagnosis is on fresh gill scrapes; standard proprietary treatments can be tried but often more powerful treatment (praziquantel bath) is necessary
- Bacterial infection (typically *Cytophaga* spp.; many other bacteria can infect damaged gills) may cause problems but the bacteria are usually secondary. Besides antibacterial treatment, any underlying cause of gill damage should be thoroughly investigated.

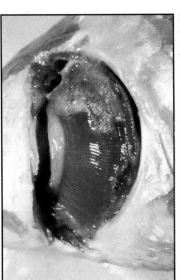

Figure 22.12 The gill of this koi shows a large area of necrosis which is infected with *Saprolegnia* and has a green appearance due to algae trapped in the fungal hyphae. (© W.H. Wildgoose.)

Ulcers

Ulcers (Figure 22.13) may be secondary to septicaemia or to wounds (damage from parasites or physical trauma) that become infected. While ulcers may not initially be a bacterial problem, they will become one, and appropriate antibacterial medication is necessary – at the very least to limit the rise in bacterial challenge in the water. The underlying cause must also be remedied if possible.

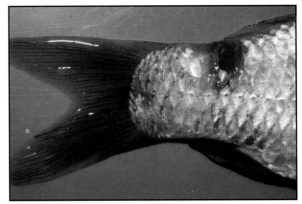

Figure 22.13 Koi ulcer. Ulcerations on koi and other coldwater fish are common and often caused by bacterial infections with *Aeromonas* or *Pseudomonas*. (© W.H. Wildgoose.)

Ulcers are often the main manifestation of an outbreak of pathogenic bacteria (septicaemia outbreak) in a group, with other signs such as dropsy and exophthalmos occurring in a proportion of fish. Possible underlying causes include water quality problems (nitrogenous wastes or other pollutants), physical trauma (e.g. a rough/sharp projection, attack from a heron or other predator), parasites, and any other factor that depresses the fish's immune status – including, significantly, spring viraemia of carp, a notifiable viral disease that should always be considered when an outbreak follows the introduction of new fish.

In investigation of an ulcer, microbiological analysis is always advisable if feasible. Treatment of an ulcer problem should involve use of a proprietary antibacterial preparation in the water to limit spread of the bacteria. For affected fish, appropriate antibiotics should be administered and the ulcers debrided if feasible.

'Dropsy'

Fish keepers, relying on various books, often present 'dropsy' as a diagnosis. It is not a diagnosis; it is only a sign – theoretically coelomic fluid accumulation, though often loosely applied to any coelomic swelling. All it means is that there is coelomic fluid, with a range of differentials as wide as ascites in more familiar species, e.g. liver, kidney, circulatory or gastrointestinal problems, tumours or infection. In theory, similar principles of investigation apply, possibly involving radiography, blood sampling, coelomic centesis, ultrasound, endoscopy, exploratory surgery, MRI and CT scanning. Figure 22.14 shows a goldfish with 'dropsy'.

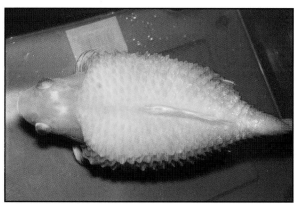

Figure 22.14 Dropsy. This goldfish was severely affected and exhibited raised scales, a swollen body and a moderate amount of exophthalmos. Histopathology confirmed renal disease as the underlying cause. (© W.H. Wildgoose.)

A practical approach for an individual fish depends on the owner's wishes and the species of fish involved. As a simple initial step, coelomic centesis can usually be carried out with relative ease and the fluid assessed for possible microbial agents and microscopy.

In practice, it is often a case of giving therapeutic trials and observing response. A standard therapeutic trial in koi or goldfish might consist of anti-inflammatories, anabolic steroids, B vitamins and antibiotics, which covers most of the possible medical causes. Diuretics may also be used, but only in selected cases as they require twice-daily injections.

Dropsy may occur in a certain proportion of fish in a septicaemia outbreak (see ulcers).

One important differential is constipation. If this is suspected (typically in tank goldfish fed nothing but flake food), offering live foods such as *Daphnia* or bloodworms, or even oral dosing with liquid paraffin, may help to relieve it.

Supportive care

Hospitalization

Hospitalization is rarely recommended (other than possibly for surgery) and for many tropical species it may not be realistically possible to set up a short-term tank that provides suitable conditions. For sensitive tropical species, owners should be asked to supply the water required, as they will be able to provide the conditions to which the fish is accustomed.

To set up a hospital tank for koi and goldfish, the requirements are for a suitably sized container, a water conditioner and preferably an air pump and air stone. Filters are not feasible for short-term hospitalization (because biological filters take weeks to establish efficacy) and so relatively frequent water changes will be required. As a rough guide, well fed fish will require about 20% of the water changed daily but this should be checked with daily ammonia and nitrite readings.

Drug administration

The relative benefits of each route are set out in Figure 22.15.

Route	Benefits	Drawbacks
Injection	Most reliable method of getting the desired dose into the fish	Stressful (the stress may be more detrimental than the injection is beneficial)
Oral	Minimal stress to fish. May be the only feasible method for some drugs in some systems (e.g. big pond, or multiple fish affected)	Unreliable dosage, depending on appetite and mixing of food/drug. Useless if fish not eating
Water treatment	Standard method for proprietary medicines. Generally useful for external parasites and infection; much less so for internal problems. May be only feasible method	Efficacy dependent on prevailing water conditions. May affect biological filters (or be affected by them). For bath treatments (i.e. short-term), will involve stress of catching fish

Figure 22.15 Routes for medication: comparative benefits and drawbacks.

Injection

- The needle should be inserted between scales and not through them
- Fish skin is inelastic. Finger pressure should be applied on withdrawing the needle, both to limit immediate leakage and to prevent scales being pulled off by the needle
- Preferred site is intramuscular into the fillets cranial to the dorsal fin (Figure 22.16). Relatively safe; usually easiest site in conscious fish; seems to work well clinically
- Another possible site is into the tail muscles, caudal to vent. Safe, but the greater muscle movement in this area will probably cause greater leakage or expulsion of the drug.

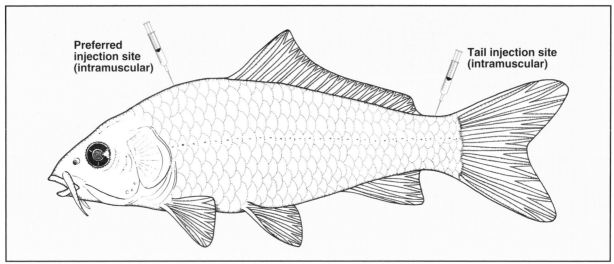

Figure 22.16 Injection sites.

- Intracoelomic injection is possible but not generally recommended. Has the potential to cause internal damage – especially in koi and goldfish, which have tightly packed organs filling their coelomic cavity.

Oral

1. Mix the calculated dose of drug thoroughly with an appropriate amount of (powdered) food.
2. Solidify with gelatin in a refrigerator.
3. Break off cubes of appropriate size and feed to the fish.

This method is susceptible to large losses into the water and so the food should be fed in such a way as to minimize the time in the water before it is eaten: little and often, added in small amounts to the water rather than in big handfuls.

Water treatments

These may be by bath (timed, generally minutes to hours, in a relatively concentrated solution of drug) or by tank/pond treatment.

Water treatments can be affected by various other water quality parameters, particularly pH and hardness. In practice, there is insufficient information to allow for these realistically in most cases. The set-up should be as clear of organic material as possible. This is particularly important for antibiotic treatments, most of which are neutralized to a greater or lesser extent by organic material in the water.

Where feasible it may be preferable to treat a small proportion of a fish collection first (especially in the case of bath treatments), warning the owner of the possibility of problems. When water baths are carried out, a container of fresh clean water should be available into which the fish can be transferred if they show signs of distress.

Units for water treatments are:

- ppm (part per million) = 1 mg/l (or 1 ml/l)
- 1 in 1000 = 1 g/l.

Advice to the client with regard to the use of proprietary aquarium and pond treatments (see later) includes the following:

- Mix well. For example, mix the dose in some pond water in a watering can and distribute it over the surface, or add the dose into water flow from an inlet pipe or fountain for rapid distribution
- Switch off any ultraviolet sterilizer.

General supportive treatments

Salt (sodium chloride)

Pure sodium chloride is useful in two quite common situations: as a supportive treatment in ulcer cases; and as an astringent to strip off mucus that might be compromising gill function.

- Maintaining a water concentration of 0.6% (6 g/l) NaCl will help fish with ulcers immensely by acting as osmotic support (reducing the osmotic gradient between the fish and the surrounding water)
- Use as an astringent involves a short-term bath treatment and must be considered in the context of stress to the fish.

It is important to use as pure a sodium chloride as possible. Table salt should be avoided (cooking salt is generally acceptable). Care must be taken that the owner does not use one of the 'healthy' salts that are primarily potassium chloride.

Benzalkonium chloride

Benzalkonium chloride is useful as an astringent, with the added benefit of being antiseptic. A bath in this can reduce mucus on the fish and can increase efficacy of subsequent water treatments, notably antiparasitic treatments.

Anaesthesia

Due to the potential effects of stress, anaesthesia is sometimes advisable for examinations and simple clinical procedures such as injections.

For short-term anaesthesia, the agents may be added to the water. Methane tricainesulphonate (MS 222) is the licensed and recommended drug. Depending on depth of anaesthesia, the fish will remain anaesthetized for several minutes out of the water for short surgical procedures (up to 5 minutes). Anoxia is unlikely to be a problem for this period. Longer-term anaesthesia is possible with various circulation systems but is beyond the scope of this chapter.

Before anaesthesia is carried out, the following should be assembled:

- Water (of known volume) in which to anaesthetize the fish
- A recovery container of fresh water (same temperature and source as the anaesthetic water)
- A wet towel or similar on which to place the fish
- All instruments required for the procedure (to minimize the time taken).

The fish is placed in a container of known volume. The calculated amount of drug is weighed or measured out and then added gradually to the water, with mixing, until the desired level of anaesthesia is obtained.

Stages of anaesthesia will vary but essentially there is a gradual loss of balance and reaction to stimuli, which the fish will initially be able to override if roused but which will become more profound. The operculum (gill cover) movements will slow. When the fish is unable to react to stimuli with any attempt to move or right itself but is still alive, surgical anaesthesia has been achieved.

Recovery (in clean water) may be aided by gently moving the fish forward through the water to encourage flow over its gills. It should not be moved backwards, as this may damage the gills.

Common surgical procedures

A major problem in fish is that suturing is impossible or impractical in most cases. Most wounds, whether surgical or traumatic, are treated open (basically as ulcers, below).

While the fish is out of water, it should be kept wet (laid on a wet towel and further moistened as necessary) and if possible the head should be covered with a wet towel. Surgical time needs to be minimized.

Ulcers

In individual fish, ulcers should be debrided (under anaesthesia). Microbiological samples such as swabs and smears may be taken at this time. Following debridement, the ulcer should be treated with antiseptic, possibly packed with a protective agent such as dental paste. Further care involves antibiotics and

supportive treatments. Povidone–iodine is the best general choice of antiseptic. If there is doubt over the effectiveness of any surgical debridement, a more caustic agent such as potassium permanganate may be appropriate.

Removal of external lumps

Where necessary, lumps may be excised level with the skin (Figure 22.17) and the remaining skin surface cauterized with potassium permanganate or treated with milder antiseptics. A mouth ulcer treatment paste may be applied to seal the wound.

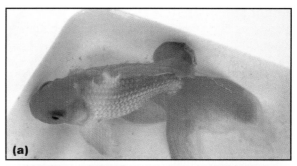

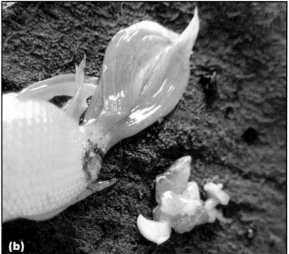

Figure 22.17 (a) Goldfish with a large mass on the caudal flank. (b) Mass excised.

Euthanasia

If the fish can be brought into the surgery, an overdose of anaesthetic (either MS222 or intracoelomic pentobarbitone) can be used. After deep anaesthesia is achieved, it should be followed by freezing or pithing to ensure death.

Where transport to the surgery would involve severe stress to an already ill fish, physically striking the fish hard on the head is effective and humane if carried out properly, though many people will find this difficult to perform or to permit. In another procedure described as effective and humane and widely known in the fish trade, clove oil is gently heated to allow dispersion and is then added to the water until the fish is unresponsive (again preferably followed by freezing). Failing this, every effort should be made to euthanase the fish humanely by overdose of anaesthetic, as above.

Therapeutics

Proprietary remedies

The components of proprietary aquarium and pond treatments are discussed only briefly here; various authors give more details (especially Bishop, 2001), including the use of base chemicals. It is not generally advisable to make up treatments from base chemicals, nor to recommend this to clients, as the chemicals involved are generally quite toxic to humans. Commercial preparations are much safer and less susceptible to miscalculations of dosage.

Antibacterial treatments

Many proprietary remedies for fish claim to treat bacteria or ulcers. As a general rule, they may help to treat external bacterial infections and are useful in reducing the water load of any potentially pathogenic bacteria (and so are advisable as supportive treatment when there is a bacterial problem in the fish) but they are generally ineffective in treating any internal infections. Proprietary antibacterial treatments may contain several chemicals, including acriflavine, proflavine, malachite green and formalin.

Antifungal treatments

Most superficial fungal infections can be readily dealt with by proprietary remedies, possibly in combination with physical debridement of lesions, but internal fungal infections are unlikely to be diagnosed under normal circumstances. Malachite green is a major component of antifungal preparations.

Antiparasitic treatments

Many parasitic problems can be satisfactorily dealt with by proprietary remedies, which are usually based on some combination of formaldehyde and malachite green. Certain external metazoan parasites (particularly gill flukes) and many sporozoan parasites may require prescription drugs.

With many skin parasites, the thick reactive mucus produced by the fish may in fact protect the parasite from water medications to some extent. Preceding any antiparasitic treatments by bathing in benzalkonium chloride may be useful, though as always the stress to the fish must be considered.

Proprietary remedies for parasites may contain the following chemicals:

- Chloramine-T – moderately effective against some protozoans
- Formaldehyde – widely effective against ectoparasites; often used in combination with malachite green
- Malachite green/formaldehyde – broad-spectrum mixture (known sometimes as Leteux–Meyer mixture) against parasites and also fungi and bacteria
- Methylene blue – effective antiprotozoal and moderately strongly antibacterial but tends to knock out bacterial filters, so rarely recommended. Recommended dose is 1–2 mg/l in the main water. May also be used as emergency treatment for nitrite toxicity at this dose but movement to fresh water is a much safer option unless the situation is very bad.

Drug formulary

This drug formulary is far from exhaustive; it includes only those drugs used commonly in small animal practice. Very few, if any, of the drugs mentioned are backed by pharmacokinetic data.

Drug	Route	Dosage	Comments
Anaesthetics			
MS 222	Water	1 g/10 l for anaesthesia; 1 g per 20 or 30 l may be used for sedation	Build up gradually to this level
Benzocaine	Water	25–50 mg/l	Use stock solution 40 g in 1 litre acetone (in dark bottle for max 3 months) at 5.5–11 ml per 9 litres of water
Antibacterials			
Trimethoprim–sulphadiazine	Injection i.m. (intramuscular)	30 mg/kg i.m. every 48 hours (dosage is combined substance)	Resistance is not uncommon
	In food	6 g per kg of food	
	In water	240 mg per 50 l	Must be in set-up free of organic matter
Enroflaxacin	Injection i.m.	15 mg/kg i.m. every 48 hours	
	In food	1 g per kg of food	
Gentamicin	Injection i.m.	3 mg/kg every 48 hours	Assumed to be as relatively toxic as in higher vertebrates, so generally not first choice
Oxytetracycline	Injection i.m.	10 mg/kg i.m. sid	Resistance very common
	In food	10 g per kg of food	
Ampicillin	Injection i.m.	10 mg/kg i.m. sid	
Antifungals			
Ketoconazole	Injection i.m.	5 mg/kg i.m. sid	

Figure 22.18 Drug formulary for ornamental fish. (continues) ▶

Drug	Route	Dosage	Comments
Antiparasitics			
Praziquantel	Water; a 3 hour bath	10 mg/l for 3 hours; repeat in 2–3 weeks	Very useful for gill flukes, which might be resistant to other treatments
	In food	4 g/kg of food for 1 week	This will probably be very expensive
Levamisole	Water – treat tank	Treat water tank: 10 mg/l	For tropical fish with nematodes
Metronidazole	Water – treat tank	Treat water tank: 7–15 mg/l	For protozoal parasites, especially *Hexamita*
Dichlorvos (NOT generally recommended)	Water	0.2 mg/l in permanent bath	Health and safety problems for person administering and for patient. May be only effective treatment for certain parasites, but rarely recommended!
Miscellaneous			
Salt (sodium chloride)	Water permanent bath	6 g /l as permanent bath	Build up over several days in steps of 1.5 g/l per day
	Water bath	10 g/l for up to 10 minutes	Observe for signs of distress, especially in smaller fish
Benzalkonium chloride	Water bath	5 mg/l for 30 minutes	Toxicity is increased in soft water
	Water	1 mg/l as permanent bath	Only when the only treatment, as it persists in the water and cannot be directly followed by other water treatments
Dexamethasone (short-acting)	Injection i.m.	5 mg/kg i.m. once	Anti-shock dose; may help to counter the stress of initial handling
	Injection i.m.	0.25 mg/kg i.m.	Anti-inflammatory dose; possible part of treatment regime for undiagnosed CNS disease or intracoelomic fluid
Flunixin meglumine	Injection i.m.	0.3 mg/kg i.m.	
Frusemide	Injection i.m.	3 mg/kg i.m. bid	As part of the treatment regime for intracoelomic fluid
Vitamin B complex	Injection i.m.	0.1 ml/kg i.m. once	As part of treatment for coelomic fluid of unknown cause
Thiamine	Injection i.m.	25 mg/kg i.m. once	As part of treatment for CNS disease of unknown cause
Nandrolin	Injection i.m.	2.5 mg/kg i.m. once (possible every 10–14 days)	As part of treatment for coelomic fluid of unknown cause

Figure 22.18 continued Drug formulary for ornamental fish.

In theory, the dose should be varied depending on species of fish, age, reproductive status, husbandry system and water temperature, but this information is not available. Water temperature is a particular concern but in practice the only advice that can be given is to be wary of using any (particularly injectable) drugs below 14°C: the possibility of side effects is vastly increased with the slowing of the fish's metabolism of the drugs. Moving the fish to a warmer situation may be part of the treatment regimen in any case but the metabolism will take some time (probably days) to adapt fully.

Resistance to antibiotics is not uncommon in fish pathogens. Many antibiotics, especially oxolinic acid and tetracyclines, have been readily available to fish keepers and grossly overused, leading to widespread resistance problems. These drugs are therefore poor choices for first-line treatment, unless sensitivity is indicated by bacteriological tests.

Imported fish (especially koi) may have had courses or single treatments of more modern antibiotics, such as enrofloxacin or gentamicin. Bacteriological testing is strongly recommended, especially for group problems. It should be stressed that this section refers to pet fish; different legal considerations may be applicable in dosing any fish destined for human consumption.

References and further reading

Andrews C, Exell A and Carrington N (1988) *Interpret Manual of Fish Health*. Salamander Books, London *(useful basic book, especially for the large number of photographs)*

Bishop Y (2001) *Veterinary Formulary*, 5th edn. Pharmaceutical Press, London

Butcher RL (1992) *Manual of Ornamental Fish*. BSAVA Publications, Cheltenham

Dawes JA (1986) *The Tropical Freshwater Aquarium*. Hamlyn, London

Mills D (1986) *You and Your Aquarium*. Dorling Kindersley, London

Stoskopf MK (1993) *Fish Medicine*. WB Saunders, Philadelphia *(excellent reference text covering all fish species)*

Wildgoose W (2001) *Manual of Ornamental Fish*, 2nd edn. BSAVA Publications, Gloucester

Useful sources

There are many fish resources on the Internet, including newsgroups and mailing lists. The sites below are a few of those available on fish health and disease, and all have many links to other relevant sites. It should be remembered that many items published on the Internet have not been refereed.

http://www.netvet.wustl.edu/fish.htm
Massive list of links to a wide variety of aquaculture resources on the internet – a good place to start

http://www.geocities.com/CapeCanaveral/Lab/7490/index
Large list of aquaculture health references

http://www.aqualink.com/disease/sdisease.html
Useful summary of some common diseases

23

Invertebrates

David L. Williams

Introduction

The very first organism definitively linked to disease was the fungus *Beauvaria bassiana* affecting silkworms in 1835. Louis Pasteur's first disease investigation concerned disease in the same insect in 1870, preceding his and others' scientific study of disease in vertebrates. For many years invertebrate medicine was overshadowed by veterinary work in vertebrates but now the investigation and control of invertebrate disease is again coming to the fore. The introduction of a veterinary licensed product for the treatment of varoosis in bees and the growing numbers of members in the Veterinary Invertebrate Society show that invertebrates are indeed becoming more important.

Invertebrate diversity

Many species of invertebrate are kept in captivity (Figure 23.1) but these are a minute proportion of the total invertebrates, which comprise well over 90% of all living species and the great majority of the biomass on Earth. In addition to the relatively few species kept as pets, invertebrates may be kept: for laboratory research, e.g. *Octopus vulgaris*; commercial production, e.g. bees and silkworms; or for conservation purposes, e.g. the field cricket *Gryllus campestris*.

Husbandry

Housing

As with the vast majority of exotic species, incorrect husbandry and dietary provision is at the heart of much invertebrate disease. There are some general considerations for housing invertebrates:

- The accommodation should be sufficiently spacious to allow the animal full movement, including that required when moulting
- The environment should provide the optimal temperature, light and humidity ranges and, in doing this, should in most cases mirror the natural habitat of the invertebrate
- Housing should be readily cleaned and disinfected
- The accommodation should be arranged such that no damage can occur to the invertebrate through burning close to heat sources, drowning in water provided for vegetation, or congregating too close to ultraviolet light sources.

Temperature and humidity

Invertebrates are ectothermic, and thus a correct ambient temperature is essential for maintaining healthy populations. It is important to ensure that the heating element, where provided, cannot cause damage.

Invertebrates have varying requirements for humidity: molluscs such as snails and slugs require a damp environment whereas arthropods, with their tough exoskeletons, can survive in drier environments. Where a damp environment is necessary, hygiene can be difficult to maintain and there is then the possibility of a significant build-up of Gram-negative organisms. In the wild, the area inhabited and the water turnover mitigate against such a bacteriological build-up. Cage hygiene is important but there should not be a toxic build-up of detergent cleaning agents. Decreased humidity can result in moulting problems in arthropods.

Size

A cause of dysecdysis in some arthropods such as phasmids and mantids is inappropriately small cages;

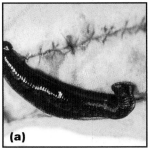
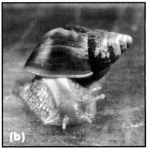
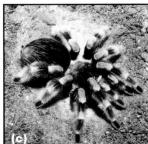
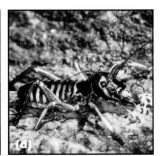

Figure 23.1 Examples of invertebrates kept in captivity: (a) medicinal leech *Hirudo medicinalis,* used in medical treatment; (b) Giant African land snail *Achatina fulica;* (c) Mexican red-kneed tarantula *Euathlus smithi;* (d) Weta cricket.

these long insects require a vivarium height at least twice their length to allow successful moulting.

Diet

Nutritional requirements are similarly highly varied: molluscs need a high calcium intake; silkworms require a high protein intake for silk production; spiders are obligate carnivores, requiring live prey (Cooper *et al.,* 1991); stick insects feed on certain plants only; the larvae of certain moths and butterflies will feed on only one food plant. Part of the interest in keeping pet invertebrates is understanding the requirements and preferences of different species. Such variations can be seen across the invertebrate world and show the importance of defining dietary preferences in the wild or by investigation of a number of foods in captivity. Other invertebrates, such as cockroaches, are noted for feeding on any dietary item.

General rules for feeding invertebrates include:

- Herbivorous species should receive fresh food at regular intervals, with foliage kept in water to discourage wilting but suitably protected to prevent the animal from falling in and drowning. Growing shoots should be provided since these have the highest protein levels and are sources of the most easily digestible carbohydrate
- Live food should be given with care as prey items can all too easily cause damage to the invertebrate to which they are fed (Figure 23.2).
- While wild plants can be a valuable food source, it should be ensured that no herbicide or pesticide has been used on the plant. As genetically modified crops may be toxic to insect pests, they should not be used as invertebrate food
- Except for species where it is known that one food source is preferred or required, a wide variety of foodstuffs should be offered, especially at the beginning of captive husbandry when it is not clear which food is preferred.

Captive breeding

A serious invertebrate keeper will be keen to attempt breeding of captive invertebrates. Sexing individual invertebrates can be difficult, and providing the correct environment to stimulate reproduction may be particularly taxing. Some invertebrate species show sexual dimorphism: the male Macleay's spectre *(Extatosoma tiaratum)* has wings while the female does not; the female American cockroach *Periplaneta americanum* has a distinct ovipositor and egg sac.

Reproductive patterns differ significantly among invertebrate species, though most lay eggs. These may develop into adults by incomplete metamorphosis, where the first instar resembles the adult closely, or through complete metamorphosis, where the young invertebrate passes through larval and pupal stages. Some invertebrates, such as snails, are hermaphrodite. Others, such as the Indian stick insect *Carausius morostus*, are parthenogenetic, with females laying fertile eggs without the intervention of males. Other stick insects demonstrate a more conventional reproductive strategy, which shows the importance of understanding each individual species rather than attempting to extrapolate from one to another.

Handling and restraint

Again, much depends on the species involved. The key feature is to avoid injury to the animal or to the handler. Some species, such as snails, millipedes and crabs, will tolerate grasping with the hand and present no hazard if carefully handled. Others, such as large arachnids, may respond to inappropriate handling by biting or releasing urticarial hairs from their dorsum. These hairs, as their name suggests, provoke an inflammatory dermal reaction but can result in more serious injury if inhaled or in contact with eyes.

If any doubt exists about handling the animal, it should be viewed while restrained by plastic wrapping film on a sheet of glass (Figure 23.3), thus allowing visualization of the dorsum and ventrum simultaneously. A plastic container can be useful (Cooper, 1987). Sedation is possible, as is the use of a light anaesthetic (see below). Hypothermia can be used to facilitate handling; 30 minutes at 4°C is sufficient for most animals but has no analgesic effect.

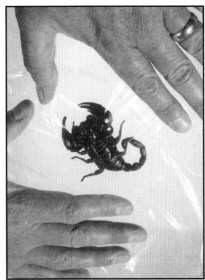

Figure 23.3 Use of a plastic sheet and glass plate to restrain a *Hetrometrus* scorpion.

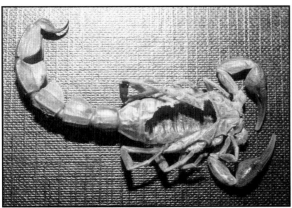

Figure 23.2 Damage to a scorpion cuticle caused by tenbrionid beetles initially introduced as mealworms but not removed when uneaten.

> Under no circumstances should hypothermia be used for immobilization for surgical procedures.

Diagnostic approach

It may be argued that the clinical examination of an arthropod or mollusc cannot be as detailed as that of a cat or dog. However, this should not prevent the documentation of observations such as swellings, discolorations or exudates. It also highlights the importance of thorough history taking and evaluation of the environment. Samples can be taken to allow investigations such as the haemocytological examination of snail haemolymph (Cooper, 1997) or the bacteriological evaluation of exudates from orifices in arachnids (Williams, 1992). The paucity of normal data on cell counts in haemolymph or the normal bacterial flora of mygalomorph mouthparts in these two cases may seem a barrier to the interpretation of information from such samples. It merely signals, however, the importance of taking samples from normal animals of the same species for comparison. Only in that way will invertebrate medicine progress, as indeed psittacine or reptile medicine has over the last 10 years.

A key factor in the approach to the clinical case is a knowledge of the normal animal and its behaviour. A particular example of this is the spider presented motionless in dorsal recumbency in its vivarium. Far from being ill, this animal is in the early stages of moulting and should be observed but on no account moved or touched. To gain a greater understanding of the wide range of invertebrate species, it is recommended that veterinary surgeons should be involved in local and national interest groups and, in particular, join the Veterinary Invertebrate Society. Details of organizations are provided at the end of this chapter.

Common conditions

Infectious diseases

Viral infections

Viral disease occurs across the range of invertebrate species but has been particularly studied in insects. The Baculoviridae include nuclear polyhedrosis virus (NPV), cytoplasmic polyhedrosis virus (CPV) and granulosis virus (Rivers, 1976).

NPV forms particles occluded in protein crystals within the nuclei of infected cells. These polyhedra are visible on light microscopy as non-staining crystals against a stained background in Giemsa-stained haemolymph. High numbers of the virus are produced: a dying cabbage moth larva yields 10^{11} virus particles from 4×10^9 inclusion bodies that develop in skin, fat-body and ovarian tissues.

Larvae with CPV infection hang head downwards and there is complete liquefaction of the body contents. CPV attacks gut cells and larvae die through inanition and failure to thrive. Leipodoptera may develop wing malformations through dysecdysis or abnormal oocyte development (Neilsen, 1965). The caterpillars regurgitate and excrete viral inclusion bodies for some time before they die, emphasizing the critical importance of quarantine and hygiene in dealing with an outbreak in an environment such as a butterfly farm.

The granulosis virus multiply sufficiently to cause a colour change in the infected host. Some caterpillars turn white (e.g. cabbage white butterfly *Pieris rapae*), some turn pink (e.g. codling moth *Carpocapsa pomonella*) and others turn yellow (e.g. *Harrisina brillans*) (Smith *et al.*, 1973).

The iridescent viruses again produce huge quantities of virus, giving up to 25% by weight of the dried weight of the larva. The virus crystals can be seen through the skin of the insect, resulting in an intense white coloration to infected larvae. Culture techniques can be invaluable in investigating viral disease of insects.

Bacterial infections

Bacterial infections of invertebrates are common but the main problem in diagnosing disease is the differentiation of a potential pathogen from the normal flora in any given species. It is only when the range of organisms normally present as commensals or symbionts is known, that the potential pathogen can be correctly isolated. Yet, in many species the normal flora have never been investigated.

The organism *Bacillus thuringiensis* is widely reported as a pathogen, as it has the ability to invade normal tissue in many circumstances and to cause disease. Defining whether an isolated organism is pathogenic can be difficult.

A bacterium of direct importance to veterinary surgeons is the Gram-positive organism *Paenibacillus larvae,* which causes the extremely contagious disease 'American foulbrood', which affects the European honeybee *Apis mellifera* (Bailey and Ball, 1991; Williams, 2000). While antibiotics have been used in other countries, with tylosin shown to be effective at reducing the effect of the disease but not in eliminating the organism completely, the disease is notifiable in the UK under the Bee Diseases Control Order (1982) and affected hives must be destroyed by burning. The disease produces a characteristic viscous ropey thread (Figure 23.4) but is best definitively diagnosed by a test using PCR.

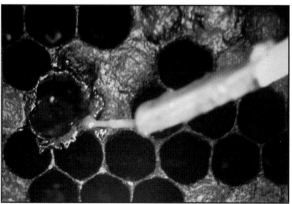

Figure 23.4 The pathognomonic ropey thread seen in American foulbrood in the European honey bee.

Another less contagious bacterial disease of bees is 'European foulbrood'; this kills larvae in the early summer, after which spontaneous recovery normally occurs. The disease produces a characteristic appearance of the brood, with larvae becoming flaccid and decomposing to leave a dry scale in the comb cell (Figure 23.5). The disease is caused by *Melissococcus pluton*, another Gram-positive organism. It is a notifiable disease but, unlike American foulbrood, mild cases can successfully be treated with oxytetracycline under the supervision of a DEFRA (formerly MAFF) bee disease officer (MAFF, 1996).

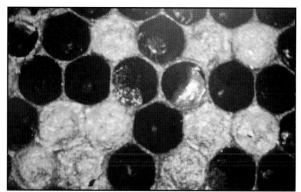

Figure 23.5 European foulbrood leaves a dry scale in the cell.

Fungal infections

Fungal infections are a significant problem throughout the arthropod world but the diagnosis of fungal disease is a major problem. The mere presence of a fungal spore, which may be identified through fungal culture, is in no way proof that the fungus is the cause of any lesions. The growth of a fungal mycelium on a dead or dying invertebrate is likely to be the entrance of a saphyrophytic species rather than the result of a pathogen. Nevertheless, the finding of large numbers of fungal spores in an affected animal at postmortem examination or in the environment is strongly suggestive that an association with disease may be made. A good example is the detection of fungal infection in populations of the wart-biter cricket *Decticus verrucivorus*, where fungal spores in a humid environment caused increased mortality (Pearce-Kelly, 1997). While the eggs were in a dormant phase the rearing room was fumigated, which entirely eliminated the disease. Such measures are very important given the intention to release crickets back into the wild; such reintroductions must be made using healthy animals, so as not to introduce disease into an already threatened population.

Some fungal species are noted more as true pathogens than as saprophytes. *Beauvaria bassiana*, the cause of muscardine in silkworms has been shown to affect over 500 insect species (Figure 23.6) and many other invertebrate hosts. Efforts at culturing these fungi to produce sexual bodies are notoriously difficult. Modern techniques of molecular biology are used in the identification of invertebrate fungal disease: samples may be evaluated and pathogenic species differentiated by techniques such as defining isoenzyme characteristics by electrophoresis or by RAPD (random amplified polymorphic DNA) analysis (Castrillo and Brooks, 1998).

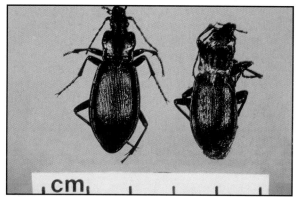

Figure 23.6 Fungal infection by *Beauvaria bassiana* in the jewel wasp (right). A normal wasp is shown on the left.

Fungi, more than any other infectious agent, however, do have marked effects on many invertebrates. Chitinolytic fungi such as *Cordyceps* and *Gibellula*, for instance, produce toxins that hydrolyse the chitinous exoskeleton, with subsequent death of the organism (Nentwig, 1985). Other fungi, such as the Hyphomycetes, *Aspergillus* and *Fusarium,* grow around superficial wounds on many species of invertebrate and appear to be opportunist colonizers. The differentiation between frank pathogens and these opportunist invaders is an important one in defining true disease from secondary fungal growth.

In other cases the fungus involved is clearly seen as a pathogen. For example, the most important fungal pathogen of oysters in the USA is *Labyrinthomyxa marina,* which causes fatal epizootics with impaired gonadal development in infected individuals, multifocal abscess formation in others, and general emaciation in many.

Parasites

Invertebrate hosts are used by a substantial number of parasites, including microsporidial protozoans (e.g. *Nosema apis),* nematodes (e.g. mermithid worms), flies and wasps. While a protozoan, nematode or mite may be sampled from an invertebrate host this by no means defines it as a parasite. It may be a commensal organism, as for instance are many of the rhabditid and diplogasterid nematodes associated with scarab beetles, or a true symbiont, as are the mites associated with the hissing cockroach *Gromphadoryna potentosa.*

The parasitic organism may be using the invertebrate as an intermediate host and thus not have the full adult characteristics that allow full identification. This is the case with mermithid nematodes: at the time of emergence from an invertebrate such as a spider all mermithid nematodes are still juveniles; they must be held for 3–4 weeks before moulting to the adult stage at which time a species identification can be made.

A gregarine protozoan parasite has been demonstrated in the British field cricket; however, it is not known whether this is part of the normal gastrointestinal flora or a pathogen (Zuk, 1987). Nematode parasites may be seen in arthropod hosts; as many of the hosts are relatively small arachnids or flies, the nematode grows to take up a substantial proportion of the coelomic volume of the host. No treatment is possible by this stage.

A significant problem in several invertebrate species is parasitism by insects such as the sphecid wasp or acrocerid flies. These lay their eggs inside the developing arthropod and the larvae gradually feed off the inside of the animal. All that may be noted for a time is an increased size of the coelom of the host, until the larvae eat their way out of the host (Figure 23.7). No treatment is possible, although hypothetically early diagnosis by ultrasound examination and removal through coeliotomy may be possible.

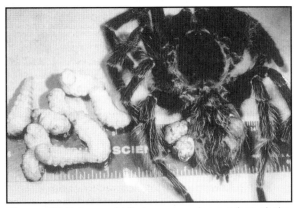

Figure 23.7 Acrocerid fly larvae passing out through the body wall of a mygalomorph spider.

A wide variety of mites is found on arthropods; while some may be truly parasitic (Figure 23.8), others may be in a phoretic relationship whereby the host is used merely as a method of transport. Others may have a commensal relationship, as has been suggested for the mites living around the mouthparts of the African hissing cockroach *Gromphadorina potentosa*.

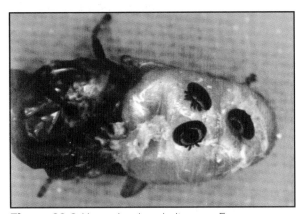

Figure 23.8 *Varroa jacobsoni* mites on a European honeybee.

Control of infectious diseases
Control of any infectious disease in invertebrates relies on prevention rather than treatment. Several factors are involved in successful management.

Hygiene: Regular cleaning of cages is important, especially as many invertebrates are kept in warm humid conditions and prefer rotting fruit as a dietary item, all of which makes the environment as much a haven to the infective organisms as to the hosts they seek to colonize. Cages and vivaria should be depopulated on a regular basis and thoroughly cleaned with agents such as cetrimide, hypochlorite or formalin, followed by meticulous flushing with plain water to remove any toxic cleansing agent before the animals are reintroduced.

Quarantine: Any new invertebrates should be housed separately from established inhabitants for 4–6 weeks to ensure, as much as is possible, that no new infectious agent or disease is being introduced. Enquiries must be made about the health of the population from which the individual to be introduced has originated.

Sampling or sacrifice of affected animals: In many cases invertebrates are kept in groups. It is always advisable not only to take samples from diseased animals but also to sample healthy animals of the same species to determine which pathogens are associated with diseased as opposed to healthy animals. In cases where a number of animals are affected by a condition which is increasing mortality among the population, it may also be appropriate to sacrifice an affected animal before it dies to submit it for postmortem examination in an attempt to determine the cause of disease.

Therapeutics: Relatively little is known about the safety or efficacy of chemotherapeutic agents in invertebrates. Sulphonamides have been used in grasshoppers (Henry, 1968) while trimethoprim and sulphadiazine was used successfully in a case of *Serratia marcescens* infection in a colony of the cricket *Gryllus assimilis*. Interestingly, in that case, where medicated food was used, efficacy of the drug dropped when a granular form was used rather than a powdered formulation (Callis and Zwart, 1999). Wallach (1972) recommended several agents for use in colonies of the mealworm *Tenebrio molitor*. Use of chlortetracycline or oxytetracycline solutions in invertebrates has been recommended previously. Where invertebrates are still eating, a useful way of providing medication is by standing shoots of vegetation in water containing the drug, although the exact dose ingested is not clear.

Physical injury
Physical injury may result in damage to the soft tissues of the animal, to the exoskeleton or to the shell where present. In many cases these self-heal remarkably quickly. However, problems occur in breaches to the exoskeleton in arthropods where loss of haemolymph occurs. Loss of more than 1–5% bodyweight of haemolymph is deleterious, while loss of less than this can generally be tolerated. Use of paraffin wax, plasticine or a plastic skin preparation has been advocated in repair of such defects (Cooper, 1998), as has cyanoacrylate tissue glue. A particular problem occurs when a moulting spider is disturbed, since a rupture in the new exoskeleton can result in substantial loss of haemolymph. Talcum powder liberally applied can reduce haemolymph loss but the prognosis is poor.

Some injuries in invertebrates appear serious but are well tolerated; loss of a limb is one such trauma. Natural closure of the entrance to the coelomic cavity can prevent substantial loss of haemolymph and the limb regenerates with each moult in a growing arthropod. In cases where haemolymph does not coagulate to prevent further loss, tissue glue or sterile talcum powder can be used to close the wound. Many arthropods exhibit autotomy, where they shed limbs in response to adverse stimuli. Autotomy has been shown on administration of wasp venom; this venom causes pain in higher vertebrates but what this indicates regarding invertebrate pain reception is unclear.

Stress

Effects of stress, especially from overhandling, are often overlooked in invertebrates. One instance which does lead to obvious signs is the tendency of the so-called 'tarantula' mygalomorph spiders to release urticarial hairs or setae from their backs as a defensive reaction. This causes obvious alopecia on the dorsum of the abdomen (Figure 23.9), which may be mistaken for a pathological lesion (Williams, 2001).

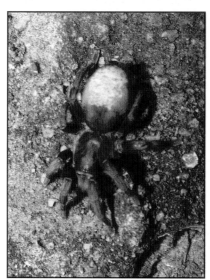

Figure 23.9 Alopecia caused by excessive release of urticarial hairs in the stressed mygalomorph spider.

Environmental problems

As noted above, the environment is critical in invertebrate health and inappropriately low temperature or humidity can be deleterious. The small size of many invertebrates gives them a very high surface area-to-volume ratio, maximizing trans-surface loss of both heat and water. Perhaps more than any other group of exotic species, the invertebrates live on a 'knife edge' of existence; any deviation from their optimal temperature or humidity range can be rapidly lethal.

Effects of changes in environment are species-specific. Mild cooling, for instance, generally has little long-term effect on invertebrates, although in the short term it produces immobility and reduction in metabolic rate. Yet in the Solifugidae (sun or camel spiders), used to desert conditions, even a reduction in temperature in a refrigerator for a few minutes may result in death (Cooper, 1998).

Ice crystal formation at low temperatures is avoided in some species through naturally occurring antifreeze compounds. In others, particularly molluscs, ice crystals cause irritation preceeding death.

Nutritional diseases

The most prevalent nutritional problem in invertebrates is failure to eat. This may occur as a secondary effect of an infectious disease or parasitic infestation, and in such cases may be responsible for the majority of the signs of the disease. Alternatively, and more commonly, captive invertebrates will fail to feed through the agency of what in 'lower vertebrates' has been termed the maladaptation syndrome.

A number of non-specific inappropriate environmental conditions lead to failure to thrive. Because of their small size and high surface area-to-volume ratio, many invertebrates need to feed regularly. When kept correctly they usually feed voraciously, but if for various reasons they do not feed, their condition can rapidly deteriorate.

Neoplasia

It may be supposed that neoplasia in invertebrates would be a very under-researched topic. Indeed, solid tumours in species such as arthropods are uncommon and often difficult to differentiate from inflammatory or fibroblastic lesions. Nevertheless, neoplasia is by no means unknown in invertebrates and indeed haemopoietic neoplasia is a significant problem in marine bivalves such as the clam *Mya arenaria* (Leavitt *et al.*, 1990).

Anaesthesia and analgesia

Anaesthesia

Anaesthesia may be required to immobilise an invertebrate for examination or for a surgical procedure. For examination, cooling may be appropriate but given that this has no analgesic efficacy it should *not* be used for a procedure in which any pain is anticipated.

Gaseous carbon dioxide can be used alone for anaesthesia but again gives no analgesia. Gaseous halothane, with induction at up to 10%, or isoflurane, with induction at between 3 and 5%, may be recommended for anaesthesia for surgical procedures.

Anaesthesia of aquatic species can be achieved with tricaine methanesulphonate (MS 222 Sandoz) or benzocaine at a concentration of 100 mg/l in water. Benzocaine must first be dissolved in a small volume of acetone. Carbon dioxide in aqueous solution has been used for anaesthesia of the medicinal leech, using a 50:50 dilution of soda water or an Alka-Seltzer® tablet (Cooper *et al.,* 1986).

Invertebrate pain

With regard to analgesia it may be asked whether invertebrates can feel pain. Clearly the response to pain varies across the massive range of species, from a simple withdrawal response to a tactile stimulus in a 'lower' invertebrate, to a response which shows characteristics of a pain response in a 'higher' vertebrate. Valuable work has been undertaken on *Aplysia californica*, the sea hare. Brief electrical or mechanical dermal stimulation of *Aplysia* produced defensive reactions such as siphon withdrawal and tail withdrawal reflexes. Noxious stimulation at the same site showed sensitization when the central nervous system was intact (Walters, 1987). The classical aversive conditioned response in *Aplysia* is also associated with a concomitant depression in feeding. Workers pre-eminent in this field have proposed that the similarity between these reactions and those in mammals suggests that *Aplysia* is undergoing the functional equivalent of fear (Walters *et al.*, 1981). The permanent changes in neuronal architecture and mechanisms in these animals are similar to those in 'higher' vertebrates and humans: after a noxious stimulus, an *Aplysia* individual is significantly more reactive to previously innocuous stimuli. This neuronal plasticity suggests that similar mechanisms are occurring in *Aplysia* as in vertebrates, including humans and other mammals (Woolf and Walters, 1991).

The same neuropeptides have been demonstrated in invertebrates as are involved in pain responses in higher species (Stefano *et al.*, 1998). Such findings suggest that, even in invertebrates relatively low down on the evolutionary ladder, we should be concerned regarding appropriate analgesia for surgical procedures.

Surgery

Invertebrate surgery is not a particularly well developed or reported field. Emergency treatment of wounds or avulsed appendages is a common surgical necessity, with tissue glue being particularly valuable in such cases. Experimental surgery on cephalopods has been reported (Boyle, 1991) and in these species integumental incisions heal well after standard closure with absorbable sutures.

Euthanasia

The question of whether invertebrates can feel pain again rises with regard to methods of euthanasia. The use of an anaesthetic overdose may be appropriate for 'lower' invertebrates but in 'higher' species such as the decapod crustaceans pithing is considered an optimal approach. All pithing techniques require skill to ensure instantaneous death but the alternative, immersion in boiling water, has been shown to provoke struggling and excitatory movements for up to 2 minutes before death occurs (Baker *et al.*, 1975). Euthanasia of insects has in the past been undertaken with ethyl acetate or prussic acid but these were selected because they cause no damage to the animal; whether they are humane methods is unclear (Invertebrate Working Group, 1990). For euthanasia of cephalopods, immersion in ethanol, urethane or magnesium chloride has been suggested, with the last of these yielding least apparent discomfort (Boyle, 1991). While no research has been reported on the use of injectable agents for euthanasia, it is to be assumed that pentobarbitone is acceptable.

A significant problem in some invertebrate species, such as gastropods, is identifying when an animal is dead. Recently the use of doppler ultrasound cardiovascular monitoring has been reported (Davies *et al.*, 2000); while the key use of this technique would be in monitoring anaesthesia the determination of death is another valuable use of such a technique.

References and further reading

Alicata JE and Jindrak K (1969) *Angiostrongylus* in the Pacific and Southeastern Asia. *American Lecture Series* No. 755. CC Thomas, Springfield, IL

Bailey L (1955) The epidemiology and control of *Nosema* disease of the honey bee. *Annals of Applied Biology* **43**, 379–389

Bailey L and Ball BV (1991) *Honey Bee Pathology, 2nd edition*. Academic Press, London

Baker JR, Dolan MB and Coxhill J (1975) Experiments on the humane killing of lobsters (*Homarus vulgaris*) and crabs (*Cancer pagarus*). *Scientific papers of the Humane Education Centre* **3**, 1–11

Boyle PR (1991) *The Care and Management of Cephalopods in the Laboratory*. Universities Federation for Animal Welfare, Potters Bar

Blackmore P (2000) Feeding stick insects. *Veterinary Invertebrate Society Newsletter* **16**, 12–13

Callis H and Zwart P (1999) An outbreak of disease in a colony of crickets *Gryllus assimilis:* case report. *Veterinary Invertebrate Society Newsletter* **15**, 17–20

Castrillo LA and Brooks WM (1998) Differentiation of *Beauvaria bassiana* isolates from the Darkling beetle *Alphitobius diaperinus* using isozyme and RAPD analyses. *Journal of Invertebrate Pathology* **72**, 190–196

Cheeseman V (2000) Invertebrate information sheets. *Veterinary Invertebrate Society Newsletter* **16**, 16–23

Colville RE (1987) Spider-hunting sphecid wasps. In *Ecophysiology of Spiders*, ed. W Nentwig, pp. 319–327. Springer-Verlag, Berlin

Cooper JE (1980) Invertebrates and invertebrate disease: an introduction for the veterinary surgeon. *Journal of Small Animal Practice* **21**, 495–508

Cooper JE (1987) A veterinary approach to spiders. *Journal of Small Animal Practice* **28**, 229–239

Cooper JE (1990) A veterinary approach to leeches. *Veterinary Record* **127**, 226–228

Cooper JE (1991) Invertebrates. In *Manual of Exotic Pets, 3rd edn*, ed. PH Beynon and JE Cooper. BSAVA, Cheltenham

Cooper JE (1998) Emergency care of invertebrates. *Veterinary Clinics of North America: Exotic Animal Practice* **1**, 251–264

Cooper JE and Knowler C (1991) Snails and snail farming: an introduction for the veterinary profession. *Veterinary Record* **129**, 541–549

Cooper JE and Knowler C (1992) Investigations into causes of death of endangered molluscs (*Partula* species). *Veterinary Record* **131**, 342–344

Cooper JE, Mahaffey P and Applebee K (1986) Anaesthesia of the medicinal leech. *Veterinary Record* **118**, 589

Cooper JE, Pearce-Kelly PE and Williams DL (1992) *Arachnida*. Chiron Publications, Southampton

Davies RR, Chitty JR and Saunders RA (2000) Cardiovascular monitoring of an *Achatina* snail with a doppler ultrasound probe. *Critical Care and Emergency Medicine, British Veterinary Zoological Society Proceedings, Royal Veterinary College*, November 18–19, 2000

Edwards CA and Lofty JR (1972) *Biology of Earthworms*. Chapman and Hall, London

Fiorito G (1986) Is there pain in invertebrates? *Behavioural Processes* **12**, 383–388

Henry JE (1968) *Malemeba locusta* and its antibiotic control in grasshopper cultures. *Journal of Invertebrate Pathology* **11**, 224–233

Invertebrate Working Group (1990) *Codes of Practice for the Care of Invertebrates in Captivity: Euthanasia of Invertebrates*. National Federation of Zoos of Great Britain and Ireland, London

Klowden MJ and Greenberg R (1977) Effects of antibiotics on the survival of *Salmonella* in the American cockroach. *Journal of Hygiene, Cambridge* **77**, 339–345

Leavitt DF, McDowell, Capuzzo J and Weinberg JR (1990) Hemopoietic neoplasia in *Mya arenaria*. Prevalence and indices of physiological condition. *Marine Biology* **105**, 313–321

MAFF (1996) *Foul Brood Disease of Honey Bees: Recognition and Control*. Ministry of Agriculture, Fisheries and Food Central Science Laboratory, York

Mead AR (1979) *Pulmonates: Economic Malacology*. Academic Press, London

Murphy (1980) *Keeping Spiders, Insects and other Land Invertebrates in Captivity*. Bartholomew, Edinburgh

Neilson MM (1965) Effects of a cytoplasmic polyhedrosis on adult Lepidoptera. *Journal of Invertebrate Pathology* **7**, 306–314

Nentwig W (1985) Parasitic fungi as a mortality factor in spiders. *Journal of Arachnology* **13**, 272–274

Pasteur L (1870) *Etudes sur la Maladie des Vers a Soie*. Paris, Gauthier-Villers

Pearce-Kelly P (1997) Coping with pathogen infections in captive populations of British field and wart-biter crickets. *Veterinary Invertebrate Society Newsletter* **12**, 7–8

Poinar GO (1975) *Entamophagous Nematodes*. EJ Brill, Leiden

Poinar GO (1985) Mermithid (Nematoda) parasites of spiders and harvestmen. *Journal of Arachnology* **13**,121–128

Poole T (1997) *The UFAW Handbook on the Care and Management of Laboratory Animals, 7th edn.* Blackwell Science, Oxford

Rao BR, Sagar IK and Bhat JV (1983) *Enterobacter aerogenes* infection of *Hoplochaetella suctoria*. In: *Earthworm Ecology*, ed. JE Satchell, pp. 383–392. Chapman and Hall, London

Ray SM and Chandler AC (1955) *Dermocystidium marinum*, a parasite of oysters. *Experimental Parasitology* **4**,170–200

Rivers CF (1976) Disease. In: *Moths and Butterflies of Great Britain and Ireland. Vol. 1*, ed. J Heath, pp.57–70. Curwen Press, London

Rivers CF (1991) The control of diseases in insect cultures. *International Zoo Yearbook* **30**, 131–137

Schlinger EI (1987) The biology of Acroceridae (Diptera): true endoparasitoids of spiders. In: *Ecophysiology of Spiders*, ed. W Nentwig, pp. 328–341. Springer-Verlag, Berlin

Stefano GB, Salzet B and Fricchione GL (1998) Enkelytin and opioid peptide association in invertebrates and vertebrates: immune activation and pain. *Immunology Today* **19**, 265–268

Steinhaus EA (1975) *Disease in a Minor Chord*. Ohio State University Press, Columbus, Ohio

Wallach JD (1972) The management and medical care of mealworms. *Journal of Zoo Animal Medicine* **3**, 29–33

Walters ET (1987) Site specific sensitization of defensive reflexes in *Aplysia*: a simple model of long-term hyperalgesia. *Journal of Neuroscience* **7**, 400–407

Walters ET, Carew TJ and Kandel ER (1981) Associative learning in *Aplysia*: evidence for conditioned fear in an invertebrate. *Science* **211**, 504–506

Williams DL (1992) Studies in Arachnid Disease. In: *Arachnida,* ed. JE Cooper *et al.*, pp.116–125. Chiron Publications, Southampton

Williams DL (1999) Sample taking in invertebrate veterinary medicine. *Veterinary Clinics of North America: Exotic Animal Practice* **2**, 777–801

Williams DL (2000) A veterinary approach to the European honey bee (*Apis mellifera*). *Veterinary Journal* **160**, 61–73

Williams DL (2001) Integumental disease in invertebrates. *Veterinary Clinics of North America: Exotic Animal Practice* **4**, 309–320

Woolf CJ and Walters ET (1991) Common patterns of plasticity contributing to nociceptive sensitization in mammals and *Aplysia. Trends in Neuroscience* **14**, 74–78

Zuk M (1987) The effects of gregarine parasites on longevity, weight loss, fecundity and development in field crickets. *Ecological Entomology* **12**, 349–354

Useful contact addresses

Veterinary Invertebrate Society Strathmore Veterinary Clinic, London Road, Andover, Hants SP10 2PH

Royal Entomological Society 41 Queen's Gate, London

National Bee Unit Central Science Laboratory, Sand Hutton, York YO4 1LZ

British Beekeeper's Association National Agriculture Centre, Stoneleigh, Kenilworth, Warwickshire

Acknowledgements

Dr Andrew Cunningham and Professor John E. Cooper have kindly contributed much information and several of the photographic ilustrations for this chapter. Their enthusiasm and expertise have, more than anyone, advanced the field of invertebrate veterinary medicine over the last decade.

24

British legislation

Margaret E. Cooper

Introduction

The veterinary surgeon working with exotic species can benefit greatly by being well versed in the relevant law and can pass this knowledge on to clients as part of the service provided by the practice. The legislation described in this chapter applies to England and Wales. In most cases it also applies to Scotland. Northern Ireland has its own, comparable, legal provisions. It is important to keep up-to-date with developments in the law because it can always change. Anyone following the advice in this chapter must also apprise themselves independently of the current state of the law.

Restrictions on keeping animals

A local government authority licence is required under the following legislation:

❖ **Dangerous Wild Animals Act 1976** as amended by **The Dangerous Wild Animals Act 1976 (Modification) Order 1984)**

- The keeping at private premises of the exotic species listed in the 1984 Order must be licensed. This does not apply to zoos, pet shops, circuses or establishments designated under the Animals (Scientific Procedures) Act 1986
- Most non-domesticated species that are likely to cause substantial harm are listed in the Order. They include many larger species, all primates except marmosets, most venomous snakes, some particularly poisonous spiders and the buthid scorpions. The only birds listed are the Rheidae (emu-like birds). The only UK species affected are the wild cat and the adder (viper)
- Basic standards of housing, safety and welfare are required. Insurance and an annual veterinary inspection are obligatory, and a fee is payable.

❖ **Zoo Licensing Act 1981**
❖ **Council Directive EC No 22/1999**

Some changes to the Act can be expected to bring it in line with the European Union Zoos Directive, which comes into effect in April 2002.

- The Zoo Licensing Act applies to all zoos and other collections of non-domesticated animals that are open (whether or not for a fee) to the public on more than 7 days in any 12-month period
- Zoos must be licensed and are subject to a major inspection by veterinarians, and others, every 6 years. Small zoos have reduced numbers of inspections. There are lesser inspections in other years, and fees are charged for licences and inspections
- Zoos must also comply with the Secretary of State's Standards of Modern Zoo Practice (DETR, 2000). Numerous non-statutory guidelines on husbandry have been developed to meet the needs of particular species (Macdonald and Charlton, 2000). Guidance relating to the inspection and euthanasia of invertebrates is also available (Federation of Zoological Gardens of Great Britain and Ireland, 1990a,b).

❖ **Pet Animals Act 1951**
❖ **Pet Animals Act 1951 (Amendment) Act 1983**

- A licence must be obtained to run a business (not solely the conventional pet shop in the high street) of selling domestic and exotic vertebrate animals as pets or for ornamental purposes
- Inspection may be by a veterinary surgeon or local authority official (Local Government Association, 1998).

❖ **Performing Animals (Regulation) Act 1925**
❖ **Performing Animals Rules 1968**

- Although a licence as such is not required by the trainer of any vertebrate animals used in a performance or exhibit, he or she must be registered with the local authority where they reside, and they must obtain a certificate of registration
- Local authorities can inspect relevant premises.

Responsibility for damage caused by non-domesticated animals

Civil law

- The keeper of non-domesticated animals is responsible for any damage that they cause
- Liability for death, personal injury or damage to property can give rise to claims for compensation in civil law under the heads of negligence, nuisance, trespass, strict liability for inherently dangerous animals (Animals Act 1971) and the escape of animals.

❖ Health and Safety at Work etc. Act 1974

- An employer must provide additional safety procedures to take account of any special risks involved in the care and management of exotic species. This may include the provision of specialized guidance, training and working procedures and protective equipment
- There is a specific code of practice for zoos (Health and Safety Commission, 1985).

Welfare

❖ Protection of Animals Act 1911
❖ Protection of Animals (Scotland) Acts 1912 supplemented by various subsequent Acts
❖ Protection of Animals (Amendment) Act 2000

- It is an offence to treat any domestic or captive species of animal cruelly or to cause it any unnecessary suffering. This can include the failure to provide necessary food, water, care and veterinary attention
- Killing an animal is not an offence under these Acts provided that it is carried out humanely.

❖ Protection of Animals (Anaesthetics) Acts 1954 and 1964

- Anaesthesia must be used in procedures that interfere with sensitive tissues or bones of an animal, with the exception of minor procedures such as injections
- Although these Acts expressly do not apply to birds, fish or reptiles, anaesthesia should be used to fulfil the general requirements of the main Protection of Animals Acts, which require an operation to be carried out with due care and humanity and without unnecessary suffering.

❖ Wildlife and Countryside Act 1981

- Section 8 of the Wildlife and Countryside Act provides that it is an offence to keep any bird in a cage that is not large enough to allow the bird to stretch its wings freely

- A smaller cage is permitted only for poultry, for use while transporting or exhibiting a bird or while it is undergoing examination or treatment by a veterinary surgeon.

❖ Abandonment of Animals Act 1960

- Animals should not deliberately and without good cause be abandoned in circumstances likely to cause them unnecessary suffering
- Although this Act is aimed primarily at pets, it should be taken into consideration when assessing the suitability of wild creatures for release.

❖ Wild Mammals (Protection) Act 1996

- It is an offence to carry out specified acts such as kicking, beating, burning or drowning a wild mammal with the intent to inflict unnecessary suffering.

❖ The Welfare of Animals (Transport) Order 1997

- Animals of any sort, including invertebrates, must not be transported in any way that causes or is likely to cause them injury or unnecessary suffering
- In the case of commercial or non-private transportation of animals, additional requirements apply to the provision of suitable containers and vehicles, food, water, ventilation, temperature and attendance.

Additional provisions on transport

- Public road and rail carriers may also have their own requirements
- Airlines apply the International Air Transport Association's (IATA) Live Animals Regulations
- The CITES (Convention on International Trade in Endangered Species of Wild Fauna and Flora) Secretariat has issued Guidelines for the transportation (by any means) of species covered by CITES
- The Welfare of Animals (Transport) Order 1997 makes it a legal requirement to comply with the IATA regulations and CITES guidelines where they are applicable
- Royal Mail forbids the transport by post of living animals apart from a few species of invertebrate, such as bees. Others, such as caterpillars, may be posted by prior arrangement. There are also precise requirements for the mailing of animal pathogens, including special packaging and labelling.

Wildlife

- ❖ **Wildlife and Countryside Act 1981** as amended: wild and game birds; listed wild creatures
- ❖ **Deer Act 1991; Deer (Scotland) Act 1996** and related legislation
- ❖ **Protection of Badgers Act 1992**
- ❖ **Conservation of Seals Act 1970**
- ❖ **Salmon and Freshwater Fisheries Act 1975**
- ❖ **Game Acts** (various): rabbits; hares; game birds
- ❖ **Destructive Imported Animals Act 1932:** mink; grey squirrel; others

Species protection

- The Wildlife and Countryside Act provides various degrees of protection for indigenous wild birds. There are close seasons for game birds, special penalties in respect of rare birds and complex provisions for ringing and registration with the Department of the Environment, Transport and the Regions in respect of the diurnal birds of prey and other rare species listed in Schedule 4
- The Department of the Environment, Transport and the Regions (DETR) issued information sheets providing guidance on the foregoing and other aspects of the Wildlife and Countryside Act (DETR, various dates). From June 2001, this department has been reconfigured as the Department for Environment, Food and Rural Affairs (DEFRA)
- Some mammals, reptiles, amphibians, insects and their habitats are also protected. Badgers are covered by a specific Act.

The Wildlife and Countryside Act provides that it is an offence:

- To take, injure, kill or sell a protected species
- To possess a protected species
- To deliberately release or allow to escape into the wild any non-indigenous species or a species already established in the wild that is listed in Schedule 9, Part 1 (e.g. grey squirrel, budgerigar).

Exceptions:

- To prove that possession is legal it is necessary to be able to show that the animal has been bred in captivity or has been imported, sold or taken in accordance with the Act or under a licence. In this situation the burden of proof falls on the person alleging legal possession, and it is therefore important to keep good records of any acquisition

- It is permissible to take a sick or injured protected creature from the wild to tend it until it is fit to be released. If it is injured or diseased beyond hope of recovery it may be killed. A humane method must be used (see Welfare above)
- Birds included in Schedule 4 taken under this provision must be ringed and registered forthwith unless they are held under (a) registered keepers of disabled wild birds, and RSPCA inspectors may keep disabled wild-bred Schedule 4 birds for up to15 days for rehabilitation provided that they notify the DETR (DEFRA) within 4 days of receipt and keep specified records and (b) a veterinary surgeon may keep any Schedule 4 bird that is receiving professional veterinary treatment for up to 6 weeks without registration. The veterinary surgeon must keep records of each such bird
- Many activities that are prohibited *prima facie*, such as trapping, shooting or selling, can be authorized by the grant of a licence from the appropriate authority if they are for purposes such as scientific studies, aviculture or crop protection.

Close season protection

Animals such as game birds, deer, fish and seals that are hunted are protected by close seasons and by the fact that certain methods of capture and killing are prohibited by the relevant legislation. In the case of deer:

- Nowadays they are to be found either wild, kept in parks and collections or farmed
- All species are subject to the Deer Acts and, with the exception of deer kept as livestock, are protected during their respective close seasons
- They are also protected at night, except in limited situations allowing for protection of property
- Sick or injured animals may at any time be killed or taken for care.

Unprotected species

- Many other species are not protected by the Act; neither do the Protection of Animals Acts apply to free-living wildlife, such as the hedgehog or fox
- The Wild Mammals (Protection) Act (see Welfare, above) provides some protection against certain forms of cruel treatment in respect of wild mammals
- Certain sporting and other activities are not affected by this Act
- Under pest control provisions it is illegal to import, keep or release certain species (including the grey squirrel) without a licence. Occupiers of land can be required to destroy animals that are causing damage.

Import and export

Health controls

❖ **Animal Health Act 1981**

Orders relating to the importation of:

- Animals, birds and hatching eggs
- Rabies and other diseases
- Pathogens and animals and poultry products.

Almost all imported animals (other than reptiles, amphibians and harmless invertebrates) and most animal derivatives and pathogens are subject to controls by DEFRA (or the Scottish or Welsh equivalent). These require:

- A licence to import
- Veterinary health certification
- Quarantine (for mammals and birds) after landing in the UK.

Conservation controls

❖ **Council Regulation EC No. 338/97 and associated legislation**
❖ **Commission Regulation EC No. 939/97 and associated legislation**
❖ **The Control of Trade in Endangered Species (Enforcement) Regulations 1997**

General

- Many exotic species that are listed in the Appendices to CITES are subject to import and export controls
- In the EU the provisions of CITES are directly imposed on member states by the CITES regulations
- Many species (in addition to those in the CITES Appendices) are included in Annexes A to D of the Regulation; consequently EU controls are more extensive than those required by CITES itself
- The importation of certain Annex B species into the EU (including some birds of prey and reptiles) has been suspended.

Controls on commercial use

- The Regulations contain additional restrictions on the sale (or other commercial use) and the display for any commercial purpose of Annex A species, including birds of prey and other types of tortoise including Mediterranean species
- Permits (Article 10 certificates) can be obtained to authorize commercial displays and for the sale of captive-bred Annex A species (either for a one-off sale or breeders can obtain a licence to deal in several specimens)

- Annex A species in commercial use must be permanently marked with a microchip or, in the case of birds, with a closed ring
- These, and other provisions, are described in the Guidance Notes issued by the DETR.

Customs and Excise
Animals imported into the UK will normally be subject to customs duty and value added tax.

Medical

❖ **Veterinary Surgeons Act 1966** and supplementary legislation

- Only veterinary surgeons and veterinary practitioners registered with the Royal College of Veterinary Surgeons have the right to practise veterinary surgery in respect of mammals (including marine mammals), birds and reptiles
- It is considered, however, that anyone may treat fish and invertebrates and, probably, amphibians, subject to the provisions of the Protection of Animals Acts (see Welfare, above)
- Owners of animals (and their employees and families) may provide minor medical treatment
- Anyone may give first aid in an emergency
- Veterinary nurses may carry out medical treatment and minor surgery not involving entry into a body cavity but only in respect of animals kept as pets or for companionship.

Medicines legislation

❖ **Medicines Act 1968**
❖ **The Medicines (Restrictions on the Administration of Veterinary Medicinal Products) Regulations 1994 and 1997**
❖ **The Medicines (Prescription Only) Order** and associated legislation

Points of particular importance in respect of exotic species are:

- Procedures for complying with the medicines legislation such as the requirements that apply to prescribing, supplying and labelling prescription-only medicines (POMs) also apply to exotic species, including fish and invertebrates
- Veterinary surgeons may only prescribe POMs for 'animals under their care.' This phrase is amplified in the *Guide to Professional Conduct* (Royal College of Veterinary Surgeons, 2000)
- The 'cascade' should be followed when prescribing outside the terms of the marketing authorization for a drug (British Veterinary Association, 2000; Veterinary Medicines Directorate, 1998).

Drug-dart weapons

- Possession of any firearms or weapons, such as a dart gun, crossbow or blowpipe that can be used to discharge tranquillizing drugs must be authorized by a Firearms Certificate issued by the police
- The use of a crossbow (with or without drugs) for wild animals requires a licence under the Wildlife and Countryside Act.

Conclusion

The aim of this chapter has been to remind veterinary surgeons of the British law that is particularly relevant to exotic pets. It is hoped that it will enable them to extend their existing knowledge of the legislation that is generally applicable to veterinary practice, thereby adding a further dimension to the service that they provide for their clients who present exotic species for advice. At the same time, this information should help to protect veterinary practitioners from being in breach of the law.

References and further reading

Blackman DE, Humphreys PN and Todd P (1989) *Animal Welfare and the Law.* Cambridge University Press, Cambridge

British Veterinary Association (1990) *Dangerous Wild Animals Act 1976. A Guide to Veterinary Surgeons Concerned with Inspections under this Act.* BVA Publications, London

British Veterinary Association (2000) *Code of Practice on Medicines.* BVA, London

BWRC (1989) *Ethics and Legal Aspects of Treatment and Rehabilitation of Wild Animal Casualties.* British Wildlife Rehabilitation Council, London

BWRC (undated) *Guidelines for Wildlife Rehabilitation Units.* British Wildlife Rehabilitation Council, Horsham

Brooman S and Legge D (1997) *Law Relating to Animals.* Cavendish Publishing, London

Convention on International Trade in Endangered Species of Wild Fauna and Flora (1980) *Guidelines for Transport and Preparation for Shipment of Live Wild Animals and Plants.* CITES Secretariat, Gland, Switzerland

Cooper ME (1978) The Dangerous Wild Animals Act 1976. *Veterinary Record* **102**, 457

Cooper ME (1983) The Zoo Licensing Act 1981. *Veterinary Record* **112**, 564

Cooper ME (1987) *An Introduction to Animal Law.* Academic Press, London

Cooper ME and Sinclair DA (1989) Law relating to wildlife rehabilitation. *Abstract from the Second Symposium of the British Wildlife Rehabilitation Council, Stoneleigh, 1989.* British Wildlife Rehabilitation Council, London

DETR (1996) *Wildlife Crime: A Guide to Wildlife Law Enforcement in the UK.* Stationery Office, London

DETR (1998) *A Guide to the European Wildlife Trade Regulations.* Department of the Environment, Transport and the Regions, Bristol

DETR (2000) *Secretary of State's Standards of Modern Zoo Practice.* Department of the Environment, Transport and the Regions, London

DETR (various dates) *Information Sheets* (on aspects of the Wildlife and Countryside Act). Department of the Environment, Transport and the Regions, Bristol

DETR (various dates) *Guidance Notes* (on aspects of the CITES Regulations). Department of the Environment, Transport and the Regions, Bristol

Federation of Zoological Gardens of Great Britain and Ireland (1990a) *Codes of Practice for the Care of Invertebrates in Captivity. IWG/1 Notes for Inspectors.* Federation of Zoological Gardens of Great Britain and Ireland, London

Federation of Zoological Gardens of Great Britain and Ireland (1990b) *Codes of Practice for the Care of Invertebrates in Captivity. IWG/2 Euthanasia of Invertebrates.* Federation of Zoological Gardens of Great Britain and Ireland, London

Health and Safety Commission (1985) *Zoos – Safety, Health and Welfare Standards for Employers and Persons at Work. Approved Code of Practice and Guidance Notes.* HMSO, London

IATA (annual) *Live Animals Regulations.* International Air Transport Association, Montreal and Geneva

Local Government Association (1998) *The Pet Animals Act 1951. Model Standards for Pet Shop Licence Conditions.* Local Government Association, London

Lorton R (2000) *A–Z of Countryside Law.* Stationery Office, London

Macdonald AA and Charlton N (2000) *A Bibliography of References to Husbandry and Veterinary Guidelines for Animals in Zoological Collections.* Federation of Zoological Gardens of Great Britain and Ireland, London

North PM (1972) *The Modern Law of Animals.* Butterworth, London

Parkes C and Thornley J (1987) *Fair Game.* Pelham, London

Post Office (annual) *Post Office Guide.* Post Office, London

Radford M (2001) *Animal Welfare Law in Britain: Regulation and Responsibility.* Oxford University Press, Oxford

RCVS (2000) *Guide to Professional Conduct 2000.* Royal College of Veterinary Surgeons, London

RSPB (1998) *Wild Birds and the Law.* Royal Society for the Protection of Birds, Sandy, Bedfordshire

RSPB (undated). *Information about Birds and the Law.* Sandy, Bedfordshire

Scottish Natural Heritage (1998) *Scotland's Wildlife: The Law and You.* Scottish Natural Heritage, Perth

VMD (1998) *Guidance to the Veterinary Profession. AMELIA 8.* Veterinary Medicines Directorate, Addlestone, Surrey

Index